MEDICAL RADIOLOGY

Diagnostic Imaging and Radiation Oncology

Springer
Berlin
Heidelberg
New York
Barcelona
Hong Kong
London
Milan
Paris
Singapore
Tokyo

H. S. Thomsen · R. N. Muller · R. F. Mattrey (Eds.)

Trends in Contrast Media

With Contributions by

R. Agati · T. Albrecht · T. Almén · I. Berry · M. D. Blaufox · M. J. K. Blomley
H. Bosmans · A. A. Brayman · W. H. Bush, Jr. · C. Catalano · P. P. Chang · C. Church
M. Clanet · R. H. Cohan · B. Coley · B. Cotter · D. O. Coscrove · B. Cotter · A. N. DeMaria
J.F. Desreux · R. J. Eckersley · J. H. Ellis · A. K. Fahlvik · S. L. Fossheim · B. Frennby
D. Gilsoul · M.S. Girard · K. Golman · A. Greco · R.W. Katzberg · A. Kornerup Hansen
E. P. Krenning · G.-P. Krestin · D. J. Kwekkeboom · A. L'Abbate · A. Laghi · P. Leander
M. Leonardi · M. Lombardi · G. Manelfe · G. Marchal · R. F. Mattrey · M. T. McNamara
J. K. Moran · A. Nævestad · H.-Y. Oei · R. A. Older · P. Pavone · T. Pelura · H. M. Pollack
J. P. Ranjeva · P. A. Rinck · K.K. Shung · C. B. Sirlin · F. Stacul · G. C. Steinbach
G. Sterner · I. M. Stilbo · O. Svendsen · H. S. Thomsen · G. Torheim · R. Towart
E. C. Unger · H. J. Weinmann · E. R. Wisner · G. L. Wolf

Foreword by

A. L. Baert

With 224 Figures in 409 Separate Illustrations, 22 in Color

Springer

HENRIK S. THOMSEN, MD
Department of Diagnostic Radiology 54E2
Copenhagen University Hospital at Herlev
Herlev Ringvei 75
DK-2730 Herlev
Denmark

ROBERT N. MULLER, MD
Professor, Faculté de Médecine
Département de Chimie Organique
& Laboratoire RMN
Université de Mons-Hainaut
24, Aveneu du Champ de Mars
B-7000 Mons
Belgium

ROBERT F. MATTREY, MD
UCSD Medical Center
Department of Radiology
200 W. Arbor Drive
San Diego, CA 92109-8756
USA

MEDICAL RADIOLOGY · Diagnostic Imaging and Radiation Oncology

Continuation of
Handbuch der medizinischen Radiologie
Encyclopedia of Medical Radiology

ISBN 3-540-60924-5 Springer-Verlag Berlin Heidelberg New York

Library of Congress Cataloging-in-Publication Data. Trends in contrast media / H. S. Thomsen, R. N. Muller, R. F. Mattrey (eds.) ; with contributions by T. Albrecht ... [et al.] ; foreword by A. L. Baert. p. cm. -- (Medical radiology) Includes bibliographical references and index. ISBN 3-540-60924-5 (alk. paper) 1. Contrast media. I. Thomsen, Henrik S. II. Muller, Robert N. III. Mattrey, Robert F. IV. Albrecht, T. (Thomas) V. Series [DNLM: 1. Contrast Media. WN 160T792 1998] RC78.7.C65T74 1998 616.07'54--dc21 DNLM/DLC for Library of Congress 98-28592 CIP

Printed in Germany

Typesetting: Best-set Typesetter Ltd., Hong Kong

SPIN: 10526090 21/3135 - 5 4 3 2 1 0 - Printed on acid-free paper

Foreword

The use of contrast media within diagnostic radiology has been firmly established for many years now. Radiologic contrast media render immense services in daily clinical practice to innumerable patients all over the world. When the new cross-sectional modalities such as computed tomography and magnetic resonance imaging were introduced into clinical practice it rapidly became evident that the judicious use of contrast media allows the optimal exploitation of the great diagnostic potential of these revolutionary methods. More recently, efforts to create specific contrast media for ultrasound imaging have been successful, and the first beneficial results of their application in daily practice are now evident.

The aim of this book is to bring together the results of the tremendous research that has been performed during recent years in order to develop specific contrast media for magnetic resonance imaging and ultrasonography and also to develop safer contrast media for the classical radiologic techniques as well as computed tomography. Moreover, the book provides a comprehensive overview of the indications for and applications of these new contrast media in clinical radiology. Finally, risks, side-effects, and complications which may occur with the use of these drugs are covered appropriately.

The three editors are leading and well-known experts in their specific field. They have been very successful in ensuring the collaboration of so many internationally known specialists to cover the different topics dealt with in this book.

It is my pleasure to congratulate the editors and all the authors for their excellent contributions. I am convinced that this volume includes the latest, up-to-date information that radiologists and other clinicians are looking for in order to alow them to provide the best possible care to their patients and to maintain their standards of excellent clinical practice.

I sincerely hope that this book will meet the expectations of all those interested in updating their knowledge about radiologic contrast media and I wish this volume the same success as the previous volumes published in our series "Medical Radiology". I would appreciate every constructive criticism that might be offered.

Leuven — Albert L. Baert

Preface

During the past two decades more has happened in diagnostic imaging than during the first 8 decades following the birth of the specialty in 1895. A variety of new modalities – computed tomography, magnetic resonance imaging, ultrasonography, gamma camera imaging, and positron emission tomography – have been introduced and all have shown their importance in the workup of patients with symptoms/signs of disease. Initially it was claimed that neither magnetic resonance imaging nor ultrasonography required the use of contrast media. Today we know that this was incorrect. With all modalities, use of contrast media increases the information acquired, and accordingly there has also been enormous development with regard to contrast media during the past two decades. High-osmolar contrast media have been available since the early 1950s, but their role has now almost completely been taken over by the low- and iso-osmolar contrast media. Ultrasonography has got its bubbles. Magnetic resonance imaging uses agents distributed in the extracellular phase and organ-specific agents. Nuclear medicine has access to several pharmaceuticals attached to an isotope. More contrast media are on their way in order to improve imaging with the various modalities to the benefit of the patient. The technological development is now rapid, and sometimes it bypasses the much slower pharmaceutical projects. Therefore it is difficult to predict the future for the various old and new contrast media for diagnostic imaging. Nevertheless, diagnostic imaging has moved from being a specialty using one class of contrast media to a multipharmaceutical business. Radiologists now have many drugs on their shelves: it has not become easier to be a radiologist!

During recent years I have gained the impression that there is a strong wish among many radiologists to have an overview on the current state of the art regarding contrast media and some recommendations for daily work. Therefore this project was undertaken, with strong encouragement from Professor Albert L. Baert and Springer-Verlag. This book is devoted to the general radiologist, being designed to serve as a reference in his/her daily practice and to provide an update of current knowledge. The reader will find chapters ranging from the history of contrast media to what is going on in the laboratory, together with recommendations on doses, use, and treatment of adverse effects. The book covers iodinated contrast media used for x-ray examinations, radiopharmaceuticals employed for nuclear medicine, agents usable with magnetic resonance and echo-increasing agents for ultrasonography. It is my sincere hope that general radiologists will find it useful.

There would not have been a single word in this book without the assistance of my co-editors Prof. Mattrey and Prof. Muller as well as the authors of the chapters.

I sincerely thank them all for their excellent contributions. I am fully aware of the fact, that the project has taken the authors away from their families, clinical work, and the research laboratory, and that at some institutions it is not as rewarding to write a book chapter as it is to write an original paper published in a peer-reviewed journal. Nevertheless, the chapters were written, and I am sure that the readers will appreciate the end result.

The staff at Springer-Verlag did a tremendous job bringing the book together. Many thanks to them. Finally my wife and three boys often did not see me owing to this project; they did not complain. The book is devoted to Pia, Jannick, Michael, and Ulrik

Between Bangkok and Singapore on SK 973 HENRIK S. THOMSEN

Contents

Applications

I
Iodinated Contrast Media

1 History of Iodinated Contrast Media

H.M. POLLACK

CONTENTS

1.1 Preiodine Era (1897–1923)

1.1.1 Ureteral Catheters

It was Theodore Tuffier of Paris (Fig. 1.1a) who performed what might be called the first "contrast" study of the urinary tract. In 1897 Tuffier inserted a metal stylet into a ureteral catheter, rendering it opaque and thereby outlining the course of the ureter (Fig. 1.1b) (TUFFIER 1897; TONDREAU 1964). The idea that Tuffier merely suggested opacifying a ureteral catheter but did not actually do so himself (NESBIT 1956) is incorrect and is merely one of several myths surrounding early uroradiology that are still perpetuated. Contemporaries of Tuffier who are sometimes erroneously credited with having first demonstrated the course of the ureter roentgenographically include LOEWENHARDT (1901), who passed a flexible lead wire through a ureteral catheter, SCHMIDT and KOLISCHER (1901), who use lead wires without a catheter, and ILLYÉS (1901), who employed a silver mandrin (but who also suggested the same effect might be achieved by filling the catheter with bismuth subnitrate before inserting it). LOEWENHARDT (1901) also recommended localizing the ureters first by fluoroscopy, so as to better position them for the radiographs. KLOSE (1904) anticipated retrograde pyelography when he pointed out that a suspension of bismuth subnitrate, if injected after the catheter had passed rather than before, could also serve to fill the renal pelvis. Concerned with possible irritating effects of this suspension on the urothelium, however, Klose never attempted to do this. Ureteral catheters were nonopaque in those days, but Hurry Fenwick was able to produce radiopaque catheters by impregnating their walls with iron oxide (FENWICK 1905).

Rendering the course of the ureter radiopaque was obviously a big step forward in the ability to distinguish between ureteral calculi and phleboliths, obviating some of the problems that Leonard and others had encountered (LEONARD 1899, 1900). All of the diagnostic pitfalls were still not overcome, however, and this problem appears to have been particular sticking point among urologists.

H.M. POLLACK, MD, FACR, Professor Emeritus of Radiology and Urology, 420 Miller Rd # 408, Scottsdale, AZ 85251, USA

1.1.2 Cystography

1.1.2.1 Air

Contrast filling of a urinary viscus (bladder) was first carried out in cadavers by VON ZEISSL and HOLZKNECHT (1902) but it remained for Wittek in 1903 to attempt the same in a live patient. Wittek used air as his contrast medium and succeeded in demonstrating vesical calculi (WITTEK 1903–1904).

1.1.2.2 Bismuth

WULFF (1904) however, was the first to employ a radiopaque medium in the bladder. Filling what was in all likelihood a huge diverticulum, as well as the bladder itself, with a suspension of 10% bismuth subnitrate in starch, Wulff cautioned against the use of air: "Aside from the actual danger involved in air insufflation . . . I also believe that my procedure

a,b

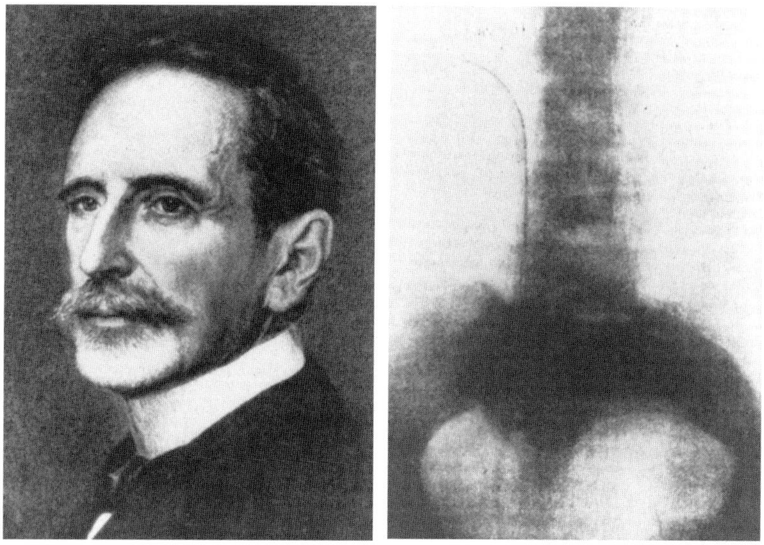

Fig. 1.1. **a** Theodore Tuffier (1859–1929), French surgeon; he first conceived of the idea of visualizing the ureter radiographically by inserting a metal stylet into a ureteral catheter. **b** First radiograph showing the course of the ureter in a living patient obtained by Tuffier in 1897. [These and following illustrations are from Pollack HM (1996) Uroradiology. In: Gagliardi R, McClennan BL (eds) History of the radiological sciences: diagnosis. Radiology Centennial, Inc., Reston, Va., USA, pp 195–253, with permission of the publisher and editors]

a,b

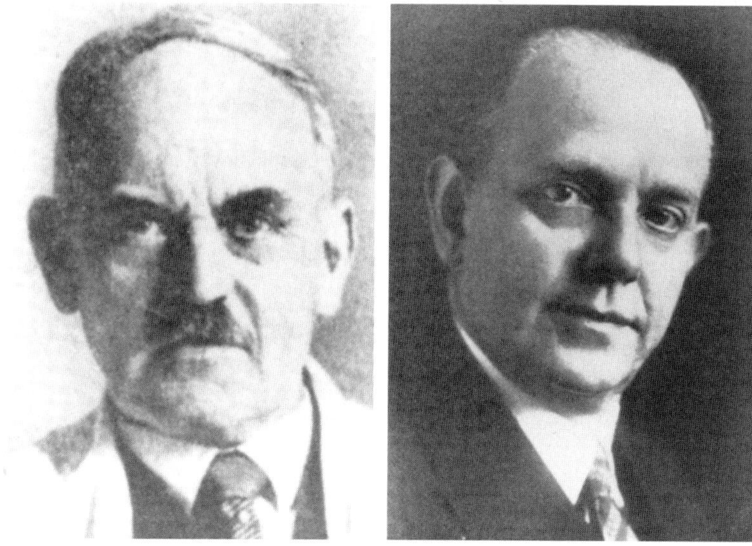

Fig. 1.2. **a** Fritz Voelcker (1872–1955), who, in conjunction with his younger associate, Alexander von Lichtenberg, revolutionized early uroradiology by introducing cystography (1905) and retrograde pyelography (1906) using colloidal silver (Collargol) as the contrast agent. **b** Alexander von Lichtenberg (1880–1949). A Hungarian by birth, a German professionally and, eventually, a Mexican by political expediency, von Lichtenberg was the dominant force in European urology for a generation. He was instrumental in introducing, with Voelcker, retrograde pyelography (1906) and, with Moses Swick, excretory urography (1929)

gives much more precise results . . ." Wulff, incidentally, was aided in his endeavor by Albers-Schönberg, who made the actual x-ray images himself. Despite Wulff's admonition, the fascination with gaseous contrast media persisted for many years (Burkhardt and Polano 1907; Pfahler 1919; Sporl 1933) and even extended to their use in the kidney (Frank 1906; von Lichtenberg and Dietlen 1911).

1.1.2.3 Colloidal Silver

In 1905, two German surgeons, Fritz Voelcker and Alexander von Lichtenberg, searching for a safe effective radiopaque contrast medium for use in the urinary tract, published the initial account of their work with Collargol, a colloidal suspension of silver. The older of the two, Voelcker, was a brilliant if sometimes moody man, and although urological surgery was his special interest[1], he was first and foremost a skilled general surgeon (Tondreau 1964) (Fig. 1.2a). His assistant, von Lichtenberg, Hungarian by birth, would spend most of his professional life in Germany, where he would eventually become one of Europe's most respected urologists (Fig. 1.2b). The

[1] He had, in fact, in association with his colleague, Joseph (1903) been the first to describe the use of indigo carmine excretion as a test of renal function.

idea of using Collargol was probably Voelcker's (NARATH 1951). As an experienced physician he knew that Collargol had been in use for some time as a local antiseptic and was undoubtedly familiar with its use in the eyes of newborns (Credé) to prevent ophthalmia neonatorum. Since the concentration used in the eye was not great enough for radiographic opacification, higher concentrations – greater than those heretofore employed clinically – would be necessary for their purposes. Concerned about the potential harmful effects of a stronger concentration of Collargol, the two surgeons tried it out first on themselves. They each instilled 2% Collargol into their own bladders and, having noticed no ill-effects, proceeded to carry out further studies on patients, again with no apparent complications (NARATH 1951; VOELCKER and VON LICHTENBERG 1905).

1.1.3 Retrograde Pyelography

1.1.3.1 Collargol

Buoyed by their success with Collargol cystography, Voelcker and von Lichtenberg extended their experiments to the kidney. In 1906, they published their near-canonical paper on pyelography (the first recorded use of this term) and thus revolutionized the diagnosis of upper urinary tract disease.

Just how epochal this discovery was is hard to appreciate today, with the vast array of technological implements now available. Using 5% Collargol, Voelcker and von Lichtenberg identified, described, and illustrated the normal renal pelvis and calyces ("cup-shaped spur"), nephroptosis, hydronephrosis, and extrinsic ureteral obstruction, and they correctly predicted that renal tumors and renal anomalies could be recognized with their technique (Fig. 1.3).

Although Collargol quickly became the contrast medium of choice for pyelography, it was by no means problem-free. Most troublesome were the reports of severe renal damage and even deaths following its use. MASON (1914) reported several cases of renal infarcts following Collargol administration, while others warned of the danger of parenchymal necrosis (BRAASCH 1913; Fig. 1.4). Several observers called attention to the persistence of silver colloid in the perinephric tissues for many days after pyelography (ZACHRISSON 1911). While it appeared that significant renal damage could be avoided by careful technique, there was no death of reported complication. RÖSSLE (1911) reported the first death after pyelography. Autopsy revealed diffuse hematogenous dissemination of silver (acute argyrosis) with necrosis of the kidney and other organs. By 1916 ZINDEL could find 11 deaths associated with Collargol pyelography and many more cases of severe renal damage. BLUM (1912) was so troubled by these complications that he rejected pyelography completely.

In addition to being dangerous, there were other objections to Collargol. It was difficult to prepare, it was quite viscous, and because it stained everything with which it came into contact, the exercise of great care was required when using it. In addition, it was expensive (ELKIN 1990; TONDREAU 1964).

1.1.3.2 Substitutes for Collargol

In an attempt to overcome some of these drawbacks, many other preparations of silver, including solutions, suspensions, emulsions, and mixtures, were tried, each with disappointing results. Formulations with such captivating names as Argyrol, Argentide, Cargentos, Dispargen, Electrogol, Intramin, Nargol, Pyelon, and Skiargen were introduced, invariably found wanting, and in short order dropped (TONDREAU 1964; NARATH 1951; BRAASCH 1915; STRAIN and BERLINER 1964; SARTORIUS and VIETHEN 1933). Clearly, silver was not the answer.

1.1.3.3 Substitutes for Silver

Attempts to replace silver with less objectionable metals resulted in trials of sodium bromide (WELD 1918), lithium iodide (Umbrenal) (JOSEPH 1921), and strontium chloride (WICHELS and BEHRENS 1924) as well as oily suspensions of bismuth (Xeroform) (DODERLEIN and KRÖNIG 1913) and iodine (Lipiodol) (SICARD and FORESTIER 1922). However, each of these agents was beset by one or more problems which prevented their use.

1.1.3.4 Thorium

In 1915 Burns introduced thorium nitrate, the first soluble salt, and since, in those days, the carcinogenic effects of thorium were not yet well appreciated, it appeared for a time that an acceptable substitute for Collargol had finally been found (BURNS 1915) (Fig. 1.5). Later, however, it was

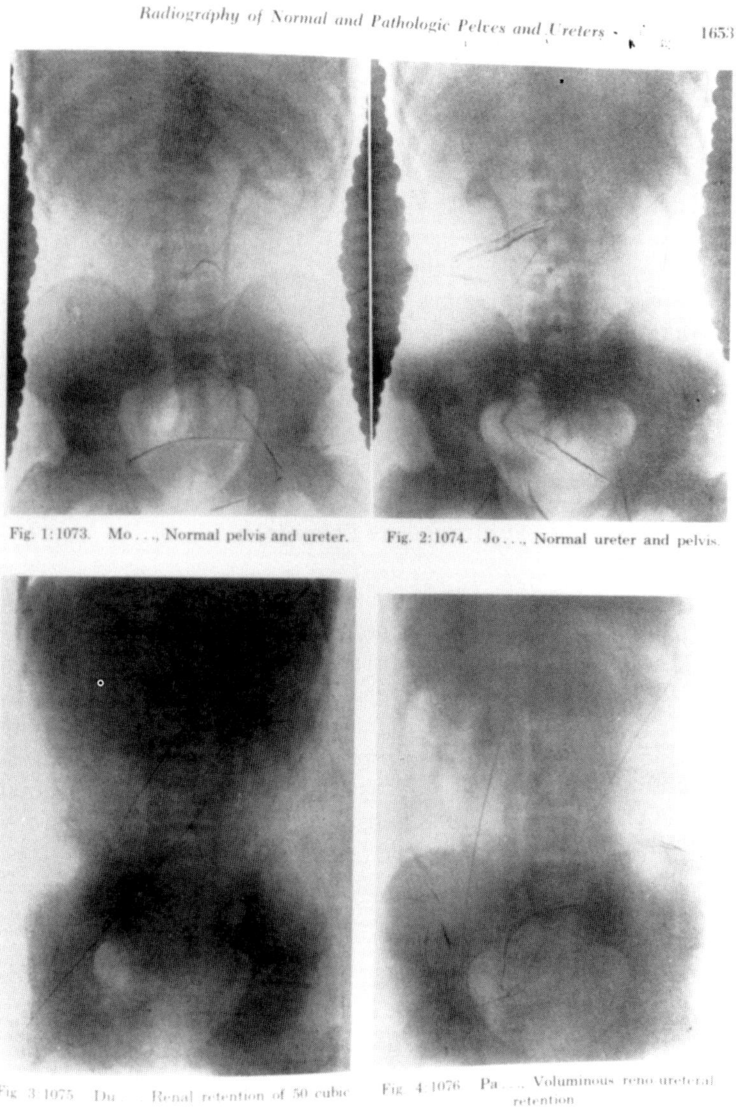

Fig. 1.3. Illustrations of some of the first retrograde pyelograms from the early paper of Professor J. Albarran of Paris, using 7% Collargol (1907)

learned that thorium nitrate caused astringent, irritant, and thrombotic problems (NARATH 1951) (probably unrelated to its radioactivity), and it was eventually abandoned after a 2- or 3-year run of popularity. Ironically this loss proved to be a blessing since the rejection of thorium nitrate prevented countless tragedies which would have undoubtedly followed its introduction on a large scale (GOLDMAN and GATEWOOD 1990). Unfortunately, thorium, in a colloidal suspension (Thorotrast), was reintroduced many years later (1928) (BLÜHBAUM et al. 1928).

Although the hazards associated with its use were known by then, they were not as well published in Europe as in America (CASPER 1967). Perhaps this explains why almost all of the reported cases of Thorotrast-related kidney neoplasms emanated from Europe (WENZ 1967). With its chemical inertness and almost total absence of acute toxicity, it is easy to appreciate Thorotrast's appeal.

Fortunately, better contrast media were available by 1928, with more on the way, and Thorotrast's time in the sun was limited. As it was, however, as many as 50 000 patients may have received it before it was finally withdrawn (JANTSCH 1984).

1.1.3.5 Iodides

The bad reputation of retrograde pyelography began to lift in 1918 when CAMERON (1920) first published his carefully detailed work showing the lack of renal

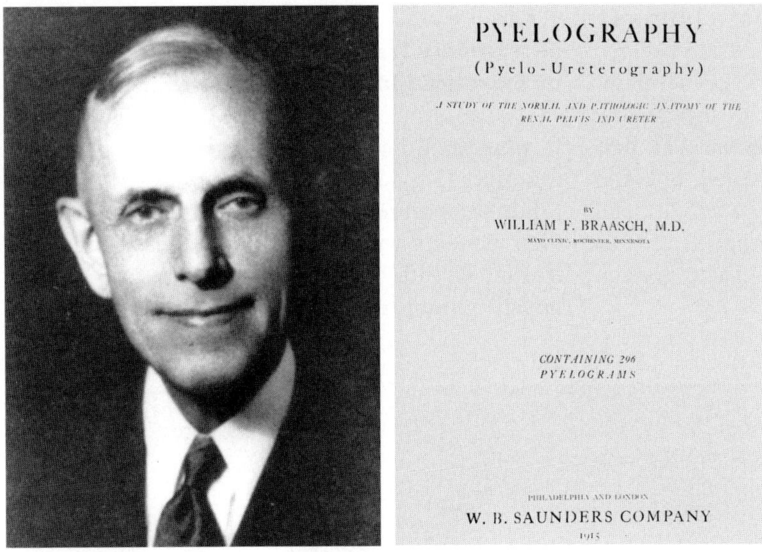

PYELOGRAPHY

(Pyelo-Ureterography)

A STUDY OF THE NORMAL AND PATHOLOGIC ANATOMY OF THE RENAL PELVIS AND URETER

BY

WILLIAM F. BRAASCH, M.D.

MAYO CLINIC, ROCHESTER, MINNESOTA

CONTAINING 296 PYELOGRAMS

PHILADELPHIA AND LONDON

W. B. SAUNDERS COMPANY

1915

a,b

Fig. 1.4. **a** William F. Braasch (1878–1975). Chairman of the Department of Urology at the Mayo Clinic for more than 30 years, Braasch was a pioneer and early advocate of retrograde pyelography. He, as much as anyone, was responsible for popularizing it. Braasch authored the first book on the subject (*Pyelography*. Saunders Philadelphia, 1915). **b** Braasch's *Pyelography* (1915) was the forerunner of a succession of texts on uroradiology by the same publisher, culminating in *Clinical urography* 75 years later

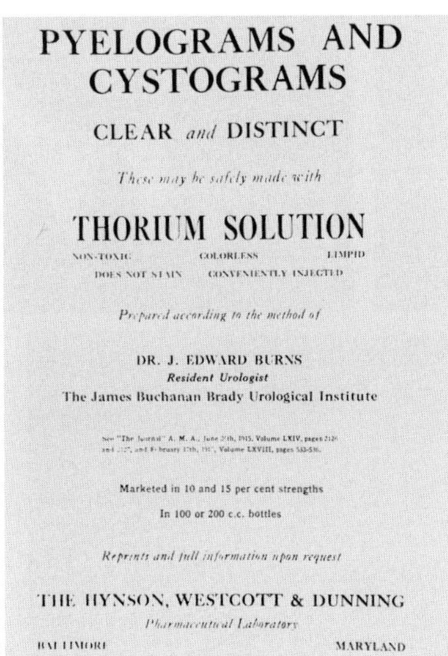

Fig. 1.5. Advertisement of thorium nitrate for use in retrograde pyelography and cystography which appeared in the *Journal of Urology* (June 1917)

toxicity of sodium and potassium iodide. He eliminated the potassium salt because of its effect on the heart. Sodium iodide in the concentrations proposed was less hypertonic than any other contrast medium. Follow-up studies in 1920 demonstrated that it produced no discernible renal changes in animals, no ill-effects followed its inadvertent entry into the circulation, and clinical experiences were extremely favorable (Maluf 1956). As the results of these and additional studies [especially those of Rubritius (1920) and Graves and Davidoff (1923)] became known, the case for sodium iodide grew stronger and the case for silver weaker. Within a few years sodium iodide had established itself as the contrast medium of choice for pyelography and it would remain so for a decade or more until replaced by a new generation of agents – the contrast media designed for excretory urography. The romance with silver was finally over.

Further historical reviews of the subject of contrast media may be found in the accounts by Narath (1951), Braasch (1927), and Goldstein and Abeshouse (1935).

1.2 The Urographic Era (1929–1975)

In spite of the fact that retrograde pyelography had become well-nigh indispensable in urological practice, it was still not an ideal diagnostic modality and could, in fact, never become one as long as it required cystoscopy, ureteral instrumentation, and, in many cases, general anesthesia for its implementation. Urologists had long appreciated the need for a less invasive, more comprehensive urological screen. The fact that it might be possible to accomplish this by means of an intravenously (or even orally) administered agent was more than fanciful. It had been known for some time, for example, that after the performance of retrograde pyelography (with sodium iodide) contrast could sometimes be detected in urine from the opposite kidney (Weld 1919) and, indeed, occasionally a pyelogram could be observed in the uninjected kidney (Narath 1951). Since pathways of backflow from the kidney to the general circulation had been demonstrated as early as 1856 by Gigon and were further elucidated by later workers such as Poirier (1891) Lewin (1897), and Marcus (1903), the concept of renal opacification by excretion of contrast media was not exactly foreign to experienced observers.

1.2.1 First Urinary Tract Visualization by Excreted Sodium Iodide

It must not have come as a great surprise to Osborne (Fig. 1.6a) and his co-workers at the Mayo Clinic to observe faintly opacified urinary tracts in their patients with syphilis who were undergoing treatment with relatively large doses of intravenously administered sodium iodide (50–250 cc of a

a,b

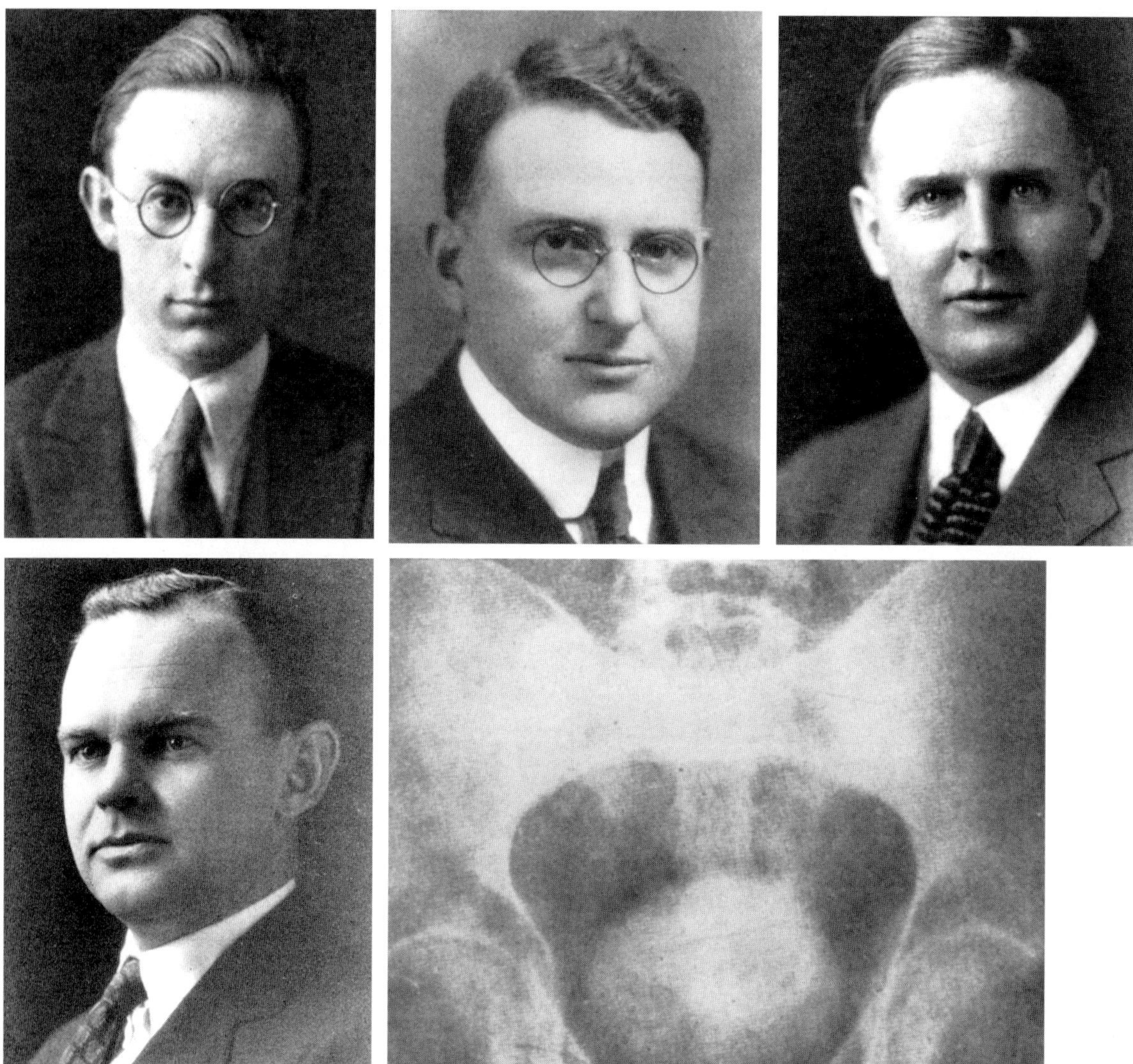

c

d

e

Fig. 1.6. **a** Earl Osborne (1895–1960), a dermatologist, was one of the Mayo Clinic group of four investigators who first noted opacification of the urinary tract following intravenous administration of sodium iodide for the treatment of syphylis (1923). **b** Leonard Rowntree (1883–1959), an acclaimed basic scientist and researcher as well as a leading Mayo Clinic internist, is generally credited with suggesting that radiography of patients receiving sodium iodide might show urinary tract opacification. **c** Charles Sutherland (1897–1951) was the radiologist member of the Mayo Clinic Team. **d** Albert Scholl (1890–1982), a urology fellow, also participated in the Mayo Clinic sodium iodide urinary tract roentgenography project. He later became one of the country's best-known urologists. **e** Illustration from original paper of Osborne et al. (1923) demonstrating opacification of the urinary bladder 2 h after an intravenous injection of 200 cc of 10% sodium iodide

10% solution) (Osborne et al. 1923). In fact the study was done prospectively with the hope that diagnostic visualization of the urinary tract would be forthcoming (Osborne et al. 1923). Credit for the notion that such opacification might be possible probably belongs to the brilliant physician and pharmacologist, Leonard Rowntree (Fig. 1.6b), although there is a small dispute about it. Grainger (1982b) states that the idea was Osborne's – a dermatologist – who allegedly serendipitously noticed that the bladder urine was roentgenographically opaque in some of his syphilitic patients who had been treated with large oral and intravenous doses of sodium iodide. Osborne himself, however, attributed the idea to Rowntree: "It occurred to one of us (L.G.R.) that if, in roentgenography of the urinary tract, advantage could be taken of the fact that sodium iodid [sic], after its introduction into the body, is normally excreted in the urine, roentgenograms of the kidneys, ureters and bladder might be secured without the need of catheterization." (Osborne et al. 1923).

Besides Rowntree and Osborne, the other participants in the study were Sutherland (Fig. 1.6c), a radiologist, and Scholl (Fig. 1.6d), a urologist. Unfortunately, the roentgenograms they obtained (some after oral administration of sodium iodide) showed only faint urinary tract opacification, never approaching the level necessary to exert a clinical impact (Fig. 1.6e). The door had been opened, however, but for some strange reason, few if any investigators – including the Mayo group – ventured through. Perhaps the doses of iodide were thought too large, but whatever the cause, for the next 5 years, essentially no further progress was made in excretory urography.

1.2.2 "Pyelognost"

To be sure, a few observers, including Rosenstein and von Lichtenberg (1924), Lenarduzzi and Pecco (1927), and Volkman (1924) repeated Osborne's work, but failed to expand upon it. Perhaps the most promising work was that of Roseno (1929a,b), who cleverly combined sodium iodide with urea (Pyelognost). Some of his films were quite impressive but the quality of the studies was inconsistent. Hryntschalk (1927–1929) tried more than 50 halides (Hryntschalk 1929) and Zeigler and Kohler (1927–1928) tried large doses by mouth (Ziegler and Kohler 1930), but neither they nor others could consistently produce diagnostic urinary tract opacification. No less a figure than von Lichtenberg himself – by now the leader of European urology and an early strong supporter of the concept of urography – was beginning to think the idea was an impossible dream (von Lichtenberg 1928). But in what was to become one of the most intriguing tales in the chronicles of radiological history, fate was about to step in.

1.2.3 Development of Organic Iodides for Urography

1.2.3.1 Selectan Neutral and Swick's Discovery

In 1928, Moses Swick (Fig. 1.7), a bright young house officer at Mount Sinai Hospital in New York City, was offered the opportunity to study abroad by his chief, Dr. Emanuel Libman (of Libman-Sack's disease fame). Dr. Swick, an aspiring urologist, chose to utilize his Libman fellowship in the clinic and laboratories of Professor Leopold Lichtwitz, a highly respected internist in Hamburg, Germany. Lichtwitz

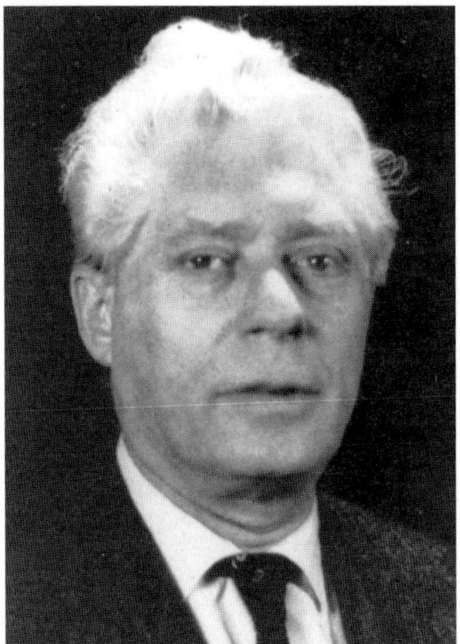

Fig. 1.7. Moses Swick (1900–1985). As a young American urologist working abroad on a Libman fellowship, Swick became absorbed in the search for a safe, effective urographic medium. In 1929, he succeeded where all before him had failed, producing diagnostic quality excretory urograms with Uroselectan (Iopax). Working in the clinic of von Lichtenberg, Swick was the discoverer of modern excretory urography although von Lichtenberg quarrelled bitterly with him over priorities to this claim

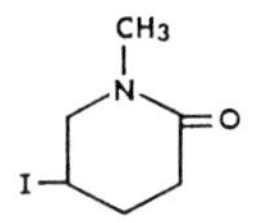

Fig. 1.8. *N*-Methyl-5-iodo-2-pyridone (54.1% I). Selectan (D), Selectan Neutral (D)

(1930), who was interested in infectious diseases, was studying the effect of newly synthesized antibacterials on local infections of the gallbladder and kidney, and Swick was anxious to help him. LICHTWITZ was fortunate to be friendly with the chemist, Arthur Binz of Berlin, who, with his associate, Curt Rath, had synthesized hundreds of compounds with potential therapeutic effectiveness and graciously provided LICHTWITZ with a smorgasbord of new and exciting agents.

Binz was to become another major player in the subsequent drama which evolved over priorities in excretory urography, and the evolution of his role is interesting. Shortly after World War I, he succeeded to the directorship of the chemical division of the State Institute for Experimental Therapy in Frankfurt, where, years earlier, Paul Ehrlich had synthesized the first chemotheapeutic agent, the antispirochetal arsenical, salvarsan 606. With his focus on preparing more effective antiluetic drugs, Binz and his associates discovered that incorporating arsenic (or other metals) into a pyridine ring markedly lessened its toxicity. Substituting iodine in place of arsenic, they created a new group of compounds which seemed to be just as antimicrobial as their arsenic-containing relatives, but less toxic. One of these compounds, SELECTAN (Fig. 1.8), was found to be particularly good in treating coccal infections of cows' udders. After altering it chemically to increases its solubility (from 4% to 10%), Binz, who by this time had moved to the Agricultural College in Berlin, forwarded the new agent, Selectan Neutral, to Lichtwitz, as well as to several other physicians (TONDREAU 1964; BINZ 1931).

During the evaluation of Selectan Neutral (Fig. 1.8) in rabbits Swick noticed that the animal's urinary iodine concentration was high and he wondered if the urine might be radiopaque (SWICK 1966, 1978). When later work in animals and man confirmed that it was, Swick persuaded Lichtwitz to let him switch his attention from the therapeutic to the diagnostic potential of Binz's drugs.

Further testing showed Selectan Neutral to be unsatisfactory for clinical use. The pyelocalyceal systems and ureters were poorly seen and distressing symptoms including nausea, vomiting, diplopia, and headache were frequent. Nonetheless, Swick and Lichtwitz were encouraged enough to press on with the search for a more suitable contrast medium. At an ensuing meeting with Binz, Swick postulated that the nature of the adverse effects of Selectan Neutral, especially the diplopia, might be attributable to its methyl radical and asked if it could be replaced. Binz offered two alternative agents, both di-iodinated compounds, but they both proved too poorly soluble for intravenous use. Trying them orally didn't work either and these two were promptly dropped. (SWICK 1978).

At this point, a decision was made which both Swick and his mentor, Lichtwitz, would later come to rue terribly (GRAINGER 1982b). Because Swick felt that the research would move along faster in a hospital with a larger urological population, he persuaded Lichtwitz to ask von Lichtenberg, whose urology service at St. Hedwig's Hospital in Berlin was probably the largest in the world (at one point it had over 250 urological beds!), if he could transfer his investigations there. Since anything having to do with urinary tract opacifications was of great interest to von Lichtenberg, Lichtwitz found a receptive ear. An added benefit of course was that moving to Berlin would put Swick closer to Binz and his arsenal of iodinated pyridones. Later, as it turned out, the work could just as well have been done in Hamburg, with the avoidance of great anguish (GRAINGER 1982a).

1.2.3.2 Uroselectan

In Berlin, another meeting with Binz took place where Swick repeated the desiderata of an acceptable contrast medium. This time Binz offered him Uroselectan (SWICK 1930, 1966, 1978), which he and Rath had actually synthesized the year before. Unknown to Swick, this compound had already made the rounds once; Hryntschalk had used it in rabbits and discarded it (HRYNTSCHALK 1928; LICHTWITZ 1930; BRAASCH and BUMPUS 1930; JACHES 1930). Because its chemical characteristics seemed to fit the bill, Swick accepted Uroselectan (Fig. 1.9) readily and tried it on a few patients at St. Hedwig's. His results were just the opposite of Hryntschalk's. The images were far better than any previously obtained (some of them appear acceptable even by today's standards!) (Fig. 1.10). Better yet, patient tolerance was high. After further testing and confirmation of the initial results, Swick excitedly cabled Libman in

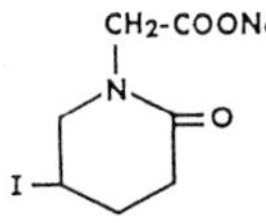

Fig. 1.9. 5-Iodo-2-pyridone-*N*-acetic acid sodium salt (42.2% I). Iopax (D), Uroselectan (D), Uro-selectan (D), Uroselektan (D)

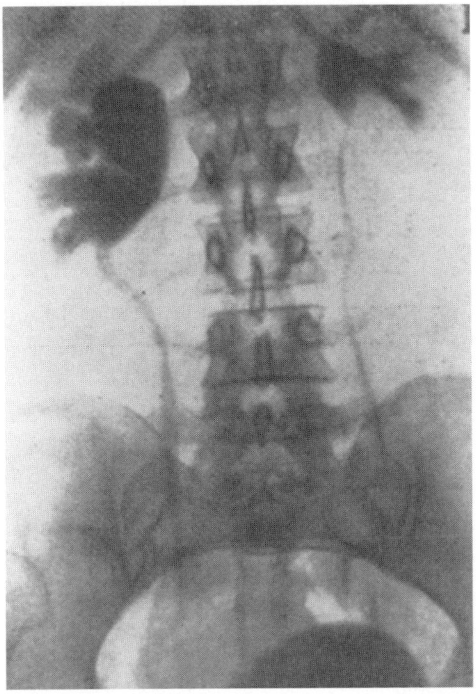

Fig. 1.10. Moses Swick's first excretory urogram with Uroselectan (1929)

New York and asked him to inform von Lichtenberg, who was lecturing in the United States. Told of the great news, von Lichtenberg returned home at once, fascinated by the prospects that his 20-year search for the holy grail of uroradiology might be over at last (Grainger 1982b).

1.2.3.3 Swick's Controversy with von Lichtenberg

There are many versions of what happened next. The facts seem only slightly hazy; it is the interpretations which vary greatly. Binz and von Lichtenberg saw things one way (Binz 1930), Lichtwitz and Swick, another (Grainger 1982b; Marshall 1977). These differences were deep and irreconcilable and would, for the rest of their lives, indelibly scar the participants. The following seems to have been the most likely scenario.

Upon reviewing Swick's results, the ebullient von Lichtenberg could hardly wait to announce the discovery to the world. He would, of course, present the results himself at the 9th German Urological Congress, in Munich, only a few months away. Having been raised in the strong Germanic tradition of *geheimrat*, wherein the Professor was the lord of the fiefdom and all others subservient to him, it never occurred to the baron that anyone else should make this presentation, or be first author on the landmark paper to follow. As the Chief, the honor belonged to him (Marshall 1977). The young American, uninhibited by the strict teutonic professional code, had other ideas. As the one whose brainchild this was, and as the one who had conducted the painstaking experiments and laborious testing (while his chief was over 3000 miles away), shouldn't he, ethically and morally, receive most of the credit for excretory urography and did he not deserve the honor of making the first oral and written presentations to the scientific community?

The dispute was heated, but was momentarily resolved at a conference attended by the protagonists, Swick and von Lichtenberg, as well as Lichtwitz, his assistant Renner, and von Salle, the editor of *Klinische Wochenschrift*, the journal in which the proceedings of the Urological Congress were to be published (Grainger 1982b; Marshall 1977). A compromise was reached. Swick would make the first presentation detailing the development of Uroselectan and would show a few roentgenograms. A joint offering, presented by von Lichtenberg, would follow, on the clinical applications of excretory urography. According to Grainger (1982b), who, with Marshall (1977), has exquisitely chronicled the details of these events, "it is probable that without Lichtwitz's support, Swick would never have been recognized as a major contributor to this work."

As scheduled, the publications appeared after the Congress. Swick's paper appeared first in *Klinische Wochenschrift* (Swick 1929) (Fig. 1.11a), followed by that of von Lichtenberg and Swick (von Lichtenberg and Swick 1929), which, by now, included data on 84 patients. Needless to say, these publications caused a furor, but they were not the only items of radiological interest in that issue. By a remarkable coincidence, the article immediately preceding Swick's was by Werner Forssmann containing the first-ever description of (self) cardiac catheterization! (Forssmann 1929) (Fig. 1.11b).

Another irony of the time concerned a paper presented by dos Santos (1929) at the 9th Congress. dos Santos' presentation, of course, was the first

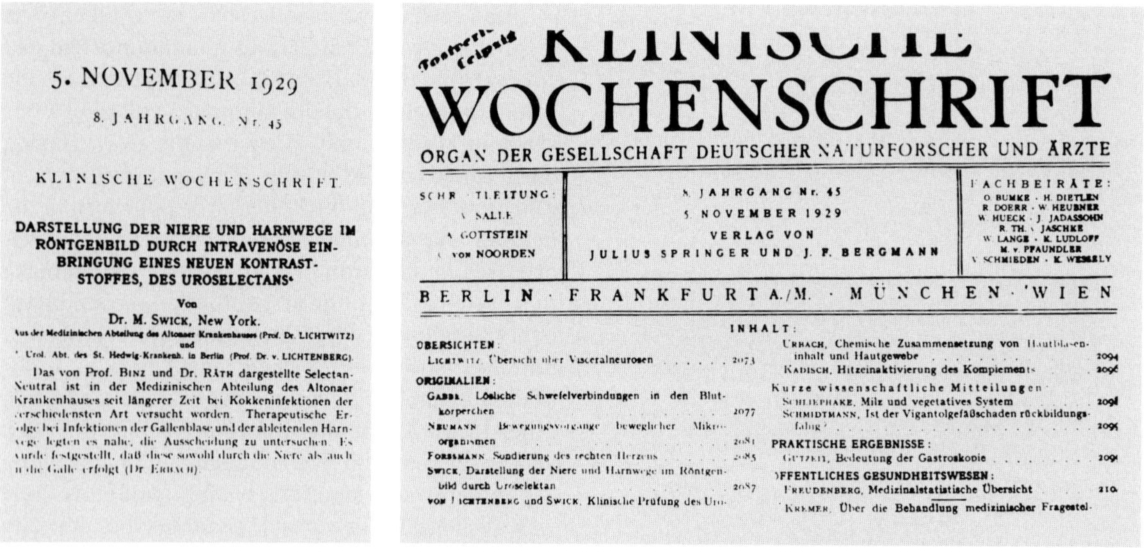

5. NOVEMBER 1929

8. JAHRGANG. Nr. 45

KLINISCHE WOCHENSCHRIFT.

DARSTELLUNG DER NIERE UND HARNWEGE IM RÖNTGENBILD DURCH INTRAVENÖSE EINBRINGUNG EINES NEUEN KONTRASTSTOFFES, DES UROSELECTANS*

Von

Dr. M. Swick, New York.

Aus der Medizinischen Abteilung des Altonaer Krankenhauses (Prof. Dr. LICHTWITZ) und * Urol. Abt. des St. Hedwig-Krankenh. in Berlin (Prof. Dr. v. LICHTENBERG).

Das von Prof. Binz und Dr. Räth dargestellte Selectan-Neutral ist in der Medizinischen Abteilung des Altonaer Krankenhauses seit längerer Zeit bei Kokkeninfektionen der verschiedensten Art versucht worden. Therapeutische Erfolge bei Infektionen der Gallenblase und der ableitenden Harnwege legten es nahe, die Ausscheidung zu untersuchen. Es wurde festgestellt, daß diese sowohl durch die Niere als auch in die Galle erfolgt (Dr. Eichach).

KLINISCHE WOCHENSCHRIFT

ORGAN DER GESELLSCHAFT DEUTSCHER NATURFORSCHER UND ÄRZTE

SCHRIFTLEITUNG: V. SALLE, A. GOTTSTEIN, C. VON NOORDEN

8. JAHRGANG Nr. 45
5. NOVEMBER 1929
VERLAG VON
JULIUS SPRINGER UND J. F. BERGMANN

FACHBEIRÄTE: O. BUMKE · H. DIETLEN, R. DOERR · W. HEUBNER, W. HUECK · J. JADASSOHN, R. TH. V. JASCHKE, W. LANGE · K. LUDLOFF, M. v. PFAUNDLER, V. SCHMIEDEN · K. WESSELY

BERLIN · FRANKFURT A./M. · MÜNCHEN · WIEN

INHALT:

ÜBERSICHTEN:
Lichtwitz, Übersicht über Visceralneurosen . . . 2073

ORIGINALIEN:
Gabbe, Lösliche Schwefelverbindungen in den Blutkörperchen . . . 2077
Neumann, Bewegungsvorgänge beweglicher Mikroorganismen . . . 2081
Forssmann, Sondierung des rechten Herzens . . . 2085
Swick, Darstellung der Niere und Harnwege im Röntgenbild durch Uroselektan . . . 2087
von Lichtenberg und Swick, Klinische Prüfung des Uro-
Urbach, Chemische Zusammensetzung von Hautblaseninhalt und Hautgewebe . . . 2094
Kadisch, Hitzeinaktivierung des Komplements . . . 2096

Kurze wissenschaftliche Mitteilungen:
Schliephake, Milz und vegetatives System . . . 2098
Schmidtmann, Ist der Vigantolgefäßschaden rückbildungsfähig? . . . 2099

PRAKTISCHE ERGEBNISSE:
Gutzeit, Bedeutung der Gastroskopie . . . 2099

ÖFFENTLICHES GESUNDHEITSWESEN:
Freudenberg, Medizinalstatistische Übersicht . . . 210
Kremer, Über die Behandlung medizinischer Fragestel-

a b

Fig. 1.11. **a** Swick's initial publication on excretory urography which appeared in *Klinische Wochenschrift* in November 1929. This was followed by a second paper, authored jointly by Swick and von Lichtenberg. **b** By an extreme coincidence the paper preceding Swick's in that same issue of the *Kliniche Wochenschrift* was Werner Forssmann's first description of his Nobel prize winning work on cardiac catheterization (with himself as the first patient)

announcement of his soon to become classic work on translumbar aortography, but unfortunately, the young Portuguese surgeon never got the recognition he deserved. His work was completely upstaged by the spectacular results of the Germans and was, for the moment, quickly forgotten. The same fate befell the Italian investigator, Roseno (1929a,b), who, 1 year after his earlier presentation at the 8th German Urological Congress in Berlin, was back with new and improved results with Pyelognost but these too were overshadowed by the reports of Uroselectan.

von Lichtenberg never forgave Swick for what he perceived as insufferable insubordination and one can only wonder how much of a hand the Berlin *uromeister* had in seeing that Swick's name was all but blotted out in future references to urography. In 1930, for example, shortly after young Swick had returned to his home town of New York, the American Urological Association held their annual meeting there. The guest of honor was von Lichtenberg, who was accorded a hero's welcome as he presented the first paper in America on "*The principles of intravenous urography*" (von Lichtenberg 1931). Swick's name was barely mentioned. In fact, he was not even invited! (Grainger 1982b).

1.2.3.4
Uroselectan B (Neo-Iopax) and Diodrast

Meanwhile, in Germany, Schering took over the commercial manufacturing of Uroselectan (now

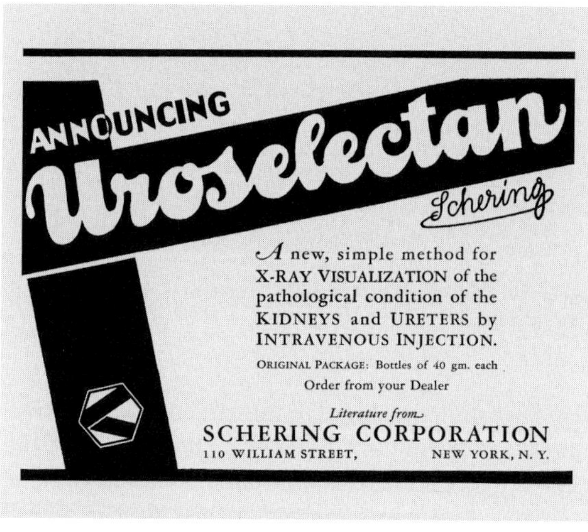

Fig. 1.12. Early advertisement for Uroselectan (later marketed as Iopax), which appeared in the *American Journal of Roentgenology*, July 1930

marketed as Iopax) (Figs. 1.9, 1.12) while Binz and Roth were busy making new iodinated pyridones. They succeeded in synthesizing two important new derivatives, Uroselectan B (Neo-Iopax) (1930) (Elkin 1990) and, 2 years later, Diodrast (Diodone) (Maluf 1956), both di-iodinated compounds with good solubility and low toxicity. Diodrast (Fig. 1.13) and Neo-Iopax (Fig. 1.14) were to become the standard contrast media for intravascular use for the next 20 years. Meanwhile, von Lichtenberg luxuriated in the limelight of intravenous urography for

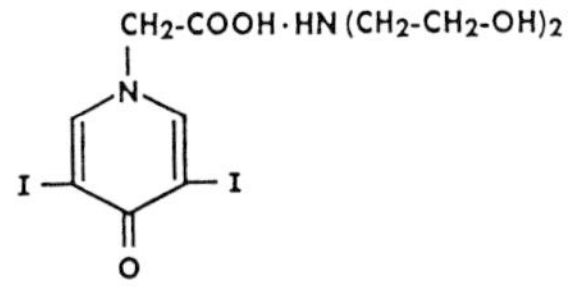

Fig. 1.13. Iodopyracet: 3,5-diiodo-4-pyridone-*N*-acetic acid diethanolamine salt (49.8% I); 35%, 50%, and 70% w/v solutions. 3203 RP, Abrogen, Arteriodone, Cardiotrast, Contraste Radiologico, D-50, Diatrast, Dijodon, Diodon, Diodone, diodone (INN), Diodrast, Diodrast Concentrated (D), Djodrast, Falitrast U, iodopyraacet (USP,XV), Iopyracil, Iopyracyl, Jodumbran, Kardiotrasta, Leodrast, Neomethioodal, Neo-Methiodal, Neo-Skiodan, Neospect, Neo-Tenebrill, Neotenebryl, Neo-Tenebryl, Nosydrast, Nosylan, Nosyland, Noviadrast, Novisdrast, Nycotrast, Ombradil, Opaarenol, Pelviranum, Pelviren D, Perabrodil, Per-Abrodil, Perhydril, Periodil, Per-Iodil, Perjodal, Per-Radiographol, Perurdil, Pielosil, Pielosyl, Pyelodrast, Pyelombrine, Pyelosil, Pyelosin, Pyelosom, Pylumbrin, Pyraceton, Savac, Umbradil, Umbragnost, Uriodone, Urognost, Urograf, Urograph, Vasiodone, Viscyazol, Yodopalina, Yoduron, Yodurone

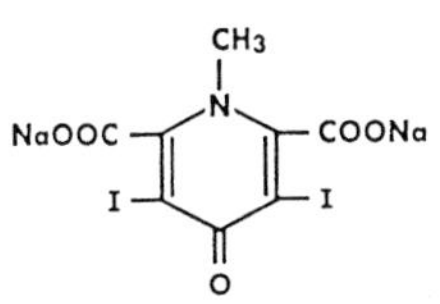

Fig. 1.14. Sodium iodomethamate: *N*-methyl-3,5-diiodo-4-pyridone-2,6-dicarboxylic acid disodium salt (51.5% I); 20%, 35%, 50%, and 75% w/v solutions. Contraste Urologico, D-40, Hypoloid Iodoxyl, Iodoxyl, iodoxyl (BP, 1958), Lumoxyd, Neo-Iopax, Neopielofanina, Neo-Pielofanina, Neo-Yopax, Nitasom, Nitaxom, Oopaxil, Pielectan, Pyelectan, sodium iodomethamate (USP,XV), Sugiuron, Ultraren, Uridognost, Urografin B, Uropac, Uropac Meurice (D), Uroselectan B (D), Uroselektan B, Urotrast, Urumbrin

which he took credit (and which was felt to have been important enough to merit consideration for a Nobel prize) (Tondreau 1964; Grainger 1982b; Schück 1950). The German professor's fame grew greater as he received countless accolades and awards from all over the world.

1.2.3.5
Benzoic Acid Derivatives (Hippuran)

What about Moses Swick? Was he relegated to oblivion after his brief moment in the sun? No, Swick was far from finished. Hurt by being shoved into the background but determined to continue his work nonetheless, he pursued other ideas for contrast media. In spite of the trials of building a urological practice, he managed to find time to team up

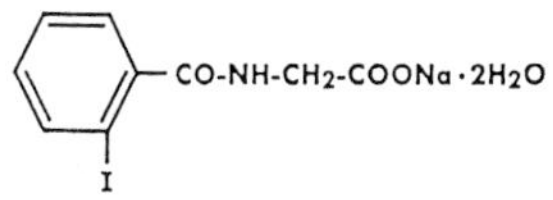

Fig. 1.15. Iodohippurate sodium: 2-iodohippuric acid sodium salt (38.8% I) dihydrate crytals; 35% and 48% w/v solutions. Hippodin, Hippuran, Iodairal, Iodairal Forte, iodohippurate sodium (NNR), Iodo-Ray Sterules, Jodairol, Jodairol Forte, Orthoiodin, Renotest, Renumbral, Urocontrast

with Vernon Wallingford, a chemist at the Malinckrodt Chemical Works in St. Louis. Abandoning the Binz pyridone-based model in favor of a new molecule configured from benzoic acid, the two brought off a biochemical tour de force; not only did they discover Hippuran, a mono-iodinated benzoic acid derivative, but they laid the chemical groundwork for the next generation of contrast media – tri-iodinated benzoic acid derivatives (Swick 1933). [It took a full 20 years, however, before Wallingford (1953) and Hoppe (1959) finally unlocked the secrets of making nontoxic tri-iodinated contrast media from benzoic acid.] Although Hippuran itself did not live up to expectations because of its low iodine content and poor tolerance in high doses, the potential impact of its synthesis was quickly appreciated. In 1933 Swick and Wallingford were awarded the prestigious Billings Gold Medal of the American Medical Association for this discovery.

1.2.3.6
Acetrizoate (Urokon), Diatrizoate (Hypaque), and Iothalamate (Conray)

Ironically, Hippuran (Fig. 1.15), nearly valueless as a radiographic contrast agent, proved to be a superb molecule for determining renal plasma flow (*para*-aminohippurate) and in its radioactive form (^{131}I-Hippuran) become a valuable agent for estimating renal tubular function (Fine and Blaufox 1990). Diodrast and Neo-Iopax dominated the urographic scene (Mullen and Hughes 1952) until 1952, when they were replaced by the first tri-iodinated contrast medium for urography, Wallingford's acetrizoate (Urokon) (Fig. 1.16) (Richardson and Rose 1950; Nesbit and Lapides 1950). The introduction of the safer compound, diatrizoate (Hypaque), in 1954 was a major advance (Moore and Mayer 1955), but later diatrizoate (Fig. 1.17) was forced to share the market with the newer and popular iothalamate (Conray), introduced in 1963 (Hoey et al. 1963). Three decades later diatrizoate and iothalamate (Fig. 1.18) are still

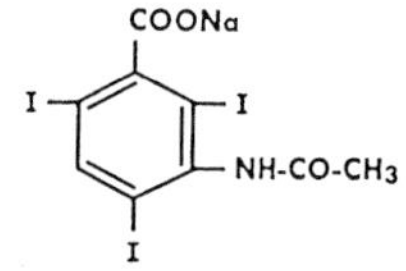

Fig. 1.16. Sodium acetrizoate: 3-acetamido-2,4,6 triiodobenzoic acid sodium salt (65.8% I); 30%, 50%, and 70% w/v solutions. Acetiodone, Contraxine, Diaginol, Iodopact, Iodopaque, Iodozoatnatrium, Jodopaque, Rheopak, sodium acetrizoate (INN), Solucotrast, Tri-Abrodil, Triiotrast, Trijodyl, Triodan, Triognost, Triopac, Triopacon, Triopaque, Triumbren, Triurol, Urokolin, Urokon Sodium (D), Uro-sombril, Vesamin, Vesamin R, Visotrast

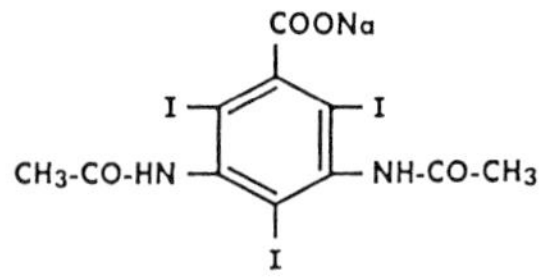

Fig. 1.17. Sodium diatrizoate: 3,5-diacetamido-2,4,6-triiodobenzoic acid sodium salt (59.9% I); 25%, 45%, and 50% w/v solutions. Hypaque Sodium, Natriumjoddiazoat 45%, sodium amidotrizoate (INN), sodium diatrizoate (USP,XVI)

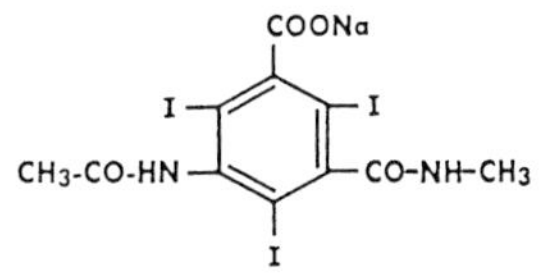

Fig. 1.18. Sodium iothalamate: 5-acetamido-2,4,6-triiodo-*N*-methylisophthalamic acid sodium salt (59.9% I); 66.8% and 80% w/v solutions. Angio-Conray (80%), Conray-400 (66.8%), iotalamic acid (INN) sodium salt, sodium iothalamate (USAN)

the dominant ionic contrast media as well as the radiopaques most commonly used for retrograde pyelography.

Who really deserved the credit for discovering excretory urography? In the minds of the embittered von Lichtenberg and Binz there was no doubt at all (Binz 1930, 1931). Swick was nothing more than a laboratory assistant out to usurp the honors rightfully belonging to them (von Lichtenberg 1931). But, realistically, could a young American doctor in a foreign country really flim-flam the tough Prussian medical establishment? Would von Lichtenberg have permitted Swick to make his presentation and author his manuscript alone if the senior professor did not feel Swick's role was primal? Probably not. Lichtwitz likened the priority issue to a three-legged stool with each man playing an indispensible role. But he reserved the main distinction for Swick: "To Dr. Swick of New York we owe the uroselectan method" (Lichtwitz 1930).

Years later, C.E. Alken, one of von Lichtenberg's last assistants and a loyal disciple, admitted that the "honors of the discovery are his (Swick's)." He argued, though, that von Lichtenberg's genius was to "recognize immediately the importance of the method" and to "successfully introduce the new method into clinical usage" (Alken 1974).

It was never clear whether the hope of discovering a practical agent for excretory urography was in Swick's mind when he came to Europe in 1928 or whether the discovery was entirely serendipitous. The available evidence would suggest the latter, but, in fact, it matters little whether it was by fortune or design. What is more important is that, when handed the opportunity, Swick, who was undoubtedly familiar with Osborne's work, was quick to make the most of it. The rest is history. Lichtwitz put it quite well:

> Important as is the existence of preparations, (i.e . . . , new compounds) they become valuable only when the right person takes them for a special purpose. The preparations of Professor Binz were tested for the same purpose before Dr. Swick began his studies (without his knowledge) by a man of great experience in research work – without sufficient results. Between the important work of chemical preparation and final success, there came the hard work of a clever and energetic man, one with the deepest devotion to and greatest passion for research work. (Lichtwitz 1930)

Perhaps Lichtwitz should also have pointed out that there was more than enough glory to go around.

1.2.3.7
Final Resolution of the Contrast Media Priority Controversy

While only a few insiders knew the truth, the vast majority of American and European physicians remained oblivious to Moses Swick's work. For many years, it appeared that this oversight would never be corrected, but finally 35 years later, the record was put straight at last. Almost entirely as a result of the diligent, persistent efforts of one man, Dr. Victor F. Marshall, of New York, the facts were unearthed and eventually disclosed (Marshall 1977). Marshall, then Professor and Chairman of the Department of Urology at Cornell Medical School, motivated by stories he had heard about Swick's role, became determined to unearth the truth and set about collecting relevant papers, documents, diaries, and first-person accounts from any and all persons with pertinent information relating to this near-forgotten tale of intrigue. After several years of painstaking research Marshall was convinced that Moses Swick had been very unfairly treated by organized medicine – urology in particular – and he undertook literally a one-man crusade to convince the leaders of American urology that they had been parties to a grave injustice. Because of the irrefutable nature of Marshall's evidence, as well as his lofty professional stature, his voice eventually fell on sympathetic ears. In 1965 as part of the award ceremony accompanying the presentation of the prestigious Valentine Award of the New York Academy of Medicine, Moses Swick finally received his just recognition. Not only did he receive the Valentine Medal, but as part of the ceremony he also received tributes – and sincere, eloquent apologies – from a number of America's leading urologists and spokesmen for organized urology including: Miley Wesson, William F. Braasch, Fred Foley (of Foley catheter fame), William P. Herbst, Hermon C. Bumpus, and Abe Goldstein: "... were it not for Dr. Swick's contributions, it is doubtful that the media used in excretory urography of today would have been discovered...." (W.F. Braasch 1965, quoted in Melicow 1966); "... my congratulations and unqualified approval of its (Award Committee) award to Dr. Swick, which at long last undoes a long standing miscarriage of justice ..." (Fred E.B. Foley 1965, quoted in Melicow 1966).

1.2.3.8 Swick's Later Career

So, at last, the tale had come full circle. Moses Swick finally received the honor so long withheld from him through bias, jealousy, politics, and just plain ignorance. He was deeply touched by the collective expression of appreciation he heard that night. Certainly it went a long way toward erasing the accumulated hurt of 35 years.

For the rest of his career, Swick remained in New York in the private practice of urology. His research activities were very limited after his work with Hippuran, but he retained an active interest in academics and clinical investigation all of his life. In later years Swick received many honors including honorary membership in the Society of Uroradiology in 1974 and an Honorary Doctor of Medicine from the Free University of Berlin in 1975. He died in 1985 at the age of 85. He is memorialized by his parent institution, Mount Sinai Medical School of New York, by an annual lecture in his name.

1.2.3.9 von Lichtenberg's Subsequent Career

von Lichtenberg, who estimated he performed more than 30 000 operations in his lifetime (Del Rio 1974), maintained his hectic surgical practice in Berlin until 1936. That year, disturbed by the political changes taking place in Germany (von Lichtenberg, who was part-Jewish, had already been forced to relinquish his teaching activities) (Del Rio 1974; Spence 1990), he moved to Budapest. Prescient as usual, he soon realized, however, that before long all Europe would be immersed in conflagration, and fearing for the welfare of his wife, who was also Jewish, and children, he emigrated with them to Mexico in 1939 (Spence 1990). von Lichtenberg died in Mexico City in 1949 having actively practiced urology there until shortly before his death, at age 69 years.

Arthur Binz continued his work on the antibacterial properties of pyridine derivatives, even after his retirement from the Berlin Agricultural College in 1935. He made several speaking tours of the United States in the late 1930s, but declined an opportunity to stay on for an extra year as a guest investigator at Philadelphia's Franklin Institute, feeling that an unfriendly atmosphere confronted all Germans in the United States at that time. He died in Germany in 1943 at the age of 75 (Tondreau 1964).

Leopold Lichtwitz's life was another casualty of the Hitler regime. Forced to leave in Germany in the early 1930s, he came to New York, where he practiced medicine at Montefiore Hospital. He died there in 1949 at the age of 69 years (Strain and Berliner 1964).

Although diatrizoate and iothalamate all but monopolized the contrast media world for nearly 30 years, that world was not perfect.

1.2.3.10 Nonionic Media

Despite their excellent safety records, occasional serious reactions accompanied the use of these agents (Katayama et al. 1990) and the search for even safer media never abated. One person who was convinced that better contrast media could be designed was Torsten Almén, a young Swedish radiologist who was particularly concerned about the pain accompanying contrast media injection during arteriography (Fig. 1.19). Almén, who liked to take an occasional dip in the Baltic, was struck by the fact that swimming under water with his eyes open in

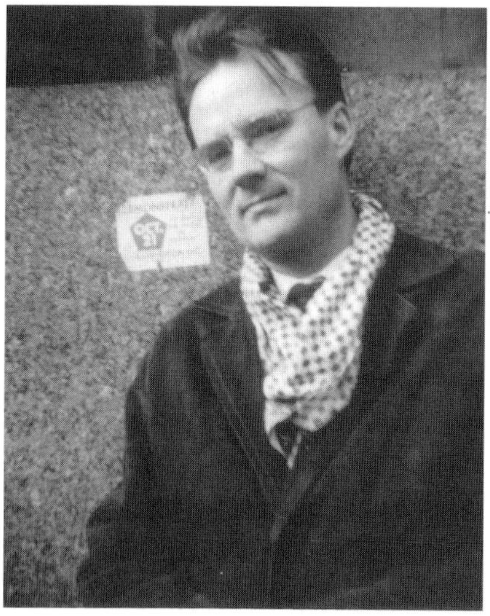

Fig. 1.19. Torsten Almén. As a postdoctoral fellow in Temple University Medical School's Departments of Radiology and Physiology, Almén conducted his epochal work on low-osmolality contrast media during the years 1967–1968. Teaching himself the requisite organic and colloidal chemistry, he proposed the chemical structure for a new class of iodinated nondisassociating sugars – the first nonionic iodinated contrast media

the isotonic Baltic Sea never caused his eyes to hurt, while the same activity performed in the hypertonic Atlantic or Mediterranean regularly produced pain. He theorized that hypertonicity damaged endothelial membranes by drawing water out of the delicate lining cells and wondered whether hypertonicity might not also be the main cause of pain during arteriography (T. ALMÉN 1992, personal communication).

The Swedish investigator soon got his opportunity to find out. Arriving in Philadelphia in 1967, as a postdoctoral Fellow in the laboratories of Professor Herbert Stauffer, then Chairman of the Department of Radiology at Temple University School of Medicine and Professor Peter Lynch of the Department of Physiology, Torsten Almén had a choice of research projects; he could either work on an improved model of a steerable angiographic catheter he had previously designed (ALMÉN 1966) or he could look into the relationship between tonicity and toxicity of contrast media. After thinking it over, he decided (quite fortunately, as it turned out) on the latter.

Torsten used bats to test his hypothesis. Working with Professor Mimi Weideman, he dripped contrast media on the very thin bat wings and studied the effects on the microcirculation (Fig. 1.20). The results proved conclusively that his osmotoxicity theory was correct. As described by Almén: "The

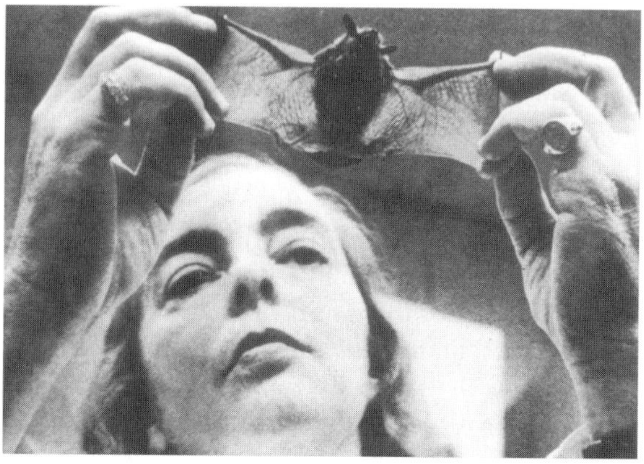

Fig. 1.20. Professor Mimi Weideman (Temple University Medical School Department of Physiology). It was in the laboratory that Torsten Almén tested the effects of contrast media on the microcirculation of blood and lymph, using the bat's wing as a model

experiments taught me the relative importance of the osmotoxicity of the contrast media: the higher the osmolality the higher the inhibiting effect on vasomotions in arteries, veins and lymphatics, and, also the higher the viscosity of the red blood cells the slower their flow through capillaries and other small vessels." (T. ALMÉN 1992, personal communication).

The demands and tedium of the laboratory were occasionally interrupted by humorous interludes as evidenced by the following episode:

> After the experiments the bats were released through an open window to fly home to their mine in New Jersey. But it was too cold to fly home that winter of 1967 and instead the bats found an open window in the basement of the medical school library. After a while the librarians did not dare enter the basement because of the bats. The culprit, me, was located and told to get rid of the bats. I found a colony of bats hanging on the backs of the *Acta Orthopaedica Scandinavia*. I did not know if this journal was the least borrowed in the library or if they were the books with the best bat temperature. I brought the bats back to my refrigerator and when spring came, they flew home to New Jersey. (T. ALMÉN 1992, personal communication)

Not being able to interest anyone in producing low-osmolality contrast media, Almén was left to his own devices. Since he was not a chemist and knew little about designing such things, he bought some organic and colloid chemistry textbooks and taught himself the essentials. He saw that replacing the carboxyl group with a nondisassociating amide would partially satisfy his requirements and he drew up a hypothetical formula for what would later become metrizamide (Amipaque), the prototype of nonionic contrast media. Poorly soluble, metrizamide (Fig. 1.21) was of limited usefulness for urography and was eventually followed by the polyhydroxylated

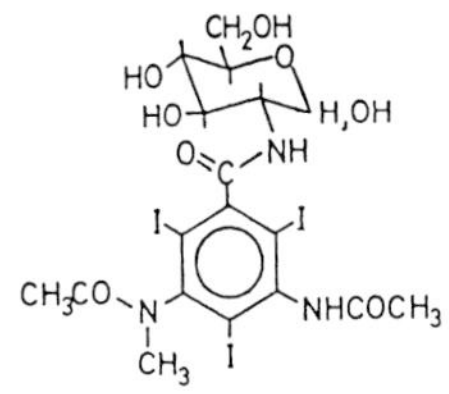

Fig. 1.21. Metrizamide

highly soluble, second-generation agents including iohexol (Omnipaque), iopamidol (Isovue), and ioversol (Optiray) (ALMÉN 1969). Unfortunately Almén was once again forced to suffer those twin maladies so common to original thinkers, rejection and frustration. It was several years before he was able to interest any pharmaceutical company in his ideas - even with a molecular blueprint in hand. Eventually, a small Norwegian company, Nyegaard A/S and Co., was persuaded to listen. The perspicacity of their director of Research and Development, Dr. Hugo Holtermann, was rewarded years later when the little known Nyegaard company evolved into the giant international Nycomed organization, largely on the strength of low-osmolality contrast media.

In addition to being the discoverer of a new and important class of biological compounds, Torsten Almén holds at least one other distinction; he was, incredible as it may seem, the first radiologist to play a major role in the synthesis of any contrast medium! (GRAINGER 1982b). And this not until 1967, 72 years after Roentgen!

Acknowledgement. The above material is extracted from the chapter "Uroradiology" by the same author, which appears as chapter 9 in "A history of the radiological sciences: diagnosis", published by Radiology Centennial Inc. Reston, Virginia, USA, 1996, and edited by R. Gagliardi and B.L. McClennan, and appears here by permission of the editors and publishers.

References

Alken CE (1974) von Lichtenberg: his life and work. Urology 3:382–384

Almén T (1966) A steering device for selective angiography and some vascular and enzymatic reactions observed in its clinical application. Acta Radiol Suppl 260

Almén T (1969) Contrast agent design. Some aspects of the synthesis of water soluble contrast agents of low osmolality. J Theor Biol 24:216–226

Binz A (1930) Discussion following: Swick M. Intravenous urography by means of the sodium salt of 5-iodo-2-phridon-n-acetic acid. JAMA 95:1403–1409

Binz A (1931) The chemistry of Uroselectan. J Urol 15:297–301

Blühbaum T, Frick K, Kalkbrenner H (1928) Eine neue Anwendungsart der Kolloide in der Röntgendiagnostik. Fortschr Geb Röntgenstr 37:18–29

Blum (1912) Über den Wert der Pyelographia und anderen Methoden zum Nachweise von Dilatationen des Nierenbeckens. Wien Med Wochenschr 62:1269–1274

Braasch WF (1913) Recent progress in uretero-pyelogaphy. J Mich Med Soc 12:189–191

Braasch WF (1915) Pyelography. WB Saunders, Philadelphia

Braasch WF (1927) Urography, 2nd edn. WB Saunders, Philadelphia, 17–39

Braasch WF, Bumpus HC Jr (1930) Report on sodium 2-oxo-5-iodo-pyridine-N-acetate (introduced as Uroselectan) to the Council on Pharmacy and Chemistry of the American Medical Association. JAMA 95:1425–1427

Burkhardt L, Polano O (1907) Die Fülling der Blase mit Sauerstoff zum Zweck der Cystoskopie und Radiographie. Münch Med Wochenschr 54:20–21

Burns EJ (1915) Thorium - a new agent for pyelography. JAMA 64:2126–2127

Cameron DF (1918) Aqueous solutions of potassium and sodium iodide as opaque mediums in roentgenography. JAMA 70:754–755

Cameron DF (1920) Comparative study of sodium iodide as an opaque medium in pyelography. Arch Surg 1:184–214

Casper J (1967) The introduction in 1928–1929 of thorium dioxide in diagnostic radiology. Ann NY Acad Sci 145:527–529

Del Rio A (1974) von Lichtenberg in Mexico. Urology 3:388–389

Doderlein ASG, Krönig B (1913) Operative Gynäkologie, 3rd edn. George Theime, Leipzig

Elkin M (1990) Stages in the growth of uroradiology. Radiology 175:297–306

Fenwick EH (1905) The value of the use of a shadowgraph ureteric bougie in the precise surgery of renal calculus. Br Med J 1:1325–1327

Fine EJ, Blaufox MD (1990) Urological applications of radionuclides. In: Pollack HM (ed) Clinical urography, Vol I. Saunders, Philadelphia, pp 519–528

Forssmann W (1929) Die Sondierung des rechten Herzens. Klin Wochenschr 8:2085–2087

Frank MF (1906) Perfectionnement du diagnostic radiographiques des affections du bassinet du rien (Referat). Ann de Malad Org Genito-urin p 1665

Gigon C (1856) Recherches sur l'ischurie;-physiologie pathologique. L'Union Médicale (Series 1) 10:8–83, 85–87, 93–94, 297–299, 301–302

Goldman SM, Gatewood OMB (1990) Neoplasms of the renal collecting system and ureter. In: Pollack HM (ed) Clinical urography. Saunders, Philadelphia, chapter 45, pp 1318–1319

Goldstein AE, Abeshouse BS (1935) A historical and practical consideration of pyelographic media. AJR 33:165–175

Grainger RG (1982a) Intravascular contrast media (letter to editor). Br J Radiol 55:251

Grainger RG (1982b) Intravascular contrast media - the past, the present and the future. Br J Radiol 55:1–18

Graves RC, Davidoff LM (1923) The choice of pyelographic mediums. JAMA 80:168–171

Hoey GB, Rands RD, DeLaMater G, Chapman DW, Weigert PE (1963) Synthesis of derivatives of isophthalamic acid as x-ray contrast agents. J Med Chem 6:24–26

Hoppe JO (1959) Some pharmacological aspects of radio-opaque compounds. Ann NY Acad Sci 78:727–739

Hryntschalk T (1928) (Discussion) Röntgenographische Nierendarstellung und Pyelographie auf intravenösem

Wege. Z Urol. Special Issue, 8th Kongress Urologie, Berlin, p 434
Hryntschalk T (1929) Studien zur röntgenologischen Darstellung von Nierenparenchym und Nierenbecken auf Intravenösem Wege. Z für Urol 23:893–904
Illyés G (1901) Uretercatherezés és radiographia. Orv Hetil 45:659–662
Jaches L (1930) Intravenous urography (Swick method). JAMA 95:1409–1412
Jantsch M (1984) Zur Geschichte der Röntgendiagnostik in der Urologie. Wien Klin Wochenschr 96:637–642
Joseph E (1921) Ein neues Kontrastmittel für die Pyelographie. Zentralbl Chir 48:707–708
Katayama H, Yamaguchi K, et al. (1990) Adverse reactions to ionic and non-ionic contrast media: a report from the Japanese Committee on the Safety of Contrast Media. Radiology 175:621–628
Klose B (1904) Radiographie eines durch das Kystoskopi diagnostizierten Falles von Kompletter Ureterenverdopplung. Deutsch 2 Chir 72:613–617
Lenarduzzi G, Pecco R (1927) Iniezioni Endovenose Di ioduro di sodio. Arch Ital Radiol 3:1055–1060
Leonard CL (1899) The roentgen ray diagnosis of renal calculus. Phila Med J 3:886–889
Leonard CL (1900) The technique of positive and negative diagnosis of ureteral and renal calculi by aid of röntgen rays. Ann Surg 31:163–179
Lewin L (1897–1898) Der Übertutt von festen Korpern aus der Blase in die Nieve und in entfernte Körperorgane. Arch Exper Pathol U Pharmakol 40:287–307
Lichtwitz L (1930) Discussion following: Swick M. Intravenous urography by means of the sodium salt of 5-iodo-2-pyridon-n-acetic acid. JAMA 95:1403–1409
Loewenhardt F (1901) Bestimmung der Lage des Ureters am Lebenden. Jahresbericht d. Schlesische Gesellsch. f. Vaterl. Kultur 79:136–137
Maluf NSR (1956) Role of roentgenology in the development of urology. AJR 75:847–854
Marcus H (1903) Experimentelle Untersuchungen über das Rückströmen von Hornblaseninhalt. Wien Klin Wochenschr 16:725–730
Marshall VF (1977) The controversial history of excretory urography. In: Witten DM, Myers GH, Utz DC (eds) Emmett's clinical urography, 4th edn, Vol I. Saunders, Philadelphia, pp 2–5
Mason JM (1914) Dangers attending injections of the kidney pelvis for pyelography. JAMA 62:839–844
Melicow MM (1966) The Fourth Ferdinand C. Valentine Medal and Award to Moses Swick. Bull NY Acad Med 42:123–127
Moore T, Mayer R (1955) Hypapaque: improved medium for excretory urography. Preliminary report of 210 cases. South Med J 48:135–141
Mullen WH Jr, Hughes CR (1952) Intravenous urographic contrast media; controlled study of diodrast and neoiopax. Am J Roentgenol 68:903–914
Narath PA (1951) Renal pelvis and ureter. Grune and Stratton, New York
Nesbit RM (1956) Radiology and its contribution to urology. AJR 75:995–996
Nesbit RM, Lapides J (1950) Preliminary report on Urokon, a new excretory pyelographic medium. J Urol 63:1109–1112
Osborne ED, Sutherland CG, Scholl AJ Jr, Rowntree LG (1923) Roentgenography of the urinary tract during excretion of sodium iodide. JAMA 80:368–373
Pfahler GE (1919) The injection of air for the roentgen diagnosis of tumors of the bladder. AJR 6:371–375
Poirier MP (1891) Sur quelque phénoménes cousécutifs aux injections uréterales. Séance et mem. Soc de Biologie 3:585–587
Richardson JG, Rose DK (1950) Clinical evaluation of Urokon. J Urol 63:113–119
Roseno A (1929a) Intravenoese pyelographie. Verhandl deutsch Ges Urol 9 Kongress, Munich, pp 337–343
Roseno A (1929b) Die intravenöse Pyelographie. Klin Wochenschr 8:1165–1170
Rosenstein P, von Lichtenberg A (1924) Intravenöse Darreichung von Jodnatrium und Pneumoradiographie des Nierenlagers. Z Urol Chir 16:225
Rössle R (1911) Tödliche Kollargolvergiftung. Münch Med Wochenschr 58:280
Rubritius H (1920) Jodkali als Kontrastmittel in der Röntgenologie der Harrwege. Z Urol 14:57–60
dos Santos R (1929) Die Arteriographie der Niere (am Lebenden) Verhandl deutsch Ges Urol 9 Kongress, Munich, pp 386–388
Sartorius F, Viethen H (1933) Klinische und experimentelle Untersuchungen zur Frage der Kontrastmittelwahl bei der retrograden Pyelographie, insbesondere über die verwendbarkeit des Thorotrastes. Z Urol Chir 36:312–342
Schmidt LE, Kolischer G (1901) Radiographie an sondierten Ureterem and Nieren. Monatsbe Urologie 6:427–431
Schück H (1950) Nobel, the man and his prizes. University of Oklahoma Press, Norman, Oklahoma
Sicard JA, Forestier J (1922) Méthode géneral d'éxploration radioligique par l'huile idoée Lipiodal. Bull et mém Soc med d'hōp de Paris 46:463–469
Spence HM (1990) The life and times of Alexander von Lichtenberg. Urology 35:464–469
Sporl HJ (1933) Über die Zulassigkeit der Gasfülling des Nierenbeckens und der Blase. Z Urol Chir 36:404–420
Steinberg I, Evans JA (1962) Conray: a new cardiovascular and urographic contrast medium. Radiology 79:395–400
Strain WH, Berliner WP (1964) Viscous and oily radiopaques. Med Radiography Photography (Suppl) 40:61–78
Swick M (1929) Darstellung der Niere und Harnwege in Röntgenbild durch intravenose Embringung eines neuen Kontraststoffes, des Uroselectans. Klin Wochenschr 8:2087–2089
Swick M (1930) Intravenous urography by means of the sodium salt of 5-iodo-2-pyridon-n-acetic acid. JAMA 95:1403–1409
Swick M (1933) Excretion urography. With particular reference to a newly developed compound: sodium ortho-iodohippurate. JAMA 101:1853–1855
Swick M (1966) The discovery of intravenous urography. Bull NY Acad Med 42:128–151
Swick M (1978) Radiographic media in urology. Surg Clin North Am 58:977–994
Tondreau RL (1964) Roentgenography of the urinary tract. In: Bruwer A (ed) Classic descriptions in diagnostic roentgenology Vol II. Charles C Thomas, Springfield, IL, pp 1605–1728
Tuffier T (1897–1899) Sonde uréterale opaque. In: Duplay, Reclus. Traite de chirurgíe, Vol VII. Masson, Paris, pp 412–413
Voelcker F, von Lichtenberg A (1905) Die Gestalt der menschlichen Harnblase im Röntgenbilde. Munch Med Wochenschr 52:1576–1578
Voelcker F, von Lichtenberg A (1906) Pyelographie Röntgenographie des Nierenbeckens nach Kollargolfulling. Munch Med Wochenschr 53:105–106
Volkman J (1924) Zur Röntgenographischen Darstellung der Harnwege durch intravenöse Verarbreichung schattenge-

bender Mittel. Deutsche Med Wochenschr 50:1413–1414
von Lichtenberg A (1928) Diskussion, 8th Kongress Urologie, Berlin 1928. Z für Urol (Special Issue) p 435
von Lichtenberg A (1931) The principles of intravenous urography. J Urol 25:249–257
von Lichtenberg A, Dietlen H (1911) Darstellung des Nierenbekens und Ureters in Röntgenbild nach Suerstoff-Füllung. Ein Beitrag zur Pyelographie. Münch Med Wochenschr 58:1341–1342
von Lichtenberg A, Swick M (1929) Klinische Prütung des Uroselectans. Klin Wochenschr 8:2089–2091
von Zeissl M, Holzknecht G (1902) Der Blasenverschluss in Röntgenbilde. Med Blätter 25:155–157
Wallingford V (1953) The development of organic iodide compounds as X-ray contrast media. J Am Pharm Assoc (Scientific Edition) 42:721–728
Weld EH (1918) The use of sodium bromide in roentgenography. JAMA 71:1111–1112
Weld EH (1919) Renal absorption with particular reference to pyelographic mediums. Med Clin North Am 3:713–731
Wenz W (1967) Tumors of the kidney following retrograde pyelography with colloidal thorium dioxide. In: Swarm RL (ed) Distribution, retention and late effects of thorium dioxide. Ann NY Acad Sci 145:806–810
Wichels P, Behrens A (1924) Ein Beitrag zur röntgenologischen Darstellung der Harnwege mit Kontrastmitteln. Z Klin Med 100:815–820
Wittek A (1903–1904) Zur Technik der Röntgenphotographie (Ledenwinbel, Blasensteine). Fortschr Röntgenstr 7:26–27
Wulff P (1904) Verwendbarkeit der X-Strahlen für die Diagnose der Blasendifformitäten. Fortschr Röntgenstr 8:193–194
Zachrisson F (1911) Fall von Kollargoinjektion in die Tubuli recti der Niere. Nordiskt Mediciniskt Arkiv 3f XI afd. 1 no 27
Ziegler J, Kohler H (1930) Perorale pyelographie. Med Klin 26:10–11
Zindel L (1916) Kritisch Sichtung der Falle von Nierenschadigungen nach Pyelographie. Z Urol Chir 3:359–404

2 Design of X-ray Contrast Agents

G.L. Wolf

CONTENTS

2.1 Introduction

In vivo imaging for diagnostic purposes began with the utilization of x-rays to penetrate the body and with film to record the differential absorption of tissues. Advances in imaging this process continue today, including digital detection of the penetrating x-rays with planar, circular, and soon volumetric detector arrays. Computer-based reconstruction of x-rays completing the journey have dramatically improved the quality and utility of imaging x-ray absorption or scatter. It is too soon to declare that further developments in radiographic imaging technologies are unlikely; for example, the time of flight methods being developed for visible light, gating or pulsing algorithms, adopting interference technologies, or building hybrid systems combining simultaneous imaging with complementary modalities could lead to new generations of medical (and non-medical) instruments. Traditionally, contrast agent enthusiasts have had to adapt their methods and materials for existing radiographic devices. Creatively, we have been analogous to mitochondria who arrive as unbidden invaders and attempt to establish an essential role that assures our reproduction by the dependent host.

G.L. Wolf, MD, PhD, Center for Imaging and Pharmaceutical Research, Massachusetts General Hospital, 149 13th Street, Charlestown, MA 02129, USA

Just as there have been cycles of rapid development of x-ray imaging devices interspersed with less dynamic periods, so also have there been cycles of development of x-ray contrast materials. These have been reviewed in Chap. 1. In this chapter, we will review the impending introduction of whole new classes of such agents with expanded roles in medical imaging. These developments will be strongly influenced by the new cost-effectiveness mind set of our current global economy.

2.2 X-ray Absorption

At the energies used for imaging – roughly 80–140 kV – most of the absorption or attenuation of the incident beam is due to the photoelectron effect. Some of the tissue electrons can be slightly more effective due to k-edge absorption, but this contributes relatively little specific attenuation of imaging energies. Rather, absorption depends upon the number of electrons per unit volume of tissue, which is approximately NZ/A times tissue density (mass per volume) where N is Avogadro's number, Z is the atomic number, and A is the atomic mass. For the elements dominating tissue composition – carbon, nitrogen, and oxygen – have Z/A ratios of about 0.5 while hydrogen has a ratio of unity. Elements with many more electrons per unit mass are present in minor concentrations in normal tissue and contribute little to differential absorption of x-rays, except for calcified structures. However, tissue density does vary widely and is mainly responsible for the four characteristic x-ray tissue contrasts: air, fat, soft tissue, and bone. Most radiopaque contrast materials would be more accurately called radiodense agents since their electron density is largely achieved by virtue of the elevations in local specific gravity rather than by Z/A enrichment. Similarly, materials that contrast soft tissue by decreasing x-ray absorption, such as CO_2, do so by lowering tissue density and should be called radiolucent materials. These considerations, already evident in Roentgen's original investigations, clarify design of x-ray contrast agents. Although iodine is often incorporated as the putative absorber in a parenteral contrast agent, we shall learn that other elements such as dysprosium or bromine are useable to create a high local density of electrons. The relative change in local tissue density caused by the radiographic contrast agent must be sustained or reestablished in vivo for a particular material to serve as a useful imaging adjunct.

Often there is more than one way to image a particular abnormal process. A general survey of imaging modalities and their companion contrast agents is shown in Table 2.1. Most imagers will recognize the considerations of the physical basis of the modality, along with considerations of spatial and temporal resolution. With new helical computed tomography (CT) instruments, radiographic imaging wins most battles where resolution dominates. On the other hand, inherent contrast, cost, and safety are handicaps for CT. Contrast agents are extremely useful in restoring tissue differentiation, whether based upon anatomy or physiology. But it takes a lot of radiographic agent to be detectable – here the radiographic modalities perform the poorest; and there is a radiographic hierarchy with plain film being worst, followed by digital methods, and then CT, where contrast sensitivity is about tenfold higher than with plain film imaging, but still orders of magnitude less sensitive than contrast detection with scintigraphy, magnetic resonance imaging (MRI), or ultrasound. Cost considerations must include the basic modality, its contrast agent, and some utility index for the clinical circumstance. All of these issues are making decision analysis and pharmacoeconomic modeling important in the use of imaging within algorithms for disease management.

Finally, the utility of a contrast agent is based upon its ability to differentially change tissue x-ray attenuation. In static or equilibrium conditions, this task usually consists in making one tissue more visible than an adjacent structure. However, with computing methods of registration and subtraction, it is possible to visualize tissue differential response in the dynamic case. Thus, processing a temporal series of images may make it possible to discern an interpretable effect of the agent when no single image in the series has diagnostic enhancement. As imaging accepts the task of depicting local function rather that local anatomy, the need for differential enhancement between two tissues may no longer pertain.

2.3 Mechanisms of Tissue Distribution

All contrast agents are designed to have a particular set of pharmacokinetic and biodistribution properties. The latter provides the easiest way to classify radiographic contrast agents while the former is key for writing the pharmacologic and imaging prescriptions. For this review, we will consider agents that distribute in extracellular spaces versus agents that distribute within the intracellular space, often with some tissue specificity. Blood pool agents are extracellular in their initial distribution but may have either an extracellular or an intracellular clearance pathway. Other classifications can also be enlightening, e.g., small versus large molecules, or targeted vs nontargeted agents.

2.3.1 The ECF Agents

The water-soluble, ionic or nonionic, monomeric, dimeric, or mixed iodinated benzene ring materials have seen a long and successful usage for radiographic enhancement. Further improvements in the

Table 2.1. Comparison of imaging modalities (modified from Wolf 1995)

Physical basis	Scintigraphy	X-ray	Ultrasound	MRI
Spatial resolution	4	1	3	2
Temporal resolution	3	1	2	1
Inherent contrast	4	3	2	1
Cost	2	3	1	1
Safety	3	3	1	1
Contrast agents				
Detection sensitivity	1	4	3	2
Targeted agents	1	3	4	2
Dose	1	4	3	2
mg/kg	10^{-5}–10^{-9}	10–10^{-2}	10^{-1}–10^{-3}	10^{-1}–10^{-3}

Note: Relative score: 1 = best, 4 = worst.

design of this class would be directed to decreasing the cost of production, improving safety, or reducing viscosity. The lowest charge per dose to the consumer has become key to market share and even extent of clinical utilization, but any advances in design for lower production costs remain proprietary. Nonionic monomers and dimers are extraordinarily safe – no other pharmaceutical is injected at grams per second into sick patients – yet concern about adverse drug responses, especially nephrotoxicity, remain a consideration in clinical use. Functional radiographic imaging would be more competitive with functional MRI if these agent were safer. If the mechanisms for adverse effects were discerned and proved preventable, then enthusiasm for new extracellular agents might wane. There are efforts underway to reduce viscosity by making the agents more compact (PETTA et al. 1998).

This class of agents had been designed to be as nonreactive as possible. Yet, a reactive agent that quickly bound to serum albumin would yield a blood pool distribution of great potential utility for minimally invasive angiography or functional characterization of abnormal vascular leakage such as occurs with neoplasms and inflammation. Alternatively, clusters of such agents that did not escape into the extracellular space for the imaging period yet broke apart into excretable subunits could accomplish a similar purpose. In like manner, these materials might be coupled to a targeting ligand directly or with a linker to gain tissue specificity. Should the targeting provide entry into the intracellular space, concerns about toxicity would increase.

2.3.2 Blood Pool Agents

If a safe ECF agent could be formulated so that it had little or no extravasation from blood to tissue, a new class of agents with exceptional clinical utility would result. It is clear that such agents would be much larger, presenting a diameter of more than 50 nm to the capillary endothelium. However, such materials could still be removed from blood by sessile macrophages that are interdigitated with endothelial cells, especially in liver, spleen, lung, bone marrow, and lymph node. This removal is via phagocytosis, which requires that the large contrast agent be trapped by the ingesting macrophage through an interaction of surfaces. Thus, the material should be protected from phagocytosis for at least the imaging period.

Several strategies have been adopted. There include encapsulation of an ECF agent within a liposome, or coating the nanoparticulate with a hydrophilic material which prevents or reduces phagocytosis (PHILLIPS and GOINS 1995). Coated nanoparticulates can be insoluble, electron-rich, dense solids or micelles. The surface of a liposome can also be coated to elude phagocytosis and the encapsulated electron-rich moiety can be bound to the inside or outside wall of the liposome.

2.3.2.1 Liposomes

Several attempts have been made to encapsulate the ECF agents in liposomes (KRAUSE et al. 1993; SCHMIEDL et al. 1995; LEANDER 1996). Formulation considerations include the amount of material that can be trapped, keeping its osmolality balanced so that the liposome does not swell and burst, and manipulating the composition of the liposomal material, formation methods, and storage. Having an equal amount of ECF agent inside and outside the liposome reduces the swelling effect but the two phases have different biodistributions in vivo. This leads to complex imaging responses. Most such formulations do not elude phagocytosis of the liposomal fraction and renal excretion of the free ECF agent. Further, adverse drug reactions (ADRs) in man have been worrisome, perhaps in part due to a macrophage activation syndrome (see below). LEANDER et al. (1997) have argued with medical persuasion that minor ADRs are acceptable in the clinical context, but this argument may be less compelling in a litigious society. Recently, Bracco reported negligible side-effects in a phase I trial of their liposomal encapsulation of iomeprol (ZACCARINI et al. 1997).

2.3.2.2 Insoluble Nanoparticulates

Insoluble esters of ECF agents such as diatrizoic acid have been milled to produce nanoparticulate suspensions with proprietary formulations containing surfactants and other additives. It has been possible to manipulate the rate of phagocytic removal of these nanoparticulate formulations, achieving preparations with blood half-lives as short as 8 min or as long as 1 h (GAZELLE et al. 1994a,b; GAZELLE and WOLF 1995; HALAVAARA et al. 1996). Figure 2.1 shows a

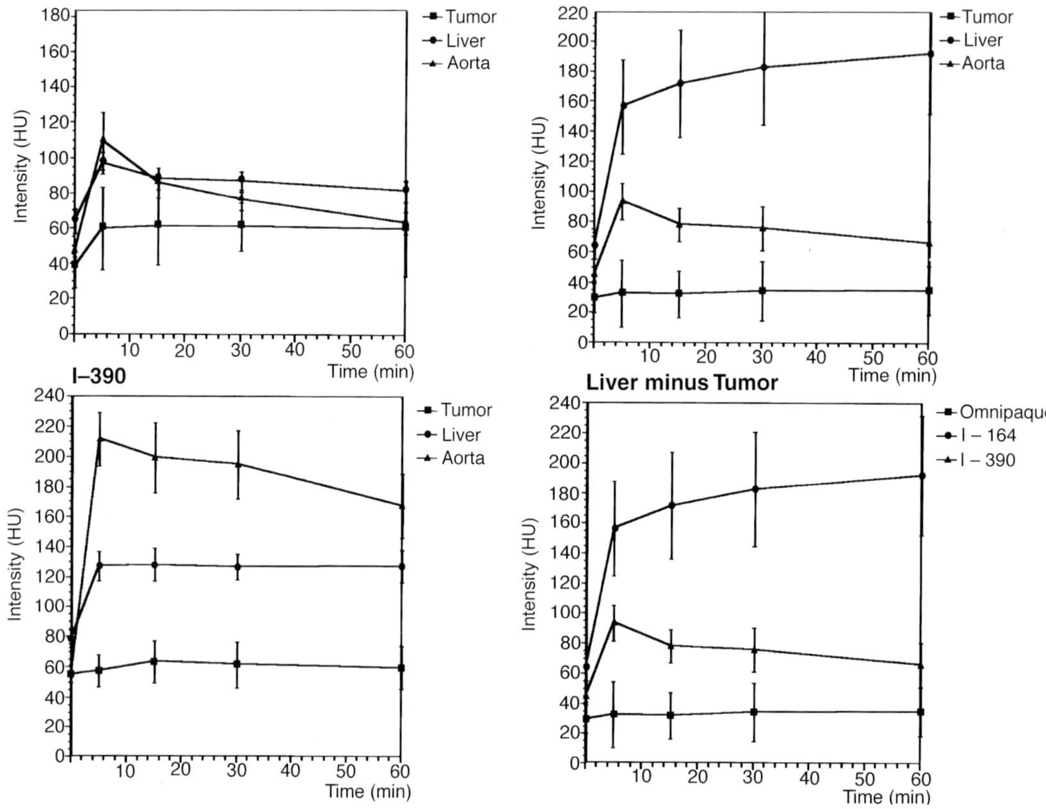

Fig. 2.1 a–d. Comparison of the time course of three x-ray contrast agents in blood, liver, and VX2 tumor in the rabbit. **a** shows the response to iohexol (Omnipaque 350). **b** shows the response to I-164, an experimental formulation of EEDA that is easily phagocytosed. **c** shows the response to I-390, an EEDA formulation protected from phagocytosis. **d** shows the liver minus tumor intensities for all three agents

quantitative time course in liver, VX2 tumor, and blood with three agents: iohexol is an ECF agent with a short blood life and early extravasation; I-164 is an ethyl ester of diatrizoic acid (EEDA) formulated to be a fair blood agent and a good MMPS agent; I-390 is formulated with the same EEDA core but different surfactants to produce a good blood agent and a fair MMPS agent (Gazelle et al. 1994a,b; Gazelle and Wolf 1995).

2.3.2.3 Micelles

Using block-copolymers of polyethylene glycol and organically iodinated polylysine, Trubetskoy et al. (1997) have created long circulating micellar formulations with an excellent blood half-life as measured in rat and rabbit. Figure 2.2 depicts both imaging efficacy and pharmacokinetics of a long-lived preparation studied in a rat. Unfortunately, imaging potency is low and safety has not been tested. These agents behave like the nanoparticulate formulations perfluorooctyl bromide (PFOB). PFOB development as a blood pool agent has been superseded due to interest in its oxygen-carrying properties. PFOB is an example of an effective radiodense parenteral where electron enhancement is achieved not with iodine but with relatively low concentrations of bromine and high specific gravity. (N.B. Density is mass per unit volume, specific gravity is mass relative to the mass of an equal volume of water. In CT, where water is the imaging reference, specific gravity is linearly related to x-ray absorption.)

2.3.3 The Intracellular Agents

Thorium dioxide (Thorotrast) and the cholegraphic agents were excellent for visualizing blood, the macrophage-monocyte system (MMPS, formerly called the reticuloendothelial system), and the liver but with unacceptable side-effects. There is little doubt that the sequestration of these agents for long times within macrophages or hepatocytes, respectively,

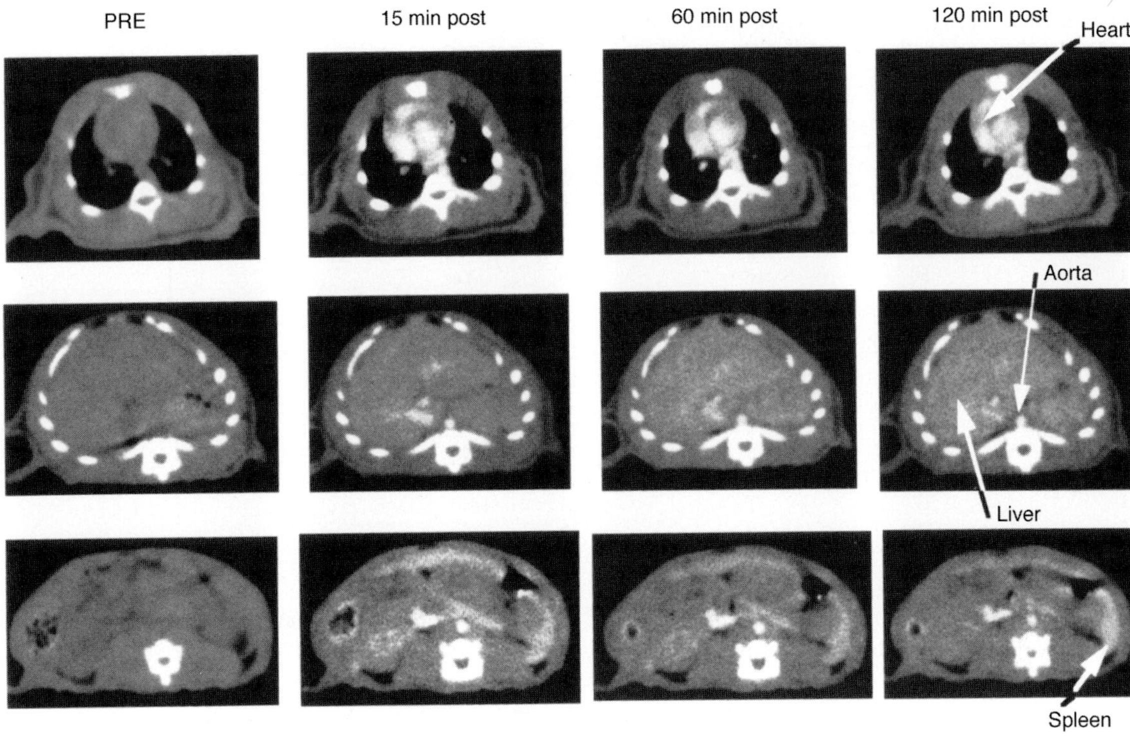

Fig. 2.2. Effects of iodine-containing polymeric micelles in rat heart, liver, aorta, and spleen. The time course of CT enhancement is shown in three separate regions. The dose was 1.4 ml of micellar solution. (Courtesy of V. TORCHILIN)

was partially responsible for this toxicity. Selective access to the intracellular space in specialized tissues will be necessary for some targeted agents, but diagnostic tasks require a much higher safety profile than pharmaceuticals with therapeutic benefit.

2.3.3.1 Macrophage Activation

Although most new intracellular agents share ADRs suggesting anaphylactoid reactions similar to extracellular agents, they have also caused an unusual constellation of delayed fever and bone or back pain, along with hypotension, headache, and malaise. These symptoms have been noted with rates of 5%–30% irrespective of whether the particulate formations were diagnostics [PFOB (BRUNETON et al. 1989; BEHAN et al. 1991), EOE-13 (MILLER et al. 1994), ferumoxide particles (DUDA et al. 1994; ROS et al. 1995)] or therapeutics [liposomal antifungals or chemotherapeutics (NEXSTAR 1996), or blood substitutes (FLAIM et al. 1994)]. Interestingly, the diagnostics also have a peculiar species sensitivity: pigs and dogs are sensitive, rodents and rabbits are not (FLAIM et al. 1991). The only other drug class causing bone or back pain and fever in man are the colony-stimulating cytokines for macrophages, G-CSF or GM-CSF (LIESCHKE et al. 1990; STERN and JONES 1992; EGUCHI et al. 1994). Macrophages can respond selectively with stimulation or inhibition of secretion of numerous cytokines, but it seems possible that ingestion of xenobiotic particulates could lead to macrophage activation and release of responsible cytokines in susceptible individuals.

Recent methodological advances have made it feasible to isolate functional macrophages from animals or man and challenge them in vitro, measuring the cytokines that they elaborate in response. Table 2.2 shows a series of such phagocytic cells collected from normal volunteers and challenged with a nanoparticulate radiopaque formulation. Four of the 14 volunteers showed markedly enhanced release of tumor necrosis factor-α (TNF-α) and/or interleukin-6. This work is preliminary but suggests that (a) macrophage activation is possible and can be measured in vitro, (b) there may be responders and nonresponders in the clinical population, and (c) the methods are suitable for screening new formulations and proposed preventative regimens prior to clinical exposure.

There are indications that some ADRs seen with particulate formulations may actually be due to the

Table 2.2. Macrophage activation screen in normal volunteers. Cultured blood monocytes challenged with a nanoparticulate radiopaque formulation in vitro. Mean cytokines released per ml of plasma (Courtesy of K. Whiteman)

Sample	Interleukin-6	Interleukin-1B	TNF-α	Responder
Activation Agent	555	134	935	
1	0	0	18	No
2	1	1.5	16	No
3	0	0	6	No
4	50	13	49	Yes
5	194	30	76	Yes
6	37	23	58	Yes
7	0	5	27	No
8	4	0	18	No
9	0	2	5	No
10	16	2	24	?
11	0	0	29	No
12	65	75	656	Yes
13	17	1	4	No
14	0	0	15	No

surfactants or endotoxin contamination. There are differences in ADR rate between similar agents, e.g., SPIO (Endorem, Feridex) causes more such reactions than USPIO (Sinerem, Combidex); indeed, a recent large clinical trial of the reformulated SPIO (Resovist) found few such ADRs (Balzer et al. 1997). Finally, some intracellular parasites seem to survive in large concentration within macrophages while causing few symptoms; perhaps this behavior could be modeled with intracellular contrast agents. Thus, there are reasons for optimism that the MMPS can be safely targeted with radiographic contrast agents.

2.3.3.2 Prototype MMPS Agents

Macrophages are widely distributed throughout the body and monitor anticipated invasion pathways in each location; the access of radiopaque or radiolucent particles is most efficient via these same pathways. Thus, the lymph nodes survey the lymph (see Chap. 14), the Peyer's patches survey small intestinal contents, skin and airway macrophages monitor those interfaces, and liver, spleen, bone marrow, and lymph node as well as circulating monocytes cleanse the blood. For radiographic contrast agents, each macrophage is capable of accumulating prodigious amounts of material from the surrounding fluid. As a consequence, a propitious route of delivery of particulate material may lead to very low effective doses and minimal unintended exposure to other tissues.

We have studied experimental formulation of nanoparticulates consisting of a core, composed of insoluble radiopaque materials such as ethyl esters of diatrizoic acid, and various coatings. The insoluble core contributes electrons and density along with excretable materials upon hydrolysis. This core can range in size from 100 to 10000 nm (Wolf et al. 1997). When coated to resist phagocytosis, these agents are good blood pool tracers while easy phagocytosis leads to deposition of systemically injected formulations in liver, spleen, and bone marrow (Figs. 2.1, 2.3, 2.4).

In Fig. 2.3, the imaging appearance of the VX2 tumor in rabbit liver is shown on CT scans taken over 1 h following the intravenous administration of iohexol (as Omnipaque 350) or a nanoparticulate agent. The tumor is easily visualized with the ECF agent on early studies, but extravasation reduces visualization at later time points.

Figure 2.4 shows another MMPS formulation that enhances the macrophages in the bone marrow of rabbits. Here, the marrow space averaged -16 ± 11 HU before and 148 ± 32 HU after intravenous administration of the experimental formulation.

2.3.3.3 Hepatocyte Agents

Weichert et al. (1996) have prepared polyiodinated triglyceride analogs which target the hepatocyte pathway for clearing chylomicron remnants from the blood. Effective analogs have particle sizes less that 200 nm and doses providing 45–100 mg I/kg body weight because more than 65% of the administered dose accumulates in the liver within 30 min. Figure 2.5 shows the response in rats bearing Morris

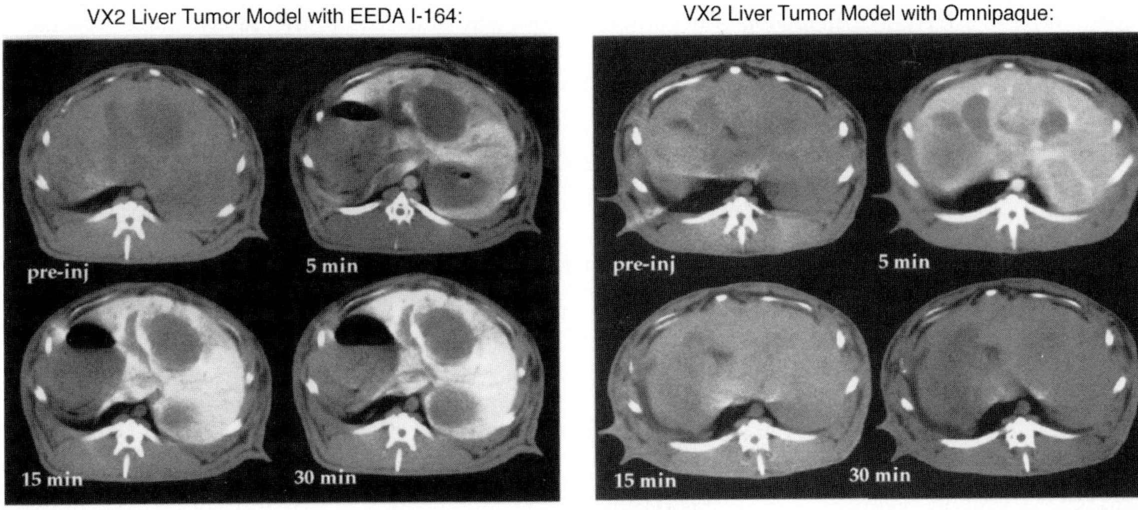

Fig. 2.3. CT images of rabbit VX2 tumors imaged with EEDA formulation (I-164) (*left*) and iohexol (Omnipaque) (*right*). The precontrast images are shown as well as images 5, 15, and 30 min later. The ECF agent improves liver visualization only for a short period, while the EEDA formulation depicts normal liver and the tumor for the entire period of study. The time course of these two agents is also shown in Fig. 2.1

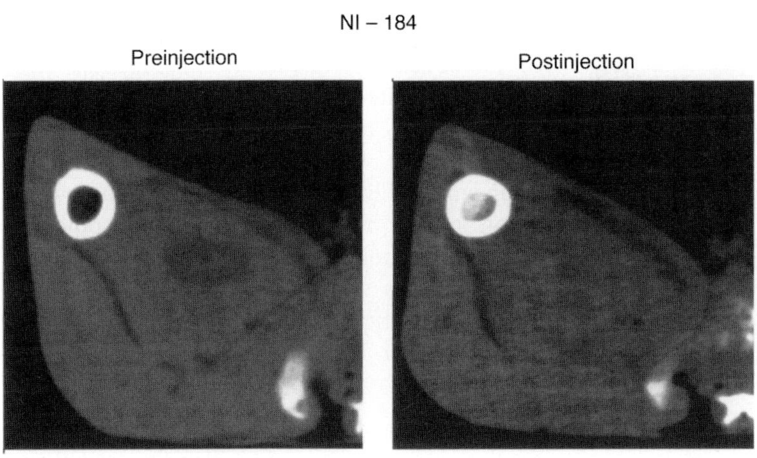

Fig. 2.4. Enhancement of bone marrow macrophages with an experimental nanoparticulate NI-184. The precontrast image is shown on the *left*; this rabbit also had a VX2 tumor in the thigh. Three and one-half hours after intravenous injection, the bone marrow enhancement is evident (*right*)

Fig. 2.5. Axial CT images of the upper abdomen in the MH-7777 rat hepatoma model. Two contiguous anatomic levels are shown 90 min after administration of 60 mg I/kg of 2-oleoylglycerol 1,3-bis [7-(3-amino-2,4-6-triiodophynyl)heptanoate] (ITG). (Courtesy of J. Weichert)

hepatoma-7777 (MH-7777), an analog of hepatocellular carcinoma.

SCHMITZ et al. (1997) and SCHUHMANN-GIAMPIERI et al. (1997) have utilized the transporter pathways (KEPPLER and ARIEA 1997) in hepatocytes that are targeted by ethoxybenzyl DTPA to show that either Gd-EOB-DTPA or Dy-EOB-DTPA can achieve CT contrast enhancement in the liver. Figure 2.6 shows an image of a normal dog liver. Effective CT doses of these compounds, designed as MRI agents (see Chap. ••), were 5–20 times higher than for MRI but still within the safety index for these compounds.

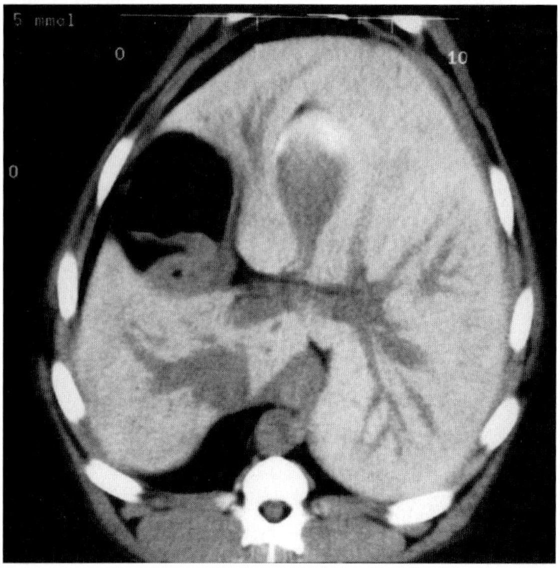

Fig. 2.6. Dy-EOB-DTPA enhanced CT study of a dog liver at 60 min following intravenous injection of 0.5 mmol Dy/kg. (Courtesy of K. RUPP, G. SCHUHMANN-GIAMPIERI, and B. HAMM, BERLIN, Germany)

At the recent CMR'97 meeting, BERGMAN et al. (1997) reported on the efficacy of a different hepatocyte agent in experimental models of diffuse liver disease in rats as well as the response in a phase I study in 24 healthy male volunteers (MAGNUSSON et al. 1997).

2.3.4 Radiopaque Agents with Therapeutic Applications

Imaging guidance is often required for minimally invasive procedures. One such intervention is therapeutic embolization. Available materials such as coils are radiopaque but these produce very proximal embolization. Large blocks of material such as polyvinyl alcohol sponge or Gelfoam embolize a little more distally, and can be rendered somewhat radiopaque by soaking them in ECF solutions. However, in vivo angiogenesis often will create collateral pathways around proximal occlusions. A capillary embolic agent has been prepared with radiopaque cores of 10 μm and suspended in dilute ECF agent to enhance visualization of the formulation at fluoroscopy. Experimental embolizations of the myocardial and renal capillaries are shown in Fig. 2.7. This material is a prototype of other radiopaques that may be designed for both diagnostic and therapeutic applications.

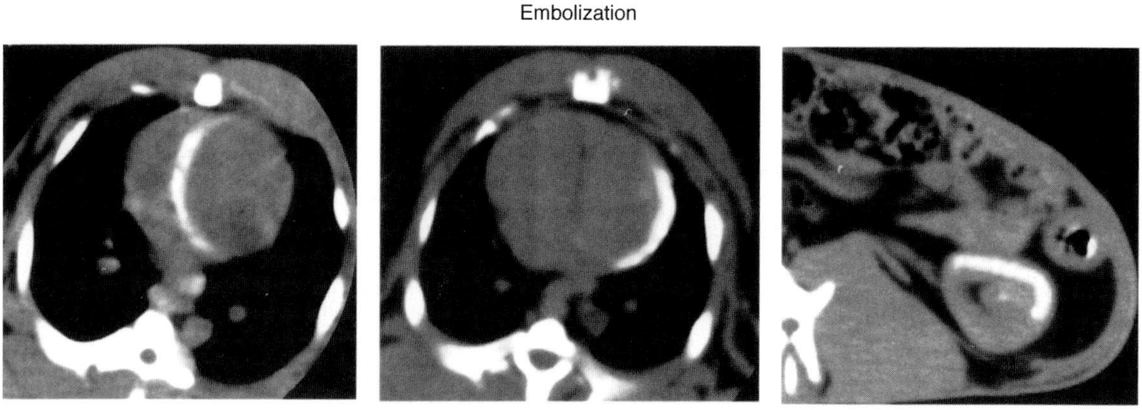

Fig. 2.7. Capillary embolization with a radiopaque formulation. Following superselective catheterization in the rabbit, 50–100 μl of the agent was injected into the left anterior descending coronary artery (*left panel*), the circumflex coronary artery (*middle panel*), and the left midventral renal artery (*right panel*). This particulate is 10 μm in diameter and is suspended in dilute iohexol

2.4 Conclusions

There are many clinical applications of x-ray imaging agents that could be improved by the design of new formulations. In some cases, the agents would make it feasible to accomplish a diagnostic task at lower cost, usually by replacing more invasive technologies. Avoiding expensive and somewhat hazardous interventions such as catheterization, surgery, or biopsy would allow new contrast agents to be cost-effective even when their frequency of use is relatively low. The intent of this brief chapter is to suggest that such new designs are feasible.

Acknowledgements. The author appreciates the work contributed by other laboratories. The experimental agents shown in Figs. 2.1, 2.3, 2.4, and 2.7 were contributed by Grey McIntire and Ed Bacon of Nycomed, USA.

References

Balzer T, Shamsi K, Kallend D, Carter EC, Niendorf HP (1997) Resovist[TM]; safety and diagnostic potential. CMP'97:76

Behan M, O'Connell D, Mattrey RF, Carney DN (1991) Perfluorooctylbromide as a contrast agent for CT and sonography: preliminary clinical results. AJR 160:399–405

Bergman A, Magnusson A, Moore K, Sundin S (1997) Efficacy of the hepatocyte-specific contrast medium FP 736-04 for CT in two experimental models of diffuse liver disease. CMR'97:28

Bruneton JN, Falewee NM, Francois E, et al. (1989) Liver, spleen, and vessels: preliminary clinical results of CT with perfluorooctylbromide. Radiology 170:179–183

Duda SH, Laniado M, Kopp AF, et al. (1994) Superparamagnetic iron oxide: detection of focal liver lesions at high-field-strength MR imaging. J Magn Reson Imaging 4:309–314

Eguchi K, Kabe J, Kudo S, et al. (1994) Efficacy of recombinant human granulocyte-macrophage colony-stimulating factor for chemotherapy-induced leukopenia in patients with non-small-cell lung cancer. Cancer Chemother Pharmacol 34:37–43

Flaim SF, Hazard DR, Hogan J, Peters RM (1991) Characterization and mechanism of side-effects of Imagent BP (highly concentrated fluorocarbon emulsion) in swine. Invest Radiol 26(Suppl):S122–124

Flaim SF, Hazard DR, Hogan J, Peters RM (1994) Characterization and mechanism of side-effects of Oxygent HT (highly concentrated fluorocarbon emulsion) in swine. Artif Cells Blood Subst Immob Biotech 22:1511–1515

Gazelle GS, Wolf GL (1995) Hepatic imaging with iodinated nanoparticles: a comparison to iohexol in an animal model. Acad Radiol 2:700–704

Gazelle GS, Wolf GL, Bacon ER, McIntire GL, Cooper ER, Toner JL (1994a) Nanocrystalline computed tomography contrast agents for blood-pool and liver-spleen imaging. Invest Radiol 29:S286–S288

Gazelle GS, Wolf GL, McIntire GL, Bacon ER, Halpern EF, Cooper ER, Toner JL (1994b) Nanoparticulate computed tomography contrast agents for blood pool and liver-spleen imaging. Acad Radiol 1:373–376

Halavaara JT, Hamberg LM, Leong FS, Hunter GJ, Gazelle GS, Wolf GL (1996) Functional CT with an experimental intravascular contrast agent in the assessment of liver vascular physiology. Acad Radiol 3:946–952

Keipert PE, Osso S, Flaim SF, et al. (1994) Influence of perflubron emulsion particle size on blood half-life and febrile response in rats. Artif Cells Blood Subst Immob Biotech 22:1169–1174

Keppler D, Ariea S (1997) Transport across the hepatocyte canalicular membrane. FASEB J 11:15–17

Krause W, Leike J, Sachse A, Schuhmann-Giampieri G (1993) Characterization of iopromide liposomes. Invest Radiol 28:1028–1032

Leander P (1996) A new liposomal contrast medium for CT of the liver: an imaging study in a rabbit tumor model. Acta Radiol 37:63–68

Leander P, Hoglund P, Kloster Y, Borseth A (1997) Efficacy of a new liposomal liver-specific contrast agent for CT; first human clinical phase I trial. CMR'97:25

Lieschke GJ, Maher D, O'Connor M, et al. (1990) Phase I study of intravenously administered bacterially synthesized granulocyte-macrophage colony-stimulating factor and comparison with subcutaneous administration. Cancer Res 50:606–614

Magnusson A, Bergman A, Carneheim C, von Scheele L, Weesen A (1997) Contrast enhancement of the liver in healthy male volunteers following intravenous administration of FP 736-04. CMR'97:27

Miller DL, Vermess M, Doppman JL, et al. (1994) CT of the liver and spleen with EOE-13: a review of 225 examinations. AJR 143:235–243

Nexstar Liposomal Daunoxome. "The Pink Sheet," 15 April 1996, pp 11–12

Petta M, Raynal I, Bourrinet P, Vadel M, Meyer D (1998) Nonionic conpace dimers; a new generation of iso-osmolar iodinated contrast media with low viscosity. Acad Radiol 5:41–49

Phillips WT, Goins B (1995) Targeted delivery of imaging agents by liposomes. In: Torchilin V (ed) Targeted imaging agents. CRC Press, Boca Ration, FL., pp 149–173

Ros PR, Freeny PC, Harms SE, et al. (1995) Hepatic MR imaging with ferumoxides: a multicenter clinical trial of the safety and efficacy in the detection of focal hepatic lesions. Radiology 196:481–488

Schmiedl UP, Krause W, Leike J, Nelson JA, Schuhmann-Giampieri G (1995) Liver contrast enhancement in primates using iopromide liposomes. Acad Radiol 2:967–972

Schmitz SA, Wagner S, Schuhmann-Giampieri G, Krause W, Wolf K-J (1997) A prototype liver-specific contrast medium for DT; preclinical evaluation of gadoxetic acid disodium, or Gd-EOB-DTPA. Radiology 202:407–412

Schuhmann-Giampieri G, Rupp K, Handreke K, Muschick P, Krause W, Hamm B (1997) Dysprosium EOB-DTPA. A new liver-specific contrast agent for CT. CMR'97:55

Stern AC, Jones TC (1992) The side-effect profile of GM-CSF. Infection 20 (Suppl 2):124–127

Sundin A, Ahlstron M, Graf W, Magnusson A (1994) Computed tomography of experimental liver metastases using an iodinated hepatocyte-specific lipid emulsion. Invest Radiol 11:963–969

Trubetskoy VS, Gazelle GS, Wolf GL, Torchilin VP (1997) Block-copolymer of polyethylene glycol and polylysine as a carrier of organic iodine; design of long-circulating particulate contrast medium for x-ray computed tomography. J Drug Targeting 4:381–388

Weichert JP, Longino MA, Spigarelli MG, Lee FT Jr, Schwendner SW, Counsell RE (1996) Computed tomography scanning of Morris hepatomas with liver-specific polyiodinated triglycerides. Acad Radiol 3:412–417

Wolf GL (1995) Targeted delivery of imaging agents: an overview. In: Torchilin V (ed) Targeted imaging agents. CRC Press, Boca Raton, Fl., pp 3–22

Wolf GL, Rogowska J, Bessin G, Trocha M, Whiteman K, Wolf D, Shore MT (1997) Visualization of renal anatomy and function with 1–10 000 nm radiocontrast agents. Acad Radiol 4

Zaccarini P, Spinazzi A, Lorusso V, Ceriate S, Pianezzola P, Fouillet X, Tournier H (1997) Safety and pharmacokinetics of BR21, a liver-specific CT agent, in healthy volunteers. CMR 97:30

3 Biological Variation, Reproducibility, and Predictability of Experimental Research in Animals

O. Svendsen and A. Kornerup Hansen

CONTENTS

3.1 Introduction

Experimental research in animals is justified due to its expected predictability for conditions in other species, primarily human beings. Only a small number of animal experiments are carried out for the benefit of the animal species involved, thereby yielding results that do not need to be extrapolated. Examples are experiments undertaken in the study of laboratory animal diseases and domestic animal diseases.

Within the same species and even within the same strain or substrain of a species the variation can be rather large. This phenotypic variation derives not only from the genotype but also from environmental factors as simple as housing conditions, feeding, and microbiology. Within recent decades a major goal has been to establish rules to control these environmental factors, to minimize the biological variation, and thereby to improve the reproducibility of animal research. Good laboratory practice (GLP) regulations, which were introduced in preclinical safety testing of new pharmaceutical agents nearly 20 years ago, have aimed to achieve standardization by description and control of environmental factors. This has led to a higher level of international acceptance of test data due to the expected reproducibility.

Integration of study results obtained by animal experimentation is generally accepted as valid. However, studies may yield contradictory results, and sometimes great difficulties have been experienced in reproducing experiments of other investigators. Although the experimental animal cannot be calibrated to the same extent as laboratory apparatus, laboratory animals have been widely characterized and broad insight into biological mechanisms has been achieved by animal experimentation.

Factors with an impact on biological variation, reproducibility, and predictability have been identified in pharmacological and toxicological research and testing. This chapter will focus on factors related to: (1) the animal, (2) the environment, and (3) the experimental procedure. These are variables which in general need to be controlled by standardization in order to reduce or eliminate their impact, if animal studies are to be reproducible and predictable.

3.2 Induction of Nephropathy in Experimental Animals by Contrast Media

Recent data suggest that nonionic low-osmolar contrast media cause fewer adverse effects on kidney

O. Svendsen, DVM, PhD, Dr.med.Sci., Professor, Department of Pharmacology and Pathobiology, Royal Veterinary and Agricultural University, 13 Bülowsvej, DK-1870 Frederiksberg C, Denmark

A. Kornerup Hansen, DVM, Dr.Vet.Sci., Professor, Department of Pharmacology and Pathobiology, Royal Veterinary and Agricultural University, 13 Bülowsvej, DK-1870 Frederiksberg C, Denmark function in normal animals than the ionic high-osmolar media (Thomsen et al. 1993). Contrast media are often used in humans with compromised renal function. In a series of studies Thomsen et al. (1991, 1993, 1995, 1996) induced specified nephropathies in rats by use of different nephrotoxic agents, each causing well-characterized nephropathy, in order to study potential contrast medium nephropathy in animals with compromised renal function. The nephrotoxic agents used were sodium maleate, glycerol, cyclosporin A, adriamycin, indomethacin, gentamicin, cisplatin, and an adrenocortical steroid. The experimental studies of diseased kidneys seemed to indicate that the nephrotoxic potential of nonionic low-osmolar contrast media did not differ from that of the ionic high-osmolar contrast media. There may, however, be minor differences in their nephrotoxic potential with respect to different nephropathies.

It is difficult to evaluate to what extent rat studies may provide new insights into nephrotoxicity in man. Comparative nephrotoxicity as such appears to have attracted little attention (Mudge 1982). Renal anatomy, biochemistry, and physiology of rats differ to some extent from those of man. In spite of this the rat is the most widely used model for studies on renal physiology and toxicology. For most renal physiological mechanisms there are qualitative similarities between rat and man. However, quantitative differences are well known. The biological turnover in rats is about 6 times faster than in man. Such differences may render the rat kidney more or less susceptible to an adverse effect of xenobiotics, including contrast media.

Renal physiology is concerned with the separate processes of filtration, reabsorption, and secretion. The most striking interspecies differences involve the medulla and the papilla. The maximal osmolarity of urine in man is about half of that in the rat, probably as a consequence of differences in the percentage of long loops and the relative medullary thickness. This osmolarity is of significance to the extent that it determines final urinary concentration and subsequent drug concentration. Renal circulation is of undoubted importance for the question of nephrotoxicity. However, renal circulation in laboratory animals appears quite uniform from one species to another and to man. The most striking differences between species are seen in dose-response relationships for pharmacological agents. A large number of extrarenal factors are involved in this variation. For radiological contrast media marked interspecies variations in susceptibility have been seen (Mudge 1980).

Nephrotoxicity in animal models appears to resemble closely the disorders seen in man. Regardless of the initiating cause there seems to be a common pathophysiological disturbance which characterizes acute renal failure once it is fully developed. This includes reduced filtration, increased tubular permeability, and tubular obstruction. Due to obvious difficulties very few comparative studies between animals and man exist. However, in cases where animal studies have indicated a nephrotoxic potential it has also been identified in man. Considerable differences in toxic dose level may be seen and differences also may be seen in toxic manifestations. Although changes in urinary profiles may indicate toxicity, the individual parameters affected may differ between rat and man, and this may also hold true for histopathological manifestations.

3.3 Animal-Related Factors

The choice of animals, i.e., species, strain, sex, etc., for an experiment is among the most important decisions to be made before initiation of an experiment with laboratory animals. Examples of information essential for the characterization of laboratory animals are given in Table 3.1. Often scientific papers fail to give this information, although essential differences exist between species, strains, substrains, and different individuals. This rather neglected fact is one of the main contributing factors in cases of difficulties with reproduction of published results.

3.3.1 Handling Laboratory Animals

Animals should be handled with care and treated as humanely as possible. Furthermore, if handling is not performed in a standardized way, this may cause an increase in variation.

In European countries that have signed a European Council convention concerning training of people participating in animal experiments, no person is allowed to take part in the practical procedures of an animal experiment if they have not passed a basic course in laboratory animal science. The course should include practical training in animal handling. Detailed instructions on several

Table 3.1. Information which, according to the British journal *Laboratory Animals*, should be given in papers submitted to the journal (Laboratory Animals 1992)

Animals
Species
Breed or designation of stock or strain
Source
Genetic status (if not obvious from stock/strain designation): strain; outbreed; hybrid; mutant
Age and/or weight at start of experiment (both should be given if possible)
Sex
Reputed microbiological status: conventional (microbiological status not specified); specified pathogen free (pathogens or groups of pathogens from which animals are free must be specified); gnotobiotic (germ-free or associated with pure cultures; all micro-organisms must be specified)
Quarantine or acclimatization period

Feeding
Feed: type and composition [according to *Journal of Nutrition* (1977) 107: 1340–1347, and *Journal of Nutrition* (1984) 114: 15–16], possibly brand name and identification number together with a reference; pretreatment; feeding schedule (quantity, frequency)

Statistical procedures
Details and references should be quoted

Husbandry during experiment
Measures to protect microbiological status: open system (no special protective measures); closed system (animals kept behind barriers or locks), isolator system
Housing equipment: type, material, dimensions; possibly cage type if a reference is included
Number of animals per cage or housing unit
Bedding: type, quality, pretreatment
Environmental temperature (°C ± range): regulated; not regulated
Relative humidity (% ± range): regulated; not regulated
Lighting: natural; artificial (time of day and intensity)
Ventilation and filtration: proportion of fresh and recirculated air or air flow speeds over cages or gas or particle concentrations in the air
Period of conditioning to husbandry conditions and procedures used during experiment

Experimental procedure
The description of the experimental procedure depends on the purpose of the experiment, but the following information must always be provided:
Number of animals and any pretreatment
Time schedule of the experiment (e.g., time of day of the investigation, time interval between sampling and processing)

techniques in various animals have been described by Iwarsson et al. (1994), e.g., as shown for oral dosing in Fig. 3.1.

Some procedures may only be performed under anesthesia. However, it should be noted that anesthesia may stress the animal more than the procedure, and therefore it may be more acceptable to use a nonstressful restraining device, e.g., as shown in Fig. 3.2 for radiography after oral dosing in the rat.

3.3.2 Genetics

The phenotype of the animal is determined by the genotype and the environmental conditions. If the environmental conditions are kept constant, the physiology, biochemistry, and behavior of the animals are primarily determined by the genotype. However, responsiveness of laboratory animals may differ in various ways due to genetic factors.

Laboratory animals may be outbred, i.e., derive from a random bred colony. Some species, especially rats and mice, may also be available as inbred, i.e., 20

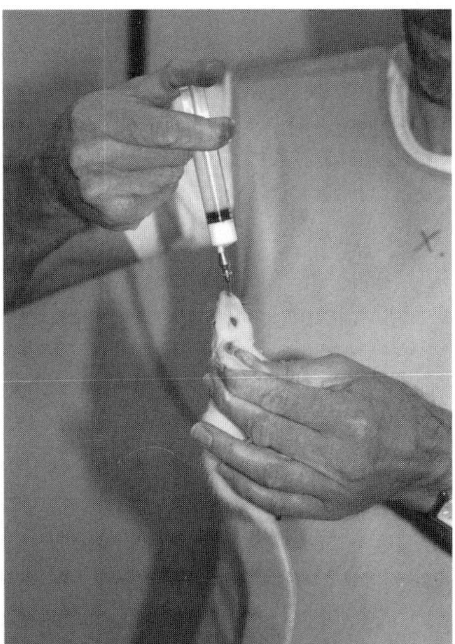

Fig. 3.1. Gastrointestinal contrast media being dosed orally to a conscious rat through a stainless steel stomaoh tube. The rat is fixed by grapping the skin on the side of neck and the stomach tube is gently passed through the esophagus into the stomach

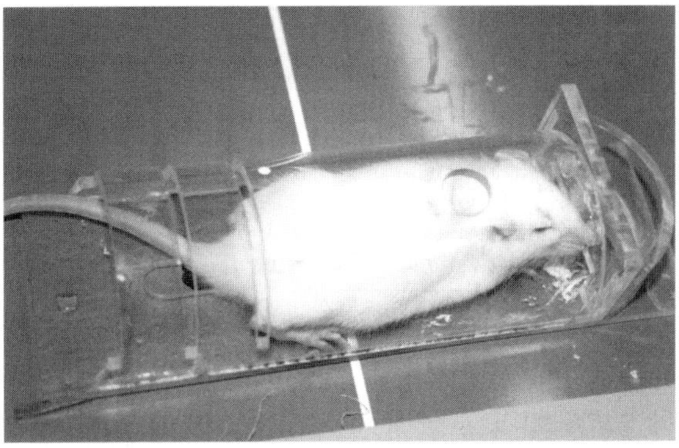

Fig. 3.2. An unanesthetized rat fixed for radiography in a restraining tube

generations of brother-sister mating have resulted in the highest achievable grade of homozygosity in the colony.

The variation of parameters in an inbred strain is smaller than that in an outbred stock. Between inbred strains there are large strain differences, some of which, e.g., histocompatibility types, are well defined, while others related to physiology, behavior, pharmacokinetics, pharmacodynamics, and toxicology must be considered on the basis of experience.

Outbred stocks are in general poorly defined and it is more the rule than the exception that there is large variation inside a colony, between different stocks, and even between stocks carrying the same name. In pharmacological and toxicological studies outbred animals are more common than inbred animals. In pharmacology outbred animals are chosen basically because they are cheaper than inbred strains. In toxicology it is sometimes argued that outbred animals are a more appropriate model for the genetically heterogeneous human. However, as the variation inside outbred strain cannot be precisely defined, and therefore cannot be differentiated in the experimental design, it should be considered that specific toxicity endpoints might be identified more precisely and with fewer animals in susceptible inbred strains (Festing 1987, 1990).

3.3.3 Sex-Related Differences

The sex of laboratory animals may seem to be of minor importance. Often only one sex of a species is included in a study protocol. This entails the risk that the results obtained will be interpreted for both sexes. Males are often preferred on the assumption that females may give results with greater variability due to the endocrine changes during the estrus cycle. In fact biochemical, physiological, and behavioral fluctuations across the estrous cycle often cause the response to an external stimulus to vary across the cycle; such variations may involve the neuronal systems, drug-induced behavioral changes and pharmacokinetics. Furthermore, males and females may react totally differently in relation to behavior, pharmacokinetics, pharmacodynamic effects, and toxicological effects. Sex differences occur over a wide range of behaviors, e.g., activity, aggression, pain and taste sensitivity, food intake and body weight regulation, the learning and retention of certain kinds of mazes, avoidance responses, taste aversion, and performance on certain schedules of reinforcement (Beatty 1979). Differences in drug metabolism and disposition may contribute to the sex differences in pharmacological and toxicological responses. Differences in receptor affinity, receptor density, and neurotransmitter systems may add to the dimorphism in the response. Sex-related differences have been described in relation to more than 200 substances. The extensive sex differences have been reviewed in relation to pharmacokinetics by Kato (1974) and in relation to toxicology by Calabrese (1984).

3.3.4 Age-Related Changes

During development numerous changes occur in the morphology, the physiology, and the biochemistry of the animal. The most extensive changes occur in the first 4–6 weeks after birth, after which maturation takes place. This is followed by a stable phase of maturity which subsequently merges into senescence over a relatively long period . These changes may result in variation in pharmacokinetics (Birnbaum 1991), pharmacodynamics, and toxicology (Calabrese 1986). Species, strain, and sex differences are important variables in age-related pharmacodynamic response. The changes in pharmacokinetics and pharmacodynamic response often lead to age dependency of toxicological effects.

Animals are often purchased from vendors according to weight, but different stocks, or the same stock from two different vendors, may have different growth curves. Therefore, animals of the same weight may have a different age, and standardization according to weight will often reduce the reproducibility of the study more than standardization according to age.

3.3.5 Stress

The stress response, including behavioral reaction and activation of autonomic and neuroendocrine functions, is the consequence of disturbance of the animal by physical or psychological stimuli. Changes in the autonomic and neuroendocrine systems may result in functional changes of different biological systems. The neuroendocrine response includes increased or decreased release of a broad range of pituitary hormones. The literature on the impact of different kinds of stress on experimental results is immense. There is a stress response to simple experimental procedures, such as cage handling, transportation, animal handling, exposure to novel situations, and emotional communication. Therefore, animals should be given time to adapt after transportation, surgery, etc. Various indices of the stress response suggest that the majority of stress effects are short-lived. However, some stress experiences may be maintained for a longer period or, in rare cases, become persistent. In general, adaptation to the stressor takes place after repeated exposure and repeated handling.

It is very important to focus on stress since differences in stress between experiments or between laboratory animal strains otherwise may become an uncontrolled factor. The neuroendocrine and autonomic reactivity of an animal is highly dependent on species and strain. Significant strain differences have been described with many examples. Animals stressed by a certain factor, e.g., transportation, may impose stress upon nearby animals not subjected to that factor (De Laat et al. 1989).

3.4 Environmental Factors

As mentioned above, the environment along with the genotype determines the phenotype of animals (Poole 1987; Reese 1991). Environmental factors include the microbiology of the animal, housing, and feeding factors. Examples are given in Table 3.1. These are critical factors in animal experimentation and should be documented in detail in any experiment involving laboratory animals.

3.4.1 Microbiological Factors

Infections in the animals may cause pathological changes and clinical disease, but they may also have an impact on the animal which is not clinically visible, e.g., on immunology, physiology, oncology, and reproduction. Infections may inhibit the induction of a certain animal model, make it difficult to interpret the final results, show a dose-related response, or increase the variation within the experiment (Hansen 1994). For example, infection with *Clostridium piliforme* in mice irreversibly changes the pharmacokinetics of warfarin (Friis and Ladefoged 1979) and mice infected with this agent will, when treated with carbon tetrachloride, develop a dose-related number of focal necroses in the liver, while uninfected mice do not show such a response (Takenaka and Fujiwara 1975). To avoid interference from infectious agents only microbiologically defined animals should be used, i.e., animals from colonies started on the basis of animals deriving from caesarean section or embryo transfer, and housed in facilities where they can be efficiently protected against infections, i.e., so-called barrier facilities. The commercial vendors should run a current screening program for infectious agents according to internationally acceptable standards (Kraft et al. 1994). Also during the experiments it is recommendable to protect the animals against infections by the adoption of certain hygiene precautions.

3.4.2 Housing Conditions

The room temperature, relative humidity, and air change should be adapted to the species housed in the room and the number of individuals, and should be adequately controlled. Normally animals are not housed at temperatures within their thermoneutral zone, i.e., small changes in room temperature will be compensated for by the animals by a change in their metabolism (Svendsen 1994). The light is normally standardized with a light-dark cycle, e.g., 12 h light and 12 h dark. The design of the animals' cage, the bedding material, the number of animals in the cage, and the subsequent microclimate in the cage may influence the animal characteristics, e.g., rats housed in dirty cages show an impaired activity of the drug-metabolizing enzymes aniline hydroxylase, cytochrome P-450, and morphine demethylase (VESELL et al. 1973). It is well known that individual contra group housing may affect pharmacological responsiveness related to behavior (aggression in particular), central depressants, and nociception, e.g., hexobarbital is metabolized faster by isolated rats than by group-housed rats (DAIRMAN and BALAZT 1970). Animals kept on pine or spruce bedding have significantly higher activity of cytochrome P-450 than animals kept on beech or aspen bedding (CUNLIFFE-BEAMER et al. 1981). The significance of housing factors has been reviewed by CLOUGH (1982).

3.4.3 Dietary Factors

The health status of animals is highly dependent on the amount and quality of the consumed food. Diet may change physiological parameters (NELSON and FELICIO 1984), induce pathological changes (MEYER et al. 1989; RITSKES-HOITINGA et al. 1989), and enhance tumor development (TUCKER 1985). In some studies a purified diet may be required, e.g., if certain ingredients have to be reduced below the levels found in natural compounds such as barley. However, most diets for experimental animals are natural ingredient diets. Animals in experiments are fed a commercial diet considered adequate for the needs of the animal, but many different commercial diets are available, and they differ quantitatively as well as qualitatively to such an extent that it may influence biological response. Mostly, the nutritional levels are calculated rather than documented by analysis, and although nutrients have been documented they may not be completely available to the animal. Within the same brands of diets often more than one type exists, e.g., one for young growing animals and one just for maintenance. Documentation of absence of contaminants such as growth promoters, pesticides, heavy metals, and biological contaminants is essential for certain types of studies where such contaminants may affect the outcome of the study.

Rodents consume their food in separate meals and both food and water intake is almost exclusively restricted to the dark phase of the light and dark cycle. The intake pattern is affected by strain, sex, and age of the animal, by the housing conditions, and by the drugs being tested.

3.4.4 Biological Rhythms

Animals show biological rhythms, i.e., parameters may differ over time. Rhythms such as pulse, respiration, etc. shorter than 24h are called *ultradian rhythms*. Body temperature, defecation, metabolism, etc. follow a 24-h rhythm, the *circadian rhythm*, while the estrous cycle, for instance, is an example of a rhythm longer than 24h, the *infradian rhythm*. Biochemical variables in blood and tissues, neuronal characteristics, pharmacodynamics and pharmacokinetics, and subsequent toxicological effects vary according to especially circadian and infradian rhythms, e.g., the normal values of the serum parameters such as glucose differ from season to season (PESSACQ et al. 1976). These variations have to be taken into consideration for the design of a study in order to obtain comparable data with minimum variation. Also, it should be noted that the environment of the animals, e.g., the length of the lighting period in the animal rooms, will have an impact on the biological rhythms, although the infradian rhythms cannot be eliminated by the use of a standardized light-dark cycle.

3.5 Experimental Factors

The responsiveness of the animal to the experimental stimuli is strongly related to the test conditions. Important experimental factors are those related to the administration of the test compound, feeding, and anesthesia.

3.5.1 Factors Related to Administration of the Test Compound

Variations in bioavailability and biological activity are mainly the consequence of differences in the drug formulation administered, and should always be considered in relation to the type of formulation and the route of administration.

3.5.1.1
Intravenous Administration

For a simple procedure such as intravenous drug administration variations can arise from the rate of drug administration by injection or infusion, the volume administered, and the tonicity of injected fluid. The rate of intravenous injection may range from a few seconds up to some minutes. With the antidepressant fluvoxamine, CLAASSEN (1994) observed a clear reduction in arterial blood pressure in the cat after a dose of 3 mg/kg given over less than 20 s, whereas no reduction took place when the same dose was given over 2 min. Slowing down the intravenous infusion rate may prolong the time before onset of the effect and reduce the total dose required for onset of effect (DANHOF and LEVY 1984). The administered volume is important in particular for intravenous injections. Hemodilution and increase in cardiac output may occur as a consequence of the acute expansion of the blood volume, e.g., a volume of 2 ml/kg to a rat corresponds to about 3% of the blood volume. By interruption of the vessel wall by intravenous injection or infusion there is a risk of inflammation and thrombus formation, especially when using chronic catheters or frequently repeated injections. Concentration and pH of the drug formulation are important determinators. Often small thrombi are released from chronic catheters into the circulation, causing subsequent pulmonary microembolization. Repeated intravenous injection into the caudal veins of the rat may result in a high rate of pulmonary emboli with fragments of hair and skin and formation of granulomatous inflammation. Blood concentrations may be lower than expected because the drugs have been absorbed by the polymer material of the applied catheters. If later sampling is done via such catheters loaded with compound, the compound may be released again, resulting in artificially high concentrations (GARRETT and CHANDRAN 1989).

3.5.1.2
Intra-arterial Administration

The possibility of pulmonary first-pass elimination is seldom recognized. However, higher plasma concentrations after intra-arterial administration versus intravenous administration may be due to pulmonary first-pass elimination, e.g., as reported for propranolol in rats (IWAMOTO et al. 1987). The first-pass elimination of serotonin and norepinephrine in the canine lungs is very high (92%), while the amines will gradually be released into the circulation if the metabolism is inhibited by a monoamine oxidase inhibitor (BAKHLE and VANE 1974).

3.5.1.3
Intramuscular Administration

While intramuscular administration is frequently used in clinical practice and in veterinary clinics, it may be of limited use in experimental studies; this is particularly true in rodents, where strict intramuscular injection is difficult due to the size of the muscles. The intramuscular administration often causes a drug deposit at the injection site with relatively low bioavailability as a consequence. Many intramuscular drug formulations have physical-chemical characteristics that are unphysiological. The muscle tissue is a rather fragile tissue sensitive to unphysiological conditions such as high or low osmolarity and high or low pH values, in particular where the solutions have a substantial buffer capacity. Such formulations cause damage to the local muscle tissue at the injection site, and this may reduce the bioavailability. The characteristics of intramuscular injections have been dealt with in detail by SVENDSEN (1988).

3.5.1.4
Subcutaneous Administration

Subcutaneous administration is frequently used in experimental studies due to the simplicity of the injection procedure. However, the rate and extent of the bioavailability of the injected drug depend on a great number of biological and biopharmaceutical factors. In contrast to the muscle tissue, the subcutaneous tissue is well supplied with lymph vessels, and lymphatic absorption may contribute significantly to the absorption process. Absorption from subcutaneous injections is also influenced by pH and osmolarity. High or low osmolarity may reduce the bioavailability (MARVOLA and LAINE 1980), as may high or low pH values. Poorly soluble substances may be solubilized in vegetable oil. In general this will slow the absorption rate, and the absorption rate may vary with volume injected and concentration of substance in oil (HIRANO et al. 1982). Absorption from aqueous suspensions varies to such an extent that any prediction is very difficult.

3.5.1.5 Intraperitoneal Administration

Intraperitoneal administration is attractive due to its simplicity. However, this route of administration in experimental work should only be used after careful consideration. In general, absorption occurs rather rapidly. It is often overlooked that parts of the substance are absorbed to the portal system and thus subject to hepatic first-pass metabolism. In addition, nonspecific side-effects may occur in response to both the vehicle and the compound.

3.5.1.6 Oral Administration

Oral administration is one of the most frequently applied routes of dosing. Oral administration results in a relatively low peak drug level in plasma in comparison to parenteral dosing. Oral dosing in rodents is either with gavage or by admixtures in the diet. They are not equivalent and the latter method is primarily used in long-term chronic toxicity studies. For most compounds absorption is limited to the nonionized form of the molecule. The rate of absorption after oral dosing may depend on the contents of the gastrointestinal lumen (NIELSEN 1997). With ad libitum feeding the stomach is never empty and the food contents parallel the eating behavior. The eating behavior depends on the light and dark cycle in the animal room. After fasting for 16 h the stomach will be empty provided that the rats are kept on a wire mesh with no access to bedding (otherwise they will eat bedding). The gastric emptying rate is fairly constant in the rat (NEWMAN and BOOTH 1981), although it may be under the influence of the circadian rhythm. Transit time in the first and second quarters of the small intestines is very short; it is considerably longer in the third and fourth quarters and very long in the cecum and large intestines.

3.5.2 Factors Related to the Chemical or Physical Form of the Test Compound

Chemical (salt form, complexes, ester) and physical (crystal form, particle size) characteristics of the test compound itself are essential factors. Absorption is influenced by, for example, the solvent in which the compound is dissolved/suspended, additional components such as co-solvents, surfactants, or suspending agents, the route of administration, and the administration procedure (choice of injection site, rate of injection, volume administered), as well as animal-related characteristics such as age, sex, feeding conditions, and circadian rhythms.

The volume of drug solution or suspension influences absorption rate. In general, the absorption rate is enhanced by dilution of the dose. This is most probably related to a reduced transit time in the stomach (TSUZUKI et al. 1984).

Viscosity-increasing agents may affect bioavailability from either drug solutions or drug suspensions. In general the availability is reduced by viscosity-increasing agents in drug solutions (SAKIYA et al. 1981a,b), whereas it is increased by viscosity-increasing agents in drug suspensions (BARZEGAR-JALALI and RICHARDS 1979).

Co-solvents such as dimethylsulfoxide (DMSO), ethanol, glycerine, polyethylene glycol, and propylene glycol may cause reversible structural and functional changes of the gastrointestinal mucosa. Drug absorption is highly dependent on the co-solvent, and promotion as well as inhibition may occur. Co-solvents may have biological properties by themselves and they may affect drug metabolism. Poorly water-soluble drugs may be dissolved or suspended in oily vehicles. They delay gastric emptying and inhibit gastric secretion as other lipids do. Orally administered triglycerides are transported as chylomicrons via the lymph and may incorporate lipid-soluble substances. This absorption route bypasses the liver and may affect the availability.

3.5.3 Feeding Factors

Fasting causes severe changes in the physiological and biochemical processes which may be observed after fasting periods as short as 16–24 h. However, it is fairly common to withdraw food from animals for a period before the experiment. This will alter the metabolic state of the animal and induce adaptational changes in the endocrine and neuronal state. Withdrawal of food will result in decreased water intake, probably altering the hydration state. Changes in pharmacokinetics and pharmacodynamics may be a consequence. Fasting of animals should therefore be limited to studies where fasting is an essential factor in the study. Animals with a vomiting reflex, e.g., dogs, cats, pigs, ruminants, and primates, have to be fasted prior to anesthesia, while rodents do not have this reflex and therefore do not need fasting before anesthesia.

Food restriction may be necessary in studies on eating behavior and operand behavior, and in certain types of toxicity studies. Biochemical an physiological functions differ between restricted food and ad libitum food regimens. Ageing, tumor development, and other types of pathology are among those characteristics which differ remarkably (BEYNEN et al. 1993a).

3.5.4 Anesthesia

Anesthetics induce a state of unconsciousness, amnesia, and pain insensitivity and at the same time interfere with numerous other life processes. These disturbances are important not only in *in vivo* experiments but also in ex vivo and post-mortem studies. Maintenance of a well-defined anesthetic depth is important for the responsiveness of the animal and for the reproduction of the data obtained. This can best be achieved with inhalation anesthesia. However, in most animal studies intravenous anesthetics are used. An uncontrolled decrease in body temperature or blood pressure during anesthesia may contribute to physiological and biochemical changes.

The cardiovascular and autonomic effects of anesthetics are complex. In addition, anesthetics influence metabolic processes, pharmacodynamics, and pharmacokinetics. The characteristics of blood and tissue samples from anesthetized animals may differ from those of conscious animals.

3.6 Experimental Design

Experimental results are accepted or rejected after statistical evaluation. Concluding that there is a difference, when this in reality is not so, is called a *type I error*, while concluding that there is no difference, when there actually is one, is called *a type II error*. The probability of avoiding a type II error is called *power*. Committing such errors will obviously not give a high level of either predictability or reproducibility of that study. Furthermore, resources may be wasted and unnecessary animal suffering caused if too many animals are used due to a poor experimental design. For example FESTING (1995) described an experiment in which a proper experimental design would have reduced the 216 rats used to 72 rats. On the other hand, using too few animals may result in too little power, and therefore a careful determination of the correct size of the experiment is important. Such determinations may be based upon either mathematical equations, previous experience, or the so-called *resource equation method*, a method for adding the numbers of animals needed due to the degrees of freedom, the environmental variation, and the error (MEAD 1988). All the factors described in this chapter will add to the variation in the study or cause error and should be eliminated, reduced, or standardized. Error may be reduced by *stratification*, i.e., dividing animals into groups based on certain known characteristics, e.g., their weights. If there is no such information the study may be totally *randomized*, i.e., the animals are randomly assigned to test or control groups, thereby equally dividing the interindividual variation between the groups. Bias in the treatment may be prevented by standardizing such factors as the housing conditions of the animals.

Table 3.2. Examples of different experimental designs usable for eliminating variation in animal experiments (BEYNEN et al. 1993b)

Experimental design	Explanation
Randomized/parallel	Each group of animals undergoes one and only one of the various treatments simultaneously
Randomized block	The animals are grouped into blocks based upon certain characteristics
Cross-over	Each treatment is applied to all animals for a predefined period followed by the next treatment
Latin square	Each group of animals is subjected to each of the treatments, but in different order

Different experimental designs may be usable for eliminating variation in animal experiments (Table 3.2). For further information the reader is referred to either BEYNEN et al. (1993b) or VØLUND (1994).

3.7 General Conclusion

The uncertainties in animal characteristics and test conditions have not hindered the insight into biological regulatory mechanisms. If animal studies are to have the highest degree of predictability and reproducibility, only animals of well-defined health status, housed under well-defined conditions should be used. The experiment should be planned in order to eliminate the variation caused by improper standardization from group to group or over time and the bias caused by erroneous techniques. This review has summarized the various factors which are critical for variation, and thereby for the reproducibility and predictability in experimental research in animals. The factors are numerous and some are more important than others. Furthermore their importance may vary with the goal and the design of the study. It is the responsibility of the scientist generating the hypothesis to be tested and designing the study to elucidate the hypothesis to take these factors into consideration in order to obtain data which present minimal biological variation and are reproducible. Taking this responsibility seriously will not only improve biological sciences involving laboratory animals but also be in accordance with the ethical obligation to gain as much information as possible whenever using animals for experiments.

References

Bakhle YS, Vane JR (1974) Pharmacokinetic function of the pulmonary circulation. Physiol Rev 54:1007–1045

Barzegar-Jalali M, Richards JH (1979) Effects of various suspending agents on the bioavailabilities of aspirin and salicylic acid in the rabbit. Int J Pharm 3:133–141

Beatty WW (1979) Gonadal hormones and sex differences in non-reproductive behaviors in rodent: organizational and activational influences. Horm Behav 12:112–163

Beynen AC, Festing MFW, van Montfort MAJ (1993a) Nutrition and experimental results. In: van Zutphen LFM, Baumans V, Beynen AC (eds) Principles of laboratory animals science. Elsevier Science, Amsterdam, pp 109–125

Beynen AC, Festing MFW, van Montfort MAJ (1993b) Design of animal experiments. In: van Zutphen LFM, Baumans V, Beynen AC (eds) Principles of laboratory animal science. Elsevier Science, Amsterdam, pp 209–239

Birnbaum LS (1991) Pharmacokinetic basis of age-related changes in sensitivity to toxicants. Ann Rev Pharmacol 31:101–128

Calabrese EJ (1984) Toxic susceptibility: male/female differences, Wiley, New York.

Calabrese EJ (1986) Age and susceptibility to toxic substances. Wiley New York

Claassen V (1994) Neglected factors in pharmacology and neuroscience research. Elsevier, Amsterdam

Clough G (1982) Environmental effects on animals used in biomedical research. Biol Rev 57:487–523

Cunliffe-Beamer TL, Freeman LC, Myers DD (1981) Barbiturate sleeptime in mice exposed to autoclaved or unautoclaved wood beddings. Lab Anim Sci 31:672–675

Dairman W, Balazt T (1970) Comparsion of live microsome enzyme systems and barbiturate sleep times in rats caged individually or communally. Biochem Pharmacol 19:951–955

Danhof M., Levy G (1984) Kinetics of drug action in disease state. I. Effect of infusion rate on phenobarbital concentrations in serum, brain and cerebrospinal fluid of normal rats at onset of loss of righting reflex. J Pharmacol Exp Ther 229:44–50

De Laat JM, van Tintelen G, Beynen AC (1989) Transportation of rats affects behaviour of non-transported rats in the absence of physical contact (preliminary communication). Zeitschr Versuchstierkunde 32:235-237

Festing MFW (1987) Genetic factors in toxicology: implications for toxicological testing. CRC Crit Rev Toxicol 18:1–26

Festing MFW (1990) Use of genetically heterogenous rats and mice in toxicological research: a personal perspective. Toxicol Appl Pharmacol 102:197–204

Festing MFW (1995) Reduction of animal use and experimental design. In: Goldberg AM, van Zutphen LEM (eds) The world congress on alternatives and animal use in the life sciences. Education Research Testing 11:43–49

Friis AS, Ladefoged O (1979) The influence of *Bacillus piliformis* (Tyzzer) infections on the reliability of pharmacokinetic experiments in mice. Lab Anim 13:257–261

Garrett ER, Chandran VR (1989) Pharmacokinetics of morphine and its surrogates. Discrepancies among infused buprenorphine plasma concentrations sampled from different veins. J Pharm Sci 78:644–647

Hansen AK (1994) Health status and the effects of microbial organisms on animal experiment. In: Svendsen P, Hau J (eds) Handbook of laboratory animal science, vol I. Selection and handling of animals in biomedical research. CRC Press, Boca Raton, Chap. 11

Hirano K, Ichihashi T, Yamada H (1982) Studies on the absorption of practically water-insoluble drugs following injection. V. Subcutaneous absorption in rats from solutions in water immiscible oils. J Pharm Sci 71:495–500

Iwamoto K, Watanaba, J, Aoyama Y (1987) High capacity for pulmonary first-pass elimination of propranolol in rats. J Pharm Pharmacol 39:1049–1051

Iwarsson K, Lindberg L, Waller T (1994) Common non-surgical techniques and procedures. In: Svendsen P, Hau J (eds) Handbook of Laboratory animal science, vol I. Selection and handling of animals in biomedical research. CRC Press, Boca Raton FL., Chap. 16

Kato R (1974) Sex-related differences in drug metabolism. Drug Metab Rev 3, 1–32

Kraft V, Deeney AA, Blanchet HM, et al. (1994) Recommendations for the health monitoring of mouse, rat, hamster, guineapig and rabbit breeding colonies. Report of the Federation of European Laboratory Animal Science Associations (FELASA) Working Group on Animal Health accepted by the FELASA Board of Management November 1992. Lab Anim 28:1–12

Laboratory Animals (1992) Notes to authors. Lab Anim 26: xxxviii–xxxix

Marvola, M, Laine T (1980) The effect of osmotic pressure on the intraperitoneal and subcutaneous absorption of sulfafurazole in the rat. Acta Pharm Fenn 89:223–229

Mead R (1988) The design of experiments. Cambridge University Press, Cambridge

Meyer OA, Kristiansen E, Wuertzen G (1989) Effects of dietary protein and butylated hydroxytoluene on the kidneys of rats. Lab Anim 23:175–179

Mudge GH (1980) Nephrotoxicity of urographic radiocontrast drugs. Kidney Int 18:540–552

Mudge GH (1982) Nephrotoxicity associated with the use of radiological contrast drugs. Monogr Appl Toxicol 1:460–473

Nelson JF, Felicio, LS (1984) Dietary modulation of estrous cyclicity in singly and multiply housed C57BL/6J mice. Lab Amin Sci 34:173–176

Newman JC, Booth DA (1981) Gastro-intestinal and metabolic consequences of a rats meal on maintenance diet ad libitum. Physiol Behav 27:929–939

Nielsen P (1997) Fodringens indflyelse på den orale biotilgœngelighed af antibiotika/kemoterapeutika hos grise. Dansk Veterinœrtidsskrift 11:495–501

Pessacq MT, Rebolledo OR, Mercer RG, Gagliardino JJ (1976) Effect of fasting on the circadian rhythm of serum insulin levels. Chronobiologia 3:20–26

Poole T (1987) The UFAW handbook on the care and management of laboratory animals. Longman Sci Techn, Edinburgh

Reese EP (1991) The role of husbandry in promoting the welfare of laboratory animals. In: Hendriksen CFM, Koeter HBWM (eds) Animals in biomedical research. Elsevier, Amsterdam, pp 155–192

Ritskes-Hoitinga J, Lemmens AG, Beynen AC (1989) Nutrition and kidney calcification in rats. Lab Anim 23:313–318

Sakiya Y, Miyauchi Y, Tsuemura Y (1981a) Influence of osmotic pressure and viscocity on intestinal absorption. I. Studies on gastric effluent following oral administration of various quinine solutions to rats. Chem Pharm Bull 29:539–544

Sakiya Y, Miyauchi Y, Tsuemura Y (1981b) Influence of osmotic pressure and viscocity on intestinal absorption. II. Quinine concentration profile in plasma after oral administration of various quinine solutions to rats. Chem Pharm Bull 29:1470–1472

Svendsen O (1988) Studies of tissue injuries caused by intramuscular injection of drugs and vehicles. Methods for quantification and effects of concentration, volume, vehicle, injection speed and intralipomatous injection. Dr.M.Sci. Thesis, Medical Faculty, Copenhagen University

Svendsen P (1994) Environmental impact on animal experiments. In: Svendsen P, Hau J (eds) Handbook of laboratory animals science, vol I. Selection and handling of animals in biomedical research. CRC Press, Boca Raton, Chap. 14

Takenaka S, Fujiwara K (1975) Effect of carbon tetrachloride on experimental Tyzzer's diseases of mice. Jpn J Exp Anim Med 45:393–402

Thomsen HS, Goldman K, Svendsen O, Skaarup P, Hemmingsen L, Larsen S (1991) Pretreatment with steroids before intravenous injection of diatrizoate or iohexol. Invest Radio 26:1083–1086

Thomsen HS, Goldman K, Hemmingsen L, Larsen S, Skaarup P, Svendsen O (1993) Contrast medium induced nephropathy: animal experiments. Front Eur Radio 9:83–108

Thomsen HS, Dorph S, Larsen S, Horn T, Hemmingsen L, Skaarup P, Golman K, Svendsen O (1995) Urine profiles and kidney histology after ionic and nonionic radiologic and magnetic resonance contrast media in rats with cisplatin nephropathy. Acad Radiol 2:657–682

Thomsen HS, Dorph S, Larsen S, Horn T, Hemmingsen L, Skaarup P, Golman K, Svendsen O (1996) Chronic cisplatin nephropathy and contrast media, and creatinine. Acad Radiol 3:444–446

Tsuzuki O, Kotsubo J, Tanaka Y, Matsumoto Y, Kouno K (1984) Effect of fluid volume on the gastric emptying and absorption of quinine in mice, rabbits and humans. Chem Pharm Bull 32:3199–3204

Tucker MJ (1985) Effect of diet on spontaneous disease in the inbred mouse strain C57B1/10J Toxicol Lett 25:131–135

Vesell ES, Lang CM, Passananti GT, Tripp SL (1973) Hepatic drug metabolism in rats. Impairment in a dirty environment. Science 179:896–897

Vølund AA (1994) Experimental design and statistical evaluation. In Svendsen P, Hau J (eds) Handbook of Laboratory animal science, vol 1. CRC Press, Boca Raton, pp 203–229

4 Experimental Testing of Iodinated Contrast Media Before Human Testing

R. Towart and K. Golman

CONTENTS

4.1 Introduction

This chapter describes the testing of iodinated angio- and urographic x-ray contrast media before clinical testing. Once a promising series of chemical compounds has been conceived, a range of physicochemical and toxicological tests will be used to select the most promising candidate(s), which then will be subjected to a wider range of tests, including stability, pharmacokinetic, and toxicological tests, in order both to make the final choice and to predict its expected safety in man before clinical testing. After a new compound has been synthesized, and has been shown to be chemically stable, the major factor determining its suitability as a contrast agent is its toxicology. Much of this chapter is therefore devoted to aspects of toxicological testing.

Contrast media comprise an unusual subset of medicinal agents. In general, and in comparison with almost all therapeutic agents, they are very inert, have little biological activity, and are administered in very high doses. Later chapters will discuss the adverse effects which are known to occur in man. Although these are typically minor effects such as feelings of warmth or pain, the large number of diagnoses (one human being is injected every second) carried out with high doses means that life-threatening events such as renal failure or ventricular fibrillation are seen every day around the world (see Chap. 11). Therefore much effort has been expended to develop relevant models of these effects, both as a means of understanding their pathophysiology and as testing methods to try to reduce their occurrence in new chemical entities (NCEs) under development. As with all drug development, no testing on animal models in vitro or in vivo can be completely predictive of human toxicity. Nevertheless, experimental testing with relevant and well-tested models is accepted as being sufficiently predictive of human toxicity to allow initial testing in humans, and has the obvious advantage of allowing the administration of either extremely high doses or long-term treatment which would not be possible in humans (see Chap. 3).

Another type of nonclinical testing comprises in vitro experiments which examine particular aspects of the pharmacology or toxicology of contrast agents with a view to unravelling the mechanisms and/or pathophysiology of the effects. In this way risk factors for clinical use of contrast agents may be predicted, or potential treatments or prophylactic methods devised. Advances in this field will be mentioned if they seem relevant to the preclinical testing of NCEs.

Earlier work on this topic has been excellently summarized in previous reviews (e.g., Sovak 1984; Swanson et al. 1986; Speck 1994). This chapter will therefore concentrate on recent work. Table 4.1 gives an overview of recently published preclinical experimental models not described in detail in this review.

R. Towart, BSc, PhD, Department of Experimental Research, Malmö University Hospital and Nycomed Innovation AB, Ideon-Malmö, S-205 12 Malmö, Sweden
K. Golman, PhD, Professor, Department of Experimental Research, Malmö University Hospital and Nycomed Innovation AB, Ideon-Malmö, S-205 12 Malmö, Sweden

Table 4.1. Some methods and models for preclinical testing of contrast agents

Topic	Description	References
Physical tests		
Angiographic opacification	Time density measurement in plastic tubes	Yang et al. 1994
Physical performance	X-ray absorption by heavy metals	Sandborg et al. 1995
Biochemical tests		
Protein binding	Equilibrium dialysis	Krause and Niehues 1996
Glucose metabolism	Glucose uptake and metabolism in rat brain	Morris et al. 1988
Enzyme inhibition	Enzyme activity measured photometrically	Krause and Niehues 1996
Cholinesterase	Enzyme activity in mice	Howell and Dawson 1985
Creatine phosphokinase	Enzyme and isoenzyme activity in canine tissues	Canillot et al. 1983
Bradykinin and ACE	Angiotensin-converting enzyme inhibition in vitro	Lasser and Lyon 1990
Serine proteases	X-ray analysis of elastase/iohexol interactions	Prange et al. 1995
Prostacyclin	PGI_2 generation in isolated rat lung	Paajanen and Uotila 1985
Leukotrienes	LTB_4 synthesis and metabolism in human PMNs	Romano et al. 1991
Toxicity testing		
Local tissue damage	Intradermal injection (mice)	Elam et al. 1991
Local tissue damage	Subcutaneous injection (rats)	Kim et al. 1990
Local tissue damage	Injection into rabbit muscle	Thomsen et al. 1991
Pulmonary toxicity	Induction of pulmonary edema (rat)	Mare et al. 1984
Mutagenicity, etc.		
Chromosomal damage	Micronucleus test in cultured human lymphocytes	Parvez et al. 1986
Spermatogenesis	Sperm head survival and abnormalities (mouse testis)	Yaghmai et al. 1993
Cardiac effects		
Impulse conduction	Intracellular microelectrodes	Fillette et al. 1988
Selective coronary perfusion	Selective perfusion of coronary arteries (rat)	Skarstein et al. 1997
Cardiac microcirculation	Fluoroscopic examination of vasomotion in vivo (rat)	Klopp et al. 1995
Blood vessels		
Endothelium	In vitro	Laerum 1987
Endothelial injury	Cultured human umbilical endothelial monolayers	Benyon et al. 1994
Microcirculation	In vivo microscopy of rat intestine	Krause et al. 1994a
Renal effects		
Endothelin release	Endothelin and renal blood flow in rats	Heyman et al. 1992
Vascular resistance	Tubuloglomerular feedback and vasoconstricting mediators	Morcos et al. 1995
Renal microcirculation	Fluorescence microscopy of kidney (mouse)	Hogstrom et al. 1993
Renal artery	Isolated renal artery (rabbit)	Drescher et al. 1995
Tubular toxicity	Renal proximal tubule cells in vitro (rabbit)	Messana et al. 1988
Vacuolization	Light and electron microscopic study (rat)	Tervahartiala et al. 1991
CNS and neural effects		
Neurotransmitter receptors	Ligand binding studies in rat brain membranes	Mennini et al. 1993
Cerebrospinal fluid	CSF production in dogs	Harnish et al. 1985, 1986
Neural toxicity	EEG recording in rats	Adams et al. 1988
Cerebral vasculature	Isolated basilar artery (rabbit)	Jansen et al. 1987
Skeletal muscle	Twitching reaction in vivo (rat)	Bååth et al. 1994
Disease states/risk factors		
Pancreatitis	Microcirculation in experimental pancreatitis (rats)	Schmidt et al. 1995
Coronary thrombolysis	Postischemic reperfusion model (dog)	Sheu et al. 1991
Congestive heart failure	CA-induced nephropathy in heart failure (dogs)	Margulies et al. 1990
Ischemic heart failure	Acute particle-induced heart failure (dogs)	Pedersen et al. 1994
Pulmonary hypertension	Effects after pulmonary embolism (dogs)	Rees et al. 1988
Ischemic renal failure	RBC trapping in renal microcirculation	Nygren et al. 1993
Renal insufficiency	Renal plasma flow and GFR in subtotal nephrectomy (dogs)	Arakawa et al. 1996
Myasthenia gravis	CA effects in autoimmune myasthenic rabbits	Eliashiv et al. 1990
Hyperthyroidism	Thyroid scintigraphy in rabbits	Steidle 1989
Diabetes	Renal morphological lesions (streptozotocin, rats)	Tervahartiala et al. 1993
Dehydration	Fatal reactions in dehydration (dogs)	Katzberg et al. 1983

Table 4.1. *Continued*

Topic	Description	References
Cell culture and tissues in vitro		
Bacteria	Effects on bacterial growth	Blake and Halasz 1995
Cellular toxicity	LDH leakage from isolated rat hepatocytes	Nordby et al. 1987
Cellular incorporation	Intracellular penetration into cultured human cells	Nordby et al. 1989
Cytotoxicity	Viability and enzyme release in MDCK cells	Haller et al. 1997
Cytotoxicity	Morphology and viability of cultured renal tubular cells	Andersen et al. 1995
Cytotoxicity	pH and intracellular acidification of human cell lines	Dascalu and Peer 1994
Cytotoxicity	Viability and permeability of renal epithelial cells	Haller et al. 1997
Cardiac myocytes	Contractility and Ca transients (chick myocytes)	Kohmoto et al. 1992
Blood, platelets, and blood coagulation		
Coagulation parameters	APTT, TT, FpA, etc. in whole blood	Corot et al. 1996
Coagulation parameters	In vitro bleeding time	Melton et al. 1996
Coagulation parameters	Effects on fibrinogen and factor VIII in vitro	Andes 1988
Coagulation	Effects on factor XII in vitro	Laurie et al. 1991
Blood clotting	Thrombin activity and fibrin polymerization	Belleville et al. 1985
Blood clotting	Platelet activation and aggregation	Hay and Bull 1995
Blood clotting	Platelet degranulation	Chronos et al. 1993
Blood clotting	Thromboplastin time and clot formation	Krause and Press 1997
Blood clotting	Kallikrein/kinin system activation	Hoffmeister et al. 1988
Thrombogenicity	Platelet adhesion to cultured endothelial cells	Grabowski et al. 1993
Thrombogenicity	Platelet deposition on isolated carotid artery (rabbit)	Riemann et al. 1993
Thrombogenicity	Laser-induced thrombosis in vivo (rat)	Aguejouf et al. 1995
Thrombogenicity	Fibrinogen accretion in jugular thrombi in vivo (rabbit)	Levi et al. 1991
Thrombin	Thrombin generation in human blood ex vivo	Parvez and Vik 1994
Complement	Activation of complement	Akagi et al. 1991
Blood rheology	Filtrability of rat blood and RBC morphology	LeMignon et al. 1988
Blood rheology	Filtrability of human blood and RBC morphology	Imai et al. 1993
Blood rheology	Blood viscosity	Smedby 1992
Serum calcium levels	Ionized serum calcium levels after CA in vitro	Hayakawa et al. 1994
Hypersensitivity and idiosyncratic reactions		
Antibody production	IgE, IgG1, IL4 measurement in mice	Miyauchi et al. 1996
Antibody production	Rabbit and mouse antibody production to CA	Siegle et al. 1988
Histamine and complement	Complement activation and histamine in human blood	Vik et al. 1995
Kinins and complement	Kallikrein and complement activation in human blood	Hoffmeister et al. 1988
Complement activation	Complement activity and C3A RIA in human plasma	Eaton et al. 1990
Granulocyte migration	Agarose chemotactic technique	Georgesen et al. 1990

(Standard tests are given in Tables 4.2 and 4.3)

APTT, Activated partial thromboplastin time; CA, contrast agent; GFR, glomerular filtration rate; LDH, lactate dehydrogenase; PMNs, polymorphonuclear neutrophilic leukocytes; RBC, red blood cell; TT, thromboplastin time.

4.2 Chemical and Physical Testing

Unlike other pharmacological agents, iodinated contrast media are selected as the compound with the *least* bioactivity. For this reason the classical technique of examining and predicting the structure-activity relationships of a series of related chemical structures is of limited value.

It is known that the low-osmolar, nonionic contrast agents produce fewer adverse events and are safer than high-osmolar ionic agents (Katayama et al. 1990; Hill et al. 1993), and the assumption is made here that new agents to be introduced in the foreseeable future will be nonionic. In designing such candidates, the chemist aims at maximising the iodine content, normally by substituting the 1, 3, and 5 positions of tri-iodobenzoic acid with polyhydroxyalkyl groups, or by devising some sort of oligomer (presently almost entirely dimers, such as iodixanol or iotrolan) of this basic subunit. The major tests in the analytical laboratory are water solubility, the osmolality, the lipophilicity, and the viscosity (see Skinnemoen 1987; Krause et al. 1994b; and Eivindvik and Sjögren 1995 for methods). Candidate compounds must be highly water soluble (>80%), and for practical reasons must not have too high a viscosity (<40 mPas·s, 20°C) at clinically useful iodine concentrations of 300–370 mg I/ml. The chemist will test stability under various conditions, especially after autoclaving (Skinnemoen et al. 1987b). In addition protein binding will normally be predictive of interaction with enzymes and proteinaceous membrane components (e.g., receptors or ion channels) and suggests toxicity (Speck 1994). All recently introduced nonionic contrast agents have very low binding to plasma proteins (Jacobsen et al. 1995); this is indicative of low toxicity, and in addition allows the agent to be removed from the body by dialysis if necessary.

In vitro incompatibility is an additional useful test (Krause 1994). As contrast agents are often introduced through an indwelling catheter used for the administration of other drugs, it should be shown that the new agent does not cause precipitation with other commonly used pharmacological agents or formulations (see Kim et al. 1992).

4.3 Toxicology – Theoretical Considerations

One can divide the toxic potential of the use of iodinated contrast agents into several categories, not all of which are entirely independent from each other:

1. Physical effects, or physicotoxicity (e.g., caused by osmolality or viscosity)
2. Chemotoxicity, normally ascribed to interactions with biological proteins and membranes
3. Possible secondary pharmacological effects at clinical doses
4. Idiosyncratic effects
5. Effects caused by the agent temporarily replacing circulating constituents of the blood
6. Effects caused by excipients, impurities, or contaminants.

The *physical effects* of *hyperosmolar* contrast agents are obvious: a hyperosmolar agent will withdraw water from a tissue to restore the osmotic equilibrium, and dehydrate the cells. This effect contributes to the vascular pain experienced during injection of hyperosmolar ionic agents. Thus today one trend is to develop formulations equiosmolar with blood, of around 290 mOsm (Almén 1995; Karlsson et al. 1995). The recent development of dimeric molecules such as iodixanol, which contain 6 atoms of iodine per molecule (see Chap. 1.6), has even allowed formulations in which a hypoosmolar solution of contrast agent can be supplemented with small amounts of physiologically vital ions such as sodium and calcium (Jynge et al. 1995).

The high *viscosity* of contrast agents has at least three disadvantages: (a) the mechanical difficulty of injection, especially if thin catheters have to be used (e.g., in infants); (b) intrarenal pressure effects in the renal tubule as water is reabsorbed, and (c) the possible problems of perfusion of the viscous solution through some vascular beds. The viscous solutions are retained for longer periods in the poorly stirred layers close to the endothelium of blood vessels.

The *chemotoxicity* of contrast agents at high concentration is much discussed but poorly understood. Certainly it can be shown that contrast agents of different structures bind to proteins to a small extent (Speck 1994; Krause and Niehues 1996), and a range of enzymes have been shown to be inhibited by the agents in vitro (Krause and Niehues 1996). Several cell culture models (especially endothelial or kidney epithelial cells) have been used to assess chemotoxicity by measuring cell viability, DNA synthesis, thymidine incorporation, or enzyme leakage as measures of cellular damage (see Sect. 4.6).

Contrast agents have been designed to have the lowest possible bioactivity, and have few direct *secondary pharmacological effects* (Morris and Fischer 1986; Pugh and Karlsson 1997). For example, standard ligand binding experiments to assess interactions with neurotransmitter receptors showed no interactions of iopamidol or iohexol up to high concentrations (Mennini et al. 1993). Nevertheless, at the high concentrations used most contrast agents are vasoactive, in general contracting resting vessels and relaxing constricted vessels (Pugh and Karlsson 1997). The exact mechanisms of these effects are unknown. Thus in addition to chemotoxic effects, most contrast agents produce local and/or general circulatory effects, which indirectly, if not directly, can stimulate the release or synthesis of counter-regulatory mediators such as eicosanoids, kinins, endothelial relaxing factors, or endothelins (see Table 4.1 for references).

Contrast agents, especially the newer nonionic agents, have very low if any allergenicity. Nevertheless, various anaphylactoid reactions or certain *idiosyncratic effects* of unknown etiology do occur (Siegle 1993). Most contrast agents release histamine and activate complement to some extent in vitro and in vivo, although this depends on tissue, species, and conditions (Krause and Niehues 1996).

Replacement effects, i.e., those caused by the agent temporarily replacing circulating constituents of the blood (e.g., ions necessary for initiation or propagation of impulses in excitable tissue), are beyond the scope of the present article, but the interested reader is referred to BESJAKOV et al. (1994) or JYNGE et al. (1995) for discussion. Many contrast agents are formulated with *excipients* such as tromethamine or EDTA to ensure stability. In the 1970s the calcium-binding effects of NaEDTA were implicated in an increased incidence of fibrillation with formulations containing it (TRÄGÅRDH et al. 1975; FISCHER and MORRIS 1980), and $Na_2CaEDTA$ is therefore used in modern contrast media.

4.4 Toxicological Testing

In classical drug development, new chemicals were screened for a certain activity, and when a compound with this activity (i.e., a "lead") was found, the lead was optimized by synthesizing similar compounds to increase the selectivity and minimize the toxicity. The iodinated contrast agents do not require screening per se, as any stable compound with a high percentage of iodine atoms will absorb x-rays and act as a contrast agent. Thus the first biological test (after measuring protein binding in vitro, see above) is a generalized toxicity test.

The classical LD_{50} test is now regarded as redundant, especially when the test is carried out uncritically with large numbers of animals. New guidelines have now been issued by most regulatory authorities (e.g., FDA 1996). However, in a reduced form the single-dose acute toxicity test is still an important initial biological test for the testing of contrast agents. The amount of contrast agent injected into humans is much larger than for almost all other pharmaceuticals, treatment may be repeated, but is never chronic, and the patients often have renal, liver, or other disease or may have suffered major trauma. It has been found that the single-dose acute toxicity test will provide a large amount of predictive information with the use of a small number of animals. The results of this test closely parallel the results of classical LD_{50} tests, which, possibly because of the general nature of physico- and chemotoxicity, are strongly predictive of the general incidence of adverse effects caused by different contrast agents in a patient population. In addition recording the animals' appearance and behavior as well as symptoms and histological analysis after death or euthanisation can give vital information as to the specific and nonspecific toxicity of the agent, and the tissues or body systems affected.

Table 4.2. Typical profile of general toxicology

Acute intravenous toxicity - Mice, rats, dogs
Acute oral toxicity - Mice
Toxicity after intracisternal injection - Rat
Subacute intravenous toxicity - Rat, dog, monkey
Local tolerance and toxicity (intravenous and perivenous, skin, intramuscular, subcutaneous, intraperitoneal) - Rabbit
Antigenicity (passive cutaneous anaphylaxis test) - Guinea-pig
Reproductive and teratogenicity studies (including peri- and postnatal development) - Rat, rabbit
Mutagenicity studies - Bacterial reverse mutation assay - Micronucleus test - Test for chromosomal aberrations - Mutation assay

A large body of historical data for the chemically related agents already used is available for comparative purposes. If the test is carried out in mice, it also has the advantage of requiring relatively small amounts of compound. [For details of the test, see standard toxicology reference works or supplements describing new agents (e.g., HEYWOOD et al. 1987; HEGLUND et al. 1995; DONADIEU et al. 1996).]

As required by current regulatory requirements, a wide range of toxicological studies must be carried out before the introduction of an agent into clinical practice. A typical profile is given in Table 4.2 (details may vary from country to country) (AULIE MICHELET et al. 1987; HEYWOOD et al. 1987, HEGLUND et al. 1995; DONADIEU et al. 1996).

4.5 Pharmacology – Testing on Animals and Isolated Organs

4.5.1 Safety Pharmacology

Given that a compound in development has an acceptably low toxicity and a good toxicological profile (see above), its pharmacological profile should next

Table 4.3. Typical profile of safety pharmacology

Cardiac effects in vitro (Langendorff heart) (Blankson et al. 1995; Jynge et al. 1995)
Cardiopulmonary effects in vivo (anesthetized dog) (Idée et al. 1996)
Effects during coronary angiography (anesthetized dog) (Klöw et al. 1995)
Vasoconstrictor and vasodilator effects (isolated blood vessels) (Karstoft and Bååth 1995)
Renal effects (various species) (Dobrota et al. 1995; Walday et al. 1995; Morcos et al. 1995)
Pulmonary effects in vitro (isolated perfused lung) (Idée et al. 1996)
Occurrence of bronchospasm in vivo (Konzett Rössler) (Idée et al. 1996)
RBC morphology, osmotic fragility, and hemolysis (human red cells ex vivo) (Hardeman et al. 1991)
Coagulation and platelet function (human blood ex vivo) (Stormorken et al. 1987)
Histamine release (human blood ex vivo) (Idée et al. 1996)
Neurological effects (intracarotid injection in rabbits) (Maly et al. 1995)
Interaction with enzymes (Krause et al. 1994b)
Cytotoxicity (cultured human fibroblasts) (Idée et al. 1996)
Receptor binding studies (Mennini et al. 1993)

be assessed. Thus a range of "safety pharmacology" experiments will be carried out to ensure that its effects (other than increasing x-ray absorption and thus contrast) are minimal. Safety pharmacology is required for international registration, but in addition will contribute to rational high-dose selection for toxicity studies, and provides a bridge between the preclinical and clinical segments of compound development (Kinter and Dixon 1995). The core studies comprise cardiovascular, CNS/neuromuscular, respiratory, renal, and gastrointestinal pharmacology, but may also contain some tests like receptor binding profiles (Table 4.3).

4.5.2 Special Pharmacological Testing

Although modern contrast agents, especially low-osmolar nonionic agents, as mentioned above, are very nontoxic and have few direct pharmacological effects, they are known to produce a certain incidence of adverse events, some of which can be modeled in preclinical testing. Because of their potential seriousness, it is worthwhile performing tests specifically to exclude renal effects, cardiodepressant or profibrillatory effects, and hematological and hypersensitivity effects. Table 4.1 gives an overview of recent methods, with selected references. Models should be carefully validated so that the contrast agent-induced lesions correspond as closely as possible to those observed in the clinic.

4.5.2.1 *Cardiovascular Testing*

The circulatory effects of contrast agents are well known from the clinic, and mimicked in standard cardiovascular models such as anesthetized rats. In addition a range of isolated organs, especially kidney and heart, have been used experimentally. A classical technique for investigating mechanisms and comparing potencies is the use of isolated blood vessels. Thus the effects of contrast agents on isolated renal (Drescher et al. 1995), cerebral (Jansen et al. 1987) and other vessels (Gomi 1992; Pugh and Karlsson 1997) has been described.

The clinical importance of contrast agents for cardiac diagnosis (e.g., coronary angiography) or intervention (e.g., coronary angioplasty), and the occasional occurrence of fibrillation during such procedures has stimulated the investigation of many effects of contrast agents on the heart, both healthy and diseased (see below), in recent years. Contrast agents affect cardiac contractility, electrophysiology (Fillette et al. 1988), and coronary flow and may influence blood clotting and coagulation (see below). These effects can be investigated using a wide range of models, from in vivo studies using large animals such as the pig or the dog (e.g., Morris 1988; Besjakov et al. 1994; Klöw et al. 1995) to isolated heart preparations such as Langendorff preparations (Bååth and Almén 1989) or perfused atria (Tande et al. 1989). Effects on cardiac metabolism in humans have been investigated by Wisneski et al. (1985), and the technique of phosphorus-31 nuclear magnetic resonance spectroscopy can be used in isolated hearts to measure intracellular pH, phosphocreatinine, and ATP (Goosens et al. 1995).

During coronary arteriography the blood in the artery being examined is temporarily replaced by contrast media, which, in addition to any intrinsic chemotoxicity, will in general contain little oxygen and few if any physiological ions. Thus there exists a danger of arrhythmias or ventricular fibrillation, especially if the injection time is prolonged or if the catheter is accidentally wedged. The susceptibility to fibrillation (and to changes in contractility, coronary hemodynamics, etc.) can be investigated either in vitro or in vivo. For testing in vitro, a rabbit Langendorff heart may be used, in which injection of 7–14 ml of contrast agent induces fibrillation (BÅÅTH and ALMÉN 1989). An interesting new model uses a specialized twin cannula to perfuse the left coronary artery selectively with contrast medium (SKARSTEIN et al. 1997). An in vivo model was developed by Morris, in which contrast agent injected into the canine right coronary artery produced fibrillation (MORRIS 1988). This model has been improved by injecting into the left coronary artery (to give more systemic hemodynamic information) and using vectorcardiography in the pig (BESJAKOV et al. 1994). Because fibrillation is probably due to a premature ventricular beat from the perfused area which occurs during the vulnerable period of the rest of the heart, the technique of programmed electrical stimulation can also be used to assess fibrillation propensity (MURDOCK et al. 1985).

4.5.2.2
Pulmonary Testing

Although generalized effects of contrast media on the lungs would be seen in the standard toxicology tests, some models exist for examining various aspects of the pulmonary hemodynamic effects of contrast agents either intravenously (pig, SORENSEN et al. 1994; rat, HAYASHI et al. 1994) or right atrially, to test the "pulmonary chemoreflex" (dog, MORETTIN et al. 1994).

LARSEN et al. (1995) have applied contrast agents intratracheally (to simulate accidental aspiration) and reviewed previous findings.

Little experimental work has been carried out on the ventilatory effects of contrast agents. The Konzett-Rössler bronchospasm model may be used (CIPOLLA et al. 1995; IDÉE et al. 1996), and LAUDE et al. (1996) have investigated effects of contrast agents on a standard respiratory analysis model in the rat.

4.5.2.3
Renal Models

Many models exist for examining contrast agent effects on the kidney (see, e.g., GOLMAN and ALMÉN 1984; THOMSEN et al. 1993; IDÉE et al. 1994; IDÉE and BONNEMAIN 1996 for reviews). Most important are whole animal models and isolated kidney models. Both have advantages, depending on the questions being asked. Interestingly, there seems to be a large species variation in the sensitivity of the kidney to contrast agents, with the rabbit being more sensitive than the rat to contrast agent-induced renal changes (BHARGAVA et al. 1990).

Conscious whole animal models have the advantage that parameters such as renal clearance, protein- or enzymuria, and histopathology can be examined at various time points. Anesthetized whole animals are frequently used in acute experiments to measure renal blood flow and glomerular filtration rate (GFR), and may be useful in comparing the nephrotoxicity of agents and in testing potential protective agents (e.g., BAGNIS et al. 1997). Isolated kidney models (normally rat) are less physiological than in vivo preparations, but allow carefully controlled perfusion conditions, and with small animals have higher testing capacity (OLDROYD et al. 1995; MORCOS et al. 1997). Again, there may be differences in sensitivity in models in vitro and in vivo (BREZIS et al. 1991). The GFR of single nephrons can be examined with micropuncture techniques (UEDA et al. 1992).

4.5.2.4
CNS and Neuromuscular Testing

Any contrast agent used in neuroangiography or myelography needs to be very safe, and LATCHAW (1993) has reviewed the experimental methods used to assess this safety. These include the ability to break the blood-brain barrier (HOLTZ et al. 1983) and effects on neurons in vivo (epileptic activity and motor coordination, SIEFERT et al. 1980) or in vitro (microelectrode studies, BRYAN et al. 1982; cerebral metabolism, EKHOLM et al. 1989). The direct effects of intrathecal (LA NOCE et al. 1996b) or intracisternal injections (SUNDGREN et al. 1995; MALY et al. 1995) can be measured by examining depressive or excitative effects in conscious animals. Electromyography can be used to detect direct effects of contrast agents on skeletal muscle (WILSON et al. 1991).

Several animal models exist to test the painfulness or other unpleasant effects of injected contrast agents (SPECK et al. 1980; SOVAK et al. 1988; ALGUACIL et al. 1994; LA NOCE et al. 1996a).

4.5.2.5
Disease Models

Contrast agents are used to help the diagnosis of diseased or traumatized individuals, who are frequently elderly. Epidemiological studies show that rates of certain adverse reactions are unsurprisingly greater in such groups. Several methods have therefore been developed to test the safety of contrast agents in animal models of human diseases, especially cardiovascular disease (e.g., heart failure or pulmonary hypertension), renal failure, or diabetes. Contrast agents themselves may be used to induce renal failure in the search for antidotes (Schwartz et al. 1994). Details can be found in the references cited in Table 4.1.

4.6 Testing In Vitro

Much of basic biology is now carried out using in vitro methods, where well-characterized cell lines are known to express particular proteins under controlled conditions. There is a trend towards the increasing use of cell culture methods in contrast agent research. Such methods have some advantages, including high reproducibility, high capacity with small amounts of newly synthesized compound, and the ability to concentrate on one type of cell without interactions from other tissues. The latter advantage, however, is also a major *disadvantage* when an agent clearly affects different cell types simultaneously. Thus, for example, kidney epithelial cells may provide interesting evidence on the accumulation of contrast agents in that type of cell (e.g., Andersen et al. 1994) but the nephropathy which is induced by high doses of contrast agents is multifactorial, and involves inter alia changes in renal blood flow, production of agents such as endothelin, reduction of glomerular filtration, and renal ischemia (Idée and Bonnemain 1996; Bagnis et al. 1997). The interplay of such factors can only be studied in isolated kidney or in vivo models. Similar considerations apply with other target tissues such as heart or vasculature.

Several cell or tissue culture methods have been developed to test the toxicity of contrast agents. Because contrast agents are frequently injected intravascularly, cultured endothelial cells are especially popular (e.g., Laerum 1987; Grabowski 1989; Morgan and Bettmann 1989), although it can be shown that endothelial cells from different vascular beds have important differences in their responses to contrast medium exposure. Hepatocytes (Nordby et al. 1987), chick myocytes (Kohmoto et al. 1992), and renal epithelial cells (Andersen et al. 1995; Idée and Bonnemain 1996; Haller et al. 1997) have also been used. Cochran et al. (1996) have used human lymphocytes to assess the role of free radicals in contrast agent toxicity.

4.7 Hematological Testing

As contrast agents generally are injected intravascularly, their effects on the blood should be minimal. Basic hematological testing therefore forms a vital part of a preclinical safety pharmacology profile (see Table 4.3). Contrast media are known to influence the coagulation system, the fibrinolytic system, the kinin system, and the complement system. In addition they alter blood rheology (Smedby 1992) and red blood cell morphology (Hardeman et al. 1991), affect platelets and the endothelium (Stormorken and Sakariassen 1995), and interact with leukocytes (Rasmussen and Georgsen 1989).

Hoffmeister and Heller (1996) and Krause and Press (1997) have recently reviewed the effects of contrast agents on blood coagulation and the complement system. Selected methods are cited in Table 4.1. The formation of platelet thrombi in rat arterioles in vivo has been described by Corot et al. 1994.

Contrast agents have many effects on erythrocytes. Effects on aggregation of human blood have recently been described (Chai et al. 1995). The effects of contrast agents on red blood cell membrane elasticity, and thus possible effects on microcirculation, have been measured and reviewed by Bucherer et al. (1994).

Rasmussen et al. (1992) have described how contrast agents affect leukocyte chemotaxis and phagocytosis; Roobottom et al. (1994) describe effects on leukocyte motility.

4.8 Hypersensitivity and Idiosyncratic Reactions

Iodinated contrast media induce mild allergic/pseudoallergic reactions in ca. 30% of patients, and potentially life-threatening reactions in ca. 0.1% (Ennis et al. 1991). Controlled studies have shown that patients with a history of allergy or asthma are especially susceptible to allergic-type reactions to contrast agents (e.g., Simon 1995). However, investigators have failed to detect specific antibodies in patients who have suffered a reaction, and have failed to induce hypersensitivity reactions in experimental animals (RASMUSSEN and GEORGSEN 1989). This suggests that the agents act as haptens, i.e., combine with some host protein, and only then induce a reaction (see KRAUSE et al. 1995). MIYAUCHI et al. (1996) have demonstrated that contrast agents can have an adjuvant effect for IgE and IgGl.

There have been many investigations of histamine release by contrast agents, either in vitro using mast cells or basophils (ENNIS et al. 1989; BAXTER et al. 1993), or in vivo (ENNIS et al. 1991) measuring plasma histamine levels (see Table 4.1). Although most agents can be shown to release histamine in vitro, the concentrations required are higher than would be expected to occur in routine clinical use (BAXTER et al. 1993). Because of the species differences in histamine release profile, it may be useful in early testing to measure histamine release in vitro in blood from animals or human volunteers (FARAJ and MARTIN 1990). However, the adverse reactions to contrast media seen in the clinical situation cannot be explained by histamine release alone.

Other mediators involved in allergic reactions are the compounds derived from arachadonic acid, the prostaglandins, thromboxane, and the leukotrienes. Contrast agents seem to have little effect on the production of these mediators (e.g., ROMANO et al. 1991). Several other approaches have been taken towards trying to predict the likelihood that a new compound could cause idiosyncratic reactions. Effects on complement or the complement cascade have been suggested to be involved in severe reactions to contrast agents (LANG et al. 1976), but a short review in KRAUSE and NIEHUES (1996) suggests that data measured in vitro has no relationship with the incidence of side-effects. Lasser's group has investigated contrast agent effects on production of several other vasoactive compounds, including bradykinin and nitric oxide (LASSER et al. 1996). Despite all these attempts to understand the idiosyncratic reactions it has not been possible to find a single good test to predict and explain what is going to happen when a new contrast agent is introduced to general clinical use.

4.9 Pharmacokinetics

The experimental pharmacokinetics of an iodinated contrast agent is normally much simpler than that of most drugs. When the compound is injected into the body, it relatively quickly distributes in the extracellular water, is metabolized to an insignificant extent (e.g., DENCAUSSE et al. 1996), and more than 98% is excreted within 24h, almost exclusively by glomerular filtration (GOLMAN 1979; LUNDQUIST and LEANDER 1991; FRENBY et al. 1996), with no tubular reabsorption. In addition the analytical methods for contrast agents (e.g., HPLC or x-ray fluorescence spectrometry) are usually uncomplicated (GRÖNBERG 1981; SKINNEMOEN et al. 1987a; JACOBSEN et al. 1995). The tests normally carried out include standard pharmacokinetic tests on rats and monkeys, measuring metabolism, elimination half-life, clearance, volume of distribution, organ distribution after 24h and 7 days, and excretion in urine, bile, and feces. Details of methods can be found in AULIE MICHELET and SKINNEMOEN (1987), KRAUSE (1994), HEGLUND et al. (1995), and DENCAUSSE et al. (1996).

A new technique of dynamic computer tomography processed by factor analysis allows detailed selective examination of renal pharmacokinetics of contrast agents, including quantification of the osmotic diuretic effect (LESNIK et al. 1996).

Because of the known risks of contrast agents in patients with preexisting renal failure, pharmacokinetic tests on animals with reduced renal capacity should be done (e.g., WALDAY et al. 1995). Finally, whole-body autoradiography studies of the distribution of radioactively labelled compound will show any unsuspected target organs and confirm absence of blood-brain barrier permeability (e.g., BOURRINET et al. 1994).

4.10 Conclusions

This review has tried to describe the main preclinical testing which should be performed to provide evidence that a potential x-ray contrast agent will be safe for use in man. We have described supplementary tests which can be used to predict that the agent will have a low incidence of specific adverse events such as nephropathy, and whether the agent is suitable for use in specific indications, e.g., urography, myelography, and coronary intervention.

We have given only an outline of the hierarchical order in which these different tests should be performed, partly because individual laboratories will have different priorities, depending on the chemistry of the agents under development and their potential applications, and also because many of the tests judged necessary can be carried out in parallel, thus decreasing the development time, and allowing a fast "time to market."

References

Adams MD, Hopkins RM, Ferrendelli JA (1988) A rat EEG model for evaluating contrast media neurotoxicity. Invest Radiol 23 (Suppl 1):S217–S219

Aguejouf O, Doutremepuich F, Azougagh-Oualane F, Doutremepuich C (1995) Thrombogenicity of ionic and nonionic contrast media tested in a laser induced rat thrombosis model. Thromb Res 77:259–269

Akagi M, Masaki S, Kitazumi K, Mio M, Tasaka K (1991) Comparative study of the adverse effects of various radiographic contrast media including ioversol a new low-osmolarity medium. II. The complement system and endothelial cells. Meth Find Exp Clin Pharmacol 13:449–454

Alguacil LF, Gonzalez C, Bohle F, Jimenez I, Alamo C, Martin JL (1994) Contrast media algogenic potential in peripheral arteriography: potentiation of bradykinin-induced pain in the rat. Invest Radiol 29:294–300

Almén T (1995) Visipaque: a step forward. A historical review. Acta Radiol Suppl 399:2–18

Andersen KJ, Christensen EI, Vik H (1994) Effects of iodinated X-ray contrast media on renal epithelial cells in culture. Invest Radiol 11:955–962

Andersen KJ, Vik H, Eikesdal HP, Christensen EI (1995) Effects of contrast media on renal epithelial cells in culture. Acta Radiol Suppl 399:213–218

Andes WA (1988) Effects of contrast media on fibrinogen and factor VIII. Invest Radiol 23 (Suppl 2):346–350

Arakawa K, Suzuki H, Naitoh A, Hatashi K, Matsuda H, Ichihara A, Kubota E, Saruta T (1996) Role of adenosine in the renal responses to contrast medium. Kidney Int 49:1199–1206

Aulie Michelet Å, Salvesen S, Renaa T (1987) Acute toxicity of iopentol in rodents. Acta Radiol Suppl 370:41–44

Aulie Michelet Å, Skinnemoen K (1987) Pharmacokinetics of iopentol in the rat. Acta Radiol Suppl 370:101–104

Bååth L, Almén T (1989) Reducing the risk of ventricular fibrillation by adding sodium to ionic and nonionic contrast media with low iodine concentration. Acta Radiol 30:207–212

Bååth L, Besjakov J, Pettersson G (1994) Effects of nonionic and dimeric contrast media on the twitching reaction of the rat. Invest Radiol 29:985–989

Bagnis C, Idee JM, Dubois M, Jacquiaud C, Maister G, Jacobs C, Deray G (1997) Role of endothelium derived nitric oxide-endothelin balance in contrast medium-induced acute renal vasoconstriction in dogs. Acad Radiol 4:343–348

Baxter AB, Lazarus SC, Brasch RC (1993) In vitro histamine release induced by magnetic resonance imaging and iodinated contrast media. Invest Radiol 28:308–312

Belleville J, Baguet J, Paul J, Glendinnen G, Elroy R (1985) In vitro study of the inhibition of coagulation induced by different radiocontrast molecules. Thromb Res 38:149–162

Benyon HLC, Walport MJ, Dawson P (1994) Vascular endothelial injury by intravascular contrast agents. Invest Radiol 29(Suppl 2):S195–S197

Besjakov J, Chai C-M, Bååth L, Almén T (1994) Comparison between oxygenated iohexol solution enriched with electrolytes and other low-osmotic contrast media. Electrophysiologic and haemodynamic effects during perfusion of the left coronary artery in the pig. Invest Radiol 29:S238–S241

Bhargava AS, Hofmeister R, Siegmund F, Schobel C, Gunzel P (1990) Effect of three non-ionic contrast media on rats and rabbits with regard to renal changes. Interspecies comparison. Arzneimittelforsch 40:822–829

Blake MP, Halasz SJ (1995) The effects of X-ray contrast media on bacterial growth. Australas Radiol 39:10–13

Blankson H, Holten T, Öksendal AN, Jynge P (1995) Changes in contractile function with low-osmolal and isoosmolal contrast media for coronary angiography. Acta Radiol Suppl 399:135–141

Bourrinet P, Dencausse A, Cochet P, Bromet-Petit M, Chambon C (1994) Whole body quantitative autoradiographic study of the biodistribution of iobitridol in rats. Invest Radiol 29:1057–1060

Brezis M, Greenfeld Z, Herman M, Meyer JJ, Heyman SN, Rosen S (1991) Experimental nephrotoxicity of the radiocontrast agents iohexol, ioxaglate and iothalamate. An in vitro and in vivo study. Invest Radiol 26:325–331

Bryan RN, Centeno RS, Hershkowitz N, Poelstra RJ, Osato MS (1982) Neurotoxicity of iohexol: a new nonionic contrast medium. Radiology 145:379–382

Bucherer C, Lacombe C, Lelievre J-C (1994) Effects of two low-osmolar contrast media, ioxaglate and iopamidol, on erythrocyte membrane elasticity. Invest Radiol 12:1026–1030

Canillot C, Etienne J, Borson F, Guidollet J, Amiel M, Louisot P (1983) Iodinated contrast agents. Effect on ATP:creatinine *N*-phosphotransferase isoenzymes in arterial wall. Invest Radiol 18:81–86

Chai C-M, Almén T, Aspelin P, Bååth L (1995) Effects on erythrocyte aggregation and blood coagulation from iohexol solutions with and without sodium chloride. Acta Radiol 36:204–209

Chronos NAF, Goodall AH, Wilson DJ, Sigwart U, Buller NP (1993) Profound platelet degranulation is an important side effect of some types of contrast media used in interventional cardiology. Circulation 88:2035–2044

Cipolla P, Castano M, Kirchin MA, de Haen C, Torine P (1995) Effects of iodinated contrast media on pulmonary airway resistance in anaesthetised guinea-pigs. Acad Radiol 2:306–312

Cochran ST, Lin V, Norman A (1996) Mechanism for contrast media toxicity. Acad Radiol 3:S207–S209

Corot C, Stucker O, Duverger J-P, Pons C, Vicaut E (1994) Effects of iodinated contrast agents on the formation of platelet thrombi in rat arterioles. Invest Radiol 29 (Suppl 2):S203–S205

Corot C, Chronos N, Sabattier V (1996) In vitro comparison of the effects of contrast media on coagulation and platelet activation. Blood Coagul Fibrinolysis 7:602–608

Dascalu A, Peer A (1994) Effects of radiologic contrast media on human endothelial and kidney cell lines: intracellular pH and cytotoxicity. Acad Radiol 1:145–150

Dencausse A, Violas X, Feldman H, Havard P, Chambon C (1996) Pharmacokinetic profile of iobitridol. Acta Radiol Suppl 400:25–34

Dobrota M, Powell CJ, Holtz E, Wallin A, Vik H (1995) Biochemical and morphological effects of contrast media on the kidney. Acta Radiol Suppl 399:196–203

Donadieu AM, Idée JM, Doucet D, et al. (1996) Toxicological profile of iobitridol a new nonionic low-osmolality contrast medium. Acta Radiol Suppl 400:17–24

Drescher P, Rauch D, Knes JM, Madsen PO (1995) Contrast medium-induced renal vasoconstriction, role of alpha receptors. Scand J Urol Nephrol Suppl 172:103–108

Eaton S, Tsay HM, Yost F, Tweedle MF (1990) Assays for plasma complement activation by X-ray contrast media Invest Radiol 25:789–792

Eivindvik K, Sjögren CE (1995) Physiochemical properties of iodixanol. Acta Radiol Suppl 399:32–38

Ekholm SE, Morris TW, Fonte D, Simon J, Marinetti GV, Leakey P, Prentice L (1989) Effects of contrast media on neural tissue glucose uptake in vitro: Invest Radiol 24:145–149

Elam EA, Dorr RT, Lagel KE, Pond GD (1991) Cutaneous ulceration due to contrast extravasation. Invest Radiol 26:13-16

Eliashiv S, Wirguin I, Brenner T, Argov Z (1990) Aggravation of human and experimental myasthenia gravis by contrast media. Neurology 40:1623–1625

Ennis M, Amon EU, Lorenz W (1989) Histamine release from canine and liver mast cells induced by radiographic contrast media. Agents Actions 27:101–103

Ennis M, Lorenz W, Nehring E, Schneider C (1991) In vitro and in vivo studies of radiographic contrast media-induced histamine release in pigs. Agents Actions 33:26–29

Faraj BA, Martin LG (1990) A simplified radioenzymatic method for the study of whole blood histamine release in patients receiving radiographic contrast media. Invest Radiol 25:1228–1231

FDA (1996) Guidance for industry: single dose acute toxicity testing for pharmaceuticals, FDA Center for Drug evaluation and Research, Federal Register 61 FR 43934, 26 Aug 1996

Fillette F, Nassif G, Aouate P (1988) Etude par microélectrodes intracellulaires des effets électrophysiologiques des produits de contraste. Arch Mal Coeur 81:801–807

Fischer HW, Morris TW (1980) Cardiovascular radiology. Possible factors in intravascular contrast media toxicity. Invest Radiol 15(Suppl 6):S232–S238

Frenby B, Sterner G, Almén T, Chai C-M, Jönsson B, Månsson S (1996) Extrarenal plasma clearance of iohexol, chromium-51 ethylenediaminetetraacetic acid, and inulin in anephric pigs. Acad Radiol 3:145–153

Georgesen J, Rasmussen F, Pedersen JO (1990) Granulocyte chemotaxis: influence of radiographic contrast media on the chemoattractive properties of serum. Acta Radiol 31:531–536

Golman K (1979) Experimental urography. Thesis, University of Oslo

Golman K, Almén T (1984) Urographic contrast media and methods of investigative uroradiography. In: Sovak M (ed) Radiocontrast agents. Springer, Berlin Heidelberg New York, pp 127–191

Gomi N (1992) Vasoconstriction by angiographic contrast media in isolated canine arteries. Br J Radiol 65:961–967

Goosens A, Elst LV, Haverbeke YV, Muller RN (1995) Mechanical and biochemical cardiac disturbances induced by bolus administration of iodinated contrast media and noniodinated solutions. Invest Radiol 30:1–9

Grabowski EF (1989) Effects of contrast media on endothelial cell monolayers under controlled flow conditions. In: Enge I, Edgren J (eds) Patient safety and adverse events in contrast medium examinations. Excerpta Medica, Amsterdam, pp 85–95

Grabowski EF, Rodriguez M, McDonnel SL (1993) Platelet adhesion/aggregation in an in vitro model of coronary artery stenosis. Cathet Cardiovasc Diagn 28:65–71

Grönberg T (1981) In vivo X-ray fluorescence analysis for medical diagnosis. Doctoral Thesis, Lund University

Haller C, Schick CS, Zorn M, Kubler W (1997) Cytotoxicity of radiocontrast agents on polarised renal epithelial cell monolayers. Cardiovasc Res 33:655–665

Hardeman MR, Goedhart PT, Koen Y (1991) The effect of low osmolar ionic and nonionic contrast media on human blood viscosity, erythrocyte morphology and aggregation behaviour. Invest Radiol 26:810–819

Harnish PP, Distefano V (1985) Pharmacological action of radiographic contrast media reduced cerebrospinal fluid production in the dog. J Pharmacol Exp Ther 232:88–93

Harnish PP, Northington FK, Distefano V, Banerjee S (1986) Mechanism of decreased cerebrospinal fluid production by radiographic contrast media: role of adenyl cyclase activation. J Pharmacol Exp Ther 236:464–469

Hay KL, Bull BS (1995) An analysis of platelet activation and aggregation produced by three classes of contrast media. J Vasc Intervent Radiol 6:211–217

Hayakawa K, Okuno Y, Fujiwara K, Shimizu Y (1994) Effect of iodinated contrast media on ionic calcium. Acta Radiol 35: 83–87

Hayashi H, Kumazaki T, Asano G (1994) Pulmonary edema induced by intravenous administration of contrast media: experimental study in rats. Radiat Med 12:47–52

Heglund IF, Michelet ÅA, Blazak WF, Furuhama K, Holtz E (1995) Preclinical pharmacokinetics and general toxicology of iodixanol. Acta Radiol Suppl 399:69–82

Heyman SN, Clark BA, Kaiser N, Spokes K, Rosen S, Brezis M, Epstein FH (1992) Radiocontrast agents induce endothelin release in vivo and in vitro. J Am Soc Nephrol 3:58–65

Heywood R, Matfield R, Allan JA, Aulie Michelet Å (1987) Summary of the toxicologic profile of iopentol. Acta Radiol Suppl 370:45–48

Hill JA, Winniford M, Cohen MB, et al. (1993) Multicenter trial of ionic versus nonionic contrast media for cardiac angiography. The Iohexol Cooperative Study. Am J Cardiol 72:770–775

Hoffmeister HM, Heller W (1996) Radiographic contrast media and the coagulation and complement systems. Invest Radiol 31:591–595

Hoffmeister HM, Fuhrer G, Pirschel J, Heller W (1988) Veränderungen des Kallikrein-Kinin- und des Komplement-Systems bei Angiographien mit nichtionischen Kontrastmitteln. Klin Wochenschr 66:760–763

Hogstrom B, Rooth P, Sunnegardh O, Hietala SO (1993) In vivo fluorescence microscopy of microcirculation in the renal cortex of mice. V. Effects of mannitol and iohexol infusions in normal, obese/hyperglycemic and diabetic mice. Acta Radiol 35:176–181

Holtz E, Golman K (1987) Experimental urography with new nonionic dimeric and monomeric contrast agents. Acta Radiol Suppl 370:49–56

Holtz E, Michelet ÅA, Jacobsen T (1983) Absorption after subarachnoid and subdural administration of iohexol, ^{51}Cr-EDTA, and ^{121}I-albumin to rabbits. AJNR Am J Neuroradiol 4:338–341

Howell MJ, Dawson P (1985) Contrast agents and enzyme inhibition II. Mechanisms. Br J Radiol 58:845–848

Idée JM, Bonnemain B (1996) Reliability of experimental models of iodinated contrast media-induced acute renal failure. Invest Radiol 31:230–241

Idée JM, Beaufils H, Bonnemain B (1994) Iodinated contrast media-induced nephropathy: pathophysiology, clinical aspects and prevention. Fundam Clin Pharmacol 8:193–206

Idée JM, Balut C, Beaufils H, et al. (1996) Pharmacologic profile of iobitridol, a nonionic iodinated contrast medium. Acta Radiol Suppl 400:35–48

Imai H, Himura H, Kumazaki T, Uyesaka N (1993) Effect of low-osmolality contrast media on red cell filterability. Acta Radiol 34:214–219

Jacobsen PB, Blindheim L, Skotland T (1995) Bioanalytical methods for iodixanol and their application to studies on metabolism and protein binding. Acta Radiol Suppl 399:61–66

Jansen I, Golman K, Edvinsson L (1987) Mechanisms of action of contrast media on cranial vessels. Comparison of diatrizoate, ioxaglate, iohexol, mannitol and NaCl on rabbit basilar and ear arteries. Invest Radiol 22:814–821

Jynge P, Blankson H, Falck G, Refsum H, Karlsson JOG, Almén T, Öksendal AN (1995) Sodium-calcium relationships and cardiac function during coronary bolus perfusion. Acta Radiol 36:Suppl 399, 122–134

Karlsson JOG, Gregersen M, Refsum H (1995) Visipaque is isotonic to human and rat blood plasma. Acta Radiol Suppl 399:39–42

Karstoft J, Bååth L (1995) Vasodilative and vasoconstrictive effects of angiographic contrast media. Acta Radiol Suppl 399:164–172

Katayama H, Yamaguchi K, Kozuka T, Takashima T, Seez P, Matsuura K (1990) Adverse reactions to ionic and nonionic contrast media. A report from the Japanese Committee on the Safety of Contrast Media. Radiology 175:621–628

Katzberg RW, Morris TW, Schulman G, et al. (1983) Reactions to intravenous contrast media. 1. Severe and fatal cardiovascular reactions in a canine dehydration model. Radiology 147:327–330

Kim SH, Park JH, Kim YI, Kim C-W, Han MC (1990) Experimental tissue damage after subcutaneous injection of water soluble contrast media. Invest Radiol 25:678–685

Kim SH, Lee HK, Han MC (1992) Incompatibility of water-soluble contrast media and intravascular pharmacologic agents: an in vitro study. Invest Radiol 27:45–49

Kinter LB, Dixon LW (1995) Safety pharmacology program for pharmaceuticals. Drug Dev Res 35:179–182

Klopp R, Niemer W, Schippel W, Krause W (1995) Changes in the microcirculation of the intact heart after iodinated and gadolinium-containing contrast media. Invest Radiol 30:69–74

Klöw NE, Jacobsen EA, Refsum H (1995) Cardioangiographic and haemodynamic effects of iodixanol. Acta Radiol Suppl 399:93–99

Kohmoto O, Matsui H, Momura S, Serizawa T, Sugimoto T, Iizuka M (1992) Effects of new intravascular contrast agents on $(Ca^{2+})_i$ transients and contraction in cultured ventricular myocytes. Heart Vessels 7:42–51

Krause W (1994) Preclinical characterisation of iopromide. Invest Radiol 29 (Suppl 1):S21–S32

Krause W, Niehues D (1996) Biochemical characterisation of X-ray contrast media. Invest Radiol 31:30–42

Krause W, Press W-R (1997) Influence of contrast media on blood coagulation. Invest Radiol 32:249–259

Krause W, Kloop R, Niemer W, Schippel W, Kulmann H (1994a) Elimination of the diatrizoate-induced effects of the microcirculation by the prostacyclin derivative iloprost. Invest Radiol 29:922–927

Krause W, Miklautz H, Kollenkirchen U, Heimann G (1994b) Physiochemical parameters of X-ray contrast media. Invest Radiol 29:72–80

Krause W, Bunte T, Schubert R, Blaszkiewicz P (1995) Lack of immunogenicity of iotrolan. Invest Radiol 30:548–551

Laerum F (1987) Cytotoxic effects of six angiographic contrast media on human endothelium in culture. Acta Radiol 28:99–105

La Noce A, Danielli A, Bertani F, Tirone P, de Haen C (1996a) Conditioned taste aversion in rats following intrathecal administration of contrast media. Acta Radiol 37:116–120

La Noce A, Lorenzon Pugiliese F, Pellechi G, Orlandini I, Tirone P (1996b) Brain penetration of intrathecal iomeprol in dogs. Acta Radiol 37:578–581

Lang JH, Lasser EC, Kolb WP (1976) Activation of serum complement by contrast media. Invest Radiol 11:303–308

Larsen LE, Grant D, Walday P (1995) Tissue reaction following intratracheal application of roentgen contrast media in rats. Acta Radiol Suppl 399:258–261

Lasser EC, Lyon SG (1990) Inhibition of angiotensin-converting enzyme by contrast media. 1. In vitro findings. Invest Radiol 25:698–702

Lasser EC, Lamkin GE, Lyon S (1996) Nitric oxide and toxicity of contrast material. Acad Radiol 3:S204–S206

Latchaw RE (1993) The use of nonionic contrast agents in neuroangiography: a review of the literature and recommendations for clinical use. Invest Radiol 28 Suppl 5:S55–S59

Laude EA, Godfrey IC, Emery CJ, Morcos SK (1996) Ventilatory effects of contrast media. Radiology Abst 1205 p 350

Laurie AJ, Lyon SG, Lasser EC (1991) The effects of contrast media on coagulation factor XII. Invest Radiol 26 (Suppl):S23–S25

LeMignon MM, Ducret MN, Bonnemain B, Donadieu AM (1988) Effect of contrast media on whole blood filterability. An in vitro study of iohexol, iopamidol and ioxaglate on rat blood. Acta Radiol 29:593–597

Lesnik A, Chabriais J, Benali H, Guinebretiere J-M, DiPaola R, Moreau J-F (1996) Early renal transit of an iodinated contrast medium: factor analytic dynamic computed tomography scanning studies in rabbits. Acad Radiol 3:S248–S250

Levi M, Biemond BJ, Sturk A, Koek J, ten Cate JW (1991) Variable effects of radiological contrast media on thrombus growth in a rabbit jugular vein thrombosis model. Thromb Haemost 66:218–221

Lundquist S, Leander P (1991) The extrarenal clearance of water-soluble iodinated contrast media: an experimental study in rabbits. Invest Radiol 26:75–79

Maly P, Sundgren P, Bååth L, Walday P (1995) Neural tolerance of the nonionic dimers iodixanol and iotrolan and the nonionic monomer iopamidol during myelography in nonanaesthetised rabbits. Acta Radiol 36:644–648

Mare K, Violante M, Zack A (1984) Contrast media induced pulmonary oedema: comparison of ionic and nonionic agents in an animal model. Invest Radiol 19:566–569

Margulies KB, McKinley LJ, Cavero PG, Burnet JC Jr (1990) Induction and prevention of radiocontrast-induced nephropathy in dogs with heart failure. Kidney Int 38:1101–1108

Melton LG, Muga KM, Gabriel DA (1996) Effects of iodixanol on in vitro bleeding time. Acad Radiol 3:407–411

Mennini T, Bernasconi P, Fiori MG (1993) Neurotoxicity of nonionic low-osmolar contrast media: a receptor binding study. Invest Radiol 28:821–827

Messana JM, Cieslinski DA, Nguyen VD, Humes HD (1988) Comparison of the toxicity of the radiocontrast agents iopamidol and diatrizoate to renal proximal tubule cells in vitro. J Pharm Exp Ther 244:1139–1144

Miyauchi T, Hirano T, Ushiyama C, Ovary Z, Okumura K, Katayama H (1996) Anaphylactic IgE and IgG1 production for hapten can be enhanced by contrast media. Br J Radiol 69:920–924

Morcos SK, Brown PWG Oldroyd S, El Nahas AM, Haylor J (1995) Relationship between the diuretic effect of radiocontrast media and their ability to increase renal vascular resistance. Br J Radiol 68:850–853

Morcos SK, Oldroyd S, Haylor J (1997) Effect of radiographic contrast media on endothelium derived nitric oxide-dependent renal vasodilatation. Br J Radiol 70:154–159

Morettin LB, Zhan X, Sant'ambrogio FB, Sant'ambrogio G (1994) Cardiorespiratory responses elicited by right atrial injections of iodinated contrast media. Invest Radiol 29:201–209

Morgan DML, Bettmann MA (1989) Effects of X-ray contrast media and radiation on human vascular endothelial cells in vitro. Cardiovasc Intervent Radiol 12:154–160

Morris TW (1988) Ventricular fibrillation during right coronary arteriography with ioxaglate, iohexol and iopamidol in dogs. Invest Radiol 23:205–208

Morris TW, Fischer HW (1986) The pharmacology of intravascular radiocontrast agents. Ann Rev Pharmacol Toxicol 26:143–160

Morris TW, Ekholm SE, Simon JH, Marinetti GV, Harnish PP, Isaac L, Fonte D, Leakey P (1988) In vitro models for testing the metabolic effects of myelographic contrast media. Invest Radiol 23(Suppl 1):S213–S216

Murdock DK, Piao ZE, Euler DE, Murdock JD, Hwang MH, Loeb HS, Scanlon PJ (1985) The use of programmed electrical stimulation to assess the fibrillatory propensity of ionic and nonionic contrast media. Invest Radiol 20:579–582

Nordby A, Hagunset J, Thostensen K, Haugen OA (1987) Short-term effects of radiographic contrast media on monolayer cell cultures and hepatocytes. Invest Radiol 22:603–607

Nordby A, Tvedt KE, Halgunset J, Kopstad G, Haugen OA (1989) Incorporation of contrast media in cultured cells. Invest Radiol 24:703–710

Nygren A, Hellberg O, Hansell P (1993) Red cell trapping in the rat renal microcirculation induced by low-osmolar contrast media and mannitol. Invest Radiol 28:1033–1038

Oldroyd S, Haylor J, Morcos SK (1995) The acute effect of ioversol on kidney function. Eur J Radiol 19:91–95

Paajanen H, Uotila P (1985) Effect of contrast media on the formation of prostacyclin in isolated rat lungs. Acta Radiol 26:777–783

Parvez Z, Vik H (1994) Intravascular contrast media and thrombin generation. Acta Radiol 35:172–175

Parvez Z, Kormano M, Moncada R, Eklund R (1986) Contrast media-induced chromosomal damage in human lymphocyte cultures. Invest Radiol 21:864–869

Pedersen HK, Jacobsen EA, Refsum H, Klöw NE (1994) Cardiac effects of coronary angiography with electrolyte addition to iohexol: a study in dogs with and without heart failure. Acta Radiol 35:77–82

Prange T, Gauey F, Ohanessien J, Avenel D, Neuman A, Corot C, Meyer D (1995) Angiography contrast agents interact with serine proteases. The molecular structure of the model system elastase/iohexol. FEBS Lett 357:247–250

Pugh ND, Karlsson JOG (1997) Vasodilator and haemorheological effects of iodinated contrast media. Drugs of Today 33:1–11

Rasmussen F, Georgsen J (1989) The influence of contrast media on leucocytes. In: Enge I, Edgren J (eds) Patient safety and adverse events in contrast medium examinations. Elsevier, Amsterdam, pp 63–71

Rasmussen F, Antonsen S, Georgsen J, Christensen JK (1992) Radiographic contrast media and release of neutrophil specific proteins in vitro and after intravenous injection. Acta Radiol 33:495–499

Rees CR, Palmaz JC, Garcia O, Alvarado R, Siegle RL (1988) The hemodynamic effects of the administration of ionic and nonionic contrast materials into the pulmonary arteries of a canine model of acute pulmonary hypertension. Invest Radiol 23:184–189

Riemann CD, Massey CV, McCarron DL, Borkowski P, Johnson PC, Ziskind AA (1993) Ionic contrast agent-mediated endothelial injury causes increased platelet deposition to vascular surfaces. Am Heart J 125:71–78

Romano M, DiBello M, Salmona M, Piovani B, Rosati G (1991) Effect of iodinated contrast media on the synthesis and metabolism of leukotriene B_4. Invest Radiol 26:348–352

Roobottom CA, Farrow R, Wells IP, Hurlock-Fimls N (1994) The effect of radiographic contrast media on leukocyte motility. Invest Radiol 29:65–67

Sandborg M, Christoffersson JO, Alm-Carlsson G, Almén T, Dance DR (1995) The physical performance of different X-ray contrast agents: calculations using a Monte Carlo model of the imaging chain. Phys Med Biol 40:1209–1224

Schmidt J, Hotz HG, Foitzik T, Ryschich E, Buhr HJ, Warshaw AL, Herfarth C, Klar E (1995) Intravenous contrast medium aggravates the impairment of pancreatic microcirculation in necrotising pancreatitis in the rat. Ann Surg 221:257–264

Schwartz D, Blum M, Peer G, et al. (1994) Role of nitric oxide (EDRF) in radiocontrast acute renal failure in rats. Am J Physiol 267:F374–F379

Sheu SH, Hwang MH, Piao ZE, Hariman RJ, Loeb HS, Scanlon PJ (1991) Effects of intracoronary administration of contrast media on coronary hemodynamics in a canine post-ischemic reperfusion model. Cathet Cardiovasc Diagn 23:144–149

Siefert HM, Press WR, Speck U (1980) Tolerance to iohexol after intracisternal, intracerebral and intraarterial injection in the rat. Acta Radiol Suppl 362:77–81

Siegle RL (1993) Rates of idiosyncratic reactions. Ionic versus nonionic contrast media. Invest Radiol 28(Suppl 5):S95–S98

Siegle RL, McGuire WL, Peters JE (1988) Development of polyclonal and monoclonal antibodies to iodinated contrast media. Acta Radiol 29:737–740

Simon MR (1995) Allergic-type adverse reactions to low osmolarity contrast media in patients with a history of allergy or asthma. Invest Radiol 30:285–290

Skarstein S, Dunkel JA, Refsum H (1997) Selective coronary artery perfusion in vitro: a method to study cardiac effects of contrast media. Acad Radiol 4:483–491

Skinnemoen K (1987) Physiochemical properties and degree of protein binding of iopentol. Acta Radiol Suppl 370:33–35

Skinnemoen K, Fagervoll R, Jacobsen T (1987a) Determination of iopentol and other nonionic contrast agents in biological fluids by high-performance liquid chromatography. Acta Radiol Suppl 370:23–25

Skinnemoen K, Fagervoll R, Aanstad L, Jacobsen T (1987b) Formulation and stability of iopentol. Acta Radiol Suppl 370:37–40

Smedby Ö (1992) Viscosity of some contemporary contrast media before and after mixing with whole blood. Acta Radiol 33:600–605

Sorensen L, Sunnegardh O, Svanegard J, Lundquist, Hietala SO (1994) Systemic and pulmonary haemodynamic effects of intravenous infusion of nonionic isoosmolar dimeric contrast media. An investigation in the pig of two ratio 6 contrast media Acta Radiol 35:383–390

Sovak M (1994) (ed) Radiocontrast agents. Springer, Berlin Heidelberg New York

Sovak M, Halkovich CA, Foster SJ (1988) Current contrast media and ioxilan: comparative evaluation of vascular pain by aversion conditioning. Invest Radiol 23 (Suppl 1):S84–S87

Speck U (1994) Principles and aims of preclinical testing Invest Radiol 29(Suppl 1):S15–S20

Speck U, Siefert HM, Klink G (1980) Contrast media and pain in peripheral arteriography Invest Radiol 15(Suppl 6):S335–S339

Steidle B (1989) Iodine-induced hyperthyroidism after contrast media: animal experimental and clinical studies. Fortschr Geb Röntgenstr Nuklearmed Ergänzungsbd 128:6–14

Stormorken H (1989) Biocompatibility of contrast media as evaluated by their effects on the thrombotic and haemostatic mechanisms. In: Enge I, Edgren J (eds) Patient safety and adverse events in contrast medium examinations. Elsevier, Amsterdam, pp 73–77

Stormorken H, Sakariassen KS (1995) Contrast media effects on hemostatic and thrombotic parameters. Acta Radiol Suppl 399:173–181

Stormorken H, Testart MC, Braeke G, Sveen K, Jakobsen JÅ, Grande T, Andrew E (1987) Effect of iopentol on coagulation and platelet function in vitro and in vivo. Acta Radiol Suppl 370:93–96

Sundgren P, Bååth L, Maly P (1995) CNS effects from subarachnoid injections of iohexol and the nonionic dimers iodixanol and iotrolan in the rabbit. Acta Radiol 36:307–311

Swanson DP, Thrall HJ, Shetty PC (1986) Evaluation of intravascular low-osmolality contrast agents. Clin Pharm 5:877–891

Tande PM, Klöw NE, Refsum H (1989) Electromechanical effects of two low osmolality contrast media ioxaglate and iohexol on isolated rabbit and rat atria. Pharmacol Toxicol 65:307–311

Tervahartiala P, Kivisaari L, Kivisaari R, Virtanen I, Standertskjöld-Nordernstam C-G (1991) Contrast media-induced renal tubular vacuolisation. Invest Radiol 26:882–887

Tervahartiala P, Kivisaari L, Kivisaari R, Virtanen I (1993) Contrast media-induced renal morphologic lesions in diabetic rats. Acta Radiol 34:220–225

Thomsen HS, Golman K, Svendsen O (1991) Muscle toxicity of diatrizoate and iohexol in rabbits. A model for local tissue damage. Acta Radiol 32:182–183

Thomsen HS, Golman K, Hemmingsen L, Larsen S, Skaarup P, Svendsen O (1993) Contrast medium-induced nephropathy: animal experiments. Front Eur Radiol 9:83–108

Trägårdh B, Almén T, Lynch P (1975) Addition of calcium and other cations to ionic and nonionic contrast media. Invest Radiol 10:231–241

Ueda J, Nygren A, Hansell P, Erikson U (1992) Influence of contrast media on single nephron glomerular filtration rate in rat kidney. Acta Radiol 33:596–599

Vik H, Fröysa A, Sönstevold A, Toft K, Stahl Skov P, Ege T (1995) Complement activation and histamine release following administration of roentgen contrast media. Acta Radiol Suppl 399:83–89

Walday P, Heglund IF, Golman K, Cornacoff J, Holtz E (1995) Renal effects of iodixanol in animals. Acta Radiol Suppl 399:204–212

Wilson AJ, Guindy M, Evill CA, Sage MR (1991) Muscular reactions to femoral angiography with low osmolality contrast media. Invest Radiol 26:S115–S117

Wisneski JA, Gertz EW, Neese RA, Morris DL (1985) Absence of biochemical toxicity with a nonionic contrast agent (iopamidol). Am Heart J 110:609–617

Yaghmai V, Harapanhalli, RS, Patel YD, Baker SR, Rao DV (1993) Effects of diatrizoate and iopamidol on spermatogenesis. Invest Radiol 28:1160–1164

Yang X, Manninen H, Soimakallio S (1994) Comparison of angiographic opacification of ioxaglate and iodixanol by digital region-of-interest processing technique in an experimental circulation model. Invest Radiol 29:31–34

5 Phase I, II, III, and IV Studies: Good Clinical Practice

I.M. Stilbo

CONTENTS

5.1 Introduction

The development of new medicines, including drugs, for use in radiology has made it possible to diagnose, treat, and prevent a number of previously refractory diseases. Due to the necessary intensification of demands by the health authorities, the time required to develop new drugs has increased. Regulations have come into force regarding both production processes (Good Manufacturing Practice, GMP) and preclinical investigational programs (Good Laboratory Practice, GLP).

Demands on the conduct of clinical trials have also been intensified during recent decades. The aim has been to ensure sufficient quality and quantity of clinical documentation submitted to the regulatory authorities when pharmaceutical companies apply for marketing authorization of medicinal products. In this field a number of international guidelines and national rules have been established. It is necessary for all parties involved in the performance of clinical trials to be familiar with the present guidelines and rules.

In the EU a series of Notes for Guidance on Clinical Trials provides general guidelines and guidelines for various groups of medicinal products. A clinical trial/study is described as "any investigation in human subjects intended to discover or verify the clinical, pharmacological and/or other pharmacodynamic effects of an investigational product(s), and/or to identify any adverse reactions to the investigational product(s), and/or to study absorption, distribution, metabolism, and excretion of an investigational product(s) with the object of ascertaining its safety and/or efficacy. The terms clinical trial and clinical study are synonymous." (CPMP/ICH/135/95, 1996).

The development of new drugs demands careful planning of every individual trial as a part of the whole drug development plan. Before clinical trials in humans are carried out the results of relevant nonclinical studies (pharmacology, toxicology, pharmacokinetics and metabolism) should be available and form the basis for the studies in humans. Clinical trials in humans are generally classified into phases I–IV (Commission of the European Communities 1990; Ankier and Warrington 1989); however, it is not possible to draw distinct lines between the phases.

5.2 Phase I Studies

Phase I studies are the first trials performed with new chemical entities in humans. The investigational products are often given to a limited number of healthy volunteers in small doses for a short time, with the intention of investigating the pharmacological properties of the product. Any potential risk incurred by participating should be taken into consideration and must be minimal. This is a reason why, occasionally, patients suffering from a disease for which the drug is intended will be included in phase I trials (e.g., in trials of cytostatics).

5.3 Phase II Studies

The next step in the development of the drugs is phase II studies. These are therapeutic pilot studies

I.M. Stilbo, MD, The Danish Medicines Agency, 378, Frederikssundsvej, DK-2700 Brønshøj, Denmark and are normally performed on a limited number of patients suffering from a disease or condition for which the drug is intended. In the early stage the trials are performed without a control group, but at a later stage a comparative trial design may be relevant.

The aim of this phase is mainly to determine an appropriate dose range and regimen, and also, if possible, to estimate the therapeutic effect in comparison with the risk before the development of the drug continues with large-scale studies including many patients.

5.4 Phase III Studies

Phase III studies are performed in selected larger patient groups to determine the therapeutic effects and also the safety profile of the drugs in both short- and long-term trials. It is normally intended to show that the product under investigation is better than or equal to established treatments, if such exist. Comparison either with established drugs or methods of treatment or, if appropriate, placebo control will therefore be necessary. The design of these trials should preferably be randomized and double-blind, and the circumstances of the trials should resemble the normal conditions of use. More specific uses or characteristics of the drugs may also be examined at this phase, e.g., use in the elderly and possible interactions with other drugs.

In the EU the results of phase III studies taken in conjunction with the other clinical and preclinical documentation may lead to marketing authorization of the drugs. Also in the EU an application must be accompanied by an expert report; this has been a demand for a longer period in the United States.

5.5 Phase IV Studies

Phase IV studies on new medicinal products are performed after marketing authorization has been granted. These trials are carried out on the basis of the existing documentation regarding products in order to provide further information on the drugs, e.g., postmarketing surveillance studies, where it will be possible to observe rarer adverse drug reactions which normally will not be identified until use of the drug in question has become more widespread. Supplementary trials to appraise the therapeutic value in comparison with established treatments or possible changes in dosage regimens may also be appropriate.

By chance new indications for use may be observed after a product has been marketed. In such cases it may be necessary to complement the existing preclinical and usually also the clinical documentation from the earlier phases in drug development.

With reference to the aforementioned phases of drug development, some specific considerations with respect to trial design may be particularly applicable in the development of new drugs for use in radiology (e.g., drugs for diagnosis and exclusion of diseases). Comparative trials can often be difficult or impossible to perform using a double-blind design, either because of difficulties in performing placebo-controlled trials or because the active comparator may have an opposite effect on the radiological examination. Therefore the chosen design must be well founded to meet the demands of the authorities.

5.6 Good Clinical Practice

"Good Clinical Practice (GCP) is an international ethical and scientific quality standard for designing, conducting, recording and reporting trials that involve the participation of human subjects. Compliance with this standard provides public assurance that the rights, safety and well-being of trial subjects are protected, consistent with the principles that have their origin in the Declaration of Helsinki, and that the clinical data are credible." (CPMP/ICH/135/95, 1996) (Table 5.1).

"Good Clinical Practice" is a concept similar to GMP and GLP, despite the fact that the name has sometimes resulted in misunderstandings. It refers only to the demands of clinical drug research and not to the usual work of physicians. More descriptive terms such as "Good Clinical Research Practice" and "Good Clinical Trial Practice" have been used, but GCP has continued to be employed in recent international contexts.

5.6.1 Guidelines and Harmonization

During recent decades a number of GCP guidelines or regulations for the conduct of clinical trials of pharmaceutical products have come into force. Both

Table 5.1. Relevant terms

Clinical trial
Any investigation in human subjects intended to discover or verify the clinical, pharmacological, and/or other pharmacodynamic effects of an investigational product(s), and/or to identify and adverse reactions to an investigational product(s), and/or to study absorption, distribution, metabolism, and excretion of an investigational product(s) with the object of ascertaining its safety and/or efficacy. The terms clinical trial and clinical study are synonymous.

Good clinical practice (GCP)
A standard for the design, conduct, performance, monitoring, auditing, recording, analyses, and reporting of clinical trials that provides assurance that the data and reported results are credible and accurate, and that the rights, integrity, and confidentiality of trial subjects are protected.

Investigator
A person responsible for the conduct of the clinical trial at a trial site. If a trial is conducted by a team of individuals at a trial site, the investigator is the responsible leader of the team and may be called the principal investigator.

Sponsor
An individual, company, institution, or organization which takes responsibility for the initiation, management, and/or financing of a clinical trial.

Sponsor-Investigator
An individual who both initiates and conducts, alone or with others, a clinical trial, and under whose immediate direction the investigational product is administered to, dispensed to, or used by a subject. The term does not include any person other than an individual (e.g., it does not include a corporation or an agency). The obligations of a sponsor-investigator include both those of a sponsor and those of an investigator.

Quality control (QC)
The operational techniques and activities undertaken within the quality assurance system to verify that the requirements for quality of the trial-related activities have been fulfilled.

Quality assurance (QA)
All those planned and systematic actions that are established to ensure that the trial is performed and the data are generated, documented (recorded), and reported in compliance with Good Clinical Practice (GCP) and the applicable regulatory requirement(s).

the regulatory authorities and organizations representing the pharmaceutical industry have released GCP documents. First, the American Food and Drug Administration (FDA) prepared a set of guidelines for the conduct of clinical trials, and this initiative was soon followed by other authorities in Western countries (Ankier and Warrington 1989; Hvidberg 1994). The EEC notes for guidance with the title: "Good Clinical Practice for Trials on Medicinal Products in the European Community" came into force in July 1991 (Commission of the European Communities 1990). Since then the individual member states have been working on the implementation of the guidelines within national laws.

Parallel with the national and regional work on the preparation of the GCP documents, much effort has been put into the international harmonization of both clinical trial regulations and GCP. To provide guidance on a more world-wide basis, WHO guidelines for GCP for trials on pharmaceutical products were prepared in the early 1990s (World Health Organization 1993).

Cooperation has also been taking place between health authorities and industry in the United States Japan, and the EU. Groups of experts from these regions have been working on the preparation of a GCP document which has been a topic of discussion at the regularly arranged ICH conferences (International Conference of Harmonization of Technical Requirements for Registration of Pharmaceuticals for Human Use). Such harmonization is of importance for various reasons, including the fact that the majority of the pharmaceutical industry, and consequently the development and testing of new medicinal products, is located in these three regions. During the creation of the guidelines, current trial practices as well as relevant existing guidelines were taken into consideration.

The final ICH guidelines for Good Clinical Practice were approved in the EU in July 1996 and came into operation in January 1997 (The European Agency for the Evaluation of Medicinal Products, Human Medicines Evaluation Unit, CPMP/ICH/135/95, 1996).

5.6.2 ICH Guidelines for Good Clinical Practice

The objective of these guidelines has been to provide a unified standard for the participating regions to facilitate the mutual acceptance of clinical data by the regional authorities within their jurisdiction. In other words, the goal has been to ensure (a) more uniform regulation of the conduct of clinical trials, and (b) the validity of the collected data. The guidelines should be followed when generating clinical trial data that are intended to be used as documents accompanying applications for marketing authorizations of new drugs and to be submitted to regulatory authorities.

Adherence to the guidelines should save time and money in drug development, and also reduce the number of trial subjects who are exposed to new drugs, given that duplicate trials may no longer be needed to satisfy the demands of individual authorities.

The guidelines describe the principles of ICH GCP and thoroughly consider responsibilities, ethical aspects, relevant procedures, data handling and record keeping, quality assurance, and inspections. They also describe in detail all the essential elements and considerations which should be addressed in the trial protocol (including protocol amendments), as well as in the Investigator Brochure, which should give information on the product and preclinical and clinical data of relevance for the investigators. Essential documents for the planning, conduct, recording, and reporting of clinical trials are also mentioned to ensure that it will be possible to evaluate the compliance with GCP and all applicable regional requirements.

The existence of GCP is of importance for all parties involved in clinical trials – the ethical committees, the regulatory authorities, the investigators, the pharmaceutical industry, and the trial subjects – and as a consequence of this a closer relationship between ethics, regulations, and scientific standards has been established.

Many of the basic elements in GCP are designed to ensure optimal protection of trial subjects. It goes without saying that the investigator plays a central role, and precision during the performance of a trial is mandatory. The trial protocol has to be approved or given a favorable appraisal from at least an institutional review board (IRB) or an independent ethics committee (IEC). Also, freely given informed consent should be obtained from every subject prior to participation. Protection of the privacy of trial subjects is also an essential part of GCP.

Other elements in GCP concern the responsibilities of all the involved parties and apply to health authorities, IRBs/IECs, the pharmaceutical industry, and the responsible investigators, often physicians. Procedures for recording, handling, and evaluation of data and for record keeping and reporting are also important components in the document; all such guidelines are designed to ensure a satisfactory scientific standard of the results, which may be used as documentation in applications for marketing authorization.

Storage of essential data (source data) in trials involving, for instance, radiological examinations such as x-ray examinations, is the responsibility of the investigators and the data should be stored in such a way that they are available for review (e.g., inspection). Furthermore, certain procedures should be followed with respect to renewal/copying of material, so that the data remain intact for an appropriate period in accordance with the GCP guidelines.

Quality control (QC) and quality assurance (QA) are essential parts of GCP and are responsibilities of the sponsors – often the pharmaceutical companies. QC is undertaken to verify that the requirements for quality of the trial-related activities have been fulfilled, and QA is performed to ensure that the trial is carried out in compliance with GCP and the applicable regulatory requirements.

Other control measures include inspections of trials by regulatory authorities with the aim of undertaking an official review of documents, facilities, records, and other resources deemed to be related to the trial. The inspections can take place at the trial sites and/or at the involved companies. In the United States inspection by the FDA has long been standard practice, but in Europe this is a new field of responsibility for authorities, and the inspections have only been introduced and inserted into the regulations in a few countries (e.g., Denmark).

5.6.3 GCP Directive

Though GCP documents have been in force for years, this has not yet resulted in unified standard procedures for the evaluation and approval of clinical trials, even in limited numbers of countries such as the member states of the European Union or the Nordic countries. The cultural differences are obvious and a reason why individual national requirements are maintained. Among pharmaceutical companies there has been a tendency to plan and coordinate multinational trials and the mentioned differences in the regulations can make this very difficult (Legrand et al. 1995). During the last year the

Commission of the European Communities has been working on the preparation of a GCP Directive in order to establish a system of common trial regulation, taking into consideration the present national procedures together with the many differences in these without jeopardizing the advantages already existing in individual national regulations. Thus, harmonization may become a reality in the future.

References

Ankier SI, Warrington SJ (1989) Research and development of new medicines. J Int Med Res 17:407–416

Commission of the European Communities (1990) Good Clinical Practice for Trials on Medicinal Products in the European Community. In: The rules governing medicinal products in the European Community, vol. III, addendum July 1990, pp 57–98

Hvidberg EF (1994) Clinical trials on medicinal products (in Danish). Ugeskr Laeger 156:789–793

Legrand C, Cheix F, Dumais H, Laugel V, De Cremier F, Dupont C (1995) Clinical trial initiation procedures in Europe: the legal framework and practical aspects. Drug Information J 29:201–259

The European Agency for the Evaluation of Medicinal Products, Human Medicines Evaluation Unit (1996) Note for Guidance on Good Clinical Practice (CPMP/ICH/135/95)

World Health Organization (1993) WHO Guidelines for Good Clinical Practice (GCP) for Trials on Pharmaceutical Products. Division of drug management and policies

6 Currently Available Iodinated Contrast Media

F. Stacul

CONTENTS

6.1 Introduction

A large majority of the papers to appear in scientific journals in recent years on the subject of contrast media have focused on agents for magnetic resonance imaging (MRI) and ultrasonography (US). Iodinated contrast media have received relatively little attention in spite of their widespread use, which far exceeds that of agents for US and MRI. Possibly, scientific arguments concerning iodinated contrast media came to an end because current agents are so good that it seems unlikely that anything more than modest incremental improvements are possible (Dawson 1995). Available contrast agents are so efficacious and safe that it is becoming more and more difficult to identify significant differences among them. Possibly our methodological approach to clinical trials needs to change if such small differences are to be detected. Clinical studies could be better focused on populations that are more susceptible to contrast media toxicity, and other scientific branches, such as pharmacoepidemiology, could help us to improve the methodological approach to clinical trials (Stacul and Spinazzi 1997).

In this chapter, data concerning use of iodinated agents following intravascular injection will be discussed, the utmost attention being devoted to clinical experience. We shall focus on available iodinated contrast media, trying to avoid repetition of well-known data. In particular, emphasis will be placed on new topics and on new agents that have recently appeared on the market.

6.2 Currently Available Iodinated Contrast Media

In the early 1950s the first tri-iodinated compound was developed by Wallingford and this was the precursor of the water-soluble agents that were extensively used subsequently. These agents are ionic monomers, that is, salts consisting of a cation (sodium, methylglucamine, or a combination thereof) and an anion (benzoic acid derivative). For every three atoms of iodine, two particles in solution exist (ratio between atoms of iodine and particles in solution, 3:2 = 1.5). The osmolality of such agents is 4–7 times the osmolality of the plasma and they are usually called "high-osmolality" contrast media.

Research on contrast agents was subsequently focused on the reduction of contrast media osmolality, which appeared related to certain toxic effects of these agents. Almen, in the late 1960s, developed the first nonionic monomer, which was still a benzoic acid derivative, with three atoms of iodine per molecule but without the ionizing carboxyl group. These compounds were made soluble by including large numbers of hydrophilic groups on the side chains. They have an osmolality which is almost twice that of the plasma and a ratio between atoms of iodine and particles in solution of 3:1.

Research aimed at reduction of osmolality led to the synthesis of dimeric ionic contrast media as well,

F. Stacul, MD, Institute of Radiology, University of Trieste, Ospedale di Cattinara, Strada di Fiume 447, I-34149 Trieste, Italy

Table 6.1. Classes of currently available iodinated contrast media

	Iodine atoms	Soluted particles	I/P ratio
Ionic monomers	3	2	1.5
Nonionic monomers	3	1	3
Ionic dimers	6	2	3
Nonionic dimers	6	1	6

Table 6.2. Viscosity of currently available iodinated contrast media

	Iodine concentration (mg I/ml)	Viscosity at 37°C (cP)
Diatrizoate	370	8.4
Iothalamate	400	9.0
Ioxithalamate	380	8.5
Metrizoate	350	3.4
Ioxaglate	320	9.5
Iobitridol	350	10.0
Iohexol	350	11.2
Iomeprol	350	8.1
Iopamidol	370	9.8
Iopentol	350	12.0
Iopromide	350	9.5
Ioversol	350	8.5
Ioxilan	350	7.8
Iodixanol	320	11.1
Iotrolan	320	9.5

Table 6.3. Osmolality of currently available iodinated contrast media

	Iodine concentration (mg I/ml)	Osmolality at 37°C (mOsm/kg water)
Diatrizoate	370	2100
Iothalamate	400	2400
Ioxithalamate	380	2100
Metrizoate	350	1970
Ioxaglate	320	577
Iobitridol	350	915
Iohexol	350	823
Iomeprol	350	610
Iopamidol	370	774
Iopentol	350	810
Iopromide	350	774
Ioversol	350	790
Ioxilan	350	700
Iodixanol	320	290
Iotrolan	300	290
Blood		290

that is molecules containing six atoms of iodine but actually dissociating in solution into an anion and a cation (ratio 6:2 = 3).

Both monomeric nonionic compounds and dimeric ionic agents are named "low-osmolality" contrast media. However, while their osmolality is low in comparison to ionic monomers, it is still roughly twice that of plasma.

More recently nonionic dimers have been developed, that is molecules carrying six atoms of iodine without dissociating in solution. Their ratio is 6:1 and they are provided in solutions which are iso-osmolar with plasma.

Therefore, currently available iodinated contrast media can be divided into four classes with regard to their chemical structure (Table 6.1, Fig. 6.1). The most important physicochemical properties of these agents are their solubility, viscosity (Table 6.2), osmolality (Table 6.3), hydrophilia, and electrical charge.

Very high water solubility allows the production of highly concentrated contrast media. It should be remembered that some agents may crystallize at low temperatures, and warming is required to dissolve the crystals.

Viscosity affects injection speed. Viscosity increases markedly when concentration rises or temperature falls. Therefore use of more viscous compounds such as nonionic dimers is recommended following preheating. In fact at 37°C their viscosity is close to that of nonionic monomers.

Osmolality depends very much on concentration and to a lesser extent on temperature. Its significance derives from its direct relationship to contrast media tolerability (heat, pain) and other effects (hypervolemia, bradycardia, hypotension, endothelial damage, blood-brain barrier damage). Osmolality affects diuresis and therefore urinary iodine concentration as well.

Hydrophilia is also related to some contrast media side-effects. For instance, higher hydrophilia lowers the frequency of nausea and vomiting. However, it is interesting that nonionic agents are less hydrophilic than comparable ionic compounds; other factors are clearly responsible for better tolerance of the former.

Electrical charge is obviously a property of ionic compounds. It affects both the solubility and the hydrophilia of the agents (Speck 1994b).

6.3 Comparison Between High-Osmolality and Low-Osmolality Contrast Media

High-osmolality contrast media have a long history of efficacy and safety and have served as the standard against which low-osmolality contrast media have been compared. Such comparisons have formed the

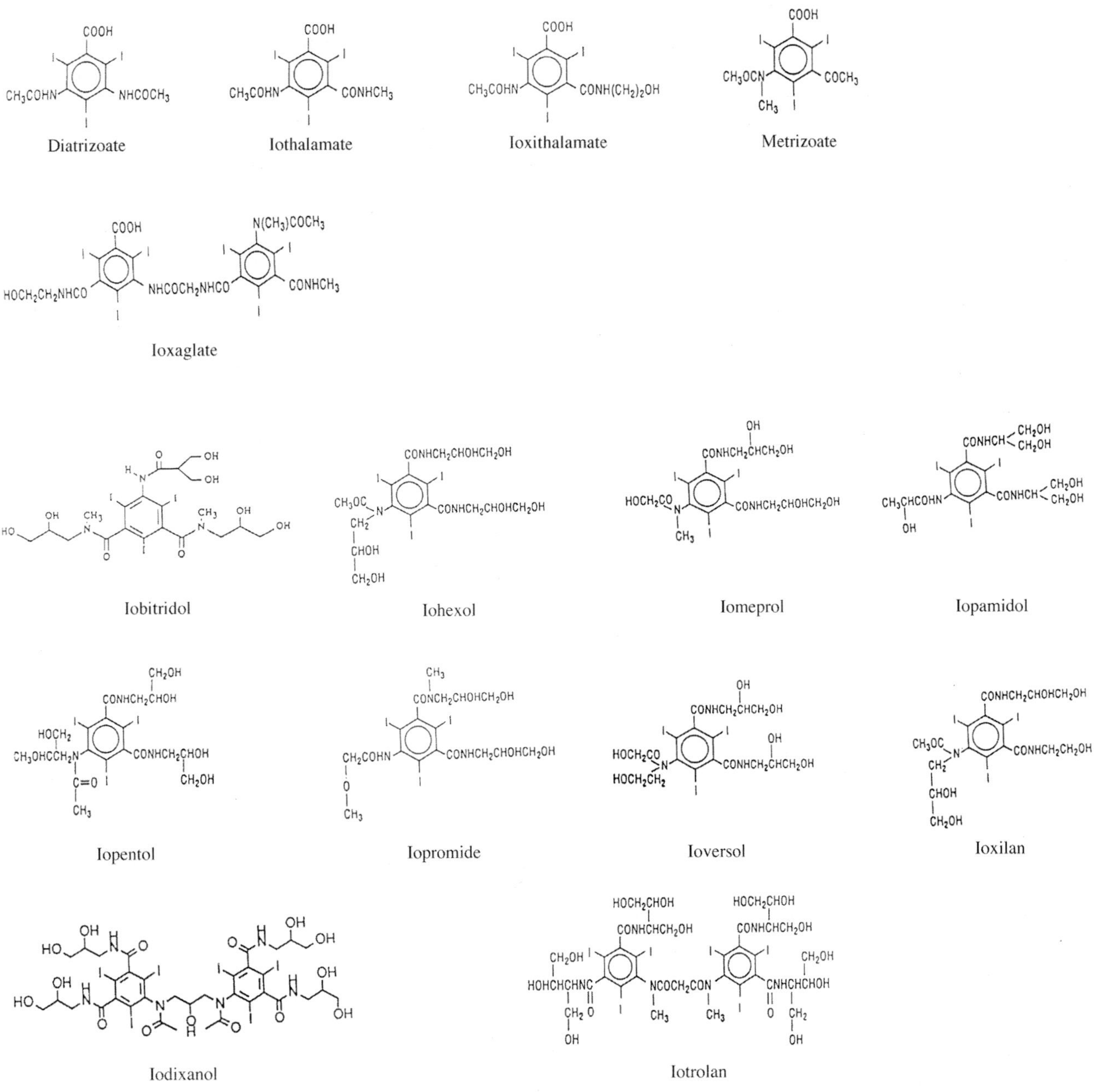

Fig. 6.1. Chemical structures of currently available iodinated contrast media

basis for hundreds of scientific papers; on the one hand it is difficult to take into account all of the different contributions, but on the other hand there is a huge amount of data that allows conclusions to be drawn on certain issues.

6.3.1 Efficacy

Following intra-arterial administration, all high-osmolality and low-osmolality agents provide similar opacification of the arterial vessels. However, improvements in patient comfort and tolerance (see below) can translate into less motion and better quality angiograms. High-osmolality agents withdraw more water through capillary and venule walls and therefore a lower iodine concentration may be expected in the venous runoff than when low-osmolality agents are used. Some such differences have indeed been described (Morris et al. 1983) but it is doubtful whether these are clinically important.

Following intravenous injection for intravenous digital subtraction angiography (DSA) or computed tomography (CT), the dilution of contrast media in the blood contained in the lungs is expected to be greater with high-osmolality agents. KORMANO (1981) showed a slightly greater aortic enhancement following iopamidol as compared with some high-osmolality agents, but the same author believes that interindividual variations are much more significant and that such minor differences in the pharmacokinetic behavior of various uroangiographic agents have no diagnostic relevance.

In urography low-osmolality contrast media produce a diuretic effect which is roughly halved in comparison with high-osmolality agents. As a result the opacification of the excretory pathway is denser; this is a distinct advantage of these agents, as many authors have reported (DALLA PALMA et al. 1982; SPATARO 1984; THOMPSON et al. 1984). However, at the same time a reduced distention of the excretory pathway is caused. Possible small filling defects could be missed because of the greater opacification and the reduced distention. Therefore the urographic technique requires routine use of ureteral compression and possibly delayed films in the case of poorly distended bladders.

6.3.2 Safety

The higher *tolerability* of low-osmolality agents has been fully demonstrated in clinical experience (KINNISON et al. 1989). Heat sensation and possible pain following administration of these contrast media are undoubtedly less pronounced, and this feature has been perceived as a distinct advantage above all in painful procedures such as peripheral arteriography. For pain caused by intra-arterial contrast agent injections there appears to be an "osmolality threshold" at around 600 mOsm (MORRIS 1993), close to the osmolality of solutions of low-osmolality agents commonly used for these studies.

There is universal consensus that *hemodynamic and cardiovascular changes* are fewer and less marked following low-osmolality contrast media injection. The intravascular injection of hyperosmolar contrast agents causes an increase in the circulating blood volume, drawing water from the extravascular compartment, and vasodilatation, causing a decrease in systemic vascular resistance and a reduction in arterial pressure. As to the heart, an elevation of cardiac filling pressure and an increase in cardiac output are shown. All these effects are directly related to the contrast material osmolality.

Following an intracoronary injection of an ionic monomer, a transient depression in left ventricular contractile function occurs (decrease in left ventricular peak systolic pressure, decrease in the maximum rate of increase in left ventricular pressure, increase in left ventricular end-systolic and end-diastolic diameter) and is related to the osmolality of the solution. Injection of ioxaglate (ionic dimer) is followed by changes that are similar but smaller in magnitude, while injection of nonionic monomers actually enhances contractile performance and increases left ventricular systolic shortening. Moreover, following intracoronary injection of contrast agents, electrophysiologic effects occur, namely a transient reduction in heart rate, a prolongation of the Q-T interval, and a reduction in the ventricular fibrillation threshold. Low-osmolality contrast media produce less pronounced changes in all these parameters as compared with high-osmolality media (HIRSHFELD 1991).

All contrast media cause red blood cell deformation, which depends both on a toxic effect on the cell membrane and, to a greater extent, on an osmotic extraction of water. This phenomenon is of uncertain clinical relevance and is less marked with low-osmolality agents.

All contrast agents are anticoagulant and this property could partially compensate for inadequacies in angiographic technique. Nonionic compounds are less anticoagulant and therefore the likelihood of clot formation in catheters and syringes containing these agents is greater (DAWSON 1991). However, these differences should be clinically unimportant if operators adhere to proper technique (HIRSHFELD 1991).

Concerning the action of contrast media on blood vessels, toxic effects on the endothelium should be mentioned. Again, this endothelial damage is higher when high-osmolality agents are employed. The possible occurrence of thrombi could be relevant above all in phlebography, when the contact time between contrast agent and vessel wall is longer.

The comparative *nephrotoxicity* of high-osmolality and low-osmolality contrast agents has been a matter of much debate. Theoretically, all the mechanisms possibly related to contrast media-induced nephrotoxicity (decrease in renal perfusion, glomerular injury, tubular injury, tubular obstruction) should be affected by low-osmolality contrast media to a lesser extent. However, some papers (GOMES et al. 1989; KINNISON et al. 1989; SCHWAB et

Table 6.4. Adverse reactions after intravenous injection of ionic and nonionic contrast media

	No. of patients		Overall rate of reactions (%)		Rate of severe reactions (%)	
	Ionic	Nonionic	Ionic	Nonionic	Ionic	Nonionic
KATAYAMA et al. (1990)	169284	168363	12.7	3.1	0.22	0.04
PALMER (1988)	79278	30268	3.8	1.2	0.1	0.01
WOLF et al. (1989)	6006	7170	4.1	0.7	0.4	0.0

al. 1989) published in the late 1980s failed to show any significant difference between the two classes in this regard and cases of renal impairment were reported following the injection of low-osmolality agents, indicating that they could not be considered as nonnephrotoxic.

More recently other studies (KATHOLI et al. 1993; TALIERCIO et al. 1991) have reported a lower nephrotoxicity of low-osmolality agents, and this result was confirmed in the meta-analysis of 31 randomized trials carried out by BARRETT and CARLISLE (1993), which showed that these agents were beneficial in patients with preexisting renal impairment. RUDNICK et al. (1995) again showed the lower nephrotoxicity of one nonionic monomer (iohexol) as compared with diatrizoate in patients with renal impairment, possibly associated with diabetes mellitus. Therefore, today, there is sufficient reason to believe that low-osmolality agents are to be preferred in patients with impaired renal function.

The issue of *adverse reactions* is no longer a matter of debate. Large observational studies (KATAYAMA et al. 1990; PALMER 1988; WOLF et al. 1989) clarified the advantages of low-osmolality agents (Table 6.4). In particular, the large study by KATAYAMA et al. on 337647 cases showed a prevalence of reactions to ionic and nonionic media of 12.66% and 3.13% respectively ($P < 0.01$), while severe reactions occurred in 0.22% and 0.04% of cases respectively ($P < 0.01$). Nonionic contrast media were estimated to be safer than ionic contrast media by a factor of 6, and therefore it could be concluded that the most effective means of increasing the safety of contrast media examinations is the use of nonionic agents. This comment is in agreement with the paradox outlined by PALMER (1988), who realized that fewer reactions occurred in at-risk patients injected with low-osmolality agents than in patients without risk factors who received high-osmolality contrast media. Therefore the advantage of low-osmolality agents in reducing adverse reactions is beyond doubt, while there is presently some discussion over the predictive value of preclinical studies on contrast media with regard to this issue.

Table 6.5. Acute toxicity of second- and third-generation contrast media after intravenous administration in mice (1 ml/min)

	LD_{50} (g I/kg)
2nd generation	5–10.2
Diatrizoate	7.7
3rd generation	18.5–22.6
Iopamidol	21.8

Comparing the acute toxicity of second- and third-generation contrast media in mice after intravenous administration (1 ml/min), the LD_{50} of the former is in the range 5–10.2 g I/kg while the LD_{50} of the latter is 18.5–22.6 g I/kg. For example, the LD_{50} for diatrizoate is 7.7 g I/kg, while iopamidol has an LD_{50} of 21.8 g I/kg (Table 6.5). Thus, in animals, nonionic monomers have about a threefold higher intravenous tolerability than ionic monomers, evaluated as intravenous LD_{50}.

In clinical intravascular use, nonionic monomers are associated with an approximately sixfold lower frequency of severe adverse reactions than are ionic monomers (KATAYAMA et al. 1990). Indeed, it seems that there is some relationship between LD_{50} in animals and the incidence of severe adverse reactions in humans, although the ratio in humans is even more favorable to nonionic agents. According to ROSATI et al. (1992), uncertainty factors such as the variability of response in humans (because of the different health status of patients), and the fact that death in animals is compared with severe reactions in man, may explain the underestimation of the toxicity ratio between ionic and nonionic compounds in animals. SPECK (1994a) agrees that a correlation between experimental results and tolerability in humans has been established. However, he feels that these relationships are vague and argues that LD_{50} for a single contrast agent is meaningless because such concentrations or doses will not be reached in clinical practice.

It should be noted that, if it is true that LD_{50} evaluation is done under conditions which are far from the clinical reality, because we are discussing LD_{50} values close to total substitution of blood or cerebral fluid in the experimental animal, it is also true that such conditions are the same for all contrast media when they are tested in the same experiment. Therefore, the differences that are observed among the products should represent an expression of the different toxicity of these molecules.

The last issue concerning the safety of these agents is the hot topic of *mortality* rates. Using meta-analysis, no statistical difference was noted in mortality rates between high-osmolality and low-osmolality contrast media. Such a comparison may not be feasible in comparative studies owing to the large sample size that would be needed (PALMER 1990). However, the comparison of severe life-threatening side-effects can represent a satisfactory substitute, and, as has been mentioned, the incidence of such side-effects is indeed lower with low-osmolality agents.

6.4 Comparison Among Low-Osmolality Contrast Media

Presently, eight nonionic monomers (iobitridol, iohexol, iomeprol, iopamidol, iopentol, iopromide, ioversol, ioxilan) and one ionic dimer (ioxaglate) are commercially available. Besides obvious differences between the two classes, these agents differ slightly from each other in terms of number of hydroxyl groups, possibility of crystallization, osmolality, viscosity, hydrophilicity, LD_{50}, and EB_{50}[1] (STACUL and THOMSEN 1996). Therefore it is important to assess whether such differences may be relevant in clinical studies.

6.4.1 Efficacy

Several clinical trials have shown that if similar iodine strengths of these uroangiographic agents and equivalent administration schemes are used, there is no way of detecting any difference in opacification or contrast enhancement. Therefore it seems that efficacy is not a parameter that can serve as a basis for selection among these agents.

6.4.2 Safety

Thus far, clinical trials have not revealed differences among nonionic monomers as to safety. Some concern has been raised over the low EB_{50} of iopromide, which might reflect a greater neurotoxicity of this agent. ROSATI et al. (1995) found a higher incidence of nervous side-effects following iopromide administration as compared with iomeprol. However, another study did not show any differences in safety between iopromide and other agents used in cerebral arteriography (HAUGHTON et al. 1994). In any case, the intrathecal injection of iopromide is presently not allowed.

As mentioned above (see Sect. 6.3.2), the intracoronary injection of ioxaglate is followed by a slight transient depression of left ventricular contractile function, while nonionic monomers actually enhance it (HIRSHFELD 1991). Moreover in comparison with nonionic monomers the injection of ioxaglate is followed by a higher frequency of some minor reactions, namely nausea and vomiting (DAWSON et al. 1983; SPATARO et al. 1987). These phenomena occur with a frequency similar to that following diatrizoate administration and may be related to the chemical structure of the molecule and the consequent cholinesterase inhibition or histamine release from basophils and mast cells (DAWSON and EDGERTON 1983). A significantly higher incidence of urticaria following ioxaglate administration, in comparison with iopamidol, was also reported by DEL FAVERO et al. (1993). These authors pooled the results from 16 comparative randomized trials and found that the incidence of adverse reactions was 5% in the iopamidol group and 18% in the ioxaglate group.

BRISMAR et al. (1991), commenting on the higher incidence of adverse events following ioxaglate in comparison with nonionic monomers, reported that this was a reason why the real difference in safety between high-osmolality and low-osmolality contrast media was actually partially obscured by pooling studies using nonionic monomers and ioxaglate.

[1] EB_{50} = Effective dose for disturbing behavior in 50% of the animals (reflecting the direct neurotoxicity)

6.5 Comparison Between Low-Osmolality and Iso-osmolality Contrast Media

Research on iodinated contrast media has assessed the relation between osmolality and safety of compounds, as has already been underscored in the discussion of trials comparing ionic and nonionic monomers. On the basis of such evidence, one research line was oriented towards the synthesis of nonionic dimers, which are provided in solutions which are iso-osmolar with plasma at around 300 mg I/ml. Two agents (iodixanol and iotrolan) recently appeared on the market and there is now sufficient data from clinical trials to offer some comments on their efficacy and safety following intravascular injection in comparison with nonionic monomers. More limited data are available on the comparison between ionic and nonionic dimers.

6.5.1 Efficacy

The efficacy of nonionic dimers in comparison with nonionic monomers in cardiovascular procedures has been a matter for claims and counterclaims. According to Dawson (1996), the iso-osmolality of nonionic dimers, possibly combined with a slower diffusion of the larger molecules across vessel walls and out of the vascular space, may play a significant role in producing better quality venous phase images following arteriography and arterial phase images following venous injection. The author emphasized the implications for i.v. DSA, the venous phase of arteriography, CT portography, and spiral CT arteriography.

No doubt these considerations are in favor of nonionic dimers, but unfortunately no single comparative study has shown a greater cardiovascular efficacy of these agents as compared with nonionic monomers. All studies have demonstrated equivalent results with the two classes of compounds (Grynne et al. 1995). Possibly better focused trials could provide different evidence.

It has also been claimed that nonionic dimers may provide similar results to nonionic monomers at lower doses and therefore might be preferred. This argument is based on the evidence that clinical trials have usually compared (a) nonionic monomers at a concentration of 350–370 mg I/ml with 320 mg I/ml nonionic dimers or (b) 300 mg I/ml nonionic monomers with 270–280 mg I/ml nonionic dimers. That is, the concentration of the dimers has usually been slightly lower in these comparative trials which failed to show differences in cardiovascular efficacy. However, we believe that it is not scientifically correct to argue for a greater efficacy of nonionic dimers following the comparison of solutions with small iodine concentration differences using gross methods for image quality assessment (such as rating the vessel opacification as poor, good, or excellent).

The use of nonionic dimers for arteriography has raised another criticism relating to the higher viscosity of these compounds, as a consequence of which hand injection, particularly through long thin catheters, could be a significant problem. However, Gmeinwieser and Wenzel-Hora (1995) showed that iotrolan 280 mg I/ml could be injected at room temperature with a flow rate of 20 ml/s through 100-cm-long 5F pigtail catheters. Klow et al. (1993) realized that iodixanol 320 mg I/ml was indistinguishable from iohexol 350 mg I/ml during hand injection in cardioangiography. Moreover, at 37°C there are only small differences in viscosity between the most concentrated contrast media, thus suggesting that preheating of nonionic dimers before use may minimize difficulties arising from viscosity. Overall, therefore, the viscosity problem looks minor in clinical practice.

The urographic efficacy of nonionic dimers has been claimed to be greater by some authors because comparative trials of these agents and nonionic monomers injected at slightly higher iodine concentrations showed no significant differences. Again, this comment is not acceptable, as we already clarified with regard to the cardiovascular efficacy. It is more relevant to remark that the iso-osmolality of nonionic dimers induces lower osmotic diuresis in comparison with low-osmolality agents. As a consequence, a greater opacification of the excretory pathway may be achieved, which may represent an advantage particularly in patients with impaired renal function. On the other hand, poorer distention of the excretory pathway might be forecast, which could be perceived as a limitation. Indeed, greater opacification of the excretory pathway following administration of nonionic dimers has been shown in some series of patients with normal renal function (Adolph et al. 1995; Narimatsu and Hiramatsu 1995) A single study (Sundgren et al. 1996) showed that iodixanol permitted more frequent detection of collecting ducts and papillary blush and provided poorer bladder distention as compared with iohexol, again supporting theoretical expectations. It should be mentioned that detection of collecting ducts and papillary blush might lead to the erroneous diagnosis of medullary sponge kidney. However, SAXTON (1989) stated that if the opacified tubules are slender, measuring 0.3 mm or less, and are densely radiopaque for their size, then there is little likelihood of sponge kidney disease.

Clinical experience concerning the use of nonionic dimers in urography in patients with impaired renal function is limited, possibly because of the infrequent need for urography in such patients. We carried out a clinical trial in 100 patients with hematuria or stone disease and serum creatinine values between 1.5 and 3.0 mg/dl who underwent urography with iodixanol or iopromide. Iodixanol showed better filling and density of the calyces (p=0.004), more frequent detection of papillary blush (p=0.003) and better opacification of the renal pelvis (p=0.006) (STACUL et al. 1998).

6.5.2 Safety

The *tolerability*, which depends on the incidence of pain or heat sensation following intravascular contrast media administration, is a definite point in favor of nonionic dimers in comparison with nonionic monomers. A large number of clinical trials have unanimously reached this conclusion. Here reference is made to the two largest trials to focus on this issue. SILVAY-MANDEAU et al. (1995) reported the results of a multicenter clinical study in Europe, comparing iotrolan with nonionic monomers in 2410 patients following intra-arterial or intravenous injection of the contrast material. During intra-arterial procedures a lower incidence of heat ($P = 0.0001$) and pain ($P = 0.0001$) was recorded following iotrolan, and a lower incidence of heat ($P = 0.0038$) following iotrolan was shown during intravenous procedures as well. Another multicenter clinical study (JUSTESEN et al. 1997) assessed the tolerability of iodixanol in comparison with iopromide in 2490 patients who underwent DSA and conventional arteriography. Pain and/or severe heat was reported by 4.1% of patients injected with iodixanol and by 19.8% patients who received iopromide. We can definitely conclude that use of nonionic dimers entails a significantly lower incidence of pain in peripheral angiography than is experienced with nonionic monomers. Furthermore a significantly lower frequency and/or intensity of heat sensation is shown in arteriography, phlebography, urography, and CT. A few comparative studies have also reported a lower intensity of heat sensation with iodixanol than with ioxaglate (ANDERSEN et al. 1993; TVEIT et al. 1994).

Assessment of the *cardiovascular safety* of nonionic dimers includes analysis of their cardiac effects as well as their effects on large vessels and the microcirculation.

With regard to cardiac effects, preclinical data suggest less pronounced electrophysiological disturbances with nonionic dimers than with nonionic monomers. Unfortunately there is a lack of clinical data on this subject; however it appears evident that nonionic dimers and nonionic monomers are both well tolerated. In one study systolic pressure and heart rate seemed less influenced by iodixanol than by iopromide during left ventriculography (MANNINEN et al. 1995). Moreover left ventricular contractile function was found to be less influenced by iodixanol than by ioxaglate (ANDERSEN et al. 1993; FINET et al. 1992; TVEIT et al. 1994).

PUGH et al. (1993) evaluated the effects of iodixanol on large vessels and showed that a transient increase in femoral blood flow in aortofemoral arteriography followed the injection of both iodixanol and iopromide but was clearly less pronounced following iodixanol administration. However, it is interesting that the iso-osmolar solution of iodixanol still produced a detectable vasodilation, thus suggesting that osmolality is not the only factor responsible for this effect.

The possible effects of nonionic dimers on microcirculation have been a matter of debate. It has been shown (HAGEN and WENZEL-HORA 1989; MORRIS et al. 1982; PALMERS et al. 1993) that a more viscous contrast material solution mixed with blood can cause a transient slowing of the blood flow through microcirculation. Nonionic dimers constitute a highly viscous bolus and in addition are iso-osmolar, with the consequence that they do not withdraw water from the interstitium. The result could be a prolongation of the anoxia time. This argument is undoubtedly of interest, but its clinical relevance looks minor. In fact, on the basis of these premises, signs or symptoms of ischemia could be forecast following the injection of nonionic dimers whereas the opposite is actually true: pain in femoral arteriography is lower after the administration of nonionic dimers.

The *nephrotoxicity* of contrast media can still be a problem, particularly in certain groups of patients, and therefore the potential nephrotoxic effects of nonionic dimers deserve special attention.

The effects of these agents both on glomeruli and on tubules have been discussed. In rats, UEDA et al.

(1993) found a more evident reduction in the single nephron glomerular filtration rate in superficial nephrons with iotrolan than with ionic and nonionic monomers. However, the urine of rats is much more concentrated than that of humans and these results should therefore be validated by clinical trials. Several clinical studies evaluated possible changes in serum creatinine during the 24 h after contrast material administration, comparing iodixanol and different nonionic monomers. Serum creatinine was usually unaffected and no study showed any difference between the investigated compounds. Furthermore, trials comparing iotrolan with nonionic monomers did not suggest higher nephrotoxic effects of this agent on glomerular function. On the contrary, in 697 patients CLAUSS et al. (1995) reported smaller changes in serum creatinine following iotrolan administration than after iohexol, iopamidol, and iopromide.

Concern has been expressed regarding the effects of nonionic dimers on tubular cells because the higher concentrations reached by these agents in the tubules could be perceived as a cause of higher nephrotoxicity.

Another consideration militating against nonionic dimers is the higher retention of these agents in the proximal tubular cells, as shown by detectable vacuoles. Vacuoles containing contrast material can be identified following intravascular injection of any contrast agent. However, this phenomenon is clearly more evident after administration of nonionic dimers, and evidence that more iodine is retained in the kidney after injection of nonionic dimers than after nonionic monomers is provided by CT attenuation values as well (JAKOBSEN et al. 1992). Nevertheless, such higher iodine retention in the kidneys has not been found to correlate with changes in tubular parameters. Several trials comparing the urinary excretion of tubular enzymes following administration of iodixanol and nonionic monomers were unable to show higher urinary excretion of tubular enzymes following injection of the dimer; indeed, in some trials the opposite was true.

The aforementioned studies compared nephrotoxicity of nonionic dimers and monomers in patients with normal renal function. Obviously it is of interest to assess the nephrotoxic effects of these agents in patients with impaired renal function, i.e. in a high-risk group.

We compared iodixanol with iopromide in urography in 64 patients with mild to moderate impairment of renal function (serum creatinine 1.5–3.0 mg/dl) and were unable to detect any difference between the agents as to serum creatinine and the excretion of several tubular enzymes from baseline, in spite of the long observation time (7 days) (CARRARO et al. 1998). The same was true in another study carried out by JACOBSEN et al. (1994) in 16 patients with severe nondiabetic renal failure who underwent pretransplantation angiography with iodixanol or iohexol.

Therefore it actually appears that no significant clinical difference in renal safety can be detected when comparing nonionic monomers and dimers.

Until 1995, the type and frequency of *adverse events* following intravascular administration of nonionic dimers seemed comparable to those occurring with nonionic monomeric agents; moreover it was considered that conclusive data would be impossible to obtain because of the very low incidence of adverse events with both classes of compounds, such that enrolment of an extremely large number of patients would be required to obtain conclusive results in a comparative trial. However, in October 1995 Schering, the company manufacturing iotrolan, decided to temporarily suspend sales of this agent as a precautionary measure and reported that the reason for the decision was that, following more widespread use of the contrast medium, there had been an increased number of reports from physicians of delayed reactions, in particular allergy-like skin reactions. This temporary suspension still applies, and therefore a deeper insight into this problem seems required. One supplement to *European Radiology* and one "Insert for Radiologists" in the same journal have extensively discussed this matter. In this chapter the more relevant clinical issues will be discussed. It is to be emphasized that we are dealing with delayed adverse events, that is with onset 60 min or more after contrast agent administration. It is worthwhile underscoring that the reported frequency of such events with commonly employed contrast media varies remarkably, from 0.4% to 18%.

Comparative data on the frequency of delayed reactions following use of iotrolan and nonionic monomers also vary between countries (NIENDORF 1996). European studies in 2890 patients showed the rate of reactions following iotrolan (2.4%) to be slightly lower than that following nonionic monomers (3.6%). The frequency of delayed reactions was comparable (0.62% and 0.83% respectively), with delayed skin reactions occurring in 0.41% and 0.28% of cases, respectively. On the other hand in the Japanese studies (670 patients) the overall rate of reactions was 4.8% and 6.8% respectively, but the rate of delayed reactions following iotrolan proved substantially higher than that following nonionic monomers (3.00% vs 1.19%) and these results were largely due to the reported rate of skin manifestations (2.40% vs 0.30%). The U.S. trials confirmed the Japanese data and therefore it was concluded that delayed allergy-like reactions occur 2–5 times more often with iotrolan than with the nonionic monomers. This evidence was supported by spontaneous reporting by physicians on the frequency of adverse events in Germany and Japan following iotrolan administration. It turned out that there were as many acute reactions as delayed ones and that skin reactions (generalized or localized urticaria, edema, exanthema, pruritus) mainly occurred as a delayed event. Such delayed skin reactions are usually a minor clinical event, but they were perceived by Japanese groups as a new problem that usually requires at least the consultation of the referring physician. Besides this, spontaneous reporting in Germany and Japan identified 26 serious delayed reactions (shock, hypotension with anaphylactic reactions, Quincke edema, dyspnea, glottis edema), the majority of them occurring between 6 and 24 h after injection. However, it should be stressed that during the time these reports were collected, roughly 300 000 patients received iotrolan in these two countries.

Of course, the different frequency of delayed reactions in Europe and Japan has been a matter of extensive discussion. One interesting explanatory hypothesis relies on racial differences, namely on the deficiency of acetaldehyde dehydrogenase in 43% of Japanese patients; this deficiency might result in the accumulation of acetaldehyde, which could potentiate the ability of contrast agents, especially of dimers, to bridge proteins, thus promoting reactions to contrast agents.

Again on this topic, it is important to underscore that results should be analyzed with great caution. For instance, one study reported in the mentioned "Insert for Radiologists" compared the frequency of delayed reactions in three groups of patients undergoing CT (the first receiving iotrolan, the second injected with iopromide, and the third undergoing plain CT only) and showed that the highest frequency of delayed symptoms actually occurred in the group which did not receive any contrast agent! These results clearly show that there is a significant "background noise" to these events.

On the basis of all these data it is tempting to state that it was perhaps an overreaction to withdraw iotrolan from the European market on the basis of the reports from Japan.

The evidence concerning iotrolan stimulated research on this topic with the other available nonionic dimer, iodixanol. Presently available results are still unpublished. In one study, concerning 2973 patients, the rate of reactions following iodixanol was 6.0%, the same as that in the group which did not receive any contrast, while it was 8.6% in the group receiving nonionic monomeric compounds. Delayed reactions were slightly more frequent following iodixanol (2.1%) than in the "plain" group (1.6%) and in the group injected with nonionic monomers (1.5%), while the incidence of delayed skin reactions was 1.5% (iodixanol), 0.7% (nonionic monomers), and 0.4% (no contrast). Somewhat similar results were collected in a multicenter study in 4427 patients: the overall frequency of reactions was comparable (iodixanol 11.6%, nonionic monomers 12.5%), while the frequency of delayed reactions was 4.6% and 2.9% respectively.

Nycomed, the company manufacturing iodixanol, reported that delayed adverse events in response to this agent were mostly mild allergy-like skin and mucosal reactions, and that no serious delayed reactions had been reported.

6.6 Concluding Remarks

Low-osmolality and iso-osmolality contrast media are more comfortable for the patient and safer than high-osmolality agents. This debate has come to an end, and very few European radiologists still administer high-osmolality agents intravascularly (Thomsen 1994). The major obstacle to total conversion is the price difference between high-osmolality agents and the new contrast media. In the United States this difference is even higher, and therefore cost-effectiveness analyses there do not demonstrate the feasibility of universal use of low-osmolality contrast media (Ellis et al. 1996). In the United States selective use of low-osmolality agents is still considered the best available approach and this raises the question of which patients should receive the new agents. Of course, the answer is complex and does not involve scientific features only. The expected appearance of generic agents on the market could lower the prices and therefore expedite the conversion process in some countries.

The relative merits of low-osmolality and iso-osmolality agents are still a subject of scientific debate. However, possible improvements achieved with any agent among the nonionic monomers and dimers are likely to be marginal and do not justify significant price differences.

References

Adolph JMG, Engelkamp H, Herbig W, Peters PE, Wenzel-Hora BI (1995) Iotrolan in urography: efficacy and tolerance in comparison with iohexol and iopamidol. Eur Radiol (Suppl 2) 5:S63–S68

Andersen PE, Bolstad B, Berg KJ, Justesen P, Thayssen P, Kloster YF (1993) Iodixanol and ioxaglate in cardioangiography. A double-blind randomized phase III study. Clin Radiol 48:268–272

Barrett BJ, Carlisle EJ (1993) Metaanalysis of the relative nephrotoxicity of high- and low-osmolality iodinated contrast media. Radiology 188:171–178

Brismar J, Jacobsson BF, Jorulf H (1991) Miscellaneous adverse effects of low- versus high-osmolality contrast media: a study revised. Radiology 179:19–23

Carraro M, Malalan F, Antonione R, Stacul F, Ceva M, Petz S, Assante M, Grynne BJ, Haider T, Dalla Palma L, Faccini L (1998) Effects of dimeric versus monomeric nonionic contrast media on renal function in patients with mild to moderate renal insufficiency: a double-blind, randomized clinical trial. Eur Radiol :144–147

Clauss W, Dinger J, Meissner C (1995) Renal tolerance of iotrolan 280 – a meta-analysis of 14 double-blind studies. Eur Radiol (Suppl 2) 5:79–84

Dalla Palma L, Rossi M, Stacul F, Agostini R (1982) Iopamidol in urography: comparison between ionic and nonionic contrast media in patients with normal and impaired renal function. Urol Radiol 4:1–3

Dawson P (1991) Contrast agents in clinical angiography. Relevance to thromboembolic phenomena. Front Eur Radiol 8:53–59

Dawson P (1995) Design plays major role in new contrast media. Diagn Imaging Eur June:3–4

Dawson P (1996) The non-ionic isotonic contrast agents. Perspectives and controversies. Eur Radiol (Suppl) 6:S20–S24

Dawson P, Edgerton D (1983) Contrast media and enzyme inhibition. I. Cholinesterase. Br J Radiol 56:653–656

Dawson P, Grainger RG, Pitfield J (1983) The new low-osmolar contrast media: a simple guide. Clin Radiol 34:221–226

Del Favero C, Rossini G, Martegani A (1993) A comparison of iopamidol and ioxaglate in CT enhancement. Eur Radiol 3:77–82

Ellis JH, Cohan RH, Sonnad SS, Shafiroff Cohan N (1996) Selective use of radiographic low-osmolality contrast media in the 1990s. Radiology 200:297–311

Finet G, Roriz R, Nantois C, Borch KW, Revel D, Beaune J, Amiel M (1992) Iodixanol in ventriculography and coronary angiography. A double blind parallel phase III comparison with ioxaglate. Cardiovasc Intervent Radiol (Suppl) 15:S48

Gmeinwieser JK, Wenzel-Hora BI (1995) Peripheral and penile angiography with iotrolan 280 versus non-ionic monomers: results of the European clinical phase II and III trials. Eur Radiol (Suppl 2) 5:S30–S38

Gomes AS, Lois JF, Baker JD, McGlade CT, Bunnell DH, Hartzman S (1989) Acute renal dysfunction in high risk patients after angiography. Comparison of ionic and nonionic contrast media. Radiology 170:65–68

Grynne BJ, Nossen JO, Bolstad B, Borch KW (1995) Main results of the first comparative clinical studies on Visipaque. An overview of 18 clinical studies. Acta Radiol 36(Suppl 399):265–270

Hagen B, Wenzel-Hora BI (1989) Initial experience with a nonionic, dimeric contrast medium (Iotrolan) in direct and indirect arteriography: a randomized intraindividual double-blind study in 60 patients. In: Taenzer V, Wende S (eds) Recent developments in nonionic contrast media. Thieme, Stuttgart, pp 54–60

Haughton VM, Papke A, Hyland D, Drayer BP, Osborn AG, Maravilla K, Hilal SK (1994) Safety and efficacy of iopromide in cerebral arteriography. Invest Radiol (Suppl) 29:S94–S97

Hirshfeld JR (1991) Radiographic contrast agents. In: Marcus ML, Skorton DJ, Schelbert HR, Wolf GL (eds) Cardiac Imaging. Saunders, Philadelphia, pp 162–181

Jakobsen JA, Lundby B, Kristoffersen DT, Borch KW, Hald JK, Berg KJ (1992) Evaluation of renal function with delayed CT after injection of nonionic monomeric and dimeric contrast media in healthy volunteers. Radiology 182:419–424

Jakobsen JA, Berg KJ, Nossen JO (1994) Renal function and contrast retention after angiography in patients with severe renal failure. Acta Radiol (Suppl 394) 35:S38

Justesen P, Downes M, Hougens Grynne B, Lang H, Rasch W, Seim E (1997) Injection associated pain in femoral arteriography: a European multicentre study comparing safety, tolerability and efficacy of iodixanol 270 mg I/ml (Visipaque) and iopromide 300 mg I/ml (Ultravist). Cardiovasc Intervent Radiol 20:251–256

Katayama H, Yamaguchi K, Kozuka T, Takashima T, Seez P, Matsuura K (1990) Adverse reactions to ionic and nonionic contrast media: a report from the Japanese Committee on the safety of contrast media. Radiology 175:621–628

Katholi RE, Taylor GJ, Woods WT, Womack KA, Katholi CR, McCann WP, Moses HW, Dove JT, Mikell FL, Woodruff RC, Miller BD, Schneider JA (1993) Nephrotoxicity of nonionic low-osmolality versus ionic high-osmolality contrast media: a prospective double-blind randomized comparison in human beings. Radiology 186:183–187

Kinnison ML, Powe NR, Steinberg EP (1989) Results of randomized controlled trials of low- versus high-osmolality contrast media. Radiology 170:381–389

Klow NE, Levorstad K, Berg KJ, Brodahl U, Endressen K, Kristoffersen DT, Laake B, Simonsen S, Tofte AJ, Lundby B (1993) Iodixanol in cardioangiography in patients with coronary artery disease. Acta Radiol 34:72–77

Kormano M (1981) Kinetics of contrast media after bolus injection and infusion. In: Felix R, Kazner E, Wegener OH (eds) Contrast media in computed tomography, Proceedings International Workshop Berlin, January 14–17. Excerpta Medica, Amsterdam, pp 38–45

Manninen M, Tahvanainen K, Borch KW, Wallén T, Soimakallio S, Matsi P, Suhonen M (1995) Iodixanol, a new non-ionic dimeric contrast medium in cardioangiography: a double-masked parallel comparison with iopromide. Eur Radiol 5:364–370

Morris TW (1993) X-ray contrast media: where are we now, and where are we going? Radiology 188:11–16

Morris TW, Kem MA, Katzberg RW (1982) The effects of media viscosity on hemodynamics in selective arteriography. Invest Radiol 17:70–76

Morris TW, Harnish PP, Reece K, Katzberg RW (1983) Tissue fluid shifts during renal arteriography with conventional and low osmolality agents. Invest Radiol 18:335–340

Narimatsu Y, Hiramatsu K (1995) A Japanese multicenter comparison of iotrolan 280 with iopamidol 300 in intravenous urography. Eur Radiol (Suppl 2) 5:S58–S62

Niendorf HP (1996) Delayed allergy-like reactions to X-ray contrast media. Problem statement exemplified with iotrolan (Isovist) 280. Eur Radiol (Suppl) 6:S8–S10

Palmer FJ (1988) The RACR survey of intravenous contrast media reactions. Final report. Australas Radiol 32:426–428

Palmer FJ (1990) Morbidity and mortality with intravenous contrast media: ionic and nonionic. Invest Radiol (Suppl) 25:S18–S19

Palmers Y, DeGreef D, Grynne BH, Smits J, Put E (1993) A double-blind study comparing safety, tolerability and efficacy of iodixanol 320 mg I/ml and ioxaglate 320 mg I/ml in cerebral arteriography. Eur J Radiol 17:203–209

Pugh PD, Sissons GRJ, Ruttley MST, Berg KJ, Nossen JO, Eide H (1993) Iodixanol in femoral arteriography (phase III): a comparative double-blind parallel trial between iodixanol and iopromide. Invest Radiol 17:70–77

Rosati G, Morisetti A, Tirone P (1992) Toxicity in animals and safety in humans. The predictive value of animal studies. Toxicol Lett 64:705–715

Rosati G, Davies A, Spinazzi A (1995) Predictable and unpredictable adverse reactions to iomeprol and iopromide. Acad Radiol (Suppl) 2:S210–S213

Rudnick MR, Goldfarb S, Wexler L, Ludbrook PA, Murphy MJ, Halpern EF, Hill JA, Winniford M, Cohen MB, VanFessen DB (1995) Nephrotoxicity of ionic and non-ionic contrast media in 1196 patients: a randomized trial. Kidney Int 47:254–261

Saxton HM (1989) Opacification of collecting ducts at urography. Radiology 170:16–17

Schwab SJ, Hlatky MA, Pieper KS, Davidson CJ, Morris KJ, Skelton TN, Bashore TM (1989) Contrast nephrotoxicity: a randomized controlled trial of a non-ionic and an ionic radiographic contrast agent. N Engl J Med 320:149–153

Silvay-Mandeau OM, Meissner C, Wenzel-Hora BI (1995) Clinical safety assessment of iotrolan 280 in European clinical trials. Eur Radiol (Suppl 2) 5:S85–S88

Spataro RF (1984) Newer contrast agents for urography. Radiol Clin North Am 22:365–380

Spataro RF, Katzberg RW, Fisher HW, McMannis MJ (1987) High-dose clinical urography with the low-osmolality contrast agent Hexabrix: comparison with a conventional contrast agent. Radiology 162:9–14

Speck U (1994a) Principles and aims of preclinical testing. Invest Radiol 29 (Suppl 1):515–520

Speck U (1994b) Physicochemical properties of contrast media: osmotic pressure, viscosity, solubility, lipophilicity, hydrophilicity, electrical charge. In: Dawson P, Clauss W (eds) Contrast media in practice. Springer, Berlin Heidelberg New York, pp 20–26

Stacul F, Spinazzi A (1997) Is it possible to choose the safest contrast media through the results of clinical studies? Eur Radiol 7:532–533

Stacul F, Cova M, Assante M, Hougens Grynne B, Halder T (1998) Comparison between the efficacy of dimeric and monomeric non-ionic contrast media (iodixanol vs iopromide) in urography in patients with mild to moderate renal insufficiency. Br J Radiol 71:918–922

Stacul F, Thomsen H (1996) Non ionic monomers and dimers. Eur Radiol 6:756–761

Sundgren PC, Baath L, Tornquist C, Hougens Grynne B, Kjaersgaard P, Almen T (1996) Image quality and safety after iodixanol in intravenous urography; a comparison with iohexol. Br J Radiol 69:699–703

Taliercio CP, Vliestra RE, Ilstrup DM, Burnett JC, Menke KK, Stensrud SL, Holmes DR (1991) A randomized comparison of the nephrotoxicity of iopamidol and diatrizoate in high risk patients undergoing cardiac angiography. J Am Coll Cardiol 17:384–390

Thompson WM, Foster WL Jr, Halvorsen RN, Dunnick NR, Rommel HJ, Bates M (1984) Iopamidol: new non ionic contrast agent for excretory urography. AJR 142:329–332

Thomsen HS (1994) Universal use of low-osmolar contrast media: a European perspective. Acad Radiol 1:295–297

Tveit K, Bolz KD, Bolstad B, Haugland T, Berg KJ, Skjaerpe T, Kloster YF (1994) Iodixanol in cardioangiography. A double-blind parallel comparison between iodixanol 320 mg I/ml and ioxaglate 320 mg I/ml. Acta Radiol 35:614–618

Ueda J, Nygren A, Hansell P, Ulfendahl HR (1993) Effect of intravenous contrast media on proximal and distal tubular hydrostatic pressure in the rat kidney. Acta Radiol 34:83–87

Wolf GL, Arenson RL, Cross AP (1989) A prospective trial of ionic vs nonionic contrast agents in routine clinical practice: comparison of adverse effects. AJR 152:939–944

7 Clinical Doses of Contrast Media

R.A. OLDER

CONTENTS

7.1 Introduction

Iodinated contrast media are used in a multitude of examinations, intravenously, intra-arterially, intrathecally, directly into various anatomic structures such as the gastrointestinal tract, urinary tract, or joint spaces, and into abnormal structures such as fistulous communications. The majority of the discussion in this chapter will relate to procedures in which the contrast material is administered intravenously, which is the most common route of administration. Angiographic doses will be presented in chart form.

Currently, the most common use of intravenous iodinated contrast material is for computed tomography (CT). Excretory urography, although not used as often as previously, is also a major indication for intravenous contrast material.

Factors important in determining contrast media dose are:

1. What dose is effective
2. What is the cost of this dose
3. What is the toxicity, if any, of this dose

R.A. OLDER, MD, Professor of Radiology and Urology, University of Virginia, Health Sciences Center, Department of Radiology, Box 170, Charlottesville, VA 22908, USA

There is no significant difference in the optimal dose for a particular study whether high-osmolality or low-osmolality contrast media (HOCM and LOCM, respectively) are used. There has, however, been a significant cost differential, with LOCM to HOCM cost ratios as high as 20:1. This has led to selective use policies for LOCM as well as methods to reduce the amount of LOCM for a particular study without reducing its effectiveness. These dose reduction methods are included in this chapter, but it is likely that they will be less of an issue by the time this chapter is in print. Recent changes in pricing have reduced the cost ratio to approximately 5:1 (PALMISANO 1997; RADENSKY and CAHILL 1997). Whether or not there remains an impetus to reduce LOCM doses to below the HOCM levels will depend on a balance between costs and available funds.

7.2 Excretory Urography

7.2.1 High-Osmolality Contrast Media

To produce a satisfactory urogram sufficient iodine is needed to provide visualization of both the renal parenchyma and the collecting structures. Excessive contrast, however, is to be avoided because of the potential for contrast nephrotoxicity. The easiest method of establishing contrast dose is to consider grams of iodine. This allows comparison of multiple contrast products having varying concentrations and available in differing sizes. For a patient who weighs approximately 150 lb (68 kg) a recommended contrast dose is 20–22 g of iodine. This is a well-established dose, which has changed little over the past 20 years (MCCLENNAN 1978, 1988). Because of similarities in concentration the three most commonly used HOCM for urography would yield this 20- to 22-g dose with essentially the same volume. Hypaque 60, Renografin 60, and Conray 60 would produce 21 or 22 g of iodine with a 75-ml dose (Table

Table 7.1. HOCM dose for excretory urography in a 150-lb patient

Product	ml	Iodine (g)	ml/lb
Hypaque 50 (diatrizoate) (Nycomed)	75	22.5	0.5
Renografin 60 (diatrizoate) (Bracco)	75	21.9	0.5
Conray 60 (iothalamate) (Mallinckrodt)	75	21.2	0.5
Conray 400 (iothalamate) (Mallinckrodt)	50	20.0	0.33

7.1). Although the standard dose of 75 ml will suffice for most adult patients, adjustments can be made for extremely small or large patients. As is seen from Table 7.1, the dose per body weight is 0.5 ml per lb for the commonly used agents and this can be used in making adjuxtments.

7.2.2
Low-Osmolality Contrast Media

A dose of approximately 22 g of iodine is considered optimal for LOCM as well as HOCM (Table 7.2). Initially, LOCM were marketed primarily in 50-ml vials for urography, producing a 25 ml waste of contrast if only 75 ml was given. One hundred milliliters, therefore, was often used, which gave approximately 30 g of iodine.

From a diagnostic and toxicity standpoint this was not a problem and produced excellent studies. However, 100 ml of LOCM did add significant cost to an examination, leading several authors to evaluate the effectiveness of a 50-ml dose, which would provide approximately 15 g of iodine. Gavant et al. (1992) found a 50-ml dose of iohexol to produce adequate examinations with no overall diagnostic difference. The smaller dose, however, did produce a decrease in both the nephrographic and the ureteral phases of the study when compared with larger doses of either iohexol or diatrizoate, which were based on body weight (Gavant et al. 1992). Others also found that lower doses of LOCM could be used in urography with satisfactory studies being obtained, but did acknowledge lower quality in some aspects of the examination (Kennan et al. 1990). Our own experience was that a 50-ml dose of Omnipaque 300 was inconsistent in opacification of the collecting structures. This may have been related to the lack of consistent fluid restriction prior to examinations, but lack of fluid restriction is now common.

Table 7.2 LOCM dose for excretory urography in a 150-lb patient

Product	ml	Iodine (g)	ml/lb
Omnipaque 300 (iohexol) (Nycomed)	75	22.5	0.5
Optiray 320 (ioversol) (Mallinckrodt)	75	24	0.5
Isovue 300 (iopamidol) (Bracco)	75	22.5	0.5
Omnipaque 350 (iohexol) (Nycomed)	66	23.1	0.44
Ultravist 300 (iopromide) (Berlex)	75	22.5	0.5
Oxilan 300 (ioxilan) (Cook)	75	22.5	0.5
Visipaque 320 (iodixanol) (Nycomed)	75	24	0.5

Multiple forms of contrast packaging for LOCM are now available and provide greater flexibility in dosage without waste. A single multiuse bag of Omnipaque 350 can provide three 23-g (66-ml) doses at a unit cost similar to a 15-g dose from a single-use vial. At the time of writing, the 23-g dose of Omnipaque 350 costs approximately $23 at the University of Virginia, a marked decrease from just a few years ago. If, therefore, there were financial constraints our recommendation would be to maintain the standard recommended dose of approximately 22 g of iodine through the use of a higher concentration (350 mg I/ml) and multiusage packaging.

7.3
Abdominal Computed Tomography

As with urography, the best way to consider contrast dosage for CT is in terms of grams of iodine. This allows easy cross-comparison of multiple products with varying concentrations. Unlike urography, in which a standard dose has been accepted for many years, there is considerable controversy regarding contrast dose and methods of administration for abdominal CT. Changing technology with evolution from dynamic nonspiral CT to spiral CT further complicates this. As with urography, both HOCM and LOCM are used. For the HOCM, there is little cost concern and strategies can be developed strictly on the basis of optimal visualization of abdominal structures. For LOCM cost is still a consideration in some countries and multiple articles have compared dosages to determine whether dose reduction can be achieved without significant loss in diagnostic information. As the cost of LOCM continues to decline, dose reduction strategies will be less of an issue.

As expected, larger doses of HOCM and LOCM, in terms of grams of iodine, have been found to produce better visualization of the abdominal structures and in particular greater enhancement of the liver, which is often used as the determining criterion (ALLEN et al. 1994; BREE et al. 1994; FREENY et al. 1995). A dose of 45–48 g of iodine is generally used as the maximal dose or gold standard against which other doses are compared (ALLEN et al. 1994; BREE et al. 1994; FREENY et al. 1995). If there is no significant concern regarding either cost or toxicity, the optimal dose would be in this range. HOCM typically have 28–30 g of iodine per 100 ml. Any of these media (Table 7.1), therefore, would give a total dose of 42–45 g of iodine for a 150-ml dose. This is a reasonable choice for HOCM.

Because LOCM have fewer side-effects they are preferred for CT, especially when rapid injection rates are used. There is no difference in optimal dose if cost is not a consideration. It is, however, cost which has motivated many authors to develop reduced dosage schedules for LOCM. BREE et al. (1994) used quantitative and qualitative analysis to establish the best contrast dose during *nonspiral* scanning as 44–45 g of iodine. Quantitative analysis was obtained with hepatic enhancement measurements. Doses of 44 g (125 ml iohexol 350) and 45 g (150 ml iohexol 300) gave the highest average enhancement of approximately 50 Hounsfield units. Doses in the 35–37 g range gave variable results depending on the combination of volume and concentration used. Studies using a 240 mg I/ml contrast media were not satisfactory regardless of the total grams of iodine. These authors concluded that the appropriate dose would be 125 ml of iohexol 350, which would yield 44 g of iodine and be slightly less expensive than 150 ml of iohexol 300 (BREE et al. 1994).

CHAMBERS et al. (1994a) compared differing volumes of Isoview 300 in the same patient during *nonspiral* CT and found a substantial decrease in hepatic enhancement when reducing from a 150-ml dose (45 g) to a 100-ml dose (30 g). Increasing the injection rate only partially compensated for this difference (CHAMBERS et al. 1994b). ALLEN et al. (1994) also found doses below 35 g to reduce *nonspiral* study quality. The dose, however, could be decreased from a maximal level of 48 g to 75% of this, 36 g, without significant loss of quality (ALLEN et al. 1994).

FREENY et al. (1995) similarly found that dose reduction below 45–48 g of iodine produced a decrease in hepatic contrast and a decreased contrast enhancement index (CEI) during *spiral* CT. These authors, however, used a large dose reduction by going from 45–48 g to 30–32 g. They did not evaluate the intermediate 36–38 g range.

BRINK et al. (1995) used an increase of 50 Hounsfield units as an acceptable maximal hepatic enhancement to evaluate the feasibility of dose reduction during *spiral* CT. With a uniphasic injection the total iodine dose could be reduced from 44 g to 38 g of iodine without a statistically significant difference in contrast enhancement. For very thin patients a dose as low as 26 g could be used and still exceed the threshold for adequate enhancement of the liver (BRINK et al. 1995). Previous animal models have predicted that the lower limit of contrast dose for *spiral* CT should be approximately 429 mg of iodine per kilogram. Using an average weight of 183 lb (83 kg), which was the average patient weight for Brink's study, a 38-g dose would have produced 457 mg iodine per kilogram and exceeded this predicted level. A suggested dose for heavy patients was 38 g of iodine given as 125 ml of a 300 mg I/ml solution and for thin patients 26 g given as 75 ml of a 350 mg I/ml solution (BRINK et al. 1995). HOEFFEL et al. (1996), using a biphasic injection and *spiral* CT, also found a dose of 37.5 g of iodine to produce acceptable enhancement.

HEIKEN et al. (1995) approached the problem of contrast dose by developing a normogram which took into account both the patient's body weight and the desired mean hepatic enhancement. Using their normogram and selecting 50 Hounsfield units as the desired increased enhancement, the iodine dose for a 150-lb (68-kg) patient would be approximately 35 g of iodine.

The above data show that contrast doses up to 45–48 g of iodine produce the best results in terms of hepatic enhancement. Doses in the 35–38 g range, however, are satisfactory and reasonable to use in order to maintain cost at a level where LOCM can be used more routinely. We use 100 ml of Omnipaque 350, yielding 35 g of iodine, for an abdomen or abdomen/pelvis study. When a chest study is combined with an abdomen and pelvis study, we use the same dose but begin scanning with the chest so that we reach the liver at approximately the optimal time of 70 s.

7.4
Computed Tomography of the Chest

The recommended dose for chest CT varies with the specific question to be answered as well as whether scanning is spiral or nonspiral. In the Roentgen Ray 1994 categorical course on body CT a dose of 120 ml of a 300 mg I/ml contrast (36 g I) was recommended for *spiral* evaluation of the thoracic aorta and 90 ml of 300 mg I/ml contrast (27 g I) for survey studies as well as evaluation of the pulmonary arteries (Foley 1994). A similar dose in terms of iodine (28.8 g I), but using a higher volume (120 ml) of a 240 mg I/ml contrast medium, was also suggested (Sagel 1994). For *nonspiral* studies of the thorax a larger dose of 150 ml of 300 mg I/ml contrast (45 g I) was used as a biphasic injection (Sagel 1994).

As with body CT, dose reduction schedules have been evaluated. Costello et al. (1992) compared a 60-ml dose of 300 mg I/ml contrast (18 g I) during *spiral* CT with 120 ml (36 g I) during *nonspiral* studies. Better results were obtained with the spiral study despite the reduced dose. Storto et al. (1994) found that 70 ml of a 300 mg I/ml nonionic media (21 g) gave satisfactory results when injected at 3 ml/s for *spiral* CT.

Rubin et al. (1996) reduced the dose even further from 22 g of iodine to 15 g. In addition, they diluted the solution either at a 1 : 1 or a 3 : 1 ratio with normal saline. The best results were produced using 15 g of iodine diluted in a 1 : 1 solution. This provided satisfactory visualization of the vascular structures and reduced the perivascular artifact often produced by the very high density contrast material in the central vessels.

Spiral CT, therefore, facilitates a reduction in dose from the 36–45 g range used for *nonspiral* CT to doses of 15–27 g of iodine. For nonionic media use of the lower end of each dose range will result in cost savings. At the University of Virginia 75 cc of Omnipaque 240 (18 g I) is used for a chest CT when not combined with other studies, whereas 100 cc of Omnipaque 350 is used when combined with abdominal CT (Fig. 7.1).

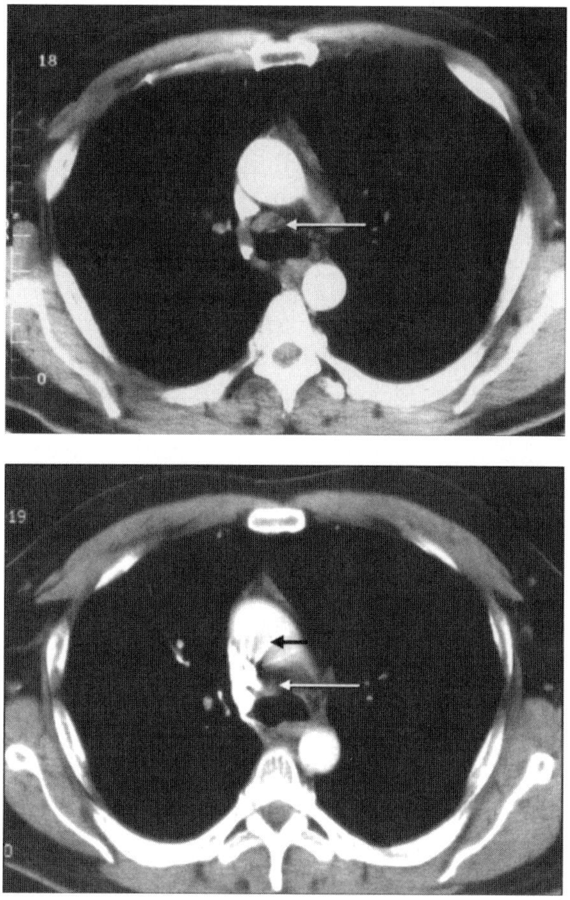
a

b

Fig. 7.1. Comparison of use of 75 cc Omnipaque 240 as part of a chest protocol (**a**) versus a higher dose of 100 cc Omnipaque 350 (**b**) as part of a chest-abdomen protocol. The chest protocol significantly reduces artifact (*black arrow*) and allows better visualization of adjacent soft tissue structures (*white arrows*)

7.5
Computed Tomography of the Head and Neck

7.5.1
Neck

Gay et al. (1991) evaluated dynamic *nonspiral* neck CT with doses ranging from 36 to 55 g of iodine. Although the largest doses scored slightly better, the lowest dose of 36 g produced good to excellent studies. As with abdominal CT, the amount of contrast needed for an examination is generally reduced by using spiral CT. Spiral CT doses can be reduced to 27 g of iodine and still give excellent results (Foley 1994; Suojanen et al. 1992). For routine neck examinations at the University of Virginia we use 24 g I given as 100 ml of Omnipaque 240 (Table 7.3).

Table 7.3. Contrast dose for neuro-CT[a]

Examination	Contrast	Total volume (ml)
Head	Omnipaque 350	100
Neck	Omnipaque 240	100
Neck/extracranial CTA	Omnipaque 350	125
Intracranial CTA	Omnipaque 350	125
Spine	Omnipaque 350	100

CTA, Computed tomographic angiography.
[a] Derived from protocols at the University of Virginia.

7.5.2 Head

Hammer et al. (1995) evaluated four dose regimens of ioversol 320 for enhanced cranial CT: 50 ml (16 g I), 75 ml (24 g I), 100 ml (32 g I), and 120 ml (38 g I). No significant difference in vessel enhancement was seen between 100 and 120 ml, but there was a statistically significant increase between 75 and 100 ml. 100 ml (32 g I) was considered the optimal dose for most patients. Lower doses, although satisfactory for vessel enhancement, may not be as effective in detecting intracranial lesions such as multiple sclerosis and higher doses may be needed in these patients if MRI cannot be performed (Hammer et al. 1995). For intracranial studies at the University of Virginia we use 100 cc of Omnipaque 350 (35 g I) (Table 7.3), a dose comparable to the higher dose levels used by Hammer et al. (1995).

7.6 Pediatric Dose

Because of the weight variability of children of different ages, doses for all studies are typically weight based. For contrast media with an iodine concentration of approximately 300 mg/ml the intravenous dose for excretory urography is 1 ml per lb (2 ml/kg) up to 50 ml (Smith and Franken 1992). The dose is essentially the same for CT. In a comparison of HOCM and LOCM in children undergoing multiple types of CT a standard dose of 2.2 ml/kg was used for all studies (Cohen et al. 1992). Roche et al. (1996) used a 2 ml/kg dose of ioversol (320 mg I/ml) in developing injection protocols for spiral and nonspiral CT.

Table 7.4. Angiographic contrast dose: arterial-body[a]

Examination	Contrast	Total volume (ml)
Abdominal midstream	Omnipaque 350	40
Abdominal midstream AAA	Omnipaque 350	60
Celiac	Omnipaque 350	60
Femoral runoff	Omnipaque 350	90–120
Gastroduodenal	Omnipaque 350	15–20
Hepatic	Omnipaque 350	20–25
Inferior mesenteric	Omnipaque 350	24–32
Inferior vena cava	Omnipaque 350	40
Pelvis (transplant and stenosis)	Omnipaque 350	45
Pulmonary (main)	Omnipaque 350	70
Pulmonary selective	Omnipaque 350	40–50
Renal selective	Omnipaque 350	10–15
Thoracic aortogram (arch)	Omnipaque 350	70–80

[a] Derived from protocols at the University of Virginia.

Table 7.5. Angiographic contrast dose: venous[a]

Examination	Contrast	Total volume (ml)
Arm venogram (lower)	Omnipaque 300	50
Leg venogram	100 ml Omnipaque 350 mixed with 50 ml normal saline	150
Superior vena cava (upper arm venogram)	Omnipaque 300	50, each arm

[a] Derived from protocols at the University of Virginia.

Table 7.6. Neuroangiographic contrast dose: digital subtraction angiography[a]

Examination	Contrast	Total volume (mL)	Rate (mL/s)
Arch aortogram	Iohexol 300	30	15
Common carotid	Iohexol 300	9	7
Internal carotid	Iohexol 300	8	6
Vertebral	Iohexol 300	7	5

[a] Derived from protocols at the University of Virginia.

7.7 Angiographic Studies

Because of the wide range of injection rates and dosage schedules for adult angiographic procedures I have included these in chart form based on the dosage schedules at the University of Virginia (A. Matsumoto, personal communication). Doses for these specialized procedures are operator dependent and the charts serve only as a guideline (Tables 7.4–7.6).

References

Allen DA, Stoupis C, Torres G, Call GA, Litwiller TL, Ros PR (1994) Dose optimization of nonionic contrast agent in dynamic computed tomography scanning of the abdomen and pelvis. Clinical Imaging 18:72–74

Bree RL, Parisky YR, Bernardino ME, Costello PH, Leder R, Brown PC (1994) Cost-effective use of low-osmolality contrast media for CT of the liver: evaluation of liver enhancement provided by various doses of iohexol. AJR 163:579–583

Brink JA, Heiken JP, Forman HP, Sagel SS, Molina PL, Brown PC (1995) Hepatic spiral CT: reduction of dose of intravenous contrast material. Radiology 197:83–88

Chambers TP, Baron RL, Lush RM (1994a) Hepatic CT enhancement. I. Alterations in the volume of contrast material within the same patients. Radiology 193:513–517

Chambers TP, Baron RL, Lush RM (1994b) Hepatic CT enhancement. II. Alterations in contrast material volume and rate of injection within the same patients. Radiology 193:518–522

Cohen MD, Herman E, Herron D, White SJ, Smith JA (1992) Comparison of intravenous contrast agents for CT studies in children. Acta Radiol 33:592–595

Costello P, Dupuy DE, Ecker CP, Tello R (1992) Spiral CT of the thorax with reduced volume of contrast material: a comparative study. Radiology 183:663–666

Foley WD (1994) Technology/contrast: current state of the art. In: American Roentgen Ray Society body CT categorical course syllabus. April, pp 1–4

Freeny PC, Gardner JC, vonIngersleben G, Heyano S, Nghiem HV, Winter TC (1995) Hepatic helical CT: effect of reduction of iodine dose of intravenous contrast material on hepatic contrast enhancement. Radiology 197:89–93

Gavant ML, Ellis JV, Klesges ML (1992) Diagnostic efficacy of excretory urography with low-dose, nonionic contrast media. Radiology 182:657–660

Gay SB, Pevarski DR, Phillips CD, Levine PA (1991) Dynamic CT of the neck. Radiology 180:284–285

Hammer G, Kuhn MJ, Meis DM, Meis LC (1995) Quantitative contrast media dose evaluation for cranial computed tomography. Comput Med Imaging Graph 19:287–293

Heiken JP, Brink JA, McClennan BL, Sagel SS, Crowe TM, Gaines MV (1995) Dynamic incremental CT: effect of volume and concentration of contrast material and patient weight on hepatic enhancement. Radiology 195:353–357

Hoeffel C, Legmann P, Girardot C, Bunoff P, Mezzi K, Bonnin A (1996) Contrast material injection for hepatic helical computed tomography. Invest Radiol 31:467–471

Kennan RJ, List A, Kengsakul C (1990) Low dose intravenous urography: results and technique modifications. Australas Radiol 34:137–141

McClennan BL (1978) Syllabus categorical course in genitourinary tract radiology. Radiology Society of North America, Chicago, November 26-December 1

McClennan BL (1988) Urography: anatomy and technique. In: Puttman CE, Raven CE (eds) Textbook of diagnostic imaging. Saunders, Philadelphia, pp 1161–1168

Palmisano SM (1997) Low-osmolality contrast media in the 1900s: prices change. Radiology 203:309–315

Radensky PW, Cahill NE (1997) Universal use of low-osmolality contrast media for the 1990s. Radiology 203: 310–311

Roche RJ, Genieser NB, Ambrosino MM (1996) Pediatric hepatic CT: an injection protocol. Pediatr Radiol 26:502–507

Rubin GD, Lane MJ, Bloch DA, Leung AN, Stark P (1996) Optimization of thoracic spiral CT: effects of iodinated contrast medium concentration. Radiology 201:785–791

Sagel SS (1994) CT of vascular mediastinal lesions. American Roentgen Ray Society body CT categorical course syllabus. April, pp 29–35

Smith WL, Franken EA (1992) Pediatric contrast agents. In: Katzberg RW (ed) The contrast media manual. Williams & Wilkins, Baltimore, pp 207–221

Storto ML, Ciccotosto C, Patea RL, Spinazzi A, Bonomo L (1994) Spiral CT of the mediastinum: optimization of contrast medium use. Eur J Radiol 18 (Suppl 1):S83–S87

Suojanen JN, Mukherji SK, Dupuy DE, Takahashi JH, Costello P (1992) Spiral CT in evaluation of head and neck lesions: work in progress. Radiology 183:281–283

8 Determination of Glomerular Filtration Rate with Contrast Media

T. ALMÉN, B. FRENNBY, and G. STERNER

CONTENTS

T. ALMÉN, MD, PhD, Professor emeritus, Institute of Diagnostic Radiology, Malmö University Hospital, S-20502 Malmö, Sweden

B. FRENNBY, MD, PhD, Department of Diagnostic Radiology, Malmö University Hospital, S-20502 Malmö, Sweden

G. STERNER, MD, PhD, Division of Nephrology, Department of Vascular and Renal Diseases, Malmö University Hospital, S-20502 Malmö, Sweden

8.1 Introduction

The review concerns the trend toward using nonradioactive contrast media as markers of glomerular filtration when determining the glomerular filtration rate (GFR). Scientific papers comparing contrast media and other markers of GFR are reviewed, as are papers comparing different techniques for the determination of GFR.

8.1.1 History of Contrast Media for Urography

Urography was born in the late 1920s when Swick injected some iodinated organic compounds intravenously in urology patients and found that within a few minutes one of the compounds had reached a high concentration in the renal pelvis and calyces, which became visible on x-ray films (SWICK 1929). In the preceding years a group of chemists headed by BINZ had synthesized the iodine compounds used by SWICK for the purpose of creating chemotherapeutic agents (BINZ 1937).

Since the 1950s research on contrast media for urography has been focused on compounds with three iodine atoms covalently bound to a benzene ring. The intention has been to minimize both their toxicity and their binding to plasma proteins. The media thus created have a plasma clearance dominated by glomerular filtration, while their tubular excretion and reabsorption and also their extrarenal plasma clearance are small. The pharmacokinetic profile of the urographic contrast media has thus been similar to those of conventional markers for the determination of GFR, such as inulin. Consequently the media developed for urography, first the ionic monomers and dimers, created in the 1950s–70s, and then the nonionic monomers and dimers, created in the 1970s–90s, have pharmacokinetic properties that allow their use for both urography and determination of GFR.

8.1.2 Indications for the Determination of GFR

To preserve GFR is an important task for nephrologists and urologists, who need repeated measurements of GFR to evaluate the degree of renal disease and follow its course. Furthermore, GFR is determined in order to assist in the selection of a proper dosage of pharmaceuticals with mainly glomerular excretion. Due to the great need for GFR determination, method(s) for this purpose should be simple to perform, be accurate, and have a low risk of adverse effects. Simple methods, such as determinations of serum creatinine and also renal creatinine clearance, which requires urine collection, may not be sufficiently accurate in all clinical situations (see Sect. 8.2.2). Other GFR methods which require long intravenous infusions of marker and in addition control of possible residual urine with ultrasound or bladder catheterization may be too cumbersome to be commonly used. Therefore much effort has gone into creating new methods with the right combination of simplicity and accuracy for various clinical situations.

8.1.3 Radioactive Urographic Contrast Media for Determining GFR

The main use of the ionic monomeric contrast media, such as diatrizoate, iothalamate, metrizoate, iodamide, and ioxythalamate, has been for diagnostic imaging, such as urography, angiography, and computed tomography (CT). For GFR determinations, radioactive media, such as diatrizoate and iothalamate labeled with iodine-125 and iodine-131, were introduced in the 1960s and are still commonly used in many countries because their concentrations in plasma and urine are easily measured in scintillation counters. Some early and later references on their use include: Morris et al. (1965), Sigman et al. (1965a,b), Nosslin (1965), Elwood et al. (1967), Hall and Rolin (1995), and Blaufox et al. (1996).

8.1.4 Nonradioactive Urographic Contrast Media for Determining GFR

In recent years there has been a trend towards using nonlabeled media, especially the nonionic monomer iohexol, to determine GFR. Other nonionic monomers, such as iobitridol, iomeprol, iopamidol, ioversol, and iopromide, may be assumed to be equally effective as GFR markers due to their similar pharmacokinetics. The reasons behind this trend are:

1. Simple and practical methods have been created to measure the concentration of iohexol in urine and plasma, including high-performance liquid chromatography (HPLC), using the absorbance of the exo- and endoforms of iohexol (Krutzén et al. 1984), or x-ray fluorescence analysis, using the characteristic radiation of the iodine atoms of the contrast medium when irradiated from an americium-241 source (Guesry et al. 1975; Grönberg 1981a,b).
2. The radiation dose to pregnant women (Krutzén et al. 1992) and children (Stake et al. 1989, 1990, 1991a,b; Stake and Monclair 1991; Stake 1992) can be decreased by using a nonradioactive GFR marker, whose concentration in plasma and urine is easy to analyze with the above methods.
3. It is more comfortable for the patients to receive only one dose of contrast medium for the dual purposes of diagnostic imaging (such as angiography, urography, or computed tomography) *and* measurement of GFR in the same clinical setting (Sjöberg et al. 1987; Boijsen 1988; Boijsen et al. 1987, 1988a,b; Stake et al. 1989, 1990, 1991a; Stake and Monclair 1991; Stake 1992; Effersöe et al. 1990; Thomsen et al. 1991, 1992a,b; Thomsen and Hvid-Jakobsen 1991; Frennby et al. 1995a; Lundqvist et al. 1994, 1996, 1997; Lundqvist 1997).

8.2 Techniques for Determining GFR

8.2.1 Terminology

Pharmacokinetically, blood, plasma, interstitial fluid, and intracellular fluid are examples of "compartments." Pharmacokinetics deals, inter alia, with measurements of the rates at which various pharmaceuticals are cleared from (removed from) anatomical or functional compartments. The clearance (ml/min) of a substance from a compartment (for example plasma) is defined as the ratio between the elimination rate (mg/min) of the substance from the compartment and the concentration (mg/ml) of the substance in that compartment (plasma) (MÖLLER et al. 1928), i.e., the clearance in this case becomes a virtual volume of plasma (ml) which in 1 min is completely cleared of the substance.

The GFR concerns the filtration of the compartment plasma through the glomeruli, which results in accumulation of the primary filtrate in Bowman's space. This filtration clears plasma of waste products and also of endogenous and exogenous GFR markers. If a substance is an ideal GFR marker (see Sect. 8.2.2) its clearance from plasma in ml/min becomes equal to the GFR in ml/min.

The definition of a clearance technique (according to tradition in pharmacokinetics) may require:

1. Definition of the compartment that is cleared (in GFR determinations that compartment is plasma).
2. Definition of the marker being cleared [inulin, chromium-51 ethylene diamine tetra-acetic acid (EDTA), technetium-99m diethylene triamine penta-acetic acid (DTPA), ^{131}I-iothalamate, iohexol, etc.].
3. The name of the organ(s) that participate(s) in the *technique chosen for the measurement* of the clearance. (The name "renal" may be used when *both* the plasma concentrations of marker *and also* the excretion rate (mg/min) of marker by the kidneys into the urine have been measured. The name "total" or "body" may be used when *only* the decrease in plasma concentrations of marker over time has been measured and consequently all the organs of the body might have contributed to that decrease in plasma concentration of marker.)
4. A description of the technique for injecting the marker (bolus injection, infusion), the timing of the plasma samples, and the method for determining the concentration of marker.

The GFR (ml/min) is determined with two different techniques. The present text describes those techniques according to tradition in nephrology and urology. The term *plasma clearance* is used when only plasma concentrations of a GFR marker have been determined and the dose of the GRF marker is known (other terms are total plasma clearance or body clearance). The term *renal clearance* is used when both plasma concentrations and urinary excretion rate of the GFR marker have been determined (another term is renal plasma clearance). GFR is expressed as ml min^{-1} 1.73 m^{-2}, which means the production of primary urine (ml) per minute normalized to 1.73 m^2 body surface.

8.2.2 Markers for Determining GFR

When determining GFR with *renal clearance* techniques the markers should be filtered through the glomeruli and have minimal binding to plasma proteins, minimal tubular reabsorption, and minimal tubular excretion. When determining GFR with *plasma clearance* techniques the markers should in addition have minimal extrarenal excretion. The most common methods of estimating GFR utilize the endogenous GFR marker creatinine. GFR is then evaluated from the plasma concentration of creatinine alone or from its renal clearance, calculated as the ratio between creatinine excretion rate in urine and creatinine plasma concentration. Due to its high tubular excretion in man, creatinine is a suboptimal GFR marker for clinical use. HOOD et al. (1971), SHEMESH et al. (1985), and GABRIEL (1986) have shown that, even at a moderately reduced GFR (30–60 ml min^{-1}1.73 m^{-2}), measurement of serum creatinine alone or measurement of the renal clearance of creatinine may overestimate "true GFR" by 50%–100% when the "true GFR" has been measured as renal clearance of an exogenous GFR marker without tubular excretion. Use of creatinine as a sole marker for determining GFR in patients with glomerular disease is "no longer justifiable in a research setting and is suboptimal in many clinical settings" (SHEMESH et al. 1985).

Examples of exogenous GFR markers are: (a) polysaccharides such as inulin and labeled inulin: (b) water-soluble labeled chelates such as ^{51}Cr-EDTA and ^{99m}Tc-DTPA; (c) urographic contrast media labeled with a radioactive isotope, such as ^{131}I-diatrizoate and ^{131}I-iothalamate, and (d) nonlabeled urographic contrast media such as ionic monomers (diatrizoate, iothalamate, or others) and nonionic monomers (iohexol, iopamidol, iopromide, or others).

8.2.3 Pharmacokinetic Models

Immediately after an intravenous bolus injection of a GFR marker, for example a urographic contrast

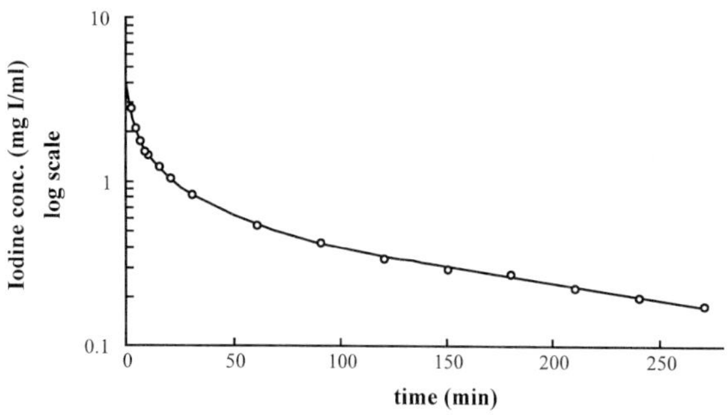

Fig. 8.1. In this subject each *small circle* represents a measured plasma concentration of iohexol as iodine (*vertical axis*, logarithmic scale) following an intravenous bolus injection of the contrast medium. Sixteen plasma samples were taken between 2 and 270 min after injection, as shown along the *horizontal axis* (linear scale). The same measurements are shown in Fig. 8.2–8.4

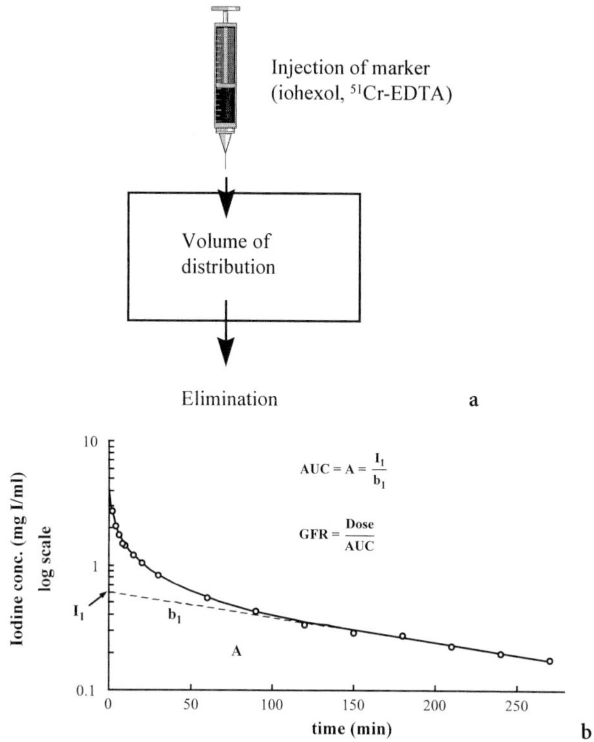

Fig. 8.2. a One-compartment kinetic model. **b** The plasma concentration of iohexol as a function of time (t) according to a one-compartment model constructed from the *dashed line* based on the four last plasma samples in the period 180–240 min after bolus injection of iohexol. The one-compartment model is mathematically described as one exponential function. $b1$ is the elimination rate constant (min^{-1}) of the GFR marker and I_1 (mg I/ml/) is the corresponding intercept on the *ordinate*. Plasma concentration of marker = $I_1\ e^{-b1\ t}$. *AUC*, Area under the curve. It is obvious that in the first 2 h after injection the measured plasma concentrations of marker (*small circles*) are far above the plasma concentration used by the one-compartment model (*dashed line*). Therefore a one-compartment model markedly overestimates clearance/GFR at high GFR levels

medium (a nonionic monomer), the plasma concentration reaches a rapid peak followed by an exponential fall (Fig. 8.1) as the medium is diluted in the circulating plasma and starts to diffuse into the extravascular space. About 70% of the injected dose may leave the plasma within 2–5 min after the injection. During the diffusion of contrast medium molecules from the plasma to the extracellular space there is a simultaneous diffusion of extracellular water (and also some contrast medium molecules) back into the plasma and an equilibrium between the intra- and extravascular fluid is slowly established. At equilibrium there is a similar concentration of contrast medium in the vascular compartment and in the extravascular compartments close to the vascular space. As the contrast medium continues to be excreted through the kidneys its concentration in the vascular space decreases and there will then be a net diffusion of contrast medium molecules from the extravascular to the vascular space.

In man, almost complete equilibration between plasma and interstitial space (sometimes named distribution) takes about 2 h at normal renal function. In patients with impaired renal function, it may take 3 h or more for equilibrium to be reached after an intravenous injection (Effersöe et al. 1990). A small fraction (<5%) of the injected contrast medium may enter "deeper compartments" and may even reach intracellular organelles in certain tissues (liver, kidney). The last few percent of the injected dose leaves the body relatively slowly (Olsson et al. 1983; Nordby et al. 1990).

In the field of pharmacokinetics mathematical models are often used to describe the distribution of a substance inside the body and its elimination from the body. For a mathematical description of changes in the plasma concentration of a GFR marker which occur in a patient or an experimental animal after an intravascular injection of the marker, the body has been divided into compartments (Figs. 8.2–8.4). The plasma concentration of marker following a bolus injection can be described (calculated) according to a one-, two-, three-, or multicompartment model (Nosslin 1965; Bröchner-Mortensen 1972; Sapirstein et al. 1955). One may consider such compartments more as mathematical tools than as defined anatomical entities. Each compartment is mathematically described as containing a marker which is already uniformly distributed at the moment of the end of injection of the marker. This early uniform theoretical concentration of marker in a compartment is described in Figs. 8.2–8.4 by the in-

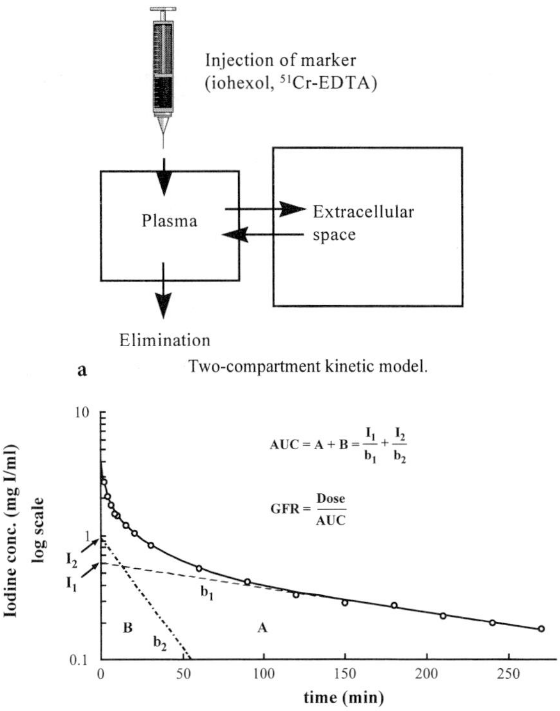

Fig. 8.3. **a** Two-compartment kinetic model. **b** The plasma concentration of iohexol as a function of time (t) based on all 16 measurements in the period 2–270 min after bolus injection of iohexol. The two-compartment model is mathematically described as the sum of two exponential functions. The elimination rate constants of the two compartments are $b1$ and $b2$ and the corresponding intercepts on the ordinate are $\mathbf{I}_1$ and $\mathbf{I}_2$ (mg I/ml). Plasma concentration of marker = $\mathbf{I}_1\, e^{-b1\,t} + \mathbf{I}_2\, e^{-b2\,t}$. *AUC*, Area under the curve

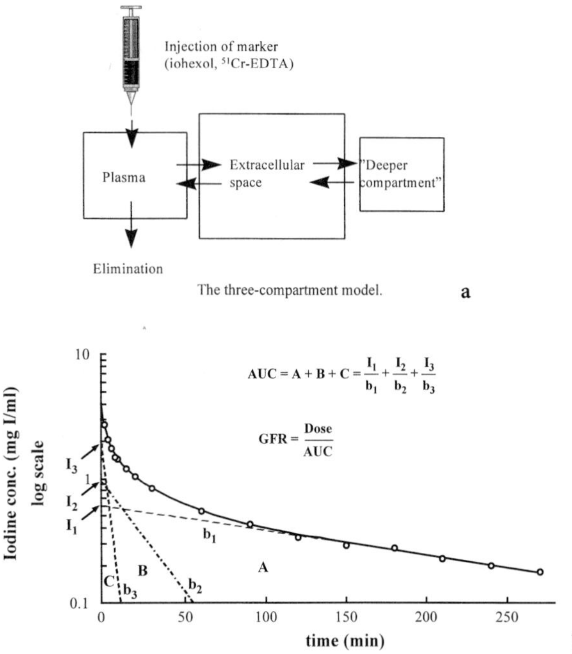

Fig. 8.4. **a** Three-compartment model. **b** The plasma concentration of iohexol as a function of time (t) based on all 16 measurements in the period 2–270 min after bolus injection of iohexol. The three-compartment model is mathematically described as the sum of three exponential functions. The elimination rate constants of the three compartments are $b1$, $b2$, and $b3$ and the corresponding intercepts on the ordinate are $\mathbf{I}_1$, $\mathbf{I}_2$, and $\mathbf{I}_3$ (mg I/ml). Plasma concentration of marker = $\mathbf{I}_1\, e^{-b1\,t} + \mathbf{I}_2\, e^{-b2\,t} + \mathbf{I}_3\, e^{-b3\,t}$. *AUC*, Area under the curve

tercept on the ordinate (vertical axis) and is symbolized by **I**, which for the contrast media has the unit [mg I (iodine)/ml]. At time t [the number of minutes after injection of GFR marker (Figs. 8.2–8.4)] the concentration of marker in a compartment (C_{comp}) in mg I/ml becomes $C_{comp} = \mathbf{I}\, e^{-b\,t}$, where b is an elimination rate constant of the marker (min^{-1}) from the compartment.

According to a *one-compartment* model the marker is injected into one compartment and is excreted from only that compartment. The marker has no communication with other spaces (Fig. 8.2a). The concentration of GFR marker (contrast medium) immediately after the end of injection (the intercept on the ordinate) is $\mathbf{I}_1$ (mg I/ml). The concentration of GFR marker (contrast medium) in that compartment (Fig. 8.2b) at time t (minutes after injection of marker) is equal to the value of *one* exponential function $\mathbf{I}_1\, e^{-b1\,t}$ (mg I/ml) ($b1$ is elimination rate constant of the marker from this compartment). The integral of this function from time of injection to infinity [the area under this concentration curve (Fig. 8.2b)] becomes $\mathbf{I}_1/b1$. It is obvious that the area under the dotted line in Fig. 8.2b (the area representing the one-compartment model and based on the last four plasma samples in Fig. 8.2b) is much smaller than the area under the real concentration curve, the uninterrupted line in Figs. 8.1 and 8.2b. Therefore, mathematical correction factors have been introduced (see Sect. 8.2.9) (Bröchner-Mortensen 1972).

The *two-compartment* model makes the assumption that immediately after injection the marker is distributed into one central compartment (plasma) and one peripheral compartment (extravascular space) with a larger volume (Fig. 8.3a). An intravenously injected marker can transfer between the plasma and the extracellular space. The elimination of the marker from the body is from plasma. In this model the plasma concentration of marker is mathematically described as the sum of *two* exponential functions with different elimination rate constants ($b1$ and $b2$) and two different intercepts ($\mathbf{I}_1$ and $\mathbf{I}_2$) (Fig. 8.3b). The concentration of GFR marker at t min ($C_{(t)}$) after injection of is $C_{(t)} = \mathbf{I}_1\, e^{-b1\,t} + \mathbf{I}_2\, e^{-b2\,t}$.

The area under this concentration curve (the integral of the previous curve from injection to infinity) becomes $I_1/b1 + I_2/b2$ (Fig. 8.3b). GFR = dose of contrast medium/area of concentration curve of marker from time of injection to infinity (Fig. 8.3b).

In the *three-compartment* kinetic model there is a communication of the intravenously injected marker from plasma not only with the extracellular space but also from the extracellular space to "deeper compartments" and from the deeper compartments back to the extracellular space and plasma. The elimination of the marker from the body is only from plasma (Fig. 8.4a). Mathematically this can be described by the sum of *three* exponential functions with different elimination rate constants ($b1$, $b2$, $b3$) and three intercepts (I_1, I_2, I_3) (Fig. 8.4b). In this model plasma concentration of the GFR marker at time t min ($C_{(t)}$) after injection of marker is $C_{(t)} = I_1 e^{-b1t} + I_2 e^{-b2t} + I_3 e^{-b3t}$. The area under this concentration curve (the integral of the previous function from time of injection to infinity) becomes $I_1/b1 + I_2/b2 + I_3/b3$ (Fig. 8.4b). Similarly, GFR = dose of contrast medium divided by area under the concentration curve of marker from time of injection to infinity. [A summary may be found in Frennby (1996, 1997).]

8.2.4 Techniques for Injection of GFR Marker

The different GFR techniques vary with regard to the injection and the sampling of the various exogenous GFR markers.

Intravenous infusion of the GFR marker to an almost *constant plasma concentration* has the effect that the disappearance rate of marker from plasma almost equals the infusion rate of marker. When measuring GFR with the renal clearance technique "the amount of marker (in gram) collected in the urine in a period of X minutes" is divided by "the average plasma concentration of marker (gram/ml), in the period when that amount of marker was filtered through the glomeruli, multiplied with the duration of the period (X minutes)." The latter "expression" is equal to "the area under the plasma concentration curve of marker during the period." When calculating GFR the time of passage of marker from glomeruli to the bladder is most commonly neglected; hence the amount of marker collected from the bladder in a period is related to its plasma concentration during the same period. But when measuring, for instance, the GFR with renal clearance in cases of severe hydronephrosis and hydroureter, that passage of time may become very long (half an hour) and neglecting it will give a falsely high GFR value. However, infusion of GFR marker to a constant plasma concentration of marker has the advantage that the time of flow of marker from glomeruli to the bladder becomes unimportant.

Intravenous bolus injection of marker is more comfortable for patient and staff than infusion. It has the disadvantage that the GFR measurement is made during a *decreasing plasma concentration* of marker. This requires calculation according to the one-, two-, or three-compartment models when plasma clearance techniques are used and requires some knowledge (or estimate) of transport time of marker from glomeruli to bladder when renal clearance is used.

8.2.5 Techniques for Determining GFR with Sampling of Marker from Plasma Alone – Plasma Clearance or Body Clearance

An advantage of this technique is that a sometimes inaccurate and tedious urine sampling is avoided. A disadvantage of plasma clearance (body clearance) is that extrarenal clearance of the GFR marker is included in the GFR measurement, though there are techniques which may decrease the effects of this error (see Sect. 8.2.9).

The number of plasma samples and the timing of the sampling may vary (see also Sect. 8.5).

8.2.5.1 Multiple Plasma Samples

The optimal period of sampling will depend on the assumed level of GFR. The lower the assumed GFR, the later the period of sampling should end (Jacobsson 1983; Bröchner-Mortensen and Rödbro 1976c; Frennby et al. 1995b, 1996a,b, 1997). When GFR is assumed to be normal, the period of sampling may end 4 h after injection of the marker. When GFR is believed to be below 20 ml min^{-1} 1.73 m^{-2}, the period of sampling may have to end as late as 24 h after injection of marker.

8.2.5.2 Single Plasma Sample

Time of sampling will depend on the assumed GFR; the lower the assumed GFR, the later the optimal time of sampling will be (Bröchner-Mortensen and Rödbro 1976; Jacobsson 1983; Boijsen et al. 1988a; Ericsson and Kallner 1991; Stake et al. 1991a; Stake and Monclair 1991; Thomsen and Hvid-Jakobsen 1991; Thomsen et al. 1992b: Nilsson-Ehle and Grubb 1994; Frennby et al. 1995b; Rydström et al. 1995; Sterner et al. 1996; Lundqvist et al. 1997). When GFR is assumed to be normal, the optimal sampling time may be 3–4 h after the injection of the marker. When GFR is, for instance, assumed to be less than 20 ml min^{-1} 1.73 m^{-2}, the ideal time of plasma sampling may be as late as 24–48 h after injection of marker.

8.2.5.3
Extrarenal Clearance of Iohexol Determined as Plasma Clearance in Anuric Patients

In 12 anuric patients (diuresis less than 10 ml/24 h) the plasma clearance of iohexol (six patients) and inulin (six patients) were determined in the 44-h period between two dialysis sessions (Frennby et al. 1995b, 1996a). The extrarenal clearance of both iohexol and inulin had a median value of 2 ml min^{-1} 1.73 m^{-2} (iohexol range 1–2, inulin range 1–3). With regard to their extrarenal clearance, the two GFR markers were equally suitable for plasma clearance techniques.

8.2.6
Techniques for Determining GFR with Sampling of Marker from Both Urine and Plasma – Renal Clearance

Renal clearance has the advantage that extrarenal clearance of GFR marker is excluded from the GFR determination. Renal clearance has the disadvantage/risk of inaccurate sampling with regard to urine volume (see Sect. 8.2.7).

8.2.7
Renal Clearance of a Nonionic Monomer Determined with Classical Techniques

When two markers such as a nonionic monomeric contrast medium and inulin are compared regarding their suitability as GFR markers, they should be compared with identical injection and sampling techniques.

Classical inulin clearance is regarded as the "gold standard" of GFR determinations. It includes renal clearance of marker during continuous infusion of inulin to approximately constant plasma concentration. Originally this classical technique required urine sampling via a catheter in the bladder; however, today voluntary micturition is used when determining urine production in order to avoid risk of infection from a bladder catheter. Urine sampling has the advantage that extrarenal excretion of marker can be neglected. Urine sampling after micturition has the disadvantage of risk of incomplete urine sampling (with a false GFR value) for two reasons:

1. The patient may forget to sample urine for the whole period.
2. There might be residual urine in the bladder. Such residual urine may be determined with ultrasound examination (Frennby et al. 1995b).

In 50 urologic patients with indwelling bladder catheters (Brown and O'Reilly 1991), both markers (iohexol and inulin) were injected simultaneously as a priming bolus followed by simultaneous infusion in the same patient and in the same setting. Multiple plasma and urine samples (with rinsing of the bladder) were taken. The correlation coefficient (r) between the classical technique with inulin and the classical technique with iohexol was $r = 0.99$. Iohexol clearance = 1.00 × (classical inulin clearance) – 2.31. The GFR values ranged from 10 to 125 ml min^{-1} 1.73 m^{-2}. It was therefore concluded that for GFR determinations with the renal clearance technique, iohexol is as suitable from a pharmacokinetic point of view as other markers such as inulin, ^{51}Cr-EDTA, or ^{99m}Tc-DTPA.

8.2.8
Pharmacokinetics of a Nonionic Monomeric Contrast Medium

Sixteen healthy males received iohexol intravenously in doses from 500 to 1500 mg I/kg body weight. Plasma samples were taken for 48 through 96 h (2–4 days) and plasma concentrations of the contrast medium were determined. An open three-compartment body model gave the best fit to the data. The half-lives corresponding to the alpha, beta and gamma phases were 22 min, 2.1 h and 13 h, respectively (Edelson et al. 1984).

^{99m}Tc-DTPA clearance was measured in 21 patients using a single injection technique, the day before, during, and the day after an intravenous injection of 50 ml of 350 mg I/ml iohexol (Brown and O'Reilly 1992). Iohexol plasma clearance also was measured from four samples taken in the interval 120–300 min after injection of the iohexol. The mean ^{99m}Tc-DTPA clearances before, during, and after iohexol injection were 71.2, 71.5, and 70.7 ml min^{-1} 1.73 m^{-2}, respectively. Pre-iohexol GFR was in the range 14–105 ml min^{-1} 1.73 m^{-2}. The authors conclude that there was no change in GFR during an observation period of 48 h after the urography dose of iohexol. Iohexol and ^{99m}Tc-DTPA clearances performed simultaneously agreed closely (r = 0.976; Cl_{DTPA} = 1.02 $Cl_{iohexol}$ − 1.35). In other volunteers (OLSSON et al. 1983) receiving iohexol intravenously in a dose of 500 mg I/kg, simultaneous and nonsimultaneous determinations of GFR with iohexol and ^{51}Cr-EDTA as markers gave similar values of GFR with both markers, and also with both plasma clearance technique and renal clearance technique, indicating absence of iohexol effects on GFR at the doses used.

8.2.9 Pharmacokinetic/Mathematical Strategies for Simplifying GFR Techniques

Following an intravascular bolus injection of a contrast medium or another GFR marker there is an initial peak concentration of marker in plasma and then the concentration falls with time. This change in plasma concentration over time is better described with a multicompartment model than with a single-compartment model. The higher the number of compartments in the pharmacokinetic and mathematical model, the more precisely the plasma concentration over time is described and the more precisely the area under this curve can be calculated. The more precisely this area is calculated, the more accurate will be the calculated plasma clearance or renal clearance. *However*, the higher the number of compartments, the higher will be the required number of plasma samples, which increases the inconvenience to the patient. Therefore a number of clinical materials have been collected in which one-compartment models have been mathematically normalized to multicompartment models so that a single-sample or a two-sample plasma clearance could give results closer to those of multisample or multicompartment models. In addition plasma clearance methods have been normalized to renal clearance models to compensate mathematically for the extrarenal clearance of the marker. The mean value of the total plasma clearance of a marker in anuric patients representing the average extrarenal clearance of that marker in man can be subtracted from the plasma clearance value to obtain measurements closer to the "true GFR."

In renal clearance techniques no mathematical correction factor exists for errors made in estimating urine production over time when this is determined from the volume of voided urine. Whether too little urine has been collected (i.e., when residual urine remains in the bladder after collection of voided urine) or whether too much has been collected (i.e., when residual urine from a previous sampling period has been included in the present sampling period) can only be found out by either catheterizing the bladder (which involves risk of infection) or measuring possible residual urine with ultrasound both before and after each collection of voided urine. The large literature on normalization factors between different techniques and between different markers (ARVIDSSON and HEDMAN 1990; AURELL 1994; BLAUFOX et al. 1996; BROWN 1990; BROWN and O'REILLY 1991, 1992; BRÖCHNER-MORTENSEN et al. 1969; BRÖCHNER-MORTENSEN 1972, 1985; BRÖCHNER-MORTENSEN and RÖDBRO 1976a–c; BRÖCHNER-MORTENSEN and FREUND 1981; FRENNBY et al. 1995a,b, 1996a,b, 1997; JACOBSSON 1983, NILSSON-EHLE and GRUBB 1994; REHLING and RABOL 1989; ROCCO et al. 1996; RYDSTRÖM et al. 1995; STAKE et al. 1989, 1990, 1991a,b; STAKE and MONCLAIR 1991; STAKE 1992; THOMSEN et al. 1992b) is not further reviewed here.

8.3 Contrast Medium Clearance for Determining GFR in Diagnostic Imaging

8.3.1 Determination of GFR in Adults

In Northern Sweden patients may travel 300 km to their nearest hospital. At Umeå University Hospital, Lundqvist et al. determined GFR by calculating total plasma clearance of iohexol injected for urography in 902 patients (LUNDQVIST 1997; LUNDQVIST et al. 1997). Urography was performed after iohexol injection with or without abdominal compression, and in the period 3–5 h after iohexol injection plasma samples were obtained to determine plasma clearance of iohexol, i.e., the GFR. In 172 patients plasma clearances were determined with iohexol and ^{51}Cr-EDTA simultaneously or within 14 days and the correlation between the different clearance techniques was r = 0.933. Simultaneous urography and calculation of iohexol clearance has proved a useful technique to save patient travelling time and for the comfort of paraplegic patients, patients on control after treatment of carcinoma of the urinary bladder, and patients with ovarian cancer or uterine cancer (LUNDQVIST et al. 1994, 1996, 1997). Previously the patients in these groups underwent urography one day and received ^{51}Cr-EDTA to determine GFR on another day.

M. Boijsen from Gothenburg, Sweden (BOIJSEN 1988; BOIJSEN et al. 1987, 1998a,b) has shown that GFR determinations can be made not only after single injections of iohexol for urography, but also after multiple injections of contrast media in angiography.

SJÖBERG et al. (1987), EFFERSÖE et al. (1990), and THOMSEN et al. (1991, 1992a,b; THOMSEN and HVID-JAKOBSEN 1991) have used the ionic media diatrizoate and metrizoate and the nonionic media iohexol and iopamidol as GFR markers for simultaneous urography and GFR determination.

8.3.2 Determination of GFR in Children

Gunnar Stake, a pediatric radiologist in Oslo, Norway, has used iohexol for GFR determinations in children, in most cases in connection with urography (STAKE et al. 1989, 1990, 1991a,b; STAKE and MONCLAIR 1991; STAKE 1992). Simultaneous and nonsimultaneous clearance determinations were made with iohexol and other markers (^{99m}Tc-DTPA and inulin). It was found that urography with iohexol in children had no significant influence on GFR. Valid GFR estimates from plasma clearances were obtained from two plasma samples taken 3 and 4 h after injection of iohexol when GFR was normal or moderately reduced. In children with GFR less than 20 ml min^{-1} 1.73 m^{-2}, valid GFR estimates were obtained with plasma clearance based on two samples or one sample when the last sample was taken as late as 24 h after the injection. In three uremic children the simultaneous renal clearances of iohexol and inulin were similar, 10.1 ± 0.9 and 10.5 ± 1.0 ml min^{-1} 1.73 m^{-2}, respectively (mean ± SD). The simultaneous plasma clearances of iohexol had similar values, 10.1 ± 1.2 ml min^{-1} 1.73 m^{-2}. The renal clearances of creatinine were approximately 50% higher than the inulin and iohexol clearances in these children.

Up to December 1992, iohexol had been used for GFR determinations in a total of 607 children (G. Stake, personal communication, 1992). In the year 1992, iohexol had been used for GFR determinations alone in 40 children, the majority of whom had cancer and were being treated with cytostatic drugs. This use of iohexol for GFR determinations in children outside diagnostic imaging has continued. In the years 1993–1997 combined urography and GFR determinations with iohexol has been used in another 870 children (G. Stake, personal communication, 1998).

8.3.3 Determination of the GFR of Each Individual Kidney (Split Renal Function)

In 43 patients, FRENNBY et al. (1995) used two GFR markers (iohexol and ^{99m}Tc-DTPA) to determine the relative GFR, i.e., the GFR of each kidney in percent of total GFR. The amount of marker in Bowman's space, tubuli, and renal pelvis within a few minutes after i.v. injection, before any marker had left a kidney via the ureter, was defined as proportional to the GFR of that kidney. The renal accumulation of iohexol was determined by CT using ten slices of 8 mm thickness in the period 1–4 min after injection. The renal accumulation of ^{99m}Tc-DTPA was determined with a gamma camera within 2 min after injection. The correlation coefficient between the two methods was 0.98. CT was more reliable than scintigraphy in patients with low relative GFR in the range 0%–15% due to fewer problems with background activity, which could be mathematically removed by the CT method. It was concluded that due to the higher radiation dose from CT than from ^{99m}Tc-DTPA injection, relative GFR determination should be performed with CT only when there is a diagnostic need to reveal morphology (e.g., aneurysm of abdominal aorta, morphology of kidneys).

8.4 Contrast Medium Clearance for Determination of GFR Outside Diagnostic Imaging

8.4.1 Determination of GFR in Adults and Children

In Lund, Sweden, Krutzén and Bäck have developed a high-performance liquid chromatography technique to determine the plasma clearance or the renal clearance of an intravenous bolus of iohexol (KRUTZÉN et al. 1984, 1990, 1992; BÄCK 1988; BÄCK et al. 1988a,b, 1989). By December 1992 (P. Nilsson-Ehle, personal communication), approximately 3000 GFR determinations had been made with iohexol as the GFR marker with a common dose of 5–10 ml iohexol 300 mg I/ml. To that date no "adverse reactions" had been reported in the following clinical setting: the physician on duty had a telephone in his pocket and would have been called on if there had been an "adverse reaction" during the iohexol injections or in the hours until the last sampling of marker. Several patients who had shown moderate adverse reactions (nausea, vomiting) after iohexol injections with the larger doses for angiography (one or several hundred ml), did not show any symptoms when they received the lower iohexol dose for GFR determination (5–10 ml). The normal values of iohexol GFR at different ages have been reported (Bäck et al. 1988a). Iohexol, like other GFR markers, detects a decrease in GFR with increasing patient age.

A measurement of GFR with determination of total plasma clearance of a nonionic monomer based on capillary sampling of plasma has also been developed for use in children (Krutzén et al. 1990). GFR determinations with plasma clearance have been performed in a group of 100 children (P. Nilsson-Ehle, personal communication, 1992). The group includes children with lymphoma or cancer. Iohexol clearance has been used to establish the dose of cytostatic drug required with regard to the level of GFR in these children.

In 1998, Brändström et al. performed simultaneous determinations of plasma clearances with iohexol and ^{51}Cr-EDTA in adults with GFR >40 ml min^{-1} 1.73 m^{-2} with both a single sample and multiple samples and found the two markers to correlate highly (*r* varied between 0.91 and 0.95 in the different comparisons) (Brändström et al. 1998).

Hall and Rolin (1995) described the use of ^{125}I-iothalamate as a GFR marker in large-scale clinical trials (Modification of Diet in Renal Disease, Diabetes Control and Complications Trial, African-American Study of Kidney Disease and Hypertension). Myers et al. (1995) described the use of unlabeled iothalamate in a clinical trial (on the progression of overt nephropathy in non-insulin-dependent diabetes).

8.4.2 Determination of GFR in Pregnancy

The GFR has been determined with iohexol in pregnancy, both in normal subjects and in patients with hypertension, preeclampsia, and diabetes (Krutzén et al. 1984, 1992). In normal pregnancy GFR increased by 40% throughout the pregnancy and during the first week postpartum, and thereafter decreased within a month to levels similar to those in nonpregnant women. The increase in GFR in diabetic pregnant women and in women with gestational hypertension was similar to that recorded in normal pregnancy. In subjects with preeclampsia, the increase in GFR observed in normal pregnancy was absent and no change in GFR was recorded after delivery. It was concluded that the development of proteinuria and fluid retention typical of preeclampsia is accompanied by a decrease of GFR.

8.4.3 Determination of GFR in a Pharmacodynamic Study of Cyclosporin A

Lewis et al. (1989, 1990, 1993) have used iohexol GFR as a research tool. In 34 patients with transplanted kidneys, the GFR of the allografts was measured at 4-month intervals for 1 year, while the patients were on long-term treatment with cyclosporin A (Lewis et al. 1993). They were divided into four groups according to GFR level at entrance (range 20–60 ml min^{-1} 1.73 m^{-2}). There were no signs of decrease in GFR at the four GFR measurements during the 1-year period. There were no signs of progressive toxic nephropathy due to cyclosporin A in the material.

8.4.4 Determination of GFR in Patients on Cytostatic Drugs

Iohexol is used to determine GFR as an aid to calculate appropriate doses and plasma levels of cytostatic pharmaceuticals with predominantly renal excretion. As mentioned above, iohexol is used for this purpose in children with malignant disease in Lund, Sweden and in Oslo, Norway. Iohexol is also used for the same purpose in adults (Lindegaard et al. 1991).

8.4.5 Determination of Residual Renal Function in Patients in Dialysis and Determination of Dialysis Clearance of Contrast Medium

The removal of nonionic contrast media from patients in chronic renal failure has been studied following hemodialysis (HD) (Kierdorf et al. 1989; Waaler et al. 1990; Moon et al. 1995; Furukawa et al. 1996) and following peritoneal dialysis (Donelly et al. 1992; Moon et al. 1995). In patients on HD with end-stage renal disease there is an increasing interest in measuring both residual renal function and quantity and quality of dialysis because insufficient dialysis increases mortality. In two studies (Swan et al. 1996; Sterner et al. 1998) a bolus of iohexol was given at the end of an HD session and a number of plasma samples were taken in the period to the next HD about 44 h later. The plasma clearance (total body clearance) of iohexol was calculated for the interdialysis period. In each study residual renal function was calculated by subtracting an average extrarenal plasma clearance value which had been obtained in a group of anuric patients from the plasma clearance value. Both studies showed that single-sample plasma clearance based on the sample at the start of the next HD gave values close to the multiple sample clearance. Patient comfort was increased by using only a single pre-HD sample for measurement of residual renal function.

Sterner et al. (1998) used the injected contrast media [the nonionic monomer iohexol (molecular mass 821 u) and the nonionic dimer iodixanol (1550 u)] also to measure dialysis clearance by determining contrast medium concentration in plasma at the end of dialysis. While the two contrast media gave the same value on residual renal function, iodixanol (the larger contrast medium molecule) was, as expected, subject to approximately 25% lower clearance through the dialysis membranes due to their cut-off effect on the passage of larger molecules, as also observed by Furukawa et al. (1997).

8.5 Choice of Method for Determining GFR with Contrast Media

In our opinion most, if not all, contrast media and other markers with similar pharmacokinetics such as inulin, ^{51}Cr-EDTA, and ^{99m}Tc-DTPA, are suitable for determining GFR. What *is* important is using the appropriate technique, and the right choice of number and timing of plasma samples.

According to an international committee that has reported on radiolabeled GFR markers (Blaufox et al. 1996), plasma clearance based on the single-sample technique is adequate in patients with GFR >30 ml min^{-1} 1.73 m^{-2}. If the GFR is <30 ml min^{-1} 1.73 m^{-2}, the technique should include urine collection, i.e., the renal clearance technique is preferred at this lower level of GFR. Urine collection is also considered to be indicated in patients with ascites or edema. But in patients in renal failure the committee may allow the plasma clearance technique provided that late sampling times are used. The alternatives (according to the committee) are:

- Estimated GFR 15–30 ml min^{-1} 1.73 m^{-2}: plasma sampling between 3 and 5 h postinjection
- Estimated GFR <15 ml min^{-1} 1.73 m^{-2}: plasma sampling between 5 and 24 h postinjection or only 24 h postinjection

With this provision that delayed plasma sampling must be used in subjects with marked renal function impairment, there is much experience in using plasma clearance of contrast medium to determine GFR. For example, Sterner et al. (1996) reported 65 patients with varying degrees of renal insufficiency who received 10 ml iohexol (300 mg I/ml) i.v. Plasma samples were collected 4 times during the following 3–24 h for determination of plasma iodine concentrations. Predicted creatinine clearance was used to choose one of the samples for determination of single-sample clearance. A single plasma specimen collected at 4 h for predicted GFR above 50 ml/min, at 7 h for predicted GFR between 20 and 50 ml/min, and at 24 h for predicted GFR below 20 ml/min gave clearance values in good agreement with those derived from a four-sample slope clearance based on samples collected 4–24 h postinjection. For subjects with very low estimated GFR <5 ml min^{-1} 1.73 m^{-2}, a sampling time 48–72 h after injection of marker was suggested by Nilsson-Ehle and Grubb (1994). They had then (1994) made 4000 GFR determinations with iohexol.

Single-sample techniques with contrast media as GFR markers have been used inter alia by Boijsen et al. (1988a), Stake et al. (1991a,b), Thomsen et al. (Thomsen and Hvid-Jakobsen 1991; Thomsen et al. 1992b), Nilsson-Ehle and Grubb (1994), Frennby et al. (1995b), Rydström et al. (1995), Sterner et al. (1996, 1998), Swan et al. (1996), Lundqvist et al. (1997), and Brändström et al. (1998).

Different nonionic monomeric contrast media may be assumed to be equally effective as GFR markers due to similar pharmacokinetics. Gaspari et al. (1995) found a highly significant correlation between the plasma clearances of iohexol and iopromide.

Acknowledgement. The revision of the English text by Rob Towart, PhD is gratefully acknowledged.

References

Arvidsson A, Hedman A (1990) Plasma and renal clearance of iohexol - a study on reproducibility of a method for glomerular filtration rate. Scand J Clin Lab Invest 50:757–761

Aurell M (1994) Accurate and feasible measurements of GFR - is the iohexol clearance an answer? Nephrol Dial Transplant 9:1222–1224

Bäck SE (1988) Contrast media markers for glomerular filtration. Methods of determination, pharmacokinetics, and clinical applicability. Thesis, The University of Lund, Lund, Sweden

Bäck SE, Krutzén E, Nilsson-Ehle P (1988a) Contrast media and glomerular filtration rate: dose dependence of clearance for three agents. J Pharm Sci 77:765–767

Bäck SE, Krutzén E, Nilsson-Ehle P (1988b) Contrast media as markers for glomerular filtration: a pharmacokinetic comparison of four agents. Scand J Clin Lab Invest 48:247–253

Bäck SE, Ljungberg B, Nilsson-Ehle I, Borgå O, Nilsson-Ehle P (1989) Age dependence of renal function: clearance of iohexol and *p*-aminohippurate in healthy males. Scand J Clin Lab Invest 49:641–646

Binz A (1937) Geschichte des Uroselectans. Z Urol 31:73–84

Blaufox M, Aurell M, Bubeck B, et al. (1996) Report of the Radionuclides in Nephrourology Committee on Renal Clearance. J Nucl Med 37:1883–1890

Boijsen M (1988) Determination of glomerular filtration rate and cardiac output in connection with routine radiological examinations. X-ray fluorescence analysis of iodinated media. Thesis, University of Gothenburg, Gothenburg, Sweden

Boijsen M, Jacobsson L, Tylén U (1987) Renal function measured by X-ray fluorescence analysis. A comparison between contrast medium clearance and a non-simultaneous ^{51}Cr-EDTA clearance. Acta Radiol 28:581–585

Boijsen M, Jacobsson L, Tylén U (1988a) Glomerular filtration rate estimated from a single plasma sample after contrast enhanced radiological examinations. Clin Physiol 8:309–316

Boijsen M, Granerus G, Jacobsson L, Björnfeld L, Aurell M, Tylén U (1988b) Glomerular filtration rate estimated after multiple injection of contrast medium during angiography. Acta Radiol 29:669–674

Brändström E, Grzegorczyk A, Jacobsson L, Friberg P, Lindahl A, Aurell M (1998) GFR measurement with iohexol and ^{51}Cr-EDTA. A comparison of the two favoured GFR markers in Europe. Nephrol Dial Transplant 13:1176–1182

Bröchner-Mortensen J, Giese J, Rossing N (1969) Renal inulin clearance versus total plasma clearance of ^{51}Cr-EDTA. Scand J Clin Lab Invest 23:301–305

Bröchner-Mortensen J (1972) A simple method for the determination of glomerular filtration rate. 30:271–274

Bröchner Mortensen J, Rödbro P (1976a) Selection of routine method for determination of glomerular filtration rate in adult patients. Scand J Clin Lab Invest 36:35–43

Bröchner-Mortensen J, Rödbro P (1976b) Comparison between total and renal plasma clearance of ^{51}Cr-EDTA. Scand J Clin Lab Invest 36:247–249

Bröchner-Mortensen J, Rödbro P (1976c) Optimum time of blood sampling for determination of glomerular filtration rate by single injection of ^{51}Cr-EDTA plasma clearance. Scand J Clin Lab Invest 36:795–800

Bröchner-Mortensen J, Freund LG (1981) Reliability of routine clearance methods for assessment of the glomerular filtration rate in advanced renal insufficiency. Scand J Clin Lab Invest 41:91–97

Bröchner-Mortensen J (1985) Current status on assessment and measurement of glomerular filtration rate. Clin Physiol 5:1–17

Brown SC (1990) Radiographic contrast media for the measurement of glomerular filtration rate: evaluation of an X-ray fluorescence technique. Thesis, University of London, London, England

Brown SC, O'Reilly PH (1991) Iohexol clearance for the determination of glomerular filtration rate in clinical practice; evidence for a new gold standard. J Urol 146:675–679

Brown SC, O' Reilly PH (1992) The estimate of glomerular filtration rate during urography: acceptability of a nonionic contrast medium as a marker of renal function. Invest Radiol 27:774–778

Donelly PK, Burwell N, McBurney A, Ward J, Walls J, Watkin E (1992) Clearance of iopamidol, a nonionic contrast medium by CAPD, in patients with end-stage renal failure. Br J Radiol 65:1108–1113

Edelson J, Shaw D, Palace G (1984) Pharmacokinetics of iohexol, a new nonionic radiocontrast agent in humans. J Pharm Sci 73:993–995

Effersöe H, Rosenkilde P, Groth S, Jensen LI, Golman K (1990) Measurement of renal function with iohexol. Invest Radiol 25:778–782

Elwood CM, Sigman EM, Treger C (1967) The measurement of glomerular filtration rate with ^{125}I-sodium iothalamate (Conray). Br J Radiol 40:581–583

Ericsson CG, Kallner A (1991) Glomerular filtration rate: a comparison between ^{51}Cr-EDTA clearance and a single sample technique with a non-ionic contrast agent. Clin Biochem 24:261–264

Frennby B (1996) Use of iohexol to determine glomerular filtration rate. Thesis, University of Lund, Lund, Sweden

Frennby B (1997) Use of iohexol clearance to determine glomerular filtation rate. A comparison between different clearance techniques in man and animal. Scand J Urol Nephrol 31, Suppl 182:1–64

Frennby B, Almén T, Lilja B, et al. (1995a) Determination of the relative glomerular filtration rate of each kidney in man. Comparison between iohexol CT and ^{99m}Tc-DTPA scintigraphy. Acta Radiol 36:410–417

Frennby B, Sterner G, Almén T, Hagstam KE, Hultberg B, Jacobsson L (1995b) The use of iohexol clearance to determine GFR in patients with severe chronic renal failure - a comparison between different clearance techniques. Clin Nephrol 43:35–46

Frennby B, Sterner G, Almén T, Chai CM, Jönsson BA, Månsson S (1996a) Extrarenal plasma clearance of iohexol, chromium-51-ethylenediaminetetraacetic acid, and inulin in anephric pigs. Acad Radiol 3:145–153

Frennby G, Sterner G, Almén T, Chai CM, Jönsson BA, Månsson S (1996b) Clearance of iohexol, chromium-51-ethylenediaminetetraacetic acid, and creatinine for determining the glomerular filtration rate in pigs with normal renal function. Comparison of different clearance techniques. Acad Radiol 3:651–659

Frennby B, Sterner G, Almn T, Chai CM, Jönsson BA, Månsson S (1997) Clearance of iohexol, ^{51}Cr-EDTA and endogenous creatinine for determination of glomerular filtration rate in pigs with reduced renal function. A comparison between different clearance techniques. Scand J Clin Lab Invest 57:241–252

Furukawa T, Ueda J, Takahashi S, Sakaguchi K (1996) Elimination of low-osmolality contrast media by hemodialysis. Acta Radiol 37:966–971

Furukawa T, Ueda J, Higashino K, Takahashi S, Sakaguchi K, Imai T (1997) Permeability of contrast media through hemodialysis membrane. Acta Radiol 38:918–921

Gabriel R (1986) Time to scrap creatinine clearance? Br Med J 293:1119–1120

Gaspari F, Perico N, Ruggenenti P, Mosconi L, Amuchastegui CS, Guerini E, Daina E, Remuzzi G (1995) Plasma clearance of non-radioactive iohexol as a measure of glomerular filtration rate. J Am Soc Nephrol 6:257–263

Grönberg T (1981) In vivo X-ray fluorescence analysis for medical diagnosis. A noninvasive method for determination of kidney function after radiographic examinations with iodinated contrast media. Thesis, University of Lund, Lund, Sweden

Grönberg T, Almén T, Golman K, Lidén K, Mattsson S, Sjöberg S (1981) Non-invasive estimation of kidney function by X-ray fluorescence analysis. Method for in-vivo measurements of iodine-containing contrast media in rabbits. Phys Med Biol 26:501–506

Guesry P, Kaufman L, Orloff S, Nelsom J, Swann S, Holliday M (1975) Measurement of glomerular filtration rate by fluorescent excitation of non-radioactive meglumine iothalamate. Clin Nephrol 3:134–138

Hall P, Rolin H (1995) Iothalamate clearance and its use in large-scale clinical trials. Curr Opin Nephrol Hypertens 4:510–513

Hood B, Attman PO, Ahlmén J, Jagenburg R (1971) Renal hemodynamics and limitations of creatinine clearance in determining glomerular filtration rate in glomerular disease. Scand J Urol Nephrol 5:154–161

Jacobsson L (1983) A method for the calculation of renal clearance based on a single plasma sample. Clin Physiol 3:297–305

Kierdorf H, Kindler J, Wintersheid R, Hollman H, Voorwerk D, Speck U (1989) Elimination of the non-ionic contrast medium iopromide in end-stage renal failure by hemodialysis. RÖFO Suppl 128:119–123

Krutzén E, Bäck SE, Nilsson-Ehle I, Nilsson-Ehle P (1984) Plasma clearance of a new contrast agent, iohexol: a method for the assessment of glomerular filtration rate. J Lab Clin Med 104:955–961

Krutzén E, Bäck SE, Nilsson-Ehle P (1990) Determination of glomerular filtration rate using iohexol clearance and capillary sampling. Scand J Clin Lab Invest 50:279–283

Krutzén E, Olofsson P, Bäck SE, Nilsson-Ehle P (1992) Glomerular filtration rate in pregnancy. A study in normal subjects and in patients with hypertension, preeclampsia and diabetes. Scand J Clin Lab Invest 52:387–392

Lewis R, Kerr N, van Buren C, et al. (1989) Comparative evaluation of urographic contrast media, inulin and ^{99m}Tc-DTPA clearance methods for determination of glomerular filtration rate in clinical transplants. Transplantation 48:790–796

Lewis RM, Knight R, Katz S, Kerman RH, van Buren CT, Kahan BD (1990) Attrition of renal allograph function associated with longterm maintainance of cyclosporin therapy reflects chronic immunologic injury not toxic nephropathy. J Nephrol Suppl 1:23–29

Lewis R, Podielski J, Spraybarry S, et al. (1993) Stability of renal allograph glomerular filtration rate associated with longterm use of cyclosporin A. Transplantation 55:1014–1017

Lindblad HG, Berg U (1994) Comparative evaluation of iohexol and inulin clearance for glomerular filtration rate determinations. Acta Paediatr 83:418–422

Lindegaard MW, Aass N, Bue E, Theodorsen L, Fosså S (1991) Glomerular filtration rate, ^{131}I-hippuran clearance and estimated creatinine clearance in cancer patients. Br J Cancer 64:401–405

Lundqvist S (1997) Contrast medium clearance in radiologic imaging. Experimental and clinical studies. Umeå University medical dissertations. New Series No 506. ISSN 0346-6612, Umeå, Sweden

Lundqvist S, Hietala SO, Berglund C, Karp K (1994) Simultaneous urography and determinations of glomerular filtration rate. A comparison of total plasma clearances of iohexol and ^{51}Cr-EDTA in plegic patients. Acta Radiol 35:391–395

Lundqvist S, Edbom G, Stendahl U, Hietala SO (1996) Iohexol clearance for renal function measurement in gynaecologic cancer patients. Acta Radiol 37:582–586

Lundqvist S, Hietala SO, Groth S, Sjödin JG (1997) Evaluation of single sample clearance calculations in 902 patients. A comparison of multiple and single sample techniques. Acta Radiol 38:68–72

Möller E, McIntosh JF, Van Slyke DD (1928) Studies of urea excretion. II. Relationship between urine volume and the rate of urea excretion by normal adults. J Clin Invest 6:427–465

Moon SS, Bäck SE, Kurkus J, Nilsson-Ehle P (1995) Hemodialysis for elimination of the nonionic contrast medium iohexol after angiography in patients with impaired renal function. Nephron 70:430–437

Morris AM, Elwood C, Sigman EM, Catanzaro A (1965) The renal clearance of ^{131}I labelled meglumine diatrizoate (Renografin) in man. J Nucl Med 6:183–191

Myers B, Nelson R, Tan M, Beck G, Bennet P, Knowler W, Blouch K, Milch W (1995) Progression of overt nephropathy in non-insulin-dependent diabetes. Kidney Int 47:1781–1789

Nilsson-Ehle P, Grubb A (1994) New markers for determination of GFR: iohexol clearance and cystatin C serum concentration. Kidney Int 46 (Suppl 47):S17–S19

Nordby A, Tvedt K, Halgunset J, Haugen O (1990) Intracellular penetration and accumulation of radiographic contrast media in the rat kidney. Microscopy 4:651–666

Nossen JO, Jacobsen JA, Kjaersgaard P, Andrew E, Jacobsen PB, Berg KJ (1995) Elimination of the non-ionic X-ray contrast media iodixanol and iohexol in patients with severely impaired renal function. Scand J Clin Lab Invest 55:341–350

Nosslin B (1965) Determination of clearance and distribution volume with the single injection technique. Acta Med Scand Suppl 179:97–101

Olsson B, Aulie Å, Sveen K, Andrew E (1983) Human pharmacokinetics of iohexol, a new nonionic contrast medium. Invest Radiol 18:177–182

O'Reilly PH, Brooman PJC, Martin PJ, Pollard AJ, Farah NB, Mason GC (1986) Accuracy and reproducibility of a new contrast clearance method for determination of glomerular filtration rate. Br Med J 293:234–236

O'Reilly PH, Jones DA, Farah NB (1987) Measurement of plasma clearance of urographic contrast media for the determination of glomerular filtration rate. J Urol 139:9–11

Rehling M, Rabol A (1989) Measurement of glomerular filtration rate in adults: accuracy of five single sample plasma clearance methods. Clin Physiol 9:171–182

Rocco MV, Buckalew VM, Moore LC, Shihabi ZK (1996) Measurement of glomerular filtration rate using nonradioactive iohexol: comparison of two one-compartment models. Am J Nephrol 16:138–143

Rydström M, Tengström B, Cederquist I, Ahlmén J (1995) Measurement of glomerular filtration rate by single-injection, single sample techniques, using ^{51}Cr-EDTA or iohexol. Scand J Urol Nephrol 29:135–139

Sapirstein L, Vidt D, Mandel M, Hanusek G (1955) Volumes of distribution and clearances of intravenously injected creatinine in the dog. Am J Physiol 181:330–336

Shemesh O, Golbetz H, Kriss J, Myers B (1985) Limitations of creatinine as a filtration marker in glomerulopathic patients. Kidney Int 28:830–838

Sigman EM, Elwood CM, Knox F (1965a) The measurement of glomerular filtration rate in man with sodium iothalamate ^{131}I (Conray). J Nucl Med 7:60–68

Sigman E, Elwood C, Reagan M, Morris A, Catanzanio A (1965b) The renal clearance of I^{131} labelled sodium iothalamate in man. Invest Urol 2:432–438

Sjöberg S, Hellsten S, Almén T, Golman K, Grönberg T (1987) Estimating kidney function during urography. Comparison of contrast medium clearance and simultaneous ^{51}Cr-EDTA clearance. Acta Radiol 28:587–592

Stake G (1992) Estimation of the glomerular filtration rate in infants and children using iohexol and X-ray fluorescence technique. Thesis, Univerity of Oslo, Oslo, Norway

Stake G, Monclair T (1991) A single plasma sample method for estimation of the glomerular filtration rate in infants and children using iohexol. I. Establishment of a body weight related formula for the distribution volume of iohexol. Scand J Clin Lab Invest 51:335–342

Stake G, Monn E, Rootwelt K, Golman K, Monclair T (1989) Influence of urography on renal function in children. A double blind study with metrizoate and iohexol. Acta Radiol 30:643–646

Stake G, Monn E, Rootwelt K, Grönberg T, Monclair T (1990) Glomerular filtration rate estimated by X-ray fluorescence technique in children. Comparison between plasma disappearance of ^{99m}Tc-DTPA and iohexol after urography. Scand J Clin Lab Invest 50:161–167

Stake G, Monn E, Rootwelt K, Monclair T (1991a) A single plasma sample method for estimation of the glomerular filtration rate in infants and children using iohexol. II. Establishment of the optimal plasma sampling time and a comparison with the ^{99m}Tc-DTPA method. Scand J Clin Lab Invest 51:343–348

Stake G, Monn E, Rootwelt K, Monclair T (1991b) The clearance of iohexol as a measure of the glomerular filtration rate in children with chronic renal failure. Scand J Clin Lab Invest 51:729–734

Sterner G, Frennby B, Hultberg B, Almén T (1996) Iohexol clearance for GFR-determination in renal failure – single or multiple plasma sampling? Nephrol Dial Transplant 11:521–525

Sterner G, Frennby B, Månsson S, Ohlsson A, Prutz KG, Almén T (1998) Assessing residual renal function and efficiency of hemodialysis – an application for urographic contrast media. Submitted for publication

Swan SK, Halstenson CE, Kasiske BL, Collins AJ (1996) Determination of residual renal function with iohexol clearance in hemodialysis patients. Kidney Int 49:232–235

Swick M (1929) Darstellung der Niere und Harnwege im Röntgenbild durch intravenöse Einbringung eines neuen Kontraststoffes, des Uroselectans. Klin Wchr 8:2087–2089

Thomsen H, Hvid-Jakobsen K (1991) Estimation of glomerular filtration rate from low-dose injection of iohexol and a single blood sample. Invest Radiol 26:332

Thomsen H, Vestergaard A, Nielsen SL, Fogh-Andersen N, Golman K, Dorph S (1991) Renal clearance of an ionic high osmolar and a nonionic low osmolar contrast medium. Invest Radiol 26:564–568

Thomsen H, Vestergaard A, Dorph S (1992a) Quality of urography and renal clearance of ionic and nonionic contrast media. Invest Radiol 27:40–44

Thomsen H, Vestergaard A, Golman K, Dorph S (1992b) One or two samples for determination of total plasma clearance of a nonionic contrast medium in patients undergoing enhanced CT. Acta Radiol 33:588–591

Waaler A, Svaland M, Fauchald P, Jacobsen J, Kolmannskog F, Berg KJ (1990) Elimination of iohexol, a low osmolar nonionic contrast medium, by hemodialysis in patients with chronic renal failure. Nephron 56:81–85

9 Neurotoxicity

M. LEONARDI and R. AGATI

CONTENTS

9.1 Introduction

Neurotoxicity is the degree of toxicity produced by molecules of contrast media in contact with the central nervous system following intracisternal or intrathecal injection. Like systemic toxicity, neurotoxicity is expressed as LD_{50} (in g I/kg or in mmol/kg) and corresponds to the intrathecal dose inducing death in 50% of experimental animals after injection. The neurotoxicity index is defined as the ratio between intravenous LD_{50} and intrathecal LD_{50}.

It is essential to establish the neurotoxicity of a contrast agent whenever direct contact with nerve tissue is envisaged following intrathecal injection, or, as is more common, whenever there is a danger of indirect contact by intravenous administration in cases of damage to the blood–brain barrier. Neurotoxicity is also an extremely important factor in the overall assessment of contrast material since the degree of neurotoxicity of various commercially available contrast media differs far more widely than that of general toxicity (LD_{50} values following intravenous injection are much closer together than values for intrathecal injection).

Animal studies have shown that ionic contrast media are from 400 to 1400 times more toxic after intracisternal rather than intravenous injection (HOPPE and ARCHER 1960). According to some authors (LALLI 1980), all adverse reactions are the result of nervous system activation by the limbic system: the contrast medium combined with the patient's anxiety triggers the limbic system and the centres responsible for homeostasis, giving rise to adverse reactions.

Since contrast media were first developed, there has been ongoing progress in the formulation of these substances, as witnessed by the constant rise in their relative diagnostic index defined as the ratio between LD_{50} and the amount of contrast medium required to perform myelography, due to both the increase in LD_{50} and the larger number of iodine atoms per particle in solution. Moreover, the introduction of nonionic contrast media has led to a four- to sixfold reduction in the frequency of adverse reactions (KATAYAMA et al. 1990; THOMSEN and DORPH 1993).

The toxic effects of contrast media depend on the chemical-physical properties of the solutions in which they are formulated and the specific chemical characteristics of their molecules (CORSICO and TIRONE 1988). The following features are particularly important:

- Osmotic characteristics, i.e., the capacity to stimulate the passage of water through cell membranes, which play an important role in determining possible temporary damage to the blood-brain barrier
- Viscosity, which not only has a negative effect on how the product is administered, but also affects the ischemia time in the area to be injected and the duration of contact between the contrast material and endothelia
- Chemical features, namely a product's capacity to bind to proteins, block enzymes, and stimulate the

M. LEONARDI, MD, Professor and Chairman, Servizio di Neuroradiologia, Ospedale Bellaria, Via Altura 3, I-40139 Bologna, Italy
R. AGATI, MD, Servizio di Neuroradiologia, Ospedale Bellaria, Via Altura 3, I-40139 Bologna, Italy

release of vasoactive substances correlated with the contrast agent's hydrophilicity
- Ionic characteristics which may interfere with cell function

9.2 Chemical Formulation and Physicochemical Properties

Currently available contrast media can be divided into four groups on the basis of their chemical formulation:

- Ionic monomers (e.g., diatrizoate, iothalamate, iodamide, metrizoate)
- Monoacidic ionic dimers (e.g., ioxaglate)
- Nonionic monomers (e.g., iopamidol, iohexol, metrizamide, iopromide, iopremol)
- Nonionic dimers (e.g., iotrolan, iodixanol)

The first step in a comparative analysis of the structure of these molecules should be to consider the number of iodine atoms per molecule which are responsible for the primary effect of contrast media, the absorption of x-rays. Plainly, the larger the number of iodine atoms, the greater the absorption and hence the need to administer a smaller amount of contrast material.

Ionic contrast agents are so called because they are made up of two ions: the negatively charged anion, which may be the diatrizoate, iodamide, iothalamate, or metrizoate ion, and the positively charged cation, the sodium or meglumine ion. As the osmotic pressure depends on the number of particles in solution, ionic contrast media naturally have a greater osmolarity, double that of nonionic contrast agents.

The ratio between the number of iodine atoms and the number of particles in solution is termed the CM ratio and is fundamental in the chemical analysis of contrast material. Clearly, this parameter provides no information on the chemotoxicity of a molecule, which is the main factor responsible for neurotoxicity.

The chemical composition of monomers is a single benzene ring while dimers have two rings. Ionic contrast agents contain carboxyl groups (COO^-) which on the one hand are essential to the molecule's structure and confer its weak hydrophilicity and on the other are the main factors responsible for neurotoxicity. Nonionic ccontrast media contain numerous hydroxyl groups (OH) which give the products their high degree of hydrophilicity.

Ionic monomers have the highest osmolarity, over 1000 mOsm per iodine concentration of 300 mg/ml (CM ratio = 1.5), the lowest tolerance for intravenous (LD_{50} = 5–10 g I/kg) and subarachnoid (LD_{50} < 200 mg I/kg) administration in animals, and the lowest viscosity; they are weakly hydrophilic and have three iodine atoms per molecule.

Ionic dimers have an intermediate osmolarity, 500–600 mOsm per iodine concentration of 300 mg/ml (CM ratio = 3), intermedite tolerance levels for intravenous (LD_{50} = 10–15 g I/kg) and subarachnoid (LD_{50} = 200 mg I/kg) administration in animals, intermediate viscosity, an intermediate hydrophilicity between that of ionic and nonionic monomers, and six atoms of iodine per molecule.

Nonionic monomers have an intermediate osmolarity, 500–600 mOsm per iodine concentration of 300 mg/ml (CM ratio = 3), the highest tolerance level for intravenous (LD_{50} = 20–25 g I/kg) and subarachnoid (LD_{50} = 1500 mg I/kg) administration in animals, intermediate viscosity, and elevated hydrophilicity with three atoms of iodine per molecule.

Nonionic dimers have the lowest osmolarity (CM ratio = 6), the highest tolerance level for intravenous and subarachnoid administration in animals, the highest viscosity, and highly elevated hydrophilicity with six atoms of iodine per molecule.

9.3 Neurotoxicity in Relation to Chemical Formulation

As discussed above, marked differences exist in the chemical structure of the various contrast agents and these are accompanied by major differences in their relative toxicity for the systemic and central nervous systems, expressed as LD_{50}. It is the molecular structure of a contrast agent that is responsible for its neurotoxicity, modifying its osmotic characteristics, viscosity, and chemical and ionic features (Almén 1989).

A product's *osmotic characteristics* depend on the number of particles in solution. For every molecule in solution ionic contrast agents are made up of two particles (ions) and hence exert a greater osmotic pressure. In theory, the osmolarity of nonionic monomers should be equal to half that of ionic monomers; in practice it is slightly less given the possible aggregation between molecules.

A comparison of the osmolarity of different types of commercially available contrast media should consider the fact that the high osmolarity of ionic monomers is exacerbated by the small number of iodine atoms per molecule (CM ratio = 1.5). This means that more molecules need to be administered to obtain the same effect in terms of x-ray absorption as that of ionic dimers or nonionic monomers (CM ratio = 3) and nonionic dimers (CM ratio = 6).

A completely different standpoint is required to compare ionic dimers and nonionic monomers. Even though ionic dimers are composed of two particles (ions), while nonionic monomers have only one (the molecule), dimers have six iodine atoms per molecule while monomers have only three. This means that x-ray absorption being equal, the osmotic pressure exerted will be similar because the number of particles in solution is the same.

Lastly, comparing non-ionic dimers with non-ionic monomers or ionic dimers, given the same x-ray absorption effect, the osmotic pressure exerted will be less because of the nonionic nature of the product and the presence of six iodine atoms per molecule.

The *viscosity* of a contrast agent is correlated to the size of its molecule:

- Ionic monomers have smaller molecules, being made up of one anion [a single benzene ring, three iodine atoms, and one carboxyl group (COO^-)] and one cation (sodium or methylglucamine).
- Ionic dimers [one cation with two benzene rings, six iodine atoms, one carboxyl group (COO^-), one hydroxyl group (-OH), and one anion (sodium or methylglucamine)] and nonionic monomers [a single benzene ring, three iodine atoms and from four to six hydroxyl groups (-OH) per molecule] have medium-sized molecules.
- Nonionic dimers [two benzene rings, six iodine atoms, over eight hydroxyl groups (-OH) per molecule] have the largest molecules.

Hydrophilicity, a key feature for intrathecal administration, is correlated to the presence of hydroxyl groups. Some authors claim that the interactions of contrast agents with biological molecules are proportional to their lipid solubility (Rapoport and Levitan 1974; Facino et al. 1979), probably due to the possible interactions between cell proteins and lipophilic areas of the benzene ring. The distribution of hydrophilic groups is also deemed important since they should be arranged in such a way as to block access to the benzene ring by biological molecules situated above and alongside the ring to ensure the lowest possible chemotoxicity (Bonnemain et al. 1990).

The number of hydroxyl groups and their distribution within the molecule affects the substance's chemotoxicity following intravenous and subarachnoid administration. Metrizamide, for example, a nonionic monomer with four hydroxyl groups located at one end of the molecule, has a chemotoxicity (after both intravenous and subarachnoid administration) greater than two other nonionic monomers, iopamidol and iohexol, which respectively have five and six hydroxyl groups distributed within the molecule. New molecules like ioversol have a reduced neurotoxicity (an LD_{50} of 3.9 mmol/kg per intracerebral administration in cat) in that they were developed in the laboratory with safety in mind.

Chemotoxicity, and more specifically neurotoxicity, is not only correlated to the hydroxyl groups in the molecule, but also the presence of the carboxyl group (COO^-) characterizing ionic contrast agents (monomers and dimers). Eliminating the carboxyl groups reduces the product's neurotoxicity also by ruling out the likelihood of *ionic interactions* with cellular biochemical processes by bringing about the passage to a nonionic molecular structure. This is demonstrated by the fact that although metrizamide (a nonionic monomer) has an osmolarity equal to half that of metrizoate (an ionic monomer), its toxicity following subarachnoid administration in animals is at least tenfold lower than that of metrizoate.

9.4 Neurotoxicity in Relation to the Physical Properties of Contrast Media

The osmotic characteristics of a contrast material are determined by the number of particles in solution; osmosis is measured in mOsm per 300 mg/ml iodine concentration (blood has an osmotic pressure of 300 mOsm).

The role of osmolarity in determining the neurotoxicity of a contrast agent is still unsettled. However, this characteristic affects the possiblility of direct contact between molecules of contrast material and nerve tissue, but only in the case of intra-arterial injection. This is because hyperosmolaric solutions can temporarily damage the blood-brain barrier, probably triggering the contraction of cells in the endothelia of cerebral vessels following opening of the intercellular occluding junctions and passage of contrast medium into the extracellular perivascular space (Rapoport et al. 1980; Corsico and Tirone 1988). When a contrast medium is injected intravenously, changes in plasma osmolarity do not affect the blood-brain barrier and material will only penetrate if the barrier has already been damaged prior to administration.

The role of contrast medium osmolarity in impairing the homeostatic mechanisms of nerve cells is a matter of debate. Inert hyperosmolaric solutions injected into experimental animals exert a depressive effect on the electrical activity of nerve cells. This would account for the depressive neurotoxic effects produced by administration of only slightly hypertonic solutions of contrast media, but it does not explain the excitatory effects such as epileptic seizures (SPECK et al. 1988).

A product's viscosity determines the length of contact between the vascular endothelium and the contrast material.

The hyperosmolaric properties of contrast agents are probably responsible for secondary neurotoxicity which gives rise to bradycardia and hypotension following intra-arterial administration. This is thought to be due to the toxic effects on receptors in the carotid sinus, the carotid vascular bed, and the nerve centres which regulate cardiovascular activity (HIGGINS and SCHMIDT 1979).

9.5 Neurotoxicity in Relation to Route of Administration

The degree of neurotoxicity depends on the route of contrast administration. Following intravenous injection, water-soluble iodate contrast media all have the same pharmacokinetic behavior: plasma concentration decreases exponentially; the half-life in the body is about 2 h. Migration through the blood-brain barrier depends, as we have seen, on existing damage to the barrier, the contrast agent's osmolarity, and also the chemotoxicity of its molecules, as demonstrated by the following experimental evidence:

- Disruption of the blood-brain barrier by a contrast medium is always more severe than that caused by the administration of saline or mannitol solutions with the same osmolarity (SAGE et al. 1982, 1983).
- Iotrolan and iodixanol have a similar osmolarity to blood (320 and 272 mOsm/kg versus 300 mg I/ml) but they both penetrate the blood-brain barrier, albeit to a limited extent (EVILL et al. 1990; HAYAKAWA et al. 1990).
- The threshold osmotic level for damage to the blood-brain barrier seems to be 1600 mOsm/kg (RAPOPORT et al. 1980).
- Following intracarotid injection of iohexol (690 mOsm/kg vs 300 mg I/ml) and iodixanol (272 mOsm/kg vs 300 mg I/ml), damage to the blood-brain barrier is the same (WILCOX et al. 1987).

In the case of ionic contrast administration, the type of cation present in the product's molecule seems to determine its chemotoxicity. The sodium ion has a more severe toxic effect on the blood-brain barrier than that of meglumine (SAGE et al. 1989).

The greater the osmolarity and amount of the injected contrast agent, the greater the damage to the blood-brain barrier. Under normal conditions the blood-brain barrier is repaired in 5–120 min after contrast administration. Repeated injections of contrast material at high concentrations, as occurs during angiography, especially in interventional therapeutic procedures (JEPPSON and OLIN 1970), therefore cause more damage to the barrier and nerve tissue. Intravenous injection of contrast material seldom produces plasma osmolarity changes great enough to rupture the blood-brain barrier unless the barrier has already been damaged by tumor or brain infarction. In any case, administration of contrast medium by infusion is preferable to a bolus injection, which is more likely to penetrate the blood-brain barrier, giving rise to greater changes in plasma osmolarity. The risk of neurotoxic effects following intra-arterial and intravenous administration is always exacerbated when the blood-brain barrier is already damaged, as in the case of metastases or cerebral expansive lesions.

In assessing the role of osmolarity of contrast agents in disrupting the blood-brain barrier, it is noteworthy that all contrast media can penetrate the barrier, even those in iso-osmolar solutions (AULIE 1980). This experimental evidence suggests that in practice chemotoxicity plays a more important role in determining neurological manifestations than osmolarity.

Intrathecal injection of contrast medium leads to a massive diffusion of material in nerve tissue given the lack of closed junctions in the ependymal and pial cells so that contrast penetrates all the most superficial layers of the cortex (DUNKER et al. 1976). The degree of contrast migration is similar for nonionic monomers (LA NOCE et al. 1996), but nonionic dimers penetrate brain tissue less than nonionic monomers, probably because their molecules are larger (CASTEL et al. 1987). Experiments in dog (SAGE et al. 1983) have disclosed an inhomogeneous dispersion of contrast medium in the most superficial layers of the cerebral cortex as early as 15 min after intracisternal injection. Contrast diffusion peaks after an hour with subcortical penetration to 13 mm depth. The time required for the clearance of contrast material from the brain cortex by diffusion through the meninges and transport along the CSF pathways varies depending on the product's molecular structure. For example, iotrol (a nonionic dimer) is eliminated more swiftly than iopamidol or metrizamide (nonionic monomers). Plainly, impaired CSF circulation (blockage or incomplete occlusion of the subarachnoid spaces) significantly delays contrast clearance.

In addition, the site of intrathecal injection is important. Cervical injection in man causes more frequent and more severe complications than lumbar administration, probably due to the enhanced diffusion of the contrast agent at the intracranial level (MOSCHINI et al. 1983).

9.6 Manifestations of Neurotoxicity

The possible clinical manifestations of neurotoxicity are listed in Table 9.1. Symptoms appear from 2 to 12 h after contrast injection depending on the time required for the material to penetrate the cerebral cortex. Many literature reports have investigated neurotoxic manifestations following intrathecal or intravenous injection of contrast agents in man and animals (ADAMS et al. 1988, 1990; CAILLÉ and ALLARD 1988; FLORAS et al. 1990; LA NOCE et al. 1994; LARSEN et al. 1995; LUZZANI et al. 1996; MALY et al. 1995; ROSATI and LETO DI PRIOLO 1992; SPECK et al. 1988; THOMSON et al. 1990; TORVIK and WAKDAY 1995; WHISSON et al. 1990; ZWEIFLER and ROTHROCK 1995).

Ionic contrast media have not been used for intrathecal injection since the 1970s, given their high rate of neurotoxicity demonstrated by rare cases of accidental administration (ROSATI and LETO DI PRIOLO 1992). However, wide differences exist in the frequency of neurological manifestations even with the newer nonionic contrast agents.

Table 9.1. Neurological manifestations following contrast medium administration (from TORVIK 1995)

Headache	Cortical blindness
Nausea	Scotomas
Vomiting	Drowsiness
Dizziness	Depressions
Meningism	Agitations
Seizures	Paranoid states
Myoclonus	Hallucinations
Diplopia	Memory loss
Nystagmus	Aphasia
Cranial nerve paresis	Arachnoiditis

A number of adverse effects have been reported following intrathecal injection of metrizamide, including headache in 50%, vomiting in 20%, transient mental disorders in 2%, epileptic seizures in 1%, and EEG changes in 34% of cases (BUCHMAN et al. 1987; JUNCK and MARSHALL 1983; SCHMIDT 1980). The frequency of such reactions is much lower following administration of monomers or nonionic dimers by the same route: headache has been reported in 15%–20% of cases and vomiting in 5%–20%, while more severe complications such as epileptic seizures or aseptic meningoencephalitis are rare (CAILLÉ and ALLARD 1988; ELKIN et al. 1986; LEVEY et al. 1988; NAKSTAD et al. 1984; TAHTA et al. 1993; VESTERGAARD et al. 1991; ZWEIFLER and ROTHROCK 1995).

The frequency of neurological complications following intravenous injection is around 7%–8% for ionic contrast media and 1%–4% for nonionic contrast agents (CARCHETTI 1988). In particular, intravenous injection of ionic contrast media in patients with existing damage to the blood-brain barrier triggered epileptic seizures in 6%–15% of patients (AVRAHMI et al. 1989; SCOTT 1980). In addition the prognosis of patients with cerebral infarction significantly deteriorated after ionic contrast administration (PULLICINO and KENDALL 1980).

Neurotoxic manifestations following administration of nonionic contrast material are so rare that they are statistically negligible (LEONARDI et al. 1989).

Intra-arterial administration of ionic contrast media (vertebral angiography) has given rise to epileptic seizures in 0.2%–0.4% of cases, cortical blindness in 0.3%–1%, global amnesia, and other mental disorders (JUNCK and MARSHALL 1983). On the other hand, intra-arterial injection of nonionic material has only caused sporadic cases of transient global amnesia and transient cortical blindness (GIANG and KIDO 1989; JUNI et al. 1992; LANTOS 1989).

9.7 Choice of Contrast Medium

The introduction of the more expensive nonionic contrast media in clinical practice has raised the ethical issue of cost-benefit: if and when would the use of the cheaper ionic contrast agents still be feasible despite the fact that they carry a much greater risk of systemic and neurological toxicity?

First and foremost, there exists a good correlation between animal models and clinical practice in terms of the neurotoxicity of contrast material (MALY et al. 1995).

As discussed above, the intrathecal administration of ionic contrast media should be ruled out because of the high neurotoxicity of these agents (Table 9.2). Many claim, however, that ionic contrast media should be abandoned altogether even in the case of intravenous injection as their use cannot be justified by ethical or economic considerations. Others (CAILLÉ and ALLARD 1988) have proposed to differentiate low- and high-risk patients, recommending ionic or nonionic media accordingly for reasons of cost. However, since the introduction of nonionic contrast media has led to a sixfold reduction in the incidence of adverse systemic reactions, some rebut this argument on the grounds that patient selection would be difficult to implement epidemiologically, ethically, and rationally as it would entail a threefold greater risk of adverse reactions in low-risk patients (Table 9.3), who by far outnumber those at high risk (PALMER 1990).

From the economic standpoint, recent evidence has shown that unlike ionic contrast material, the use of nonionic contrast media does not require the costly laboratory investigations frequently prescribed in Italy prior to contrast administration. The higher cost of the contrast agent itself would therefore be offset by savings elsewhere (LEONARDI et al. 1995).

Even though magnetic resonance (MR) imaging is gradually replacing myelography, the problem of which nonionic contrast medium to inject intrathecally still needs to be addressed for the following reasons:

- In many countries MR has not yet entered clinical practice.
- Not all patients are candidates for MR (owing to claustrophobia, pacemakers, or ferromagnetic implants).

Nonionic contrast agents have different acute neurotoxicity levels (Table 9.4) and hence only some of them are suitable for intrathecal injection. Fortunately there is a general consensus in the literature even though findings vary as some authors gauge acute neurotoxicity on the basis of animal studies (rat, mouse, cat, dog, rabbit), while others use models based on behavioral and electrophysiological changes after subarachnoid administration at sublethal doses, and yet others utilize electrophysiological or clinical changes encountered in man.

Among the nonionic monomers, ioversol is currently the contrast agent with the least neurotoxicity (ADAMS et al. 1990; LUZZANI et al. 1996), followed by iomeprol and iopamidol (LA NOCE et al. 1994, ROSATI 1994). Iopromide, iopentol, and above all, iohexol present a higher neurotoxicity.

The nonionic dimers (iofratol, iotrolan, iodixanol) have a greater neurotoxicity than nonionic monomers and hence there is no reason to opt for one of these products as against a nonionic monomer when intrathecal injection is envisaged,

Table 9.2. Median lethal dose (LD_{50}) and confidence limits ($P < 0.05$) of ionic contrast media in mice after intracerebral administration (modified from ROSATI and LETO DI PRIOLO 1992)

Compound	LD_{50} [g (iodine)/kg b.w.]
Methiodal sodium	0.060 (0.040–0.070)
Diatrizoate meglumine	0.055 (0.040–0.070)
Iodamide meglumine	0.097 (0.070–0.140)
Iothalamate meglumine	0.193 (0.160–0.230)
Ioxitalamate meglumine	0.145 (0.130–0.160)
Iocarmate meglumine	0.280 (0.200–0.390)

Table 9.3. Frequency of adverse reactions in an Australasian (RACR) survey (from PALMER 1990)

Reactions	Mild	Moderate	Severe
Low-risk/ionic CM	3.65% (SD 0.13)	0.40% (SD 0.02)	0.09% (SD 0.02)
High-risk/nonionic CM	1.26% (SD 0.09)	0.14% (SD 0.03)	0.03% (SD 0.03)
Difference	2.39% (SD 0.22)	0.26% (SD 0.07)	0.06% (SD 0.04)

CM, Contrast media.

Table 9.4. Median lethal dose (LD_{50}) and confidence limits of nonionic contrast media in mice after intracerebroventricular administration (modified from LUZZANI 1996)

Compound	LD_{50} [g (iodine)/kg b.w.]	LD_{50} (mmol/kg. b.w.)
Iomeprol	1.44 (1.26–1.64)	3.78 (3.31–4.31)
Iopamidol	1.49 (1.37–1.61)	3.91 (3.60–4.23)
Iohexol	0.84 (0.69–1.00)	2.21 (1.81–2.63)
Ioversol	1.63 (1.51–1.77)	4.28 (3.96–4.65)
Iopentol	1.23 (1.11–1.42)	3.23 (2.91–3.73)
Iopromide	1.40 (1.26–1.57)	3.68 (3.31–4.13)
Iofratol	0.95 (0.83–1.09)	1.25 (1.09–1.43)
Iotrolan	1.02 (0.87–1.20)	1.28 (1.10–1.51)
Iodixanol	0.97 (0.88–1.06)	1.27 (1.15–1.39)

especially as dimers are more difficult to administer because of their greater viscosity.

9.8 Conclusions

Given the marked sensitivity of the central nervous system, neurotoxicity is a parameter of major importance when choosing which contrast agent to administer.

Animal models are reliable indicators of neurotoxicity in clinical practice. A product's degree of neurotoxicity depends on a number of variables, some of which remain unsettled. The most important factor appears to be the molecule's chemotoxicity, which in turn correlates with the product's hydrophilicity and the osmolarity of solutions, both of which are responsible for damage to the blood-brain barrier and impaired cell function.

The intrathecal injection of nonionic contrast media has now been abandoned. Among the nonionic agents available, the least toxic monomer products are recommended (ioversol, iomeprol, iopamidol). Nonionic contrast material is also preferable for intravenous administration in view of its minor systemic and neurological toxicity.

References

Adams MD, Hopkins RM, Ferrendelli JA (1988) A rat EEG model for evaluating contrast media neurotoxicity. Invest Radiol (Suppl 1) 23:S217–S219

Adams MD, Ralston WH, Ferrendelli JA (1990) Electroencephalographic effects of intracisternally injected nonionic X-ray contrast media in rats. Invest Radiol 25:S86–S87

Almén T (1989) Relations between chemical structure, animal toxicity and clinical adverse effects of contrast media. In: Enge I, Edgren J (eds) Patient safety and adverse events in contrast medium examinations. Elsevier Science, Amsterdam, p 25

Aulie A (1980) Effect of iohexol, metrizamide and ioxaglate on the blood-brain barrier. Acta Radiol (Suppl) 362:13–16

Avrahmi E, Weiss-Peretz J, Conn DF (1989) Epilepsy in patients with brain metastases triggered by intravenous contrast medium. Clin Radiol 40:422

Belloni G, Bonaldi G, Monchini L (1988) Neurotossicità dei mezzi di contrasto iodati. Riv Neuroradiol 1:147–153

Bonnemain B, Meyer D, Schaefes M, et al. (1990) New iodinated, low-osmolar contrast media. A revised concept of hydrophilicity. Invest Radiol 25:S104–S106

Buchman AS, Klawans HL, Russell EJ (1987) Metrizamide and its neurological complications. Clin Neuropharmacol 10:1

Caillé JM, Allard M (1983) Neurotoxicity of hydrosoluble iodine contrast media. Invest Radiol 23(Suppl 1):S210

Caillé JM, Allard M (1988) Mezzi di contrasto in neuroradiologia. Riv Neuroradiol 1:129–138

Carchetti E, Baldassasare M, Penco T, Heonardi M (1988) Iopamidol 300-induced epilepsy. Intensive treatment and pathogenetic hypothesis. Neuroradiology 30:256

Castel JC, Dorcier F, Caillè JM (1987) Penetration of the brain by nonionic water soluble tri- and hexaiodinated contrast media. Experimental autoradiographic study of two contrast media: iotrol and iopamidol labelled with iodine 125. Neuroradiology 29:206–210

Corsico N, Tirone P (1988) Mezzi di contrasto iodurati ionici e non-ionici in neuroradiologia: aspetti farmacotossicologici. Riv Neuroradiol 1:155–159

Dunker RO, Harris AB, Jenkins DP (1976) Kinetics of horseradish peroxidase migration through cerebral cortex. Brain Res 118:199

Elkin C, Levan AMT, Leeds NE (1986) Tolerance of iohexol, iopamidol and metrizamide in lumbar myelography. Surg Neurol 26:542

Evill CA, Wilson AJ, Sage MR (1990) Chemotoxic effects of low-osmolar contrast media on the blood-brain barrier. Invest Radiol 25:S82–83

Facino RM, Raffaelli E, Pitre E (1979) Iopronic acid interaction with hepatic microsomal cytochrome P-450: relationship between chemical structure and binding. Pharmacol Res Commun 11:105–113

Floras P, Deliac P, Gross C, et al. (1990) Neurotoxicité de l'Iohexol vs Iopamidol dans la myélographie lombaire. Corrélations clinique, électrophysiologique et tomodensitométrique. J Neuroradiol 17:190–200

Giang DW, Kido DK (1989) Transient global amnesia associated with cerebral angiography performed with use of iopamidol. Radiology 172:195

Hayakawa K, Yamashita K, Mitsumori M, Nakano Y (1990) Iodinated contrast media. In vivo quantification of the blood-brain barrier injury using magnetic resonance enhancement. Invest Radiol 25:S80–S81

Higgins CB, Schmidt WS (1979) Identification and evaluation of the contribution of the chemoreflex in the hemodynamic response to intracarotid administration of contrast materials in the conscious dog: comparison with the response to nicotine. Invest Radiol 14:438–446

Hoppe JO, Archer S (1960) X-ray contrast media for cardiovascular angiography. Angiology 11:244

Jeppson PG, Olin T (1970) Neurotoxicity of roentgen contrast media: study of the brain-blood barrier following selective injection of contrast media into the internal carotid artery. Acta Radiol 10:17–34

Junck L, Marshall WH (1983) Neurotoxicity of radiological contrast agents. Ann Neurol 13:469

Juni J, Morera J, et al. (1992) Transient global amnesia after cerebral angiography with iohexol. Neuroradiology 34: 141

Katayama H, Yamaguchi K, Kozuka T, et al. (1990) Adverse reactions to ionic and non-ionic contrast media. A report from Japanese Committee on the Safety of Contrast Media. Radiology 175:621

La Noce A, Bertani F, Lorusso V, Luzzani F, Tirone P, De Haen C (1994) Preclinical safety assessment of iomeprol for injection as contrast medium for myelography. Eur J Radiol 18(Suppl 1):S43–S50

La Noce A, Lorenzon P, Pugliese F, et al. (1996) Brain penetration of intrathecal iomeprol in dogs. Acta Radiol 37:578–581

Lalli AF (1980) Contrast media reactions: data analysis and hypothesis. Radiology 134:1–12

Lantos G (1989) Cortical blindness due to osmotic disruption of the blood-brain barrier by angiographic contrast material. CT and MRI studies. Neurology 39:567

Larsen LE, Heglund IF, Fabian R, et al. (1995) Neural tolerability of iodixanol in mice and dogs after single and repeated intracisternal administration. Acta Radiol (1995) 36(Suppl 399):238–243

Leonardi M, Lavaroni A, Bianizzo E, et al. (1989) High-dose contrast-enhanced computed tomography (CECT) with iopamidol in the detection of cerebral metastases. Tolerance of the contrast agent. Neuroradiology 31:148–150

Leonardi M, Auxilia F, Cosmacini G, Ottomano C (1995) Impiego degli esami ematochimici preliminari all'iniezione di mezzo di contrasto: è possibile rinunciarvi? Riv Neuroradiol 8:323–327

Levey AI, Weiss H, Yu R, Wang H, Krumholz A (1988) Seizures following myelography with iopamidol. Ann Neurol 23:397

Luzzani F, Morisetti A, Bussi S, Tirone P, De Haen C (1996) Neurotolerability of nonionic X-ray contrast media. Invest Radiol 31:338–344

Maly P, Sundgren P, Baath L, Golman K, Walday P (1995) Adverse reactions in myelography. Correlation between animal research and clinical practice. Acta Radiol 36 (Suppl 399):230–237

Marder E, O'Neil M, Grossman RI, et al. (1983) Cholinergic actions of metrizamide. AJNR 4:61–65

Moschini M, Manara O, Bonaldi G, Cassinari V, Quilici N, Belloni G (1983) Iopamidol and metrizamide in cervical myelography: side effects, EEG and CSF changes. AJNR 4:848–850

Nakstad P, Helgetveit A, et al. (1984) Iohexol compared to metrizamide in cervical and thoracic myelography. A randomized double blind parallel study. Neuroradiology 26:479

Palmer J (1990) Morbidity and mortality with intravenous contrast media ionic and nonionic. Invest Radiol 25:S18–S19

Pullicino P, Kendall BE (1980) Contrast enhancement in ischaemic lesions: in relationship to prognosis. Neuroradiology 19:253–259

Rapoport ST, Levitan H (1974) Neurotoxicity of x-ray contrast media: relation to lipid solubility and blood-brain barrier permeability. Am J Roentgenol 122:186–193

Rapoport SI, Fredericks WR, Ohno K, Pettigrew KD (1980) Quantitative aspects of reversible osmotic opening of the blood-brain barrier. Am J Physiol 238:R421

Rosati G (1994) Clinical utility and safety profile of iomeprol. Eur J Radiol 18(Suppl 1):S120–S124

Rosati G, Leto di Priolo S, Tirone P (1992) Serious or fatal complications after inadvertent administration of ionic water-soluble contrast media in myelography. Eur J Radiol 15:95–100

Sage MR, Wilcox J, Evill CA, Benness GT (1982) Comparison and evaluation of osmotic blood-brain barrier disruption following intracarotid mannitol and methylglucamine iothalamate. Invest Radiol 17:276–281

Sage MR, Wilcox J (1983) Brain parenchyma penetration by intrathecal nonionic iopamidol. AJNR 4:1181–1183

Sage MR, Turski PA, Levin A (1989) CNS imaging of the brain barrier. In: Neuwelt EA (ed) Implications of the blood-brain barrier and its manipulation. Plenum, New York, vol 2, Chap. 14

Schmidt RC (1980) Mental disorders after myelography with metrizamide and other water soluble contrast media. Neuroradiology 19:153

Scott WR (1980) Seizures. A reaction to contrast media for computed tomography of the brain. Radiology 137:359

Speck U, Press WR, Mutzel W (1988) Osmolality-related effects of injections into the central nervous system. Invest Radiol 23(Suppl 1):S114–S117

Tahta K, Ozgen T, Betker M, et al. (1993) Status epilepticus following iohexol myelography. Neuroradiology 35:322

Thomsen S, Dorph S (1993) High-osmolar and low-osmolar contrast media. An update on frequency of adverse drug reactions. Acta Radiol 34:205

Thomson KR, Wells DG, O'Brien K, Tomkins DC, Dixon RG (1990) Vertebral artery injections of methylglucamine diatrizoate, 60% iopromide, and iotrolan in the rabbit. Invest Radiol 25:S88–S89

Torvik A, Wakday P (1995) Neurotoxicity of water-soluble contrast media. A review. Acta Radiol 36(Suppl 399):221–229

Vestergaard A, Dons K, Eskesen V, et al. (1991) Central nervous system reactions to cervical myelography. Acta Radiol 32:411

Whisson CC, Evill CA, Wilson AJ, et al. (1990) Muscular and central nervous system side effects of intracarotid contrast media in rabbits. Invest Radiol 25:S90–S91

Wilcox J, Wilson AJ, Evill CA, Sage MR (1987) A comparison of blood-brain barrier disruption by intracarotid iohexol and iodixanol in the rabbit. AJNR 8:769–772

Zweifler RM, Rothrock JF (1995) Aseptic meningoencephalitis following iohexol myelography. Neuroradiology 37:148–149

10 Nephrotoxicity

H.S. Thomsen

CONTENTS

10.1 Definition and Features

Contrast media nephrotoxicity refers to a condition in which impairment of renal function occurs following intravascular administration of a contrast medium in the absence of an alternative etiology (Table 10.1). The literature is conflicting with regard to the level of renal dysfunction that must be present in order to diagnose contrast media nephropathy. Some are in favor of a high sensitivity and lower specificity, requiring an increase in serum creatinine by more than 25% or 44 µmol/l (Barrett et al. 1992; Manske et al. 1990; Solomon et al. 1994). Others opt for a lower sensitivity, but a high specificity; they advocate an increase in serum creatinine by more 50% or 90 µmol/l (Parfrey et al. 1989; Rudnick et al. 1995). It is generally accepted that renal function should be monitored for at least 3 days before excluding the development of contrast media nephropathy.

The most important features of contrast media nephrotoxicity are: (a) a decrease in creatinine clearance, (b) a reduction in renal function which often resolves within 1–2 weeks, (c) an increase in serum creatinine that peaks within 3–4 days after the administration of contrast medium, and (d) oliguria. In the past a persistent nephrogram on a plain abdominal film from 6 h after contrast medium administration or on CT of the abdomen more than 24 h after the injection of contrast medium (Love et al. 1994) has been considered an important feature of contrast medium nephrotoxicity. Current literature, however, indicates that a persistent nephrogram is not an important feature of contrast medium-induced nephropathy since its presence is not always associated with a reduction in renal function (Jakobsen et al. 1992; Yamazaki et al. 1997). The detection of this sign should be followed by assessment of renal function, and the administration of further doses of contrast media is contraindicated if the results are abnormal.

10.2 The Handling of Contrast Media by the Normal Kidney

When the contrast medium molecules reach the systemic circulation, they quickly equilibrate across capillary membranes (except for an intact blood-brain barrier). During the first phase of distribution, the increase in intravascular osmolality for hypertonic agents as well as the low-osmolar contrast media causes a rapid fluid shift across capillary membranes toward the intravascular compartment. At the same time the contrast medium molecules move rapidly through capillary pores into the interstitial, extracellular space, as well as via glomerular filtration into the renal tubules.

The plasma concentration of iodine follows a biexponential decay curve like drugs which are freely distributed in the extracellular phase and excreted by pure glomerular filtration, e.g., technetium-99m diethylene triamine penta-acetic acid. The first exponential term represents the mixing of the contrast

H.S. Thomsen, MD, Department of Diagnostic Radiology, Copenhagen University Hospital at Herlev, Herlev Ringvej 75, DK-2730 Herlev, Denmark

Table 10.1. Definition of contrast medium-induced nephropathy

Contrast medium-induced nephropathy is a condition in which an impairment in renal function (*an increase in serum creatinine by more than 25% or 44 µmol/l*) occurs with 3 days following the intravascular administration of a contrast medium in the absence of an alternative etiology.

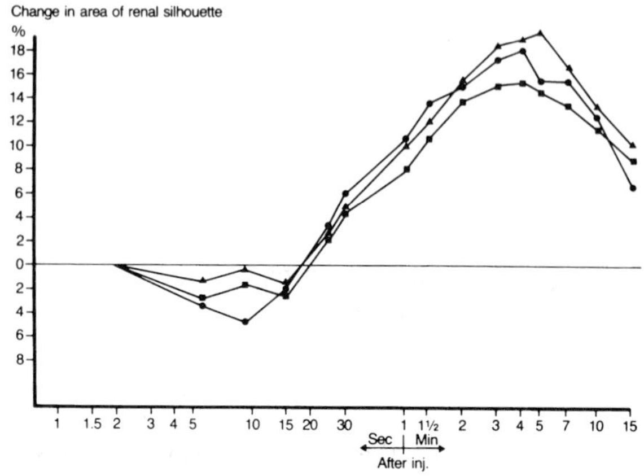

Fig. 10.1. Change in the area of the renal silhouette after renal arteriography with diatrizoate (•), iohexol (▲), or ioxilan (■) in rabbits. Within the first seconds there is a drop in the area of the renal silhouette but after 30 s it is enlarged. After approximately 5 min the area of the renal silhouette becomes smaller and within the next 15 min it approximates to normal

medium in the plasma volume and then its distribution into the interstitial space. After approximately 150 min the concentration of contrast medium decreases in a monoexponential way in patients with normal renal function; in patients with severely reduced renal function this phase is delayed (see Chap. 8).

The kidneys account for just 0.4% of the total body mass, but receive approximately 1.2–1.3 l blood each minute (20%–25% of total cardiac output). The normal glomerular filtration rate (GFR) for human beings is 125 ml or 180 l/day (60 times plasma volume) (Hollenberg 1983). Since more than 99% of the filtrate is reabsorbed, the normal urine volume is approximately 1 l/day. The glomerular membrane allows passage of substances of up to ca. 4 nm in diameter and excludes substances larger than 8 nm in diameter. The threshold for filtration is a molecular weight of around 40 000. Albumin has a molecular weight of 43 500 and a diameter of 3 nm, and approximately 22% passes through the glomerular filtration threshold (Blantz 1983; Hostetter and Brenner 1983). Subsequently it is reabsorbed in the proximal tubules of normal kidneys. Since the molecular weights of currently used iodinated intravascular media are below 2000 and since protein binding of modern urographic contrast media is negligible, the contrast medium molecules are freely filtered without hindrance.

The concentration of contrast medium within the tubule depends on the concentration in the glomerular filtrate and on the amount of water reabsorbed as the filtrate passes down the tubule. The concentration in the initial filtrate is the same as that in plasma. However, the concentration in mature urine is 50–100 times that in the plasma (Thomsen et al. 1993) since 75% of the filtered water is reabsorbed in proximal tubule, 5% in the loop of Henle, 15% in the distal tubule, and nearly 5% in the collecting ducts.

Because molecules of contrast material, like those of mannitol, are not reabsorbed, they continue to exert an osmotic force, markedly reducing reabsorption of water from the tubules. This increases pressure in the Bowman capsule and creates an acute internal hydronephrosis associated with individual nephron dilatation; this leads to global renal enlargement (Fig. 10.1). The main resistance to urine flow in the kidney is at the level of the collecting ducts, which have a total cross-sectional intraluminal area that is smaller than the total cross-sectional intraluminal area of the tubules of the nephrons (Gottschalk and Mylle 1957). The contrast-induced reductions in GFR, filtration fraction, and renal perfusion are explainable on the basis of these intratubular and intracapsular pressure changes caused by the hypertonic solution. On the basis of Sterling's law, the increase in proximal tubular hydrostatic pressure decreases the gradient for filtration from the glomerular capillary. These effects are markedly attenuated when low-osmolar contrast media and isotonic contrast media are used (Katzberg et al. 1977, 1990).

Within minutes after an intravascular osmotic diuretic is injected, the water and sodium excretion from the kidney increases markedly (Gennari and Kassires 1974; Katzberg et al. 1986). Much of the diuretic action can be accounted for on the basis of inhibition of sodium and water reabsorption in the proximal tubule, along with inhibition of sodium and water transport in the loop of Henle (Gennari and Kassires 1974). During brisk osmotic diuresis, the distal tubule and collecting duct fail to recapture any notable portion of the increased sodium and water load delivered into the early distal tubule. Increases in the rate of perfusion of the distal portion of the loop lead to a decrease in whole kidney GFR, which is a function of the so-called tubuloglomerular feedback (TGF) mechanism. This is, in part, related to the marked increase in proximal tubular pressure with increased flow rates within the nephron.

Results of micropuncture studies in rats after slow intravenous infusions of large doses of contrast medium have been useful in our understanding of the tubular handling of contrast media (UEDA et al. 1992). Monomers decrease single nephron GFR during the infusion phase. A marked pressure drop between the distal tubules and the renal pelvis has been noted and provides supporting evidence that the most distal part of the nephron, including the collecting ducts, is the main site of resistance to outflow of urine after the injection of contrast medium. The depression of single nephron GFR is attributed to the intratubular concentration, which is higher the lower the osmolality is. The higher the concentration, the higher is the tubular urine viscosity of the medium. Increased tubular urine viscosity causes a prolonged increase in tubular hydrostatic pressure and a more prolonged depression of single nephron GFR. The higher concentrations of iso-osmotic nonionic dimers, iotrolan and iodixanol, especially in the proximal tubules, where the contrast agents have a decreased osmotic force, might be due to a combination of the iso-osmotic nature and the dimeric configuration, which result in higher urine viscosity. Thus the nonionic iso-osmolar dimers produce a more prolonged depression of single nephron GFR than do the nonionic low-osmolar monomers, while the latter cause longer depression of single nephron GFR than do the ionic high-osmolar contrast media. Whether the reduction in the single nephron GFR is of clinical importance remains to be resolved. All the literature (Sect. 10.5) indicates that that monomers, which cause the shortest reduction in single nephron GFR, are the most nephrotoxic.

10.3 History

In their survey of more than 661 000 contrast-supplemented urographic procedures PENDERGRASS et al. (1942) reported 16 late deaths, including nine in patients with acute or chronic renal damage/disease. Twelve years later BARTELS et al. (1954) reported the first case of contrast-induced acute oliguric renal failure in a myeloma patient. PERILLIE and CONN (1958) reported additional cases and speculated that the cause may be the precipitation of Bence Jones protein leading to intraluminal obstruction. For many years these observations led to the conclusion that administration of contrast media is contraindicated in patients with myeloma; however, this view is no longer accepted.

In a survey of 13 207 abdominal aortograms it was noted that the most frequently reported complications were renal, with 12 uremic deaths (MCAFEE 1957). If postangiogram abnormalities of renal function were not accompanied by clinical symptoms, they were not considered as complications of the procedure. In another study it was recorded that the complications associated with renal angiography occurred in patients with coexisting renal disease (IDBOHRN 1956). It was concluded that the concentration of the contrast medium and the site of injection contributed to the risk of renal injury. Surprisingly at the same time, the classical description of oliguric renal failure by SWANN and MERRILL (1953) failed to attribute a single case to contrast media.

Simultaneously with the introduction of diatrizoate, iothalamate, and metrizoate, the logic of conducting contrast medium studies in patients with impaired renal function was questioned. Concern arose as to whether a sufficient concentration of the agents would reach the kidney and provide satisfactory imaging. This concern was answered in dramatic fashion when it was reported that 60 ml 50% sodium diatrizoate provided satisfactory visualization of the kidneys and lower urinary tract while "affecting the natural history of the renal disease" (SCHWARTZ et al. 1963). Subsequently more aggressive imaging of patients with renal insufficiency was performed using the drip-infusion technique (SCHENKER 1964). In 1972, Grainger wrote a defense of the high-dose contrast studies in patients with renal insufficiency: "Despite the occasional suspected disasters, there can be no doubt that high-dose urography has been of great value in diagnosis and assessment of patients with severe renal failure and oliguria." VAN WAES (1972) wrote an outstanding book highlighting the many advantages of high-dose urography in the workup of patients with renal insufficiency. By this means one could obtain information about (a) whether the kidney size was large, normal, or small, (b) whether the surface was smooth or irregular, and (c) whether the urinary tract was normal or dilated. This was very important information at a time when ultrasonography was not available. Simultaneously with the introduction of high-dose urography there was a growing suspicion that the standard dehydration protocol used to improve urogram quality was detrimental to patients with renal impairment (Berdon et al. 1969). A review of the outcome in 200 myeloma patients who had undergone excretory urography recommended that preurography dehydration be eliminated and abdominal compression avoided in addition to exercising care to prevent any postinjection hypotension (Myer and Witten 1973).

During the 1970s there was a steady increase in the number of cases of contrast-induced acute renal failure reported. However, uniform appreciation of this risk was lacking. As a matter of fact two reviews during the same period failed to mention nephropathy as one of the adverse consequences of contrast medium administration (Witten et al. 1973; Davis et al. 1975). Despite this inconsistency there was a growing number of studies showing that contrast medium administration in high-risk populations carried a significant incidence of post-procedure renal insufficiency (Mudge 1980; Webb et al. 1981).

A relatively high incidence of oliguric renal failure following intravascular administration of contrast media was reported in the older series, with oliguria often beginning within the first 12–24h (Byrd and Sherman 1979; Carvallo et al. 1978; Mudge 1980; Harkonen and Kjellstrand 1981). A failure to recognize the entity of nonoliguric acute tubular necrosis (acute vasomotor nephropathy) (Anderson et al. 1977) probably contributed to the mistaken impression of frequent oliguria in earlier studies. In more recent series, the vast majority of cases of contrast medium-induced nephropathy have been nonoliguric, except in patients with severely reduced renal function (Fang et al. 1980; Manske et al. 1990; Weinrauch et al. 1977; Taliercio et al. 1986).

10.4 Incidence

Intravascular administration of contrast media was claimed in the 1980s to be a common cause of hospital-acquired acute renal failure (Hou et al. 1983; Shusterman et al. 1987). However, the frequency data provided by these studies may have represented an overestimate due to bias limitations inherent in retrospective analyses. Furthermore, the awareness of contrast medium-induced nephropathy is much greater in the 1990s than it was in the 1980s, which may have lowered the incidence. However, neither a drop nor an unchanged level has been reported. Finally, in both retrospective and prospective studies the reported incidence of contrast medium-induced nephropathy can vary significantly as a result of several factors, including reporting criteria, type of radiologic procedure, use of high-, low-, or iso-osmolar contrast media, other prophylactic measures like hydration, and the presence or absence of risk factors, such as renal insufficiency, diabetes mellitus, and high volume of contrast medium. Another important factor which impacts on the incidence of contrast medium-induced nephrotoxicity is the co-administration of nephroprotective as well as nephrotoxic drugs. The insensitivity of serum creatinine as a correct measure of the GFR also affects the figures.

Patient selection is critical, since the relative risk of patients included will predictably influence the number of cases identified. For example a 0%–5% incidence was reported for studies of consecutive prospectively enrolled patients undergoing similar imaging procedures (Eisenberg et al. 1979; Kumar et al. 1981; D'Elia et al. 1982; Mason et al. 1985; Parfrey et al. 1989). Conversely, retrospectively analyzed consecutive cases involving patients undergoing similar imaging procedures yielded an incidence of 11%–12% (Martin-Paredero et al. 1983). Since the definition of contrast medium-induced nephropathy was similar for the prospective and the retrospective studies, it seems that the expected rate of change in serum creatinine of >44 µmol/l or 50% for an unselected population undergoing a contrast-enhanced imaging procedure lies between 2% and 7%. However, when the population was stratified for preprocedure serum creatinine value >120 µmol/l, a fivefold increase in the incidence was recorded (Martin-Paredero et al. 1983).

As mentioned in the introduction (Sect. 10.1), serum creatinine has become a practical parameter with which to diagnose contrast medium-induced nephropathy. However, several expressions of change in serum creatinine levels are being used, including the percent change from baseline, with the usual range being 20%–50%, and the absolute change from baseline, expressed in µmol per liter with a range from 44 µmol/l to 200 µmol/l. When five different definitions of relevant change in serum creatinine were applied on the same database, Lautin et al. (1991) found a variation in the incidence of contrast medium-induced nephrotoxicity from 2.8% to 21.2%, with the lower values reported for definitions based on absolute (µmol/l) changes and the higher values for expressions of percent change. The GFR is usually assessed indirectly by measuring serum creatinine concentration, or by measuring creatinine clearance. This operational definition greatly underestimates toxic results that are not severe enough to affect these insensitive markers of renal function (Blaufox et al. 1996). The serum creatinine concentration, the measure most often used as the indicator of renal dysfunction, depends on muscle mass and may not become elevated above the normal range until the GFR falls to 50% of normal, because of its nonlinear relation to the GFR. Creatinine clearance as a measure of the GFR is also inaccurate (Blaufox et al. 1996). This is especially the case when renal function is low, due to compensatory increase in tubular secretion, which limits its validity as a glomerular filtration marker.

Several studies have documented that the patients at highest risk for developing contrast-induced acute renal failure are those who have both diabetes mellitus and preexisting renal insufficiency or diabetic nephropathy (Fig. 10.2). Parfrey et al. (1989) and Schwab et al. (1989) found that given equal states of hydration, neither diabetes alone nor renal insufficiency alone resulted in a statistically significantly greater incidence of renal dysfunction following contrast medium administration, although patients with these conditions were at a somewhat higher risk for renal failure than the healthy population.

Katholi et al. (1993) performed a prospective double-blind randomized comparison of renal functional responses to a nonionic, low-osmolar contrast medium and to an ionic high-osmolar contrast medium in 70 patients with normal or slightly depressed renal function. They found that reductions in creatinine clearance levels were less marked after coronary angiography with low-osmolar contrast media. Creatinine clearance levels at 24 h decreased by 19% in patients who received the low-osmolar contrast medium but by 40% in patients who received the high-osmolar contrast media. In the patients who received the high-osmolar contrast medium, creatinine clearance remained depressed by 47% at 48 h, but it was normal in the low-osmolar contrast medium group.

The Iohexol Cooperative Study Group (Rudnick et al. 1995) conducted a multicenter trial to compare the renal effects of a high-osmolar medium, meglumine diatrizoate, with those of the low-osmolar medium iohexol. A total of 1194 patients undergoing elective coronary angiography were studied. Overall, nephrotoxicity was less pronounced in the iohexol group than in the diatrizoate group. However, nephrotoxicity occurred almost entirely in high-risk patients with underlying renal insufficiency (baseline serum creatinine >132 µmol/l) and diabetes. The frequency of contrast-induced acute renal failure was 27% in the diatrizoate group versus 12% in the iohexol group. The latter frequencies were based on patients who demonstrated a postcontrast increase in serum creatinine level to 88 µmol/l or more. Also, when defined as a postcontrast increase in serum creatinine to 44 µmol/l or more, the frequency of contrast medium-induced nephropathy in both contrast groups was significantly higher among the patients with renal insufficiency due to diabetes mellitus (diabetic nephropathy) (33% in the iohexol group and 48% in the diatrizoate group) than in those with renal insufficiency due to other causes (12% in the iohexol group and 27% in the diatrizoate group).

Levy et al. (1996) found a 1% incidence of contrast-induced renal failure among 16 248 inpatients undergoing procedures that involved the use of contrast material. In that study contrast-induced acute renal failure was defined as an increase in serum creatinine level of at least 25% to at least 176 µmol/l within 2 days of receiving the contrast material. The results in these patients were compared with those in 174 paired subjects in the same patient population who were matched for age and baseline serum creatinine level and who underwent similar contrast material-enhanced procedures but who did not develop renal failure. The authors found

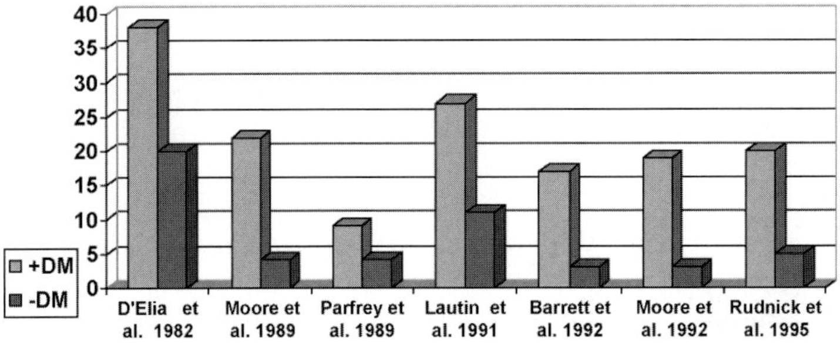

Fig. 10.2. Frequency (%) of contrast media-induced nephropathy in various prospective trials involving patients with precontrast renal insufficiency due to diabetes mellitus (+DM) and other causes (–DM)

that acute renal failure is an important disorder in its own right, noting that even apparently minor perturbations in renal function conferred excess mortality independent of any other factor. It was emphasized that only recently has it become fully recognized that apparently small decreases in renal function may greatly exacerbate the mortality caused by the underlying condition. A 25% rise in serum creatinine level may appear to be small, but it actually represents a substantial decrease in GFR because of the known exponential rise in serum creatinine level with declining GFR. They also identified major new events that are more frequent in patients with acute renal failure and that contribute to morbidity and mortality; these include acquired sepsis, bleeding, coma, and respiratory failure. Among the more than 16000 inpatients undergoing contrast-enhanced examinations, there was a 0.4% mortality, and 0.1% of the subjects required renal replacement therapy. The mortality in patients with renal failure was 34%, whereas it was 7% for those without renal failure. Contrast medium-enhanced examinations included CT of the head and body, cardiac angiography, and peripheral angiography.

It seems appropriate to conclude that in patients with diabetic nephropathy, the incidence of contrast medium-induced nephropathy averages between 15% and 35% (Fig. 10.2). In other renal diseases the incidence averages between 5% and 15%. In patients with no history or signs/symptoms of renal disease the risk is below 1%. The incidence of acute nephrotoxicity in high-risk patients is significantly less with nonionic low-osmolar contrast media compared with the conventional, higher-osmolality ionic contrast media (Fig. 10.3). Inadequate information is available for ionic low-osmolar and nonionic iso-osmolar contrast media; there are no obvious indications that they are more nephrotoxic than the nonionic low-osmolar contrast media.

There is a lack of knowledge regarding the long-term effects of contrast media in man. A recent study has shown that high-osmolar contrast medium can enhance the progression of glomerulosclerosis and renal failure in old spontaneously hypertensive male rats (Duarte et al. 1997). More research in this area is strongly warranted.

10.5 Risk Factors

Numerous studies have attempted to isolate risk factors for contrast medium-induced nephropathy. Byrd and Sherman (1979) listed various predisposing factors for contrast medium-induced acute renal failure, including preexisting renal insufficiency (serum creatinine >130 µmol/l), diabetes mellitus, dehydration per se, cardiovascular disease, the use of diuretics, advanced age (70 years or older), myeloma, hypertension, and hyperuricemia. In a retrospective study of major reports of cases of contrast medium-induced nephropathy, Berns (1989) found preexisting renal impairment (serum creatinine >132 µmol/l) to be the most compelling risk factor. Renal insufficiency was followed closely by factors like albuminuria (>2+), hypertension, age >60 years, dehydration, uric acid (>8.0 mg/dl), and multiple studies. Lower down the list he placed severe congestive heart failure, reduced effective arterial volume (as occurs in nephrosis and cirrhosis), multiple myeloma, administration of a high dose of contrast medium, and intracardiac injection. Concomitant use of certain drugs may also increase the risk; this is true of drugs that impair renal responses such as angiotensin-converting enzyme inhibitors, aminoglycosides like gentamicin, and nonsteroidal anti-inflammatory drugs. Because many patients have more than one risk factor, determining the independent contribution of each factor to the development of renal failure is not possible. It is generally accepted that coexistence of several or many of the factors increases the risk of contrast medium-induced nephropathy considerably. For example a patient with diabetic nephropathy has at least three factors: reduced renal function, albuminuria, and hypertension.

A number of patient groups have an increased risk of developing contrast-induced renal failure. Patients with preexisting renal insufficiency have been consistently demonstrated to be at increased risk by a factor of 5–10. The higher the preexisting serum creatinine, the greater the likelihood that the patient will develop contrast nephrotoxicity.

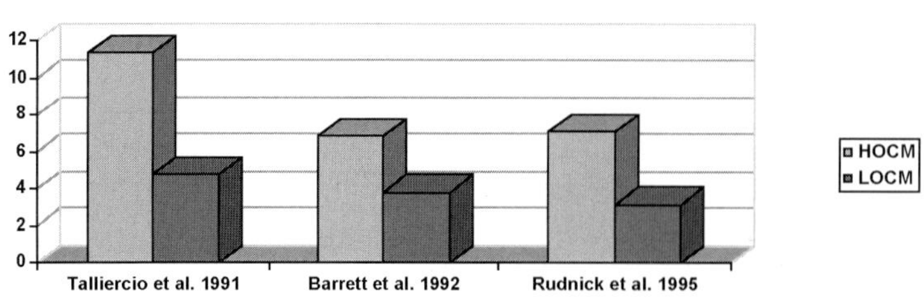

Fig. 10.3. Frequency (%) of contrast medium-induced nephropathy in three prospective randomized trials of low-osmolar contrast media (LOCM) versus high-osmolar contrast media (HOCM)

Patients whose renal failure is the result of diabetic nephropathy are at even greater risk (Fig. 10.2), and when renal failure occurs, it is more likely to be irreversible. The likelihood of irreversibility is greater, the poorer the renal function. Renal insufficiency due to hepatorenal syndrome and rapidly progressive proliferative glomerulonephritis may increase the risk of contrast medium-induced nephropathy more than the other nondiabetic diseases like obstructive nephropathy, adult dominant polycystic kidney disease, analgesic nephropathy, and other forms of glomerulonephritis.

The risk increases with increasing dose of contrast medium, independent of renal function. The threshold levels can be used as a rule of thumb (the exact threshold in man is unknown). In patients with normal serum creatinine levels, a 300 ml or higher dose of a 300 mg I/ml solution probably increases the risk factor, whereas for patients with serum creatinine levels between 130 and 300 μmol/l, the threshold dose is probably half this (150 ml). When the serum creatinine level is above 300 μmol/l, the threshold dose is probably below 100 ml of a 300 mg I/ml solution. It must be admitted that good tolerance in patients with normal renal function has been demonstrated in spite of administration of very large doses of contrast medium (Rosovsky et al. 1996). Nevertheless, a regression analysis in the same study showed a positive correlation between the dose of contrast medium and the rise in serum creatinine. Figure 10.3 shows that high osmolarity is a significant risk factor. Previous contrast medium injection is a risk factor in patients with abnormal S-creatinine levels, particularly when the injections have been given within 24 h apart.

Several preexisting conditions have probably been wrongly implicated as increasing the risk of contrast medium-induced renal failure. It is generally accepted that the presence of diabetes mellitus alone (in the absence of renal failure) is not a risk factor for contrast medium-induced nephropathy. In addition, while multiple myeloma has been listed as a risk factor for contrast-induced renal failure in the past, a recent study (McCarthy and Becker 1992) has indicated that the incidence of contrast-induced renal failure in myeloma patients is actually quite low (0.6%–1.25%). Sex is not a risk factor: no study has demonstrated a difference in frequency of contrast medium-induced nephropathy between the sexes.

The major risk factors for development of contrast medium-induced nephropathy are shown in Table 10.2.

Table 10.2. Simple guidelines of the European Society of Urogenital Radiology to diminish the risk of contrast medium nephropathy (Morcos et al. submitted)

Risk factors	**Look for**	• S-creatinine levels, particularly secondary to diabetic nephropathy. • Dehydration • Congestive heart failure • Age over 70 years old • Concurrent administration of nephrotoxic drugs, e.g. non steroid anti-inflammatory drugs.
In patients With risk factor(s)	**Do**	• Make sure that the patients is well hydrated [give at least 100 ml (oral (e.g. soft drinks) or intravenous (normal saline) depending on the clinical situation) per hour starting 4 hours before to 24 hours after contrast administration – in warm areas increase the fluid volume] • Use low- or iso-osmolar contrast media • Stop administration of nephrotoxic drugs for at least 24 hours. • Consider alternative imaging techniques, which do not require the administration of iodinated contrast media.
	Do not	• Give high osmolar contrast media • Administer large doses of contrast media • Administer mannitol and diuretics, particularly loop-diuretics • Perform multiple studies with contrast media within a short period of time.

10.6 Pathophysiology

The understanding of mechanisms responsible for the renal effects of contrast medium-induced nephropathy has improved during recent years. Direct effects on the kidney seem to be the main cause for the impairment in renal function (Brown et al. 1992, 1993; Oldroyd et al. 1994). Reduction in cardiac output, vasopressin release, and alteration in red cell morphology have also been incriminated, but the evidence for these processes is limited (Dawson 1993; Trewhella et al. 1990). It is now apparent that contrast media induce a reduction in renal function predominantly by modulating tubular regulatory mechanisms and production of renal vasoactive autacoids (Barrett 1993; Heyman et al. 1994; Morcos et al. 1995). The pronounced inhomogeneity of blood flow and oxygen supply within the kidney seems to be an important factor for the development of contrast medium-induced nephropathy.

10.6.1 Oxygen

The mechanism of contrast medium-induced nephropathy is conditioned strongly by the nature of the oxygen supply to the kidney. Total blood flow to the human kidney is high in relation to the weight of the kidney, and the arteriovenous oxygen difference between the renal artery and renal vein is low. The high renal blood flow is commonly viewed as designed to maximize flow-dependent clearance of wastes and it is often assumed that the supply of oxygen does not normally influence the ability of the kidney to function. A generous flow of blood should also protect the kidney from potential ischemic insults, by giving it a larger margin of security than other organs and making it the least likely organ in the body to be damaged by a compromise in blood flow (Morcos et al. 1996). Nevertheless, the kidney is remarkably susceptible to hypoperfusion and to toxic insults that are potentiated by ischemia. The explanation for this paradox lies in the marked inhomogeneity of blood flow and oxygen supply within the kidney. While the renal cortex is well perfused with blood, the medulla of the kidney is one of the least well perfused tissues of the body; the ambient oxygen tension in the renal medulla is habitually close to the critical pO_2 at which oxygen availability becomes a limiting factor in the work that cells can accomplish (Epstein et al. 1991).

The ability to concentrate the urine derives from the countercurrent arrangement of capillary flow in the vasa recta, permitting the diffusion of oxygen from afferent to efferent limbs of the medullary hairpin capillaries and ensuring the high oxygen supply required by the mitochondria-rich, actively transporting cells lining the medullary thick ascending limb, which absorb sodium chloride against a chemical gradient from the tubular urine into the medullary interstitium (Brezis and Rosen 1995). Almost 40 years ago it was demonstrated that the pO_2 of the medulla was strikingly lower than the renal arterial pO_2 (Auckland and Krog 1960). Within the renal medulla, under basal circumstances most of the pO_2 values are below 30 mmHg, and many measurements are obtained in the neighborhood of 10 mmHg. This contrasts with the values in the cortex, where most of the pO_2 values lie between 30 and 70 mmHg, averaging about 50 mmHg. It should be noted that the critical pO_2 of most cells is in the range of 10 mmHg. The sharp distinction between medullary and cortical pO_2, as already noted, reflects a major discrepancy in the rate of blood flow through these two regions, as well as differences in the rate of oxygen consumption by actively transporting cells. An increase in transport work (and oxygen consumption) increases the degree and extent of injury to medullary ascending cells (Brezis et al. 1984).

While all iodinated contrast media in sufficiently high concentrations appear to be directly toxic to isolated renal tubular cells in vitro, it is clear that this toxicity is highly potentiated by hypoxia. Thus the time of greatest danger to the kidney is during the first minutes after the injection of the contrast medium, when the concentration in the blood perfusing the kidney is at its highest. This is also the time when the renal vasoconstrictive response to the contrast medium is at its peak (Morcos et al. 1996). Contrast agents not only act synergistically with hypoxia in producing cellular injury, they actually increase hypoxia in the renal medulla (Heyman et al. 1991). This effect is presumably the result of the constriction of the medullary blood vessels. Immediately following the injection of a bolus of contrast medium there is a transient reduction in total renal blood flow accompanied by an even more marked decrease in blood flow to the renal medulla (Nygren et al. 1988). At the same time the tissue pO_2 of the renal medulla falls to extremely low levels (Heyman et al. 1991). The intense renal vasoconstriction is probably mediated at least in part by the release of endothelin (see Sect. 10.6.2).

10.6.2 Vasoactive Mediators

The vascular events are mainly secondary to direct renal effects of contrast media, which modulate the synthesis and release of vasoactive mediators within the kidney (Morcos et al. 1995; Morcos and el Nahas 1998). Experimental studies have shown that the endogenous vasodilators prostaglandins and nitric oxide (NO) are not directly involved in the renal hemodynamic effects of contrast media (Lund et al. 1984; Morcos et al. 1997). Nevertheless, the intrarenal production of these vasodilators is important for the maintenance of good perfusion and oxygen supply of the medulla (see Sect. 10.6.1). Renal excretion and formation of prostaglandin E_2 are increased by the administration of contrast media. Prostaglandin E_2 is a powerful dilator of medullary vessels and when its formation is inhibited by the administration of nonsteroidal anti-inflammatory drugs (NSAIDs) or similar agents, the renal vasoconstriction induced by contrast media is exaggerated and prolonged damage to medullary tubular cells is much more pronounced (Cantley et al. 1993). Nitric oxide formation may also play a role in preventing renal toxicity from contrast media, since the administration of competitive inhibitors of nitric oxide synthase greatly enhances contrast medium-induced nephropathy in rats (BREZIS et al. 1991a). In situations where the synthesis of these mediators is hampered, the renal insult caused by contrast media is accentuated.

The vasoactive substances endothelin and adenosine play an important role in mediating the renal hemodynamic effects of contrast media. The endothelins are a family of 21-amino acid peptides discovered in 1988 as a vasoconstrictor principle derived from vascular endothelial cells (YANAGISAWA et al. 1988). Contrast media can stimulate the release of endothelin by endothelial cells in culture and increase both the plasma endothelin concentration and the urinary endothelin excretion following intravascular administration (MARGULIES et al. 1991, 1992; HEYMAN et al. 1992, 1993; OLDROYD et al. 1994, 1995b). Functional studies in vitro and in vivo have shown that endothelin receptor antagonists can prevent the fall in GFR (MARGULIES et al. 1992; HEYMAN et al. 1993; TOUATI et al. 1993) and the reduction in renal perfusion induced by contrast media (HEYMAN et al. 1993; OLDROYD et al. 1994, 1995a,b). Preliminary clinical observations also indicate that endothelin may play a role in the pathophysiology of contrast medium-induced nephropathy (MARGULIES et al. 1992). Following contrast medium administration, the increase in plasma endothelin was found to be greater in patients whose renal function declined than in those whose renal function remained unchanged. In addition, patients with underlying renal insufficiency may have higher baseline levels and a greater tendency towards an increase in endothelin after exposure to contrast media (CLARK et al. 1997).

In the kidney, adenosine is a mediator of the tubuloglomerular feedback response and can induce both vasoconstriction and vasodilation through the A1 and A2 receptors. Animal studies and clinical experience indicate that adenosine is an important mediator of the reduction in GFR and renal blood flow induced by contrast media (ARAKAWA et al. 1996; ERLEY et al. 1994; KATHOLI et al. 1995). The reduction in GFR induced by contrast media in dogs with renal insufficiency can be attenuated by pretreatment with theophylline, a nonselective antagonist of the adenosine receptors, and abolished by a selective A1 adenosine receptor antagonist (ARAKAWA et al. 1996). The same study also demonstrated that the initial renal vasodilatation induced by contrast media is mediated by adenosine A2 receptors. Clinical experience, although limited, also suggests that theophylline may have some protective effect against the renal impairment associated with contrast medium administration (ERLEY et al. 1994; KATHOLI et al. 1995). However, in one study a significant reduction in creatinine clearance remained following administration of high-osmolar contrast media in spite of the prophylactic use of theophylline, suggesting that other mechanisms are involved (KATHOLI et al. 1995). The biological interaction between adenosine and endothelin in mediating the renal hemodynamic effects of contrast media is unknown and further studies are required.

10.6.3 Structural Effects of Contrast Media

Vacuolization of the epithelial cells of the proximal tubules of the kidney has been described following the intravascular administration of contrast media in both man and rats (TERVAHARTIALA et al. 1991; MOREAU et al. 1980; MORCOS et al. 1996; THOMSEN et al. 1994, 1995). In man this condition is primarily described as osmotic nephrosis (MOREAU et al. 1980). In one study more vacuoles were found after administration of low-osmolar and iso-osmolar contrast media in comparison with high-osmolar ones (MORCOS et al. 1996). In another study, by contrast, no difference was found with regard to vacuoles between high-osmolar and low-osmolar contrast media (THOMSEN et al. 1994). The vacuolar responses in the tubular cells are due to active internalization of contrast media in tubular cells causing lysosomal changes (NORDBY et al. 1990). These structural changes are reversible and resolve within a few days after contrast medium exposure (MOREAU et al. 1980). Contrast medium injection does not induce vacuoles in rats with chronic cisplatin nephropathy (THOMSEN et al. 1995). No correlation exists between the degree of vacuolization in the tubular cells and the reduction in renal function (MORCOS et al. 1996).

The morphological appearance of contrast media-induced vacuoles is rather like enlarged hyaline droplets which vary in their electron density from dense vacuoles/droplets to electron-lucent droplets associated with heavy proteinuria. The latter are more frequent when high-osmolar contrast media are given than when a contrast medium with low osmolarity is administered. This applies both to iodine-containing contrast media for x-ray and to chelates containing gadolinium for magnetic resonance (THOMSEN et al. 1994). The vacuoles are similar in appearance to the "cytoplasmic swellings" formed after in the intravenous administration of dextran (Christensen and Maunsbach 1979). Contrast media-induced vacuoles are reported to stain positively for acid phosphatase, thus confirming their association with the endosome/lysosome compartment. There is no clear experimental evidence to link the process of vacuolization with contrast media-induced nephropathy.

If there is a greater vacuolization after low-osmolar contrast media than after high-osmolar contrast media, this could be explained by the mild diuresis induced by these agents and by their viscosity, which cause a high concentration of these media in the urine and a longer exposure of the epithelial cells to the contrast media molecules (Tervahartiala et al. 1991; Morcos et al. 1996). However, vacuoles are not seen after administration of high-osmolar and low-osmolar magnetic resonance contrast media administered in the same high molar doses as radiological contrast media (Thomsen et al. 1994). Therefore, chemotoxicity of the agent must be an important factor. If the vacuolization following administration of two contrast media is identical, the one with the highest intratubular concentration must be the one with the lowest chemotoxicity. Thus, a greater vacuolization does not automatically imply that a drug is more chemotoxic.

The other structural effect of contrast media is observed in the renal medulla, which is vulnerable to ischemia (Brezis et al. 1991b; Beeri et al. 1995; Heyman et al. 1994). In vivo and in vitro studies have shown that high-osmolar contrast media can induce necrosis of the medullary thick ascending limb of the loop of Henle and that this effect is less pronounced with the low-osmolar contrast media (Brezis et al. 1991b). Extensive DNA fragmentation, a marker for programmed cell death (apoptosis), was detected selectively along thick ascending limbs of loops of Henle as early as 15 min after the administration of high-osmolar contrast media in the rat. The structural effect of contrast media in the renal medulla is due to ischemia, which is less marked with low-osmolar contrast media (Brezis et al. 1991b; Beeri et al. 1995). Activation of apoptosis might play an important role in nephron injury and renal failure induced by contrast media (Beeri et al. 1995).

10.7 Prevention

A number of measures have been recommended to prevent or reduce the risk of contrast medium-induced nephropathy (Table 10.2). They include hydration with NaCl 0.9% or NaCl 0.45%, infusion of mannitol, infusion of atrial natriuretic factor, administration of loop diuretics, calcium antagonists, theophylline, or dopamine, use of low-osmolar nonionic contrast media instead of high-osmolar ionic contrast media, hemodialysis performed rapidly after contrast administration (Younathan et al. 1994; Lehnert et al. 1998), minimization of the volume of contrast medium, and prolongation of the interval between procedures for which contrast media are used (Deray and Jacobs 1995). Of all these measures, extracellular volume expansion has repeatedly been shown to be effective and is most widely recommended. Patients with preexisting renal failure, independent of cause, should not undergo radiological procedures where contrast medium is administered without being hydrated (Solomon et al. 1994; Rudnick et al. 1995). The only exception is patients with congestive heart failure. An adequate hydration procedure includes administration of 100 ml/h of 0.9% saline from 4 h before the contrast medium administration to 24 h afterward for patients who are not allowed to drink or eat due to the fact that they are to undergo an interventional or surgical procedure. Patients who can and may drink should have at least the same volume: 500 ml of water or soft drinks before and 2500 ml during the following 24 h. This volume should cover the perspiration and secure a diuresis of at least 1 ml/min. Furthermore, nonionic low-osmolar contrast media should always be used (Thomsen 1990; Barrett and Carlisle 1993; Rudnick et al. 1995). The interval between two examinations where contrast media are administered should be at least 24 h, especially if the serum creatinine level is abnormal. Concomitant use of nephrotoxic drugs (e.g., gentamicin, NSAIDs) should be avoided.

At present the role of various drugs, e.g., calcium antagonists and theophylline, in preventing contrast medium-induced nephropathy is uncertain. It is possible that antiendothelin drugs offer better protection against the development of contrast medium-induced nephropathy in clinical practice. Hopefully we will know more during the coming decade. Clinical studies are strongly warranted.

10.8 Treatment

The treatment of contrast-induced nephropathy begins with recognition of the condition. For high-risk patients measurement of serum creatinine between the 2nd and 4th day postprocedure will identify the nonoliguric form of contrast medium-induced nephropathy, while for oliguric patients a 24-h urine volume <400 ml will trigger the diagnosis. There is no specific treatment. Hemodialysis has been tried, but this should only be done when there is a clinical need. Some patients with contrast medium-induced nephrotoxicity may require temporary dialysis support, while for those with oliguria such dialysis support often becomes permanent. The acute management of such patients is the same as that of other patients with acute renal failure and should include careful monitoring of serum electrolytes to detect hyperkalemia, meticulous attention to fluid intake and output to prevent hypovolemia or hypervolemia, daily serum creatinine measurements, daily weight determination, and adequate nutritional intake. Attempts to convert oliguric renal failure to the nonoliguric form using mannitol and furosemide have been unsuccessful. The patient should not be reexposed to contrast media before the kidney function has returned to its previous level. If contrast is to be given again, the patient must be adequately hydrated.

10.9 Lactate Acidosis in Non-Insulin-Dependent Diabetes

The biguanides, phenformin and metformin, are used in non-insulin-dependent diabetes mellitus in three ways: (a) as primary treatment in overweight patients inadequately controlled by diet, (b) as adjunct therapy when sulphonurea alone fails or (c) sometimes in combination with insulin (Monson 1993). Renal insufficiency with failure to clear metformin and failure of hepatic metabolism and excretion of phenformin leads to accumulation of these biguanides and the potential for fatal lactic acidosis (Sirtori and Pasik 1994). The use of contrast media in patients receiving metformin is currently very controversial (Dachman 1995; Rotter 1995). The potential danger of lactic acidosis exists because of accumulated metformin (i.e., from failure of renal excretion) and *not* from any interaction of contrast media and metformin. Patients at risk are those who may develop contrast medium-induced nephrotoxicity and renal insufficiency/failure. It is currently advised in Europe that metformin be stopped 48 h before and for 48 h subsequent to the administration of contrast media. Renal function, e.g., serum creatinine, should be checked to ensure that renal function has remained at the precontrast level before metformin is resumed. In the United States it is recommended that metformin administration is stopped, normal serum creatinine confirmed, contrast administered, and metformin not restarted for 48 h and then only if renal function has remained normal (=normal serum creatinine level). It is of note that the use of metformin/phenformin is contraindicated in patients with renal insufficiency in the United States. Normal renal function, defined as a normal serum creatinine level, does not totally exclude the possible occurrence of lactic acidosis, but the latter is more frequent in patients with abnormal renal function, defined as an abnormal serum creatinine level (Westberg 1995).

Recently guidelines to diminish the risk of lactic acidosis have been issued (Table 10.3)

Table 10.3. Guidelines of the European Society of Urogenital Radiology for the administration of contrast media to diabetics taking metformin (Thomsen et al. in press)

Serum creatinine level should be measured in every diabetic patient treated with biguanides prior to intravascular administration of contrast media. Low-osmolar contrast media should always be used.

2. Elective studies

a) *If the serum creatinine is normal,* the radiological examination should be performed and intake of metformin stopped from the time of the study. The use of metformin should not be resumed for 48 hrs and should only be restarted if renal function/serum creatinine remains with the normal range.

b) *If renal function is abnormal,* the metformin should be withdrawn and the contrast study should be delayed for 48 hrs. Metformin should on be restarted 48 hrs later, if renal function/serum creatinine is unchanged.

3. Emergency cases

a) *If the serum creatinine is normal,* the study may proceed as suggested for elective patients.

b) *If the renal function is abnormal (or unknown),* the physician should weigh the risks and benefits of contrast administration. Alternative imaging techniques should be considered. If contrast media administration is deemed necessary and the following precautions should be implemented:
Metformin therapy should be withdrawn.
The patient should be hydrated (E.g. at least 100 ml per hour of soft drinks or intravenous saline up to 24 hours after contrast medium administration – In warm ares more fluid should by given)
Monitor renal function (serum creatine), serum lacid acid and pH of blood
Look for symptoms of lactic acidosis (vomiting, somnolence, nausea, epigastric pain, anorexia, hyperpnea, lethargy, diarrhea and thirst). Blood test results indicative of lactic acidosis: pH<7.25 and lactic acid > 5 mmol.

References

Anderson RJ, Linas SL, Berns AS, et al. (1977) Nonoliguric acute renal failure. N Engl J Med 296:1134–1137

Arakawa K, Suzuki H, Naitoh M, et al. (1996) Role of adenosine in the renal responses to contrast medium. Kidney Int 49:1199–1206

Auckland K, Krog J (1960) Renal oxygen tension. Nature 188:671

Barrett BJ (1993) Contrast nephrotoxicity. J Am Soc Nephrol 5:125–137

Barrett BJ, Carlisle EJ (1993) Metaanalysis of the relative nephrotoxicity of high- and low-osmolality iodinated contrast media. Radiology 188:171–178.

Barrett BJ, Parfrey PS, Vavasour HM, et al. (1992) Contrast nephropathy in patients with impaired renal function: high versus low osmolar media. Kidney Int 41:1274–1279

Bartels ED, Brun GC, Gammeltoft A, Gjørup PA (1954) Acute anuria following intravenous pyelography in a patient with myelomatosis. Acta Med Scand 40:297–302

Beeri R, Symon Z, Brezis ML, Baher PH, Rosen S, Zager RA (1995) Rapid DNA fragmentation from hypoxia along the thick ascending limb of the rat kidneys. Kidney Int 47: 1806–1810

Berdon WE, Schwartz RH, Becker J, Baker DH (1969) Tamm-Horsfall proteinuria: its relationship to prolonged nephrogram in infants and children and to acute renal failure following intravenous urography in adults with multiple myeloma. Radiology 92:714–718.

Berns AS (1989) Nephrotoxicity of contrast media. Kidney Int 36:730–736

Blantz RC (1983) Glomerular filtration In: Massry SG, Glassock RJ (eds) Textbook of nephrology. Williams & Wilkins, Baltimore, pp 1.34–1.38

Blaufox MD, Aurell M, Bubeck B, et al. (1996) Report of the radionuclides in nephrourology committee on renal clearance. J Nucl Med 37:1883–1890

Brezis ML, Rosen S (1995) Hypoxia of the renal medulla – its implications for disease. N Engl J Med 332:647–655

Brezis ML, Rosen S, Silva P, Epstein FH (1984) Transport activity modifies thick ascending limb damage in the isolated perfused kidney. Kidney Int 25:65–72

Brezis ML, Heyman SN, Dinour D, Epstein FH, Rosen S (1991a) Role of nitric oxide in renal medullary oxygenation. Studies in isolated and intact rat kidneys. J Clin Invest 88:390–395

Brezis ML, Greenfield Z, Herman JJ, Meyer SN, Heyman SN, Rosen S (1991b) Experimental nephrotoxicity of radiocontrast agents iohexol, ioxoglate and iothalamate. Invest Radiol 26:323–331

Brown P, Haylor JL, Cope GH, El Nahas AM, Morcos SK (1992) Effect of diatrizoate on the function of the isolated perfused rat kidney. Eur J Radiol 65:1011–1017

Brown P, Haylor JL, El Nahas AM, Morcos SK (1993) The functional effects of contrast media on the isolated perfused rat kidney. Contrib Nephrol 101:235–240

Byrd L, Sherman RL (1979) Radiocontrast-induced acute renal failure: a clinical and pathophysiologic review. Medicine 58:270–279

Cantley LG, Spokes K, Clark B, McMahon EG, Burnett JCJ (1993) Radiocontrast increases plasma and urinary endothelin. J Am Soc Nephrol 2:1041–1045

Carvallo A, Rakowski TA, Argy WP Jr, Schreiner GE (1978) Acute renal failure following drip infusion pyelography Am J Med 65:38–45

Christensen EI, Maunsbach AB (1979) Effects of dextran on lysosomal ultrastructure and protein digestion in renal proximal tubule. Kidney Int 16:301–311

Clark BA, Kim D, Epstein F (1997) Endothelin and arterial netriutretic peptide levels following radiocontrast exposure in humans. Am J Kidney Dis 30:82–86

Dachman AH (1995) New contraindication to intravascular iodinated contrast material. Radiology 197:545

Davis P, Roberts MB, Roylance J (1975) Acute reactios to urographic contrast media. Br Med J 2:434–437

Dawson P (1993) On the nephrotic potential of the iodinated intravascular agents. Adv X-ray Contrast 1:2–9

D'Elia JA, Gleason RE, Alday M, et al. (1982) Nephrotoxicity from angiographic contrast material: a prospective study. Am J Med 72:719–722

Deray G, Jacobs C (1995) Radiocontrast neprotoxicity: a review. Invest Radiol 30:221–225

Duarte CG, Zhang J, Ellis S (1997) The SHR as a small animal model for radiocontrast renal failure. Relation of nephrotoxicity to animal's age, gender, strain and dose of radiocontrast. Ren Fail 19:723–743

Eisenberg RL, Bank WO, Hedglock MW (1979) Renal failure after major angiography Am J Med 68:43–46

Epstein FH, Brezis ML, Rosen S (1991) Role of the medulla in acute renal failure. In: Bihari D, Neild G (eds) Acute renal failure in the intensive therapy unit. Springer, Berlin Heidelberg New York, pp 91–102

Erley CM, Duda SH, Schlepckow S, et al. (1994) Adenosine antagonist theophylline prevents the reduction of glomerular filtration rate after contrast media application. Kidney Int 45:1425–1431

Fang LS-T, Sirota RA, Ebert TH, Lichtenstein NS (1980) Low fractional excretion of sodium with contrast media-induced acute renal failure. Arch Intern Med 140:531–533

Gennari FJ, Kassires JP (1974) Osmotic diuresis. N Engl J Med 291:714–720

Gottschalk CW, Mylle M (1957) Micropuncture study of pressures in proximal and distal tubules and peritubular capillaries of the rat kidney during osmotic diuresis. Am J Physiol 189:323–328

Harkonen S, Kjellstrand C (1981) Contrast nephropathy. Am J Nephrol 1:69–77

Heyman SN, Brezis ML, Epstein FH, Spokes K, Silva P, Rosen S (1991) Early renal medullary hypoxic injury from radiocontrast and indomethacin. Kidney Int 40:632–642

Heyman SN, Clark BA, Kaiser N, et al. (1992) Radiocontrast agents induce endothelin release in vivo and in vitro. J Am Soc Nephrol 3:58–65

Heyman SN, Clark BA, Cantley L, et al. (1993) Effects of ioversol versus iothalamate on endothelin release and radiocontrast nephropathy. Invest Radiol 28:313–318

Heyman SN, Rosen S, Brezis M (1994) Radiocontrast nephropathy: a paradigm for synergism between toxic and hypoxic insults in the kidney. Exp Nephrol 2:153–157

Hollenberg NK (1983) Renal circulation. In: Massry SG, Glassock RJ (eds) Textbook of nephrology. Williams & Wilkins, Baltimore, pp 1.28–1.33

Hostetter TH, Brenner BM (1983) Determinants of the glomerular filtration of macromolecules In: Massry SG, Glassock RJ (eds) Textbook of nephrology. Williams & Wilkins, Baltimore, pp 1.39–1.41

Hou SH, Bushinsky DA, Wish JB, Cohan JJ, Harrington JT (1983) Hospital acquired renal insufficiency: a prospective study. Am J Med 74:243–248

Idbohrn H (1956) Tolerance to contrast media in renal angiography. Acta Radiol 45:141–154

Jakobsen JA, Lundby B, Kristoffersen DT, Borch KW, Hald JK, Berg KJ (1992) Evaluation of renal function with delayed CT after injection of nonionic monomeric and dimeric contrast media in healthy volunteers. Radiology 182:419–424
Katholi RE, Taylor GJ, Woods WT, et al. (1993) Nephrotoxicity of nonionic low osmolality contrast media: a prospective double-blind randomized comparison in human beings. Radiology 186:183–187
Katholi RE, Taylor GJ, McCann WP, et al. (1995) Nephrotoxicity from contrast media: attenuation with theophylline. Radiology 195:17–22
Katzberg RW, Morris TW, Burgener FA, et al. (1977) Renal renin and hemodynamic responses to selective renal artery catheterization and angiography. Invest Radiol 12:381–388
Katzberg RW, Pabico RC, Morris TW, et al. (1986) Effects of contrast media on renal function and sub-cellular morphology in the dog. Invest Radiol 21:64–70
Katzberg RW, Donahue LA, Morris TW, et al. (1990) Ioxilan, a third generation low osmolality nonionic contrast medium: systemic and renal hemodynamic effects. Invest Radiol 25:46–51
Kumar S, Hull JD, Lathi S, Cohen AJ, Pletka PG (1981) Low incidence of renal failure after angiography. Arch Intern Med 141:1268–1270
Lautin EM, Freeman NJ, Schoenfeld AH, et al. (1991) Radiocontrast-associated renal dysfunction: a comparison of lower osmolality and conventional high-osmolality contrast media. AJR 157:59–65
Lehnert T, Keller E, Gondolf K, Schäffner T, Pavenstädt H, Schollmeyer P (1998) Effect of hemodialysis after contrast medium administration in patients with renal insufficiency. Nephrol Dial Transpl 13:358–362
Levy EM, Viscoli CM, Horwitz RI (1996) The effect of acute renal failure on mortality: a cohort analysis. JAMA 275: 1489–1494
Love L, Johnson MS, Bresler ME, et al. (1994) The persistent computed tomography nephrogram: its significance in the diagnosis of contrast-associated nephrotoxicity. Br J Radiol 67:951–957
Lund G, Einzig J, Salomonowitz E, et al. (1984) Effect of prostaglandin inhibition on the renal vascular response to ionic and non-ionic contrast media in the dog. Acta Radiol 25: 407–410
Manske CL, Sprafka JM, Strony JT, Wang Y (1990) Contrast nephropathy in azotemic diabetic patients undergoing coronary angiography. Am J Med 89:615–620
Margulies KB, Hildebrand FLJ, Neublein DM, Burnett JCJ (1991) Radiocontrast increases plasma and urinary endothelin. J Am Soc Nephrol 2:1041–1045
Margulies KB, McKinley LJ, Burnett JC (1992) Endothelin in human and canine radiocontrast-induced nephropathy. J Vasc Res 3:58–65
Martin-Paredero V, Dixon SM, Baker D, et al. (1983) Risk of renal failure after major angiography. Arch Surg 118:1417–1420
Mason RA, Arbeit LA, Giron F (1985) Renal dysfunction after arteriography JAMA 253:1001–1004
McAfee JG (1957) A survey of complications of abdominal aortography. Radiology 68:825–838
McCarthy CS, Becker JA (1992) Multiple myeloma and contrast media. Radiology 183:519–521
Monson JP (1993) Selected side-effects. II. Metformin and lactic acidosis. Prescribers Journal 33:170–173
Moore RD, Steinberg EP, Powe NR, et al. (1989) Frequency and determinants of adverse reactions induced by high-osmolality contrast media. Radiology 170:727–732
Moore RD, Steinberg EP, Powe NR, et al. (1992) Nephrotoxicity of high-osmolality versus low-osmolality contrast media: randomized clinical trial. Radiology 182:649–655
Morcos SK, El Nahas AM (1998) Advances in the understanding of the nephrotoxicity of radiocontrast media. Nephron 78:249–252
Morcos SK, Brown PWG, Oldroyd S, El Nahas AM, Haylor J (1995) Relationship between the diuretic effect of radiocontrast media and their ability to increase renal vascular resistance. Br J Radiol 68:850–853
Morcos SK, Epstein FH, Haylor J, Dobrota M (1996) Aspects of contrast media nephrotoxicity. Eur J Radiol 23:178–184
Morcos SK, Oldroyd S, Haylor J (1997) Effect of radiograohic contrast media on endothelium derived nitric oxide-dependent renal vasodilatation. Br J Radiol 70:154–159
Morcos SK, Thomsen HS, Webb JAW and members of Contrast Media Safety Committee of the European Society of Urogenital Radiology (ESUR) (submitted) Contrast media induced nephrotoxicity: A consensus report.
Moreau JF, Droz D, Noel LH, Leibovitch J, Jungers P, Michel JR (1980) Tubular nephrotoxicity of water soluble iodinated contrast media. Invest Radiol 15:54–60
Mudge GH (1980) Nephrotoxicity of urographic radiocontrast drugs. Kidney Int 18:540–552
Myer GH, Witten DM (1978) Acute renal failure after excretory urography in multiple myeloma. AJR 133:583
Nordby A, Tvedt KE, Halgunset J, Haugen OA (1990) Intracellular penetration and accumulation of radiographic contrast media in the rat kidney. Scanning Microsc 4:651–666
Nygren A, Ulfendahl HR, Hansell P, Erikson U (1988) Effects of intravenous contrast media on cortical and medullary blood flow in the rat kidney. Invest Radiol 23:753–761
Oldroyd S, Haylor J, Morcos SK, El Nahas AM (1992) Reduced depression of renal function by iotrolan in the isolated rat kidney. Eur J Radiol 18:64–69
Oldroyd S, Slee SJ, Haylor J, Morcos SK, Wilson C (1994) Role for endothelin in the renal response to radiocontrast media in the rat. Clin Sci 87:424–427
Oldroyd S, Haylor J, Morcos SK (1995a) The acute effect of ioversol on kidney function: role of endothelin. Eur J Radiol 19:91–95
Oldroyd SD, Haylor JL, Morcos SK (1995b) Bosentan, an orally active endothelin antagonist: effect on renal response to contrast media. Radiology 196:661–665
Parfrey PS, Griffiths SM, Barrett BJ, et al. (1989) Contrast material-induced renal failure in patients with diabetes mellitus, renal insufficiency, or both. N Engl J Med 320: 143–149
Pendergrass EP, Chamberlein GW, Godfrey EW, Burdick ED (1942) A survey of deaths and unfavorable sequelae following administration of contrast media. AJR 48:741–762
Perillie PE, Conn HO (1958) Acute renal failure after intravenous pyelography in plasma cell myeloma. JAMA 167: 2186–2189
Rosovsky MA, Rusinek H, Bernstein A, Basak S, Setton A, Nelson PK (1996) High dose administration of nonionic contrast media: a retrospective review. Radiology 200:119–122
Rotter A (1995) New contraindication to intravascular iodinated contrast material. Radiology 197:545–546
Rowlands PC, Old SL, Rees JA, Harpur ES (1994) A histological investigation on contrast media induced renal proximal tubular vacuolation in rats. Hum Exp Toxicol 13:288
Rudnick MR, Goldfarb S, Wexler L, et al. (1995) Nephrotoxicity of ionic and nonionic contrast media in 1196 patients. A randomized trial. Kidney Int 47:254–261

Schwab SJ, Hlatky MA, Piper KS, et al. (1989) Contrast nephrotoxicity: a randomized controlled trial of a nonionic and ionic radiographic contrast agent. N Engl J Med 320:149–153

Schenker B (1964) Drip infusion pyelography: indications and application in urologic roentgenologic diagnosis. Radiology 83:12–21

Schwartz WB, Hurwit A, Ettinger A (1963) Intravenous urography in the patient with renal insufficiency. N Engl J Med 269:277–283

Shusterman N, Strom BL, Murray TG, Morrison G, West SL, Maislin G (1987) Risk factors and outcome of hospital-acquired acute renal failure. Clinical epidemiologic study. Am J Med 83:65–71

Sirtori CR, Pasik C (1994) Re-evaluation of biguanide, metformin: mechanisms of action and tolerability. Pharmacol Res 30:187–228

Solomon R, Werner G, Mann D, F'Elia J, Silva P (1994) Effects of saline, mannitol, and furosemide on acute decreases in renal function induced by radiocontrast agents. N Engl J Med 331:1416–1429

Swann RC, Merrill JP (1953) The clinical course of acute renal failure 32:215–292

Taliercio CP, Vlietstra MB, Fisher LD, Burnett JC (1986) Risks for renal dysfunction with cardiac angiography. Ann Intern Med 104:501–504

Taliercio CP, Vlietsrta RE, Ilstrup DM, et al. (1991) A randomized comparison of the nephrotoxicity of iopimidol and diatrizoate in high risk patients undergoing cardiac angiography. J Am Coll Cardiol 17:384–390

Tervahartiala P, Kivisaari L, Kivisaari R, Virtanen I, Standertskjold-Nordenstam CG (1991) Contrast media-induced renal tubular vacuolisation: a light and electron microscopic study on rat kidneys. Invest Radiol 26:882–887

Thomsen HS (1990) Contrast nephropathy. Curr Opinion Radiol 2:793–802

Thomsen HS, Golman K, Hemmingsen L, Larsen S, Skaarup P, Svendsen O (1993) Contrast medium induced nephropathy: animal experiments. Front Eur Radiol 9:83–108

Thomsen HS, Dorph S, Larsen S, et al. (1994) Urine profiles and kidney histology after intravenous injection of ionic and nonionic radiologic and magnetic resonance contrast media in normal rats. Acad Radiol 1:128–135

Thomsen HS, Dorph S, Larsen S, et al. (1995) Urine profiles and kidney histology after intravenous injection of ionic and nonionic radiologic and magnetic resonance contrast media in rats with cisplatin nephropathy. Acad Radiol 2:675–682

Thomsen HS, Morcos SK and members* of Contrast Media Safety Committee of the European Society of Urogenital Radiology (ESUR) (1999) Contrast media and metformin. Guidelines to diminish the risk of lactic acidosis in non-insulin dependent diabetics after administration of contrast media. Eur Radiol 8: in press

Trewhalla M, Dawson P, Forsling M, McCarthy P, O'Donnell C (1990) Vasopressin release in response to intravenously injected contrast media. Br J Radiol 63:97–100

Touati C, Ideee JM, Deray G, et al. (1993) Modulation of renal effects of contrast media by endothelin-derived nitric oxide in the rat. Invest Radiol 28:814–820

Ueda J, Nygren A, Hansell P, Erikson U (1992) Influence of contrast media on single nephron glomerular filtration rate in rat kidney. Acta Radiol 33:596–599

Van Waes PFGM (1972) High-dose urography in oliguric and anuric patients. Excretion of urographic contrast media in advanced renal failure. Excerpta Medica, Amsterdam pp 1–150

Webb JAW, Reznek RH, Cattell WR, Kelsey-Fry I (1981) Renal function after high dose urography in patients with renal failure. Br J Radiol 54:479–483

Weinrauch LA, Healy RW, Leland OS, et al. (1977) Coronary angiography and acute renal failure in diabetic azotemia nephropathy. Ann Intern Med 86:56–59

Westberg G (1995) Metformin (Glucophage) och röntgenkontrastmedel orsakade njurinsufficiens (in Swedish). Info från Läkemedelsverket 3:170–171

Witten DM, Hirsch FD, Hartman GW (1973) Acute reactions to urographic contrast medium: incidence, clinical characteristics and relationship to history of hypersensitivity staes. AJR 133:832–840

Yamazaki H, Matsushita M, Inoue T, et al. (1997) Renal cortical retention on delayed CT after angiography and contrast associated nephropathy. Br J Radiol 70:897–902

Yanagisawa M, Kurihara H, Kimura S, et al. (1988) A novel vasoconstrictor peptide produced by endothelial cells. Nature 322:411–415

Yuonathan CH, Kaude JV, Cook MD, Shaw GS, Peterson JC (1994) Dialysis is not indicated immediately after administration of nonionic contrast media in patients with end-stage renal disease treated by maintenance dialysis. AJR 163:969–971

11 Adverse Reactions to Iodinated Radiographic Contrast Media

R.H. Cohan and J.H. Ellis

CONTENTS

11.1 Introduction

Mild adverse reactions to iodinated radiographic contrast media are encountered in as many as 3.7% of patients receiving intravenous injections of low-osmolality and 12.7% of patients receiving intravenous injections of high-osmolality ionic contrast agents (Katayama et al. 1990). Fortunately, the majority of these reactions are mild and clinically insignificant. Severe and very severe reactions (the latter requiring hospitalization) have been noted much less frequently, in only 0.04% and 0.004% of patients receiving intravenous injections of low-osmolality contrast media and 0.22% and 0.04% of patients receiving intravenous injections of high-osmolality contrast media, respectively (Katayama et al. 1990). The vast majority of patients who have severe, even potentially life-threatening, reactions respond to rapid and aggressive treatment (Hartman et al. 1982). Fatal reactions to both types of contrast media are exceedingly rare, having been encountered in as few as 1:170000 patients injected with either agent (Katayama et al. 1990). The safety profile of even HOCM therefore compares quite favorably with that of many widely used therapeutic drugs, such as the antibiotic penicillin. Adverse reactions resulting from nonvascular and nonmyelographic administration of contrast media are even less common, and are represented by only anecdotal published reports.

In this chapter the various types of adverse reactions to contrast material will be reviewed. Common manifestations of these reactions will be presented and their significance discussed. The types of patients who are at increased risk for these various reactions will be reviewed, as will techniques for reducing the incidence of adverse reactions.

11.2 Toxicity of Contrast Material

Adverse effects of contrast media are believed to be primarily due to osmotoxicity, chemotoxicity, ion toxicity, and dose (Almen 1994); however, other factors, such as viscosity and lipophilicity, may also play a role. Osmotoxic effects include pain and discomfort, vasodilatation with hypotension, and rigidification of red blood cells.

Chemotoxic effects are thought to increase as the number of carboxyl groups increases and the number of hydroxyl groups decreases. These effects promote the release of vasoactive substances that cause allergic-like symptoms. Ion toxicity occurs when ionic substances (either the ionic contrast media anion itself, the cation it is conjugated with, or ionic components in additives) interfere with cell function (Almen 1994).

Given these observations, it is not surprising that conventional ionic contrast media, with their high osmolality, carboxyl group, and relatively few hydroxyl groups, have greater osmotoxicity,

R.H. Cohan, MD, Department of Radiology, University of Michigan Medical Center, 1500 East Medical Center Drive, Ann Arbor, MI 48109-0030, USA
J.H. Ellis, MD, Department of Radiology, University of Michigan Medical Center, 1500 East Medical Center Drive, Ann Arbor, MI 48109-0030, USA

chemotoxicity, and ion toxicity than do low-osmolality nonionic monomeric or dimeric contrast agents.

11.3 Conventional Ionic Versus Nonionic Agents

Many studies have indicated that nonionic low-osmolality contrast media produce fewer mild, moderate, and severe reactions than do ionic high-osmolality contrast media (Palmer 1988; Wolf et al. 1989; Katayama et al. 1990; Caro et al. 1991; Lasser et al. 1997). For this reason, nonionic contrast material is now used exclusively for intravascular administration in many countries (Thomsen et al. 1997). The only reason that low-osmolality contrast agents have not completely replaced the older high-osmolality ionic agents in all nations is their increased cost. Although there have been recent reductions in the cost of nonionic contrast material in the United States (probably not fortuitously coincident with the emergence of many new competing nonionic agents), nonionic contrast material remains substantially more expensive than high-osmolality ionic agents in the United States. Policies of selective use are employed at many institutions, whereby more expensive nonionic agents are restricted to patients who at higher risk of having an adverse reaction (Ellis et al. 1996). Such policies have been supported by recent publications (Bettmann et al. 1997). Nonetheless, if the price decreases continue, it is possible that eventually nonionic contrast media will be used exclusively throughout the world.

11.4 Types of Adverse Reaction

Adverse reactions can be broadly classified as idiosyncratic or nonidiosyncratic (Cohan and Dunnick 1987). Idiosyncratic reactions have manifestations identical to those seen with true allergic reactions. Nonidiosyncratic reactions have manifestations that do not resemble allergic reactions, but instead are believed to reflect physiologic effects of contrast media or direct toxicity of contrast media on a variety of organ systems. Adverse reactions may be systemic or local, with the former affecting many organ systems and the latter primarily affecting the skin and/or subcutaneous tissues. While systemic reactions may be idiosyncratic or nonidiosyncratic, local reactions are usually nonidiosyncratic.

11.4.1 Idiosyncratic Contrast Reactions

Idiosyncratic reactions most often begin within 20 min of contrast media injection (Ansell 1987). Their occurrence is not related to the administered dose of contrast material. A severe idiosyncratic reaction can develop following injection of <1 ml of contrast media. Common idiosyncratic reactions include hives (urticaria), bronchospasm, upper airway edema, and hypotension. Although the manifestations of idiosyncratic reactions are identical to those seen in patients having true anaphylactoid reactions, reactions to contrast material are not true allergic reactions in the vast majority of patients. Researchers have been unable to identify anticontrast IgE antibodies in most acutely reacting patients, substances whose presence is required for the diagnosis of a true allergic reaction (Carr and Walker 1984). Also, patients do not have to be previously exposed (sensitized) to contrast media in order to have a reaction (as is the case with true allergens) (Shehadi 1982). Conversely, not all patients who have had a previous contrast reaction will have another reaction after repeat injection of contrast media (Shehadi 1982). For these reasons, idiosyncratic reactions to radiographic contrast material have been termed anaphylactoid rather than anaphylactic reactions.

The mechanism by which idiosyncratic reactions occur is uncertain. Lasser has suggested that these reactions may be precipitated by endothelial cell activation of the contact system, through which a cascade of potent vasoactive substances, including leukotrienes, histamine, and prostaglandins, is released (Lasser 1985, 1987).

11.4.1.1 Skin Reactions

Urticarial skin reactions (hives) are characterized by focal areas of skin and subcutaneous tissue swelling, manifested by a central pale area surrounded by erythema. Hives may be single or multiple. Usually, only a few (less than five) develop. They can occur anywhere on the body, although they seem to be more common on the face, neck, and chest. They are usually pruritic. While hives are often isolated skin reactions, patients should be closely observed in order to insure that no other signs or symptoms occur. In rare instances, hives may be large and numerous and patients may be extremely uncomfortable.

Some patients develop diffuse cutaneous erythema or diffuse cutaneous and subcutaneous edema (angioedema) after an intravascular injection of contrast material. Patients with these more generalized dermatologic reactions must be carefully monitored, since they are more likely to develop more severe manifestations, including hypotension or airway edema.

11.4.1.2
Respiratory Reactions

Idiosyncratic causes of respiratory decompensation after contrast media injection include upper airway/laryngeal edema, bronchospasm, and noncardiogenic pulmonary edema.

Patients with upper airway edema often complain of having a scratchy throat or of feeling tightness in their throat. Alterations in vocal quality (hoarseness or inability to speak) may be noted. On physical examination, patients have difficulty inhaling or inspiratory stridor. Laryngeal edema may also be accompanied with or preceded by swelling of the tongue, lips, and face.

Patients with bronchospasm often have a history of asthma. They usually have a normal speaking voice. These patients have more difficulty exhaling than inhaling. Wheezing is often audible, but may become harder to identify if the bronchospasm is severe.

While most patients who develop pulmonary edema have known cardiac disease, usually consisting of congestive heart failure, some patients may develop pulmonary edema in the adsence of such a history. Patients with pulmonary edema usually complain of chest tightness and often want to sit upright. Symptoms may be slow to develop. Rales are characteristically identified on auscultation.

11.4.1.3
Hypotensive Reactions

Hypotension refers to patients with a systolic blood pressure of less than 90 mmHg who have evidence of diminished tissue perfusion and/or altered mental status (Cummins 1994). Hypotensive patients often complain of feeling light-headed or weak. Occasionally, a patient may become unresponsive or may have a generalized seizure (due to cerebral hypoxia) before complaining about any symptoms. Idiosyncratic hypotensive reactions may be isolated or may be associated with other allergic-like manifestations, such as airway edema and bronchospasm. Hypotensive reactions may also occur as a result of nonidiosyncratic vasovagal reactions or cardiac disease. If the patient is bradycardic (pulse less than 60 beats per minute) and is not receiving β-blockers (which might prevent a normal tachycardic response in a patient having an anaphylactoid or cardiac hypotensive reaction), a vasovagal reaction is likely (see Sect. 11.4.2.2). Patients who are tachycardic and hypotensive should be suspected of having an anaphylactoid reaction.

11.4.1.4
Patients at Increased Risk of Having an Idiosyncratic Contrast Reaction

Certain groups of patients are more likely to have reactions to contrast media, often of the idiosyncratic type. Adverse reactions to ionic and nonionic contrast material are 4–7 times more common in patients who have had previous contrast reactions (Shehadi 1975; Ansell et al. 1980; Katayama et al. 1990). Shehadi (1982) was able to quantitate the number of patients with previous adverse reactions who had repeat reactions of the same type upon reinjection of the same agent. Sixty percent of patients who had developed hives after contrast administration in the past subsequently developed hives again. Adverse reactions of facial edema, difficulty breathing, and bronchospasm were repeated in 68%, 59%, and 38% of patients, respectively. These data indicate that although repeat reactions are common, they do not occur in all patients.

A number of other groups are at increased risk of having a contrast reaction, most commonly of the idiosyncratic type. Asthmatics have from 1.2 to 2.2 times the risk of the general population (Shehadi 1975; Ansell 1987; Katayama et al. 1990) and when reactions occur they are more likely to be severe. Ansell et al. (1980) and Katayama et al. (1990) found severe contrast reactions to be 5–9 times more common in asthmatics.

Patients with allergies to substances other than contrast material are also 1.5–3.0 times more likely to have an adverse contrast reaction. This even includes patients with hayfever. In Shehadi's study patients with seafood allergies had the highest incidence of contrast reactions among all allergic patients (15%); however, this frequency was only minimally higher than that observed in patients who reported allergies to eggs, milk, chocolate (14.6%), or other unspecified agents (13.1%) (SHEHADI 1975).

11.4.1.5 Diminishing the Risk of an Idiosyncratic Contrast Reaction in an At-Risk Patient

11.4.1.5.1 UNIVERSAL PROPHYLAXIS WITH CORTICOSTEROIDS

Premedication of patients with two doses of glucocorticoids (32 mg methylprednisolone) reduces the incidence of adverse contrast media reactions and adverse reactions requiring treatment from 9.0% and 2.0% to 6.4% and 1.2%, respectively, when the first dose is administered 12h prior to contrast media injection (LASSER et al. 1987). In comparison, use of only a single dose administered 2h before contrast media administration has virtually no effect on the incidence of total subsequent contrast reactions (9.4%) or reactions requiring treatment (2.0%). Universal corticosteroid prophylaxis along with use of high-osmolality contrast media has been recommended as a cost-effective alternative to universal use of low-osmolality contrast media (LASSER 1988). It has not been widely adopted (COHAN et al. 1995), however, probably because many physicians have found it difficult to make sure that the first dose can be administered 12h prior to every contrast material injection. Also, results from several series (WOLF et al. 1989; KATAYAMA et al. 1990) have led many to suspect that the protection conferred by these medications might not be as great as that obtained by using nonionic agents. Not surprisingly, a recent study has demonstrated that the safest alternative is to both premedicate patients with corticosteroids and use nonionic agents (LASSER et al. 1994).

11.4.1.5.2 CORTICOSTEROID PROPHYLAXIS LIMITED TO HIGH-RISK PATIENTS

Corticosteroids can also be used on a more limited basis, to reduce the likelihood of a subsequent adverse reaction in the selected group of patients who have had prior reactions to contrast material. Greenberger and co-workers showed that if a premedication regimen of prednisone (50 mg administered orally 13, 7, and 1h prior to injection of high-osmolality ionic contrast material) and diphenhydramine (50 mg administered intramuscularly 1h prior to the procedure) is utilized, adverse reactions in prior reactors can be reduced substantially (to 7%–9%) (GREENBERGER 1984; GREENBERGER et al. 1984, 1985, 1990). The addition of ephedrine, a potent α- and β_1-adrenergic stimulator (25 mg orally 1h prior to the procedure), reduces the subsequent reaction rate further (to 3%). While use of ephedrine appears effective, this medication has not been widely used, possibly because it can also produce adverse effects, particularly in patients with cardiovascular disease or hypertension.

Combining use of nonionic contrast media with premedication regimens using prednisone-diphenhydramine and prednisone-diphenhydramine-ephedrine results in an even lower frequency of adverse reactions in prior reactors (GREENBERGER and PATTERSON 1991). In Greenberger and Patterson's study, only one of 141 prior reactors who received the two-drug pretreatment regimen had an adverse reaction (urticaria) and none of the 41 patients who received the three-drug regimen had a reaction after nonionic contrast media injection. The authors recommended that patients who have had previous anaphylactoid reactions to contrast media should receive both premedication and nonionic agents.

At the present time, corticosteroid pretreatment is restricted by most authorities to patients who have had previous idiosyncratic adverse reactions to contrast media. Interestingly, there is wide variation in use of corticosteroids in patients who have had previous mild idiosyncratic reactions. For example, while nearly all uroradiologists premedicate patients who have previously developed respiratory problems, hypotension, or a severe skin reaction after contrast material injection, just under half would administer corticosteroids to patients whose previous reaction consisted only of one hive (COHAN et al. 1995).

Corticosteroids are usually well tolerated and produce no side-effects when only a few doses are administered. There are only a few circumstances in which they may aggravate underlying disease processes. A brief course of corticosteroids can precipitate tumor lysis syndromes in patients with leukemia and non-Hodgkin lymphoma (LUNA-FINEMAN et al. 1990) and can aggravate diabetes mellitus. It may also theoretically worsen symptoms of peptic ulcer disease and activate dormant tuberculosis.

11.4.1.5.3
PREMEDICATION WITH ANTIHISTAMINES
Premedication with H_1 antihistamines alone also appears to reduce the incidence of contrast reactions (BERTRAND et al. 1992). In one study, 400 patients were premedicated with either placebo or 100 mg of hydroxyzine 12 h prior to intravenous injection of ioxaglate. Twenty-five mild reactions (17 urticarial, six nausea and/or vomiting, one respiratory, and one of an unspecified nature) occurred in the group of patients given placebo, while only two reactions (nausea and bronchospasm, one each) occurred in the pretreated patients.

Studies evaluating the use of premedication with H_2 receptor blockers, such as cimetidine, have had conflicting results. While some have demonstrated that these agents are beneficial in lowering the number of subsequent adverse reactions (RING et al. 1985), others have observed adverse reactions to be more common when these agents are added to premedication regimens (GREENBERGER et al. 1985). Still others have failed to demonstrate either a significant adverse or beneficial effect of H_2 receptor blockers on the incidence of repeat contrast reactions in patients who have had previous adverse reactions to radiographic contrast media (MARSHALL and LIEBERMAN 1991). Although the utility of H_2 receptor blockers is questionable, these agents are well tolerated and might potentially be of benefit, particularly since they have proved effective in treating at least some allergic cutaneous reactions (MAYUMI et al. 1987). Most authorities agree that H_2 blockers should not be used without concomitant administration of H_1 antihistamines.

11.4.2 Systemic Nonidiosyncratic Contrast Reactions

Nonidiosyncratic contrast reactions are dose dependent. In other words, nonidiosyncratic reactions are less likely to occur and, if they do occur, are less likely to be severe when smaller doses of contrast material are employed. While data exclusively comparing the relative risks of nonidiosyncratic reactions in patients receiving high-osmolality ionic versus those receiving nonionic agents are sparse, it is still clear that nonionic agents are less likely to produce all types of nonidiosyncratic reactions.

11.4.2.1 Physiologic Effects of Contrast Media

Intravascular injections of contrast agents normally produce peripheral vessel dilatation as a result of a direct effect of these hyperosmolar agents on the vascular endothelium. The resulting peripheral vasodilatation is perceived by the patient as a sensation of heat or warmth. Nausea and vomiting are probably the result of a transient central nervous system effect of the contrast material. Since these symptoms are due to normal and expected actions of the contrast material, treatment is only required in the unusual cases in which they are quite severe. The physiologic effects of high-osmolality ionic contrast media are much more pronounced than are those of nonionic contrast media.

11.4.2.2 Vasovagal Reactions

Vasovagal reactions are acute nonidiosyncratic hypotensive reactions. Patients with vasovagal reactions frequently complain of nausea and are diaphoretic and anxious. Bradycardia is usually pronounced (heart rate <50 beats per minute). These reactions are most common in young to middle-aged males. Differentiation of a vasovagal from an anaphylactoid or, occasionally, even a cardiac hypotensive reaction may be difficult in patients receiving β-blockers. Most patients with cardiac disease are elderly.

11.4.2.3 Contrast-Induced Renal Failure

Contrast-induced renal failure, a nonidiosyncratic reaction, will be discussed in detail elsewhere, as will multiple risk factors for this complication. Briefly, contrast-induced renal failure usually refers to an acute elevation of serum creatinine level of >0.5 mg% or >50% of baseline. The incidence of this complication is estimated to be 2%–7% (PORTER 1994a, b). The mechanism of contrast-induced renal failure is unknown, but is suspected to be a combination of preexisting hemodynamic alterations (renal vasoconstriction) and direct cellular toxicity of contrast media (AMIN et al. 1993).

Patients taking the oral antihyperglycemic drug *metformin* (Glucophage, Bristol-Meyers Squibb, Princeton, N.J.) are potentially at increased risk for developing significant complications if they should develop renal failure of any type, including that resulting from the administration of iodinated radiographic contrast media. While metformin itself is not nephrotoxic, patients receiving metformin who become azotemic as a result of any renal insult (including contrast material administration) may rarely develop life-threatening lactic acidosis (Assan et al. 1977; Dachman 1995; Bailey and Turner 1996). The drug package insert for metformin in the United States indicated that it should be discontinued in all patients at least 48 h prior to any contrast-enhanced study. While many radiologists followed these recommendations, a new drug packageinsert and the American College of Radiology now suggests that metformin may be first withheld at the time of contrast medium injection. Metformin administration should not be resumed until at least 48 h have elapsed from the contrast-enhanced study, and then only provided that the patient's renal function has been checked and demonstrated to be normal (proving that the patient has not developed contrast-induced renal failure).

11.4.2.4
Aggravation of Diseases by Contrast Media

A variety of diseases can be aggravated by contrast media, including cardiac disease (aggravation of arrhythmias, precipitation of angina or congestive heart failure), pheochromocytomas (hypertensive crises), myasthenia gravis (acute worsening of respiratory symptoms of myasthenia), uncontrolled hyperthyroidism (thyroid storm), and sickle cell anemia (sickle cell crisis). Several specific disease entities are discussed in more detail in the following sections.

11.4.2.4.1
ARRHYTHMIAS

When injected directly into the coronary arteries, iodinated contrast material can produce severe, life-threatening arrhythmias. Arrhythmias may also occasionally occur after intravenous injection of contrast material, particularly when conventional ionic contrast material is utilized (Piao et al. 1988). These arrhythmias tend to be more frequent and worse in patients who have preexisting arrhythmias. In a report by Lawton et al. (1982), electrocardiograms were obtained in 135 consecutive patients both prior to and following intravenous injection of 60 ml of 45% sodium diatrizoate (at a rate of 1 ml/s). Six patients developed major arrhythmias following contrast material injection, including multiple premature ventricular beats, multiple premature multifocal ventricular beats, and ventricular trigeminy. Five of these six patients had had abnormal rhythm strips prior to contrast medium administration. Of a total of 13 patients with baseline arrhythmias, ten (77%) developed further arrhythmias during or after injection. In comparison, only 25 of 122 patients with normal baseline rhythm strips developed arrhythmias, only one of which was major.

11.4.2.4.2
ANGINA

Patients with angina usually present with symptoms of moderate to severe retrosternal discomfort. Patients often describe this discomfort as pressure rather than pain. The pressure may radiate to the back or shoulders, but can also be referred to the left arm and/or neck. Patients usually have a history of cardiac disease and often have had similar episodes previously. Occasionally, it can be difficult to distinguish anxiety from angina purely on the basis of patient symptoms, although the former more often occurs in younger patients with no history of heart disease.

11.4.2.4.3
PHEOCHROMOCYTOMAS

Hypertensive crises have been reported after contrast media infusion in patients with pheochromocytomas who have undergone adrenal arteriography (Meany and Buonocore 1966) and adrenal venography (Gold et al. 1972). Even more worrisome is the fact that hypertension may be observed in occasional patients with pheochromocytomas after contrast-enhanced CT, at least when high-osmolality ionic agents are employed (Geelhoed 1980). Raisanen and colleagues noted that following intravenous injection of ionic contrast medium, serum norepinephrine increased to levels high enough to cause hypertension in five of eight patients with pheochromocytomas had they not been premedicated with α-blockers (Raisanen et al. 1984). In comparison, the risk of hypertensive crisis in patients with pheochromocytomas who receive intravenous injections of nonionic contrast media appears to be considerably lower than is the risk in patients who receive high-osmolality ionic agents. Serum catecholamine levels did not increase significantly in any of ten patients with pheochromocytomas within 25–60 min of intravenous injection of the nonionic agent iohexol (Mukherjee et al. 1997). This suggests that while intravascular use of ionic agents should be avoided in patients with pheochromocytomas who are not receiving α-blockers, nonionic agents can probably be used without complication in many patients.

11.4.2.4.4
Myasthenia Gravis

Myasthenia gravis is a disease characterized by failure of transmission of nerve impulses at the neuromuscular junction. Typically, the disease affects muscles innervated by the cranial nerves (face, lips, tongue, neck, and throat), but it can affect any muscle group. When this disease involves the respiratory system, it may be life threatening. Myasthenia may occur at any age but has its highest incidence between the ages of 20 and 40 years and is more common in women than men. It frequently coexists with immunologic and thyroid disorders. Fifteen percent of myasthenic patients have thymomas.

Given the high incidence of thymoma in myasthenics, chest CT examinations are frequently requested in patients with this disease. It is advantageous in some cases to give intravenous contrast to better image the mediastinum. There have been several published reports of myasthenia gravis exacerbated by intravenously injected contrast media. Reported signs and symptoms that may occur after contrast media administration include weakness, dyspnea and cyanosis, strabismus, ptosis, and aphonia (Canal and Franceechi 1983). Acute signs of respiratory distress are sometimes severe (Rocha 1994). A few patients have become apneic and paralyzed and have required emergent intubation (Eliashiv et al. 1990). Contrast material-related myasthenic "crises" usually appear shortly after contrast material administration. Review of prior cases has indicated that all reacting patients had preexisting bulbar symptoms. Respiratory arrest has been encountered in patients with bulbar symptoms, even in cases where patients were well controlled with anticholinesterases (Chagnac et al. 1985; Frank et al. 1987).

11.4.2.4.5
Thyrotoxicosis

There have been a number of reports of patients in whom administration of iodinated ionic contrast material resulted in thyrotoxicosis. This phenomenon has been encountered in patients with nontoxic goiters (Blum et al. 1974; Shimura et al. 1990; Breadmore et al. 1995) and in patients with mild preexisting hyperthyroidism (Shetty et al. 1974). Recently, Martin et al. (1993) reported on seven geriatric patients who they believed developed transient hyperthyroidism following the intravenous injection of nonionic contrast media at total iodine doses of between 15 and 40 g of iodine. This accounted for 25% of the hyperthyroid patients who they encountered over 20 months. Hyperthyroidism was first detected during follow-up testing 2–8 weeks following contrast medium administration in these patients and produced clinically significant symptoms in six patients, significantly prolonging patient recovery from other illnesses. A clinically palpable goiter was present in only three of these seven patients.

There have also been reports of patients with apparently nonfunctioning metastases from thyroid cancer after thyroidectomy in whom thyroxine levels increased after intravenous administration of high-osmolality ionic contrast material (Yoshinari et al. 1988; Lorberboym and Mechanick 1996). In one instance, a patient developed life-threatening hyperthermia and atrial fibrillation with a rapid ventricular response (Lorberboym and Mechanick 1996).

11.4.2.4.6
Sickle Cell Anemia

Intravascular contrast media can precipitate sickling of red blood cells in patients with sickle cell anemia. This phenomenon has been demonstrated clinically with high-osmolality ionic contrast material (Cheatham and Brackett 1965; Richards and Nulsen 1971) and experimentally with both nonionic and, to a much greater extent, high-osmolality ionic agents (Rao et al. 1982). Sickling of red blood cells is first observed when the concentration of ionic contrast material in blood reaches or exceeds 3.1 g/dl (Rao et al. 1982). The increased osmolality of the contrast media results in fluid shifts from within the abnormal blood cells to the plasma. This results in an increased concentration of hemoglobin-S within the red blood cell and subsequent sickling. Contrast material may account for up to 55% of the volume of whole blood during selective arteriography or about 30 g/dl. In comparison, the concentration of contrast material in blood plasma during urography and CT is only about 0.5 g/dl, well below that which has been demonstrated to produce sickling. Thus, the risk of sickling is quite real during selective arteriography with high-osmolality ionic contrast agents, but is only theoretical when intravenous injections are performed at relatively low infusion rates, especially when nonionic agents are used.

11.4.2.4.7
PANCREATITIS
One retrospective report has found that patients with pancreatitis who undergo contrast-enhanced CT scans for evaluation of their disease have a longer mean duration of clinical illness (10.8 days) compared with patients who do not undergo this study (6.2 days) (McMenamin and Gates 1996). The authors suggest that intravenous contrast material should, therefore, not routinely be administered to patients with pancreatitis. While these results are intriguing, additional studies are needed for further investigation, particularly given the design limitations of this study.

11.4.2.5 Seizures

As previously described, seizures may result from hypoxia in severely hypotensive patients or in patients with respiratory insufficiency. Occasionally, a seizing patient may have normal vital signs and oxygenation. In these instances, a direct neurotoxic effect of contrast media is likely. Neurogenic seizures and other CNS disturbances have occasionally been encountered after contrast media injection in patients in whom the blood-brain barrier has been disrupted, such as those with central nervous system (CNS) neoplasms (Junck and Marshall 1983; Haslam et al. 1987; Lukovits et al. 1996). Seizures are also encountered in patients without CNS disease when extremely high doses are injected (Muruve and Steinman 1996). CNS toxicity of this type is rarely encountered, because such high doses of intravascular contrast media are avoided due to the fear of producing irreversible renal damage; however, high doses of contrast material may occasionally be given to patients on permanent dialysis (in whom end-stage renal disease already exists). Neurotoxicity of contrast material will be discussed in more detail elsewhere.

11.4.2.6 Hypertensive Crises

Acute hypertensive reasctions may become manifest when patients develop sudden severe headaches, nausea, vomiting, or altered mental status. A diagnosis of hypertension is made when diastolic blood pressure exceeds 120 mmHg (Bush and King 1995). Hypertensive crises may occur in patients with a history of hypertension and cardiac disease, in which case angina may also be present. As previously noted, crises may also occur in patients with pheochromocytomas after arterial or intravenous injections of contrast material. Hypertensive contrast reactions have also been reported in patients with lung metastases from renal adenocarcinomas who were treated with inhaled interleukin-2 (Heinzer et al. 1992).

11.4.2.7 Delayed Reactions Producing Nonspecific Symptoms

Delayed reactions are usually defined as reactions that occur more than 1 h after but within 3 days of contrast material injection. Many such reactions produce very nonspecific symptoms, including fever (which may be quite high), chills or rigors, rash, flushing, dizziness, pruritus, arthralgia, diarrhea, nausea, vomiting, headache, and, occasionally, hypotension (Donnelly et al. 1993; Choyke et al. 1992).

Delayed reactions have been observed after injection of both ionic and nonionic contrast media (Choyke et al. 1992; Yoshikawa 1992). Febrile reactions and chills have been encountered in 3% of patients after cardiac catheterization (Jacobson et al. 1983) and in more than 10% of patients who received high doses of meglumine-based contrast media (Smith et al. 1974). In these two studies, fevers and chills usually developed from within minutes to 6 h after contrast injection, and almost always resolved by 8 h. In most patients, symptoms resolved spontaneously. It has been speculated that this specific type of delayed reaction represents an unusual hypothalamic response to the contrast material injection. Delayed reactions of this type have also been observed in 4%–8% of patients injected with nonionic contrast media. In two recent series, symptoms related to delayed reactions to nonionic agents usually resolved within 1–2 days (Choyke et al. 1992; Yoshikawa 1992). These types of delayed reaction have been encountered with increased frequency (12%–28%) in patients who are currently receiving or who have recently (within 2 years) received intra-arterial or intravenous interleukin-2 immunotherapy for treatment of metastatic cancer (ZUKIWSKI et al. 1990; FISHMAN et al. 1991; CHOYKE et al. 1992). In one series the incidence of contrast reactions was higher (11%) in patients who had received interleukin-2 within 2 weeks in comparison to those who had received interleukin-2 more than 6 weeks prior to contrast media exposure (1.7%) (SHULMAN et al. 1993). While delayed reactions in interleukin-2 patients are similar to those in patients who have not received interleukin-2, they are generally more severe (CHOYKE et al. 1992). Interleukin-2-related delayed reactions (and perhaps some reactions not related to interleukin-2 therapy) may represent delayed hypersensitivity responses of the cell-mediated type; however, the etiology of all delayed reactions remains uncertain.

11.4.2.8
Anxiety Reactions

Anxiety reactions are a diagnosis of exclusion and should only be considered when all other types of acute reaction have been eliminated as possibilities. Patients with anxiety reactions may complain of chest tightness or of a variety of other symptoms that mimic other types of adverse reactions. In these instances, vital signs are normal (with the possible exception of a mild tachycardia). Auscultation of anxious patients fails to detect any wheezes or rales. Pulse oximetry reveals normal oxygen saturation. Some patients with anxiety reactions may develop symptoms as a result of hyperventilation.

11.4.3
Local Cutaneous or Subcutaneous Nonidiosyncratic Contrast Reactions

Local reactions to intravascular injections of contrast material usually occur at or near the site of intravascular injection, but can occur elsewhere. A variety of local reactions can be encountered, of which extravasation injuries are the most clinically significant.

11.4.3.1
Phlebitis

Chemical phlebitis has been encountered after intravenous injection of contrast material, most frequently after intravenous injection of nondilute high-osmolality ionic contrast agents for lower extremity ascending venography. Bettmann and associates noted phlebitis in more than 25% of patients undergoing venography with 60% sodium/meglumine diatrizoate, but in only 9% and 8% of patients injected with dilute (45%) ionic or dilute (200 mg I/ml) nonionic contrast material, respectively (BETTMANN et al. 1987). Symptoms of phlebitis, which may include warmth, tenderness, erythema, and mild swelling, localized to the skin and subcutaneous tissues over the affected vein, are only rarely encountered following upper extremity venous injections.

11.4.3.2
Extravasation

Extravasation of contrast media is a relatively common complication of intravenous contrast media administration. Fortunately most extravasations involve small volumes of fluid (<10 ml) and these almost always resolve without adverse sequelae. Large-volume extravasations (>50 ml) are more likely to produce significant injury to the skin and subcutaneous tissues, but still most commonly resolve within 24–48 h. Large-volume extravasations are usually encountered during dynamic bolus computed tomography (CT), at which time the patient receives an intravenous injection under pressure sometimes without being directly monitored during the entire contrast material injection. While many patients complain of pain as soon as an extravascular injection occurs, others may not have any discomfort or may believe that the pain they are feeling is an expected result of a contrast media injection (COHAN et al. 1997).

There is no widely accepted effective treatment for an extravascular injection of contrast media. The best way in which to minimize the chance of injury is therefore to prevent an extravasation from occurring in the first place, primarily by taking appropriate precautions in patients most at risk of having extravasations or significant extravasation injuries (COHAN et al. 1996). Extravasations are more frequent in the very young or very old, and those unable to communicate. They are also more common when patients are injected through indwelling peripheral intravenous lines, with metallic needles rather than plastic cannulae, through catheters placed in small peripheral veins, and distal to tourniquets that are left in place. In addition, extravasations are more likely when multiple attempts are made to establish access in the same vein (UPTON et al. 1979). Severe injuries from extravasated agents (including contrast material) are more common when extravasations occur in patients with peripheral vascular disease (due to diabetes mellitus, connective tissue disease, atherosclerosis, and prior radiation treatment to the extremity to be injected) (UPTON et al. 1979). Low-osmolality contrast media are much better tolerated by the skin and subcutaneous tissues than high-osmolality ionic contrast media in laboratory studies (COHAN et al. 1990a; KIM et al. 1990) and have been well tolerated when extravasated in humans (COHAN et al. 1990b; SISTROM et al. 1991). Therefore, it is reasonable to use nonionic media in high-risk clinical settings or patients, even in the absence of other indications for low-osmolality contrast media use. To date, we are aware of only three published reports of significant injuries developing after extravasation of low-osmolality agents (POND et al. 1992; MEMOLO et al. 1993; YOUNG 1994).

11.4.3.3
Pain at or Central to the Injection Site

Occasionally patients may complain of severe pain at an injection site in the absence of any detectable extravasation. This pain, speculated to be the result of irritation of the vascular endothelium by the contrast material, is usually transient, lasting for no more than 90–120 min. Delayed arm pain at or near the injection site is also occasionally encountered. In the series of patients reported by PANTO and DAVIES (1986), delayed arm pain was observed in 13% of patients who received injections of iodinated ionic contrast material. It was first noticed 0–8 days after injection (mean of 1.6 days) and lasted for 1–30 days (mean of 3.4 days). Delayed arm pain has also been noted in more than 10% of patients injected with nonionic agents (MCCULLOUGH et al. 1989).

11.4.3.4
Sialadenitis

Sialadenitis (also referred to as parotitis or iodide mumps) has been encountered after administration of ionic and nonionic contrast material (KOHRI et al. 1977; RIVERA et al. 1993). MCCULLOUGH et al. (1989) noted that 0.87% of patients injected with ionic agents and 1.7% of patients injected with nonionic agents complained of pain and swelling under the ear which was attributed to sialadenitis. The etiology of sialadenitis is unknown, but it may be due to a toxic effect of iodine on the salivary glands.

11.4.3.5
Ioderma

Ioderma refers to the development of tender pustules or vesicles often on the face, neck, and back (GOOD et al. 1980), but also occasionally elsewhere such as on the feet (VAILLANT et al. 1990), after iodide ingestion. These cutaneous lesions may develop within hours or after 1 or 2 days. This type of reaction is exceedingly rare after the administration of contrast material intravascularly, but has been reported. This reaction is believed to be more likely in patients with pre-existing renal disease (VAILLANT et al. 1990).

11.4.3.6
Koebner Phenomenon

The Koebner phenomenon is a very unusual cutaneous response to contrast medium injection. This consists of a localized skin reaction (often consisting of focal urticaria or rash) at a site of previous skin trauma or scarring. SHAH and HUTCHISON (1990) reported an immunocompromised renal transplant patient who developed a cutaneous reaction of pale papules with surrounding erythema (hive-like) at a variety of sites, including a median sternotomy scar, an old nonfunctional arteriovenous fistula site in an upper extremity, an antecubital venipuncture site, and a forehead scar, after intravenous injection of nonionic contrast material.

11.4.3.7
Chemical Burns

There has been a report of two children who developed severe bullous skin lesions over the buttocks after excretory urography (WOOD et al. 1988). These lesions were speculated to have resulted from a chemical burn caused by the contrast material that had been excreted into the patients' urine. The urine remained in contact with the buttocks because both patients were wearing disposable diapers for at least 1h after the procedure was performed.

11.4.4 Fetal or Neonatal Toxicity in Pregnant and Lactating Women

11.4.4.1 Mutagenic Effects in the First Trimester of Pregnancy

In general intravenous contrast material should be avoided, when possible, in pregnant women so as to eliminate any theoretical adverse effects on the fetus. In vitro experiments have demonstrated that contrast material is mutagenic to human cells (NELSON et al. 1982); however, animal studies have failed to demonstrate that this translates into any teratogenic effects in vivo (RALSTON et al. 1989; MORISETTI et al. 1994).

11.4.4.2 Third Semester Fetal or Neonatal Thyroid Toxicity

Fetal thyroid impairment has been observed after instillation of contrast material into the amniotic cavity during the third trimester of pregnancy (RODESCH et al. 1976). In addition, radiographic contrast agents injected into the maternal vascular system can cross the placenta and be absorbed by the fetus (DEAN 1977), also potentially producing transient fetal thyroid dysfunction (hypothyroidism).

Contrast material is excreted into human breast milk. Fortunately, the amount of contrast material excreted into breast milk is exceedingly small. In one study, no detectable ionic contrast material was found in the breast milk of two women between 6 and 16.5h after injection of 50ml of 34% and 37% by weight ionic iodine-containing contrast media (FITZJOHN et al. 1982). In another, it was determined that the amount of iohexol 350 ingested by a breast-fed baby within 24h of maternal contrast media injection (at a volume of 1ml/kg) would equal only 0.2% of the allowed pediatric dose for that infant (NIELSON et al. 1987).

These studies indicate that there is no definite reason for a lactating mother to stop breast feeding after a contrast media injection. Nonetheless, as an extra precaution, some researchers (and the package inserts in the United States) still recommend that infants be fed formula and that the mother use a breast pump and discard obtained milk for 24h following maternal contrast medium administration.

Since nonionic agents are, in general, better tolerated, their use is preferred over high-osmolality ionic agents in pregnant and lactating women. At least one study has demonstrated that use of nonionic agents does not compromise neonatal thyroid function (BONA et al. 1992).

11.4.5 Reactions After Nonvascular Studies

Although rare, systemic contrast reactions have been reported after direct instillation of contrast media into the renal collecting systems and bladder (DARDENNE 1995; MILLER 1995), the gastrointestinal tract (MILLER 1997), the biliary and pancreatic ductal systems (MOREIRA et al. 1985), and the spinal canal. The risks of systemic absorption of contrast media are greatest during percutaneous transhepatic cholangiography, endoscopic retrograde pancreatography, nephrostograms, and retrograde pyelography, because in these instances contrast material is injected into nonvascular structures under pressure.

11.4.5.1 Reactions After Nonvascular Urologic Studies

A high-pressure injection directly into the renal collecting system can result in pyelosinus, pyelotubular, pyelolymphatic, or pyelovenous extravasation, usually from leakage of contrast material at the tips of the calyces. Contrast material injected near the ureteral orifice may occasionally intravasate into the wall of the ureter or extravasate into periureteric fat. Extravasated or intravasated contrast material is subsequently resorbed into the lymphatic and vascular systems. Experimental studies have also demonstrated that a tiny amount of contrast material can be absorbed across intact uroepithelium in the bladder, perhaps by passive diffusion (CURRARINO et al. 1977). Factors that may increase the likelihood that such absorption will occur include: (a) use of highly concentrated contrast media (possibly by producing an inflammatory response), (b) use of large volumes of contrast media (as might be needed during cystography), (c) instillation of contrast material for more than 15 min, and (d) injection of contrast material into the collecting system under pressure rather than using gravity (Currarino et al. 1977; Weese et al. 1993).

There are published reports of five patients who developed severe reactions after retrograde pyelography. Symptoms in these patients included dyspnea, wheezing, hypotension, and respiratory and cardiac arrest (Payne et al. 1956; Schmidlapp 1961; Percy 1967; Johenning 1980). While many of these reactions may have resulted from systemic resorption of contrast material, neomycin was often mixed into the contrast material in the older studies (Schmidlapp 1961; Percy 1967; Johenning 1980). Systemic absorption of this antibiotic can also result in significant adverse allergic-like sequelae.

While contrast material injected during antegrade pyelography may leak from the collecting system into the renal sinus, collecting tubules, lymphatics, or veins, it can also track around the percutaneous tract and into the retroperitoneal and subcutaneous tissues. The contrast material can be subsequently absorbed systemically. Gaiser and Chua (1993) encountered a patient who developed bronchospasm and severe hypotension when nonionic contrast material was injected into the renal collecting system during a nephrostomy. This patient had previously developed a rash after an excretory urogram.

Since systemic reactions may occur after both retrograde and antegrade pyelography, it might be prudent to perform these studies with nonionic contrast material, at least in patients who have had previous idiosyncratic reactions to intravascular contrast media. Since only small volumes of contrast media are used, this should not add appreciably to the expense of the procedure. When patients have had previous severe idiosyncratic or anaphylactoid reactions to intravenous contrast media, premedication with corticosteroids might also be considered.

There have been three reported reactions attributed to ionic contrast media after cystography McAlister et al. 1974; Weese et al. 1993). In one instance, urticaria was noted during a cystogram which demonstrated bilateral vesicoureteral reflux in a 5-year-old girl who had previously developed urticaria after an excretory urogram (McAlister et al. 1974). The second patient was a 2-year-old girl in whom urticaria was noted during a cystogram (Weese et al. 1993): 150 ml of dilute ionic contrast material had been instilled into the patient's bladder under gravity pressure. There was no vesicoureteral reflux. The third patient was a 55-year-old man in whom 100 ml of meglumine iothalamate was instilled into the bladder via a Foley catheter (Weese et al. 1993). Extensive vesicoureteral reflux occurred. As soon as the reflux was seen, the patient became transiently but severely hypotensive.

Although we are aware of no published evidence to support our opinion, we believe that since the likelihood of systemic resorption is lower with cystography than with retrograde or antegrade pyelography, the need for nonionic media is not as compelling. While instillation of dilute nonionic contrast agents can be considered when cystograms are performed in patients who have had prior contrast reactions, nonionic contrast use (possibly along with corticosteroid premedication) should be reserved for patients requiring cystography whose previous reactions were severe. Such studies may be costly, since large volumes of nonionic contrast media may be required. We also recommend that patients be closely observed when retrograde urethrograms or cystograms are performed in the setting of acute trauma. Here, studies are performed to determine whether there is any extravasation. Time may preclude satisfactory corticosteroid preparation in patients who have had previous adverse reactions to systemic contrast media. Alternate tests such as radionuclide cystography might be considered.

11.4.5.2 Fallopian Tubes and Peritoneum

Water-soluble contrast material injected into the uterus for hysterosalpingography usually reaches the peritoneal cavity when it flows through patent fallopian tubes. Occasionally contrast material is also injected directly into the peritoneal cavity (usually through indwelling peritoneal dialysis catheters in order to identify loculated fluid collections in febrile patients). Nonidiosyncratic reactions are relatively common. The most common adverse reaction resulting from hysterosalpingography is abdominal pain. When abdominal pain occurs during the procedure it is felt to be due to instrumentation and/or hydrostatic pressure from the injected contrast material distending the endometrial cavity and fallopian tubes. When abdominal pain occurs after hysterosalpingography, it is presumed to often be due to peritoneal irritation by contrast material (Chen et al. 1995). Since peritoneal contrast material is systemically absorbed, idiosyncratic contrast material reactions may also be encountered, although they are rare. All reactions after hysterosalpingography and peritoneography appear to be less common when nonionic agents are employed than when conventional ionic agents are used (CHEN et al. 1995).

11.4.5.3 Idiosyncratic Reactions After Nonvascular Gastrointestinal Tract Studies

11.4.5.3.1 ENDOSCOPIC RETROGRADE CHOLANGIOPANCREATOGRAPHY (ERCP)

The most common adverse event occurring after ERCP is transient mild and asymptomatic hyperamylasemia (MAKELA and DEAN 1986). Allergic-like or idiosyncratic reactions are very rarely encountered (MOREIRA et al. 1985); however, systemic absorption (as demonstrated by excretion into the renal collecting systems) has been detected in as many as 8% of patients undergoing this procedure (LADAS et al. 1986). It has been speculated that the absorption probably occurs through the pancreatic ductal system rather than the intestinal mucosa (LADAS et al. 1986). Given the potential for systemic resorption, use of low-osmolality contrast material is suggested at least in patients at risk for having an idiosyncratic reaction.

11.4.5.3.2 ORAL CONTRAST MATERIAL

The most common significant adverse reaction related to oral ingestion of iodinated contrast media is aspiration pneumonitis (TRULZSCH et al. 1992). Since water-soluble iodinated oral contrast media are very poorly absorbed from the gastrointestinal tract, other adverse reactions not related to the gastrointestinal tract are uncommon. Idiosyncratic reactions to oral contrast agents are exceedingly rare. In fact, SKUCAS (1997) speculates that the average radiologist will probably not encounter a single reaction of this type in his or her career. Recently, however, MILLER (1997) reported on a 64-year-old patient who developed severe respiratory distress on two occasions following oral administration of Gastrografin. The author speculates that systemic resorption could have occurred in this instance because the patient had pseudomembranous colitis, likely with resultant disruption of bowel mucosa.

11.4.5.4 Myelography

Accidental misadministration of high-osmolality ionic contrast material into the subarachnoid space is highly toxic. Severe complications, including seizures, long-term dysfunction, and even death have been reported (RIVERA et al. 1995). The reader is referred to the chapter on neurotoxicity (Chap. 9) for additional discussion.

11.4.6 Other Reactions During Nonvascular Studies: Autonomic Dysreflexia

Patients with spinal cord injuries at or above the lower thoracic spine (at a level cephalad to the major sympathetic splanchnic outflow) who have intact lower cord segments can experience autonomic dysreflexia. An autonomic stimulus below the injured level, usually resulting from distention or instrumentation of the bladder or rectum (as would occur during insertion of a Foley catheter, or performance of cystography or a barium enema, for example), may precipitate a variety of significant signs and symptoms including excessive sweating, flushing of the face, nasal congestion, piloerection, headache, bradycardia or tachycardia, and severe hypertension (BRADDOM and ROCCO 1991; TROP and BENNETT 1991). Autonomic dysreflexia can result from a variety of other genitourinary examinations or pathologic conditions, including nephrostolithotomy (CHANG et al. 1991). Between 48% and 90% of quadriplegic or high paraplegic patients are reportedly affected (BRADDOM and ROCCO 1991). If manifestations of autonomic dysreflexia go untreated, life-threatening intracerebral or subarachnoid hemorrhage may result. For this reason, patients who have previously experienced this complication should be premedicated prior to instrumentation with the object primarily being to prevent severe hypertensive reactions (CHANG et al. 1991; TROP and BENNETT 1991).

11.5 Conclusions

An understanding of the causes and manifestations of reactions to iodinated contrast material may enable appropriate attempts to prevent reactions and more prompt recognition and treatment of any reactions that may occur. A rational approach to treatment is predicated on knowledge of the etiologies and manifestations of the different types of adverse reactions, many of which have been summarized here.

References

Almen T (1994) The etiology of contrast medium reactions. Invest Radiol 29(S1):S37–S45

Amin MM, Cohan RH, Dunnick NR (1993) Ionic and nonionic contrast media: current status and controversies. Appl Radiol 22:41–54

Ansell G (1987) An epidemiologic report on adverse reactions in urography: ionic and nonionic media. Diagnostic Imaging (Suppl) May:6–10

Ansell G, Tweedie MCK, West CR, et al. (1980) The current status of reactions to intravenous contrast media. Invest Radiol 15:S32–S39

Assan R, Heuclin C, Ganeval D, et al. (1977) Metformin-induced lactic acidosis in the presence of acute renal failure. Diabetologia 13:211

Bailey CJ, Turner RC (1996) Metformin. N Engl J Med 334:574–579

Bertrand PR, Soyer PM, Rouleau PJ, et al. (1992) Comparative randomized double-blind study of hydroxyzine versus placebo as premedication before injection of iodinated contrast media. Radiology 184:383–384

Bettmann MA, Robbins A, Braun SD, et al. (1987) Contrast venography of the leg: diagnostic efficacy, tolerance, and complication rates with ionic and nonionic contrast media. Radiology 165:113–116

Bettmann MA, Heeren T, Greenfield A, et al. (1997) Adverse events with radiographic contrast agents: results of the SCVIR Contrast Agent Registry. Radiology 203:611–620

Blum M, Weinberg U, Shenkman L, et al. (1974) Hyperthyroidism after iodinated contrast medium. N Engl J Med 291:24–25

Bona G, Zaffaroni M, Defillippi C, et al. (1992) Effects of iopamidol on neonatal thyroid function. Eur J Radiol 12:22–25

Braddom RL, Rocco JF (1991) Autonomic dysreflexia: a survey of current treatment. Am J Phys Med Rehabil 70:234–241

Breadmore R, McKenzie A, Arkles LB, et al. (1995) Hyperthyroidism after radiographic contrast in a patient with separate cervical and intrathoracic multinodular goiters. Clin Nucl Med 20:413–415

Bush WH, King BF (ed) (1995) Radiology Life Support (RAD-LS). Syllabus for American Roentgen Ray Society Instructional Course, Washington, DC

Canal N, Franceechi M (1983) Myasthenic crisis precipitated by iothalamic acid. Lancet I:1288

Caro JJ, Trindade E, McGregor M, et al. (1991) The risks of death and of severe non-fatal reactions with high- vs low-osmolality contrast media: a meta-analysis. AJR 156:825–832

Carr DH, Walker AC (1984) Contrast media reactions: experimental evidence against the allergy theory. Br J Radiol 57:469–473

Chagnac Y, Hadani M, Goldhammer Y, et al. (1985) Myasthenic crisis after intravenous administration of iodinated contrast agent. Neurology 35:1219–1220

Chang CP, Chen MT, Chang LS (1991) Autonomic dysreflexia in spinal cord injury patient during percutaneous nephrolithotomy for renal stone: a case report. J Urol 146:1601–1602

Cheatham ML, Brackett CE (1965) Problems in the management of subarachnoid hemorrhage in sickle cell anemia. J Neurosurg 23:488–493

Chen MYM, Zagoria RJ, Fayez JA, et al. (1995) Comparison of patient reactions and diagnostic quality for hysterosalpingography using ionic and nonionic contrast media. Acad Radiol 2:123–127

Choyke PL, Miller DL, Lotze MT, et al. (1992) Delayed reactions to contrast media after interleukin-2 immunotherapy. Radiology 183:111–114

Cohan RH, Dunnick NR (1987) Intravascular contrast media: adverse reactions. AJR 149:665–670

Cohan RH, Leder RA, Bolick D, et al. (1990a) Extravascular extravasation of radiographic contrast media: effects of conventional and low-osmolar agents in the rat thigh. Invest Radiol 25:504–510

Cohan RH, Dunnick NR, Leder RA, et al. (1990b) Extravasation of nonionic radiologic contrast media: efficacy of conservative treatment. Radiology 164:65–67

Cohan RH, Ellis JH, Dunnick NR (1995) Use of low-osmolar agents and premedication to reduce the frequency of adverse reactions to radiographic contrast media: a survey of the Society of Uroradiology. Radiology 194:357–364

Cohan RH, Ellis JH, Garner WL (1996) Extravasation of radiographic contrast material: recognition, prevention, and treatment. Radiology 200:593–604

Cohan RH, Bullard MA, Ellis JH, et al. (1997) Local reactions after injection of iodinated radiographic contrast material: detection, management, and outcome. Acad Radiol 4:711–718

Cummins RO (ed) (1994) Textbook of advanced cardiac life support. American Heart Association, Dallas

Currarino G, Weinberg A, Putnam R (1977) Resorption of contrast material from the bladder during cystourethrography causing an excretory urogram. Radiology 123:149–150

Dachman A (1995) New contraindication to intravascular iodinated contrast material. Radiology 197:545

Dardenne AN (1995) Anaphylactoid reactions during voiding cystourethrography. AJR 164:1551–1552

Dean PB (1977) Fetal uptake of intravascular radiologic contrast medium. ROFO Fortschr Rontgenstr Nuklearmed 127:267–270

Donnelly PK, Williams B, Watkin EM (1993) Polyarthropathy-a delayed reaction to low osmolality angiographic contrast medium in patients with end stage renal disease. Eur J Radiol 17:130–132

Eliashiv S, Wirguin I, Brenner T, et al. (1990) Aggravation of human and experimental myasthenia gravis by contrast media. Neurology 40:1623–1625

Ellis JH, Cohan RH, Sonnad SS, et al. (1996) Selective use of radiographic low-osmolality contrast media in the 1990s. Radiology 200:297–311

Fishman JE, Aberle DR, Moldawer NP, et al. (1991) Atypical contrast reactions associated with systemic interleukin-2 therapy. AJR 156:833–834

Fitzjohn TP, Williams DG, Laker MF, et al. (1982) Intravenous urography during lactation. Br J Radiol 55:603–605

Frank JH, Cooper GW, Black WC, et al. (1987) Iodinated contrast agents in myasthenia gravis. Neurology 37:1400–1402

Gaiser RR, Chua E (1993) Anaphylactic/anaphylactoid reaction to contrast dye administered in the ureter. J Clin Anesth 5:510–512

Geelhoed GW (1980) CAT scans and catecholamines. Surgery 87:719–720

Gold RE, Wisinger BM, Garaci AR, et al. (1972) Hypertensive crisis as a result of adrenal venography in a patient with pheochromocytoma. Radiology 102:579–580

Good AE, Novak E, Sonda LP (1980) Fixed eruption and fever after urography. South Med J 73:948–949

Greenberger PA (1984) Contrast media reactions. J Allergy Clin Immunol 74:600–605

Greenberger PA, Patterson R (1991) The prevention of immediate generalized reactions to radiocontrast media in high-risk patients. J Allergy Clin Immunol 87:867–872

Greenberger PA, Patterson R, Radin RC (1984) Two pretreatment regimens for high-risk patients receiving radiographic contrast media. J Allergy Clin Immunol 74:540–543

Greenberger PA, Patterson R, Tapio CM (1985) Prophylaxis against repeated radiocontrast media reactions in 857 cases. Arch Intern Med 145:2197–2200

Greenberger PA, Patterson R, Kelly J, et al. (1990) Administration of radiographic contrast media in high-risk patients. Invest Radiol 15:S40–S43

Hartman GW, Hattery RR, Witten DM, et al. (1982) Mortality during excretory urography: Mayo Clinic experience. AJR 139:919–922

Haslam RH, Cochrane DD, Amundson GM, et al. (1987) Neurotoxic complications of contrast computed tomography in children. J Pediatr 111:837–840

Heinzer H, Huland E, Huland H (1992) Adverse reaction to contrast material in a patient treated with local interleukin-2. AJR 158:1407

Jacobson JA, Schwartz CE, Marshall HW, et al. (1983) Fever, chills, and hypotension following cardiac catheterization with single and multiple-use disposable catheters. Cathet Cardiovasc Diagn 9:39–46

Johenning PW (1980) Reactions to contrast material during retrograde pyelography. Urology 4:442–443

Junck L, Marshall WH (1983) Neurotoxicity of radiologic contrast agents. Ann Neurol 13:469–484

Katayama H, Yamaguchi K, Kozuka T, et al. (1990) Adverse reactions to ionic and nonionic contrast media. A report from the Japanese Committee on the Safety of Contrast Media. Radiology 175:621–628

Kim SH, Park JH, Kim YI, et al. (1990) Experimental tissue damage after subcutaneous injection of water-soluble contrast media. Invest Radiol 25:678–685

Kohri K, Miyoshi S, Nagahara A, et al. (1977) Bilateral parotid enlargement ("iodine mumps") following excretory urography. Radiology 122:654

Ladas SD, Rokkas T, Kaskarelis J, et al. (1986) Absorption of iodized contrast media during ERCP. Gastrointest Endosc 32:376

Lasser EC (1985) Etiology of anaphylactoid responses: the promise of nonionics. Invest Radiol 20:S79–S82

Lasser EC (1987) A coherent biochemical basis for increased reactivity to contrast material in allergic patients: a novel concept. AJR 149:1281–1285

Lasser EC (1988) Pretreatment with corticosteroids to prevent reactions to IV contrast material: overview and implications. AJR 150:257–259

Lasser EC, Berry CC, Talner LB, et al. (1987) Pretreatment with corticosteroids to alleviate reactions to intravenous contrast material. N Engl J Med 317:845–849

Lasser EC, Berry CC, Mishkin MM, et al. (1994) Pretreatment with corticosteroids to prevent adverse reactions to nonionic contrast media. AJR 162:523–526

Lasser EC, Lyon SG, Berry CC (1997) Reports on contrast media reactions: analysis of data from reports to the US Food and Drug Administration. Radiology 203:605–610

Lawton G, Phillips T, Davies R (1982) Alterations in heart rate and rhythm at urography with sodium diatrizoate. Acta Radiol 23:107–110

Lorberboym M, Mechanick JI (1996) Accelerated thyrotoxicosis induced by iodinated contrast media in metastatic differentiated thyroid carcinoma. J Nucl Med 37:1532–1535

Lukovits TG, Fadul CE, Pipas JM, et al. (1996) Nonconvulsive status epilepticus after intravenous contrast medium administration. Epilepsia 37:1117–1120

Luna-Fineman S, Healy MV, Parker BR (1990) Corticosteroid pretreatment for potential contrast reactions in children with lymphoreticular cancer: a word of caution. AJR 155:357–358

Makela P, Dean PB (1986) The frequency of hyperamylasemia after ERCP with diatrizoate and iohexol. Eur J Radiol 6:303–304

Marshall JD Jr, Lieberman PL (1991) Comparison of three pretreatment protocols to prevent anaphylactoid reactions to radiocontrast media. Ann Allergy 67:70–74

Martin FI, Treiss BW, Colman PG, et al. (1993) Iodine-induced hyperthyroidism due to nonionic contrast radiography in the elderly. Am J Med 95:78–82

Mayumi H, Kimura S, Asano M, et al. (1987) Intravenous cimetidine as an effective treatment for systemic anaphylaxis and acute allergic skin reactions. Ann Allergy 58:447–451

McAlister WH, Cacciarelli A, Shackelford GD, et al. (1974) Complications associated with cystography in children. Radiology 111:167–172

McCullough M, Davies P, Richardson R (1989) A large trial of intravenous Conray 325 and Niopam 300 to assess immediate and delayed reactions. Br J Radiol 62:260–265

McMenamin DA, Gates LK (1996) A retrospective analysis of the effect of contrast-enhanced CT on the outcome of acute pancreatitis. Am J Gastroenterol 91:1384–1387

Meany TF, Buonocore E (1966) Selective arteriography as a localizing and provocative test in the diagnosis of pheochromocytoma. Radiology 87:309–314

Memolo M, Dyer R, Zagoria RJ (1993) Extravasation injury with nonionic contrast material. AJR 160:203–204

Miller KT (1995) Systemic reactions to contrast media during cystography. AJR 164:1551

Miller SH (1997) Anaphylactoid reaction after oral administration of diatrizoate meglumine and diatrizoate sodium solution. AJR 168:959–961

Moreira VF, Merono E, Larraona JL, et al. (1985) ERCP and allergic reactions to contrast media (letter). Gastrointest Endosc 31:293

Morisetti A, Tirone P, Luzzani F, et al. (1994) Toxicological safety assessment of iomeprol, a new X-ray contrast agent. Eur J Radiol 18(Suppl 1):S21–31

Mukherjee JJ, Peppercorn PD, Reznek RH, et al. (1997) Pheochromocytoma: effect of nonionic contrast medium in CT on circulating catecholamines. Radiology 202:227–231

Muruve DA, Steinman TI (1996) Contrast-induced encephalopathy and seizures in a patient with chronic renal insufficiency. Clin Nephrol 45:406–409

Nelson JA, Livingston GK, Moon RG (1982) Mutagenic evaluation of radiographic contrast media. Invest Radiol 17:183–185

Nielson ST, Matheson JN, Rasmussen N, et al. (1987) Excretion of iohexol in human breast milk. Acta Radiologica 28:523–526

Palmer FJ (1988) The RACR survey of intravenous contrast media reactions final report. Australas Radiol 32:426–428

Panto PN, Davies P (1986) Delayped reactions to urographic contrast media. Br J Radiol 59:41–44

Payne WW, Morse WH, Raines SL (1956) A fatal reaction following injection of urographic contrast medium, a case report. J Urol 76:661–663

Percy K (1967) An unusual complication of retrograde pyelography: neuromuscular blockade. Pediatrics 39:603–606

Piao ZE, Murdock DK, Hwang MH, et al. (1988) Contrast media-induced ventricular fibrillation: a comparison of Hypaque 76, Hexabrix, and Omnipaque. Invest Radiol 23:466–470

Pond GD, Dorr RT, McAleese KA (1992) Skin ulceration from extravasation of low-osmolality contrast medium: a complication of automation. AJR 158:915–916

Porter GA (1994a) Radiocontrast-induced nephropathy. Nephrol Dial Transplant 9(Suppl 4):146–156

Porter GA (1994b) Contrast-associated nephropathy: presentation, pathophysiology and management. Miner Electrolyte Metab 20:232–243

Raisanen J, Shapiro B, Glazer GM, et al. (1984) Plasma catecholamines in pheochromocytoma: effect of urographic contrast media. AJR 143:43–46

Ralston WH, Robbins MS, James P (1989) Reproductive, developmental, and genetic toxicity of ioversol. Invest Radiol 24(Suppl 1):S16–S22

Rao VM, Rao AK, Steiner RM, et al. (1982) The effect of ionic and nonionic contrast media on the sickling phenomenon. Radiology 144:291–293

Richards D, Nulsen F (1971) Angiographic media and the sickling phenomenon. Surg Forum 22:403–404

Ring J, Rothenberg KH, Clauss W (1985) Prevention of anaphylactoid reactions after radiographic contrast media infusion by combined histamine H_1- and H_2-receptor antagonists: results of a prospective controlled trial. Int Arch Allergy Appl Immunol 78:9–14

Rivera E, Hardjasudarma M, Willis BK, et al. (1995) Inadvertent use of ionic contrast material in myelography: case report and management guidelines. Neurosurgery 36:413–415

Rivera M, Teruel JL, Castano JC, et al. (1993) Iodine-induced sialadenitis: report of 4 cases and review of the literature. 63:466–467

Rocha MDS (1994) Exacerbation of myasthenia gravis by contrast media. AJR 162:997

Rodesch F, Camus M, Ermans AM, et al. (1976) Adverse effect of amniofetography on fetal thyroid function. Am J Obstet Gynecol 126:723–726

Salti IS, Kronfol NO (1977) Aggravation of thyrotoxicosis by an iodinated contrast medium. Br J Radiol 50:670–671

Schmidlapp CJ (1961) Respiratory (cardiac) arrest after retrograde pyelography with neomycin-containing medium. J Urol 85:993

Shah AM, Hutchison SJ (1990) Case report: the Koebner phenomenon—an unusual localization of a contrast reaction. Clin Radiol 42:136–137

Shehadi WH (1975) Adverse reactions to intravascularly administered contrast media: a comprehensive study based on a prospective survey. AJR 124:145–152

Shehadi WH (1982) Contrast media adverse reactions: occurrence, recurrence, and distribution patterns. Radiology 143:11–17

Shetty SP, Murphy GG, Shreeve WW, et al. (1974) Hyperthyroidism after pyelography. N Engl J Med 291:682–683

Shimura H, Takazawa K, Endo T, et al. (1990) T4-thyroid storm after CT-scan with iodinated contrast medium. J Endocrinol Invest 13:73–76

Shulman KL, Thompson JA, Benyunes MC, et al. (1993) Adverse reactions to intravenous contrast media in patients treated with interleukin-2. J Immunotherapy 13:208–212

Sistrom CL, Gay SB, Peffley L (1991) Extravasation of iopamidol and iohexol during contrast-enhanced CT: report of 28 cases. Radiology 180:707–710

Skucas J (1997) Anaphylactoid reactions to gastrointestinal contrast media. AJR 168:962–964

Smith MJG, Kendall BE, Tomlinson S (1974) Adverse general reactions to high doses of methylglucamine-based contrast media. Br J Radiol 47:566–569

Thomsen HS, Archer JW, Schiermer L, et al. (1997) A case study of the decision in Denmark to restrict use of high-osmolar contrast media in intravascular radiographic procedures. Acad Radiol 4:446–450

Trop CS, Bennett CJ (1991) Autonomic dysreflexia and its urological implications: a review. J Urol 146:1461

Trulzsch DV, Penmetsa A, Karim A, et al. (1992) Gastrografin-induced aspiration pneumonia: a lethal complication of computed tomography. South Med J 85:1255–1256

Upton J, Muliken JB, Murray JE (1979) Major intravenous extravasation injuries. Am J Surg 137:497–506

Vaillant L, Pengloan J, Blanchier D, et al. (1990) Ioderma and acute respiratory distress with leucocytoclastic vasculitis following the intravenous administration of contrast medium. Clin Exp Dermatol 15:232–233

Weese DL, Greenberg HM, Zimmern PE (1993) Contrast media reactions during voiding cystourethrography or retrograde pyelography. Urology 41:81–84

Wolf GL, Arenson RL, Cross AP (1989) A prospective trial of ionic vs nonionic contrast agents in routine clinical practice: comparison of adverse effects. AJR 152:939–944

Wood BP, Lane AT, Rabinowitz R (1988) Cutaneous reaction to contrast material. Radiology 169:739–740

Yoshikawa H (1992) Late adverse reactions to nonionic contrast media. Radiology 183:737–740

Yoshinari M, Tokuyama T, Okamura K, et al. (1988) Iodide-induced thyrotoxicosis in a thyroidectomized patient with metastatic thyroid carcinoma. Cancer 61:1674–1678

Young RA (1994) Injury due to extravasation of nonionic contrast material (letter). AJR 162:1499

Zukiwski AA, David CL, Coan J, et al. (1990) Increased incidence of hypersensitivity to iodine-containing radiographic contrast media after interleukin-2 administration. Cancer 65:1521–1524

12 Treatment of Adverse Reactions

W.H. Bush, Jr.

CONTENTS

12.1 Introduction

Acute reactions occurring after systemic administration of contrast media include: nausea and/or vomiting, scattered to extensive urticaria, laryngeal edema, bronchospasm, isolated hypotension with or without compensatory tachycardia, vagal reaction with hypotension and sinus bradycardia, generalized systemic anaphylaxis-like reaction (which may include severe bronchospasm, angioedema, laryngeal edema, and hypotension), angina, hypertension, convulsions, and cardiopulmonary arrest. These reactions occur in a variety of combinations and a life-threatening reaction may occur without specific preliminary symptoms.

12.2 Responding to a Contrast Reaction

Every radiologist injecting contrast material must be prepared to deal with acute systemic reactions. Rooms in which contrast material injections are done should have the emergency drugs necessary to initially treat a reaction and emergency equipment should be either in the room or in an immediately accessible area. It is my recommendation that a list of drugs (Table 12.1) and the dosages for treating a contrast reaction (such as are listed in Table 12.2) be posted on the wall in each room where intravascular contrast is injected.

The radiologist should remain nearby for at least the first critical 4–5 min following contrast injection and should stay in the immediate vicinity for the next 30–45 min. All intravenous contrast injections should be made through a short catheter which should be left in place to ensure venous access in the event of a major reaction.

12.3 General Principles in Treating Contrast Reactions

It is important that you, as the radiologist and responsible physician, remain in control of the situation and bring a calming influence to the patient and those personnel helping you treat a reaction. Take charge of the situation and direct those helping you to specific tasks. Basic responses include oxygen supplementation, initiation of intravascular physiological fluids, establishment of an adequate airway, and evaluation of blood pressure and heart rate. Talking with the patient as you check their pulse rate provides much initial information: breathing is assessed, the possibility of a vagal reaction (bradycardia) is determined, and a rough estimate of systolic blood pressure is gained (a palpable radial artery pulse approximates a systolic blood pressure of 80–90 mmHg).

Oxygen is important in treating almost every adverse reaction. Although oxygen delivered at a low flow rate through nasal prongs may be more comfortable for the patient, this method is the least effective in delivering high saturation. Oxygen is best

W.H. Bush, Jr., MD, FACR, Radiology Department, University of Washington School of Medicine, Box 357115, 1959 NE Pacific Street, Seattle, WA 98195, USA

Table 12.1. Emergency contrast reaction treatment kit (from Bush 1988)

Drug	Amount
Atropine 1 mg/ml vial	3
β_2-agonist metered dose inhaler (e.g., metaproterenol 1.5% 10 ml inhaler)	1
Epinephrine (1:1000) 1 mg/ml vial	1
Epinephrine (1:10000) 1 mg/10 ml (premixed emergency syringe)	1
H_1 antihistamine (e.g., diphenhydramine 50 mg/ml vial)	1
H_2 antihistamine (e.g., ranitidine 50 mg/2 ml vial)	1
Nitroglycerin 2% ointment, tube	1

Table 12.2. Acute reactions to contrast media: treatment outline

Urticaria:
Mild: observation, add H_1 antihistamine
Severe: add:
Intravenous fluids
Epinephrine i.v. (1:10000), 1 ml (0.1 mg) slowly
H_2 antihistamine i.v.

Bronchospasm (isolated):
Oxygen
β_2-agonist metered dose inhaler
Epinephrine i.v. (1:10000), 1 ml (0.1 mg) slowly

Hypotension (isolated):
Oxygen
Elevate patient's legs
Intravenous fluids (primary therapy), rapidly
If unresponsive: consider a vasopressor (dopamine or epinephrine)

Vagal reaction (hypotension and bradycardia):
Oxygen
Elevate patient's legs
Intravenous fluids: rapidly, normal saline or Ringer's solution
Atropine: 0.6–1.0 mg i.v. (adults)

Anapylaxis-like reaction (generalized):
Oxygen
Suction, as needed
Elevate patient's legs if hypotensive
Intravenous fluids: normal saline or Ringer's solution
Epinephrine i.v.: 1:10000, 1 ml (0.1 mg), slowly
Alternative therapy: isoproterenol i.v.; glucagon i.v.
Antihistamines: H_1 blocker plus H_2 blocker
β_2-agonist metered dose inhaler
Corticosteroids, e.g., hydrocortisone i.v.

Angina:
Oxygen
Intravenous fluids: very slowly
Nitroglycerin, sublingually or topically
Morphine i.v.

Hypertension:
Oxygen
Intravenous fluids: very slowly
Nitroglycerin
If secondary to pheochromocytoma: phentolamine i.v.

Seizures:
Protect the patient
Airway: suction prn, mouth airway for tongue
Oxygen
If caused by hypotension ± bradycardia, treat accordingly (per protocols for those entities)
Uncontrolled: consider diazepam, i.v.

delivered via a partial nonrebreather mask with the flow rate about 6 l/min. Since you are treating an acute life-threatening reaction, oxygen is indicated even for the patient with chronic obstructive pulmonary disease.

Intravascular fluid replacement is very important and it alone has been reported to be the most effective treatment for hypotension (Obeid et al. 1975). Therefore, early institution of intravenous fluids before starting drug therapy should be reemphasized as an axiomatic principle of high priority in treating hypotension (vanSonnenberg et al. 1987). Not to be forgotten is the positive effect of leg elevation on increasing central vascular volume. It has been estimated that leg elevation moves about 0.5 l of fluids to the central blood pool.

For drug therapy, four main categories of drugs are often chosen by the radiologist in treating contrast reactions: antihistamines, steroids, anticholinergics, and adrenergic agonists. It should be noted that these are not listed in order of preference when I select drugs to treat a serious or severe reaction, as will become evident from the discussions that follow (Bush 1996).

Although antihistamines (H_1 receptor antagonists) are, overall, the drugs used most frequently by radiologists for treatment of reactions to contrast media (Lasser et al. 1987), they should not be the first drugs selected to treat a serious or potentially life-threatening contrast reaction (Goldberg 1984). H_1 histamine receptor blockers are, however, effective in relieving pruritis. The combination of H_1 and H_2 antihistamines is more effective in treating urticaria than is an H_1 anithistamine alone (Runge et al. 1992).

Corticosteroid administration, even in high doses, for treatment of a severe anaphylactoid contrast reaction is not supported by a secure experimental background. Large doses of intravenous corticosteroids are often given empirically to treat anaphylactoid reactions; however, their value in treating an acute reaction is limited by slow onset of action

(LASSER et al. 1977, 1987; MORRIS 1985). Empirically, the dose used in the treatment of reactions is 200 mg to 1.0 g of hydrocortisone, or equivalent, intravenously.

Atropine and epinephrine are, in my opinion, the most important drugs for treating major adverse reactions occurring with the injection of contrast media. Atropine is often effective in the treatment of patients suffering bradycardia with a contrast reaction (STANLEY and PFISTER 1976). In conjunction with leg elevation and intravenous fluids, atropine is indicated specifically for treating the vagal reaction of symptomatic hypotension associated with bradycardia (CHAMBERLAIN et al. 1967; FISCHER and COLGAN 1976; BROWN 1990; BUSH et al. 1993).

Because small doses of atropine may worsen bradycardia and hypotension, a larger dose (0.6–1.0 mg) is recommended. The total dose limit of atropine is 0.04 mg/kg in adults (i.e., 2–3 mg). The pediatric dose is 0.02 mg/kg, and some recommend a single dose maximum of 0.6 mg. The total dose limit is 2 mg. If symptomatic bradycardia is unresponsive to the maximum of atropine, transcutaneous pacemaker should be considered.

Epinephrine has long been considered the drug of choice for treating acute anaphylactic reactions. Yet, no uniformly agreed upon regimen for its utilization in these circumstances is established (BARACH et al. 1984; BUSH et al. 1993). The α-agonist effects of epinephrine increase blood pressure and reverse peripheral vasodilatation. These vasoconstrictor changes also decrease angioedema and urticaria (BARACH et al. 1984). The β-agonist actions of epinephrine reverse bronchoconstriction, produce positive inotropic and chronotropic cardiac effects (increase in strength and rate of cardiac contractions), and may increase intracellular cyclic AMP. Increments in baseline cyclic AMP levels are generally considered to inhibit mediator release from inflammatory cells (IGNARRO and COLOMBO 1973; ZURIER et al. 1974).

The pros and cons of utilizing epinephrine merit careful consideration. For example, in individuals with a fragile intracerebral or coronary circulation, the α-agonist effects of a large dose may invoke a hypertensive crisis that could produce a stroke or myocardial ischemia (BARACH et al. 1984). β-Receptor sites ordinarily respond to lower doses of epinephrine than do α-sites, but if a patient is on β-blockers, the refractory response that might occur when epinephrine is administered could encourage the radiologist using epinephrine to increase the dose to the point that unwanted excessive α-effects would be generated.

Patients with asthma may simulate patients receiving β-blockers since a β-adrenergic hyporesponsiveness in this disease has long been appreciated. In such circumstances, when the patient is refractory to the usual doses of epinephrine, isoproterenol may be used as an alternative. Isoproterenol is a pure β-agonist (β_1 and β_2) and can be used to override the β-block and achieve β-effect. Epinephrine will also be required to achieve α-effect of vasoconstriction and control of edema, although the epinephrine can be given at a lower dose than usual (BUSH 1996). The combination of isoproterenol and small doses of epinephrine achieves both desired α- and β-effects yet avoids a high dose of epinephrine with excessive, unwanted α-effects.

Isoproterenol should not be used injudiciously in that it may cause arrhythmias and hypotension. The appropriate dosage can be titrated to effect, starting with the 1 : 5000 solution diluted to 10 ml and administered at 20 μg (1 ml) per minute. Another alternative for the patient taking β-adrenergic blocking drugs is glucagon, which provides both inotropic and chronotropic effects on the heart (WINBERY and LIEBERMAN 1995). Like isoproterenol, it may cause hypotension, but glucagon does not seem to cause arrhythmias (LVOFF and WILCHKEN 1972). Glucagon is given as a 1–5 mg i.v. bolus, followed by i.v. infusion of 5–15 μg/min.

Epinephrine is best administered intravenously, using the pre-packaged 1 : 10 000 solution (1 mg in 10 ml). Intravenously, the amount and rate of drug can be more regulated specifically, avoiding the sporadic or ineffective absorption that may occur when epinphrine is given subcutaneously or intramuscularly in the clinical setting of hypotension. When epinephrine is given slowly and in small doses there tends to be some preferential β-adrenergic over α-adrenergic effect (BARACH et al. 1984). My recommendation is to begin with 1 ml of the 1 : 10 000 dilution (0.1 mg) of epinephrine and administer this intravenously slowly over 2–5 min; this provides a dose rate of 20–50 μg a minute. One should vary the rate of injection depending on the effect of the drug and the patient's response. Usually an effective response is seen after 1–3 ml (0.1–0.3 mg). A total of 1 mg (10 ml) can ultimately be given, although this is quite a large dose. The pediatric i.v. dose of epinephrine is 0.01 mg/kg (repeated as needed every 5 min).

An alternative for the patient without i.v. access is the endotracheal route. Although reports vary as to the dose to be used, most recommend a dose that is 2–3 times the i.v. dose (Roberts et al. 1979; Powers and Donowitz 1984; Grauer and Cavallaro 1993), particularly when given endotracheally during cardiopulmonary resuscitation. With good dispersion in the airways, there appears to be good absorption.

Epinephrine should be avoided, when possible, in treating the pregnant patient with a severe contrast reaction and hypotension because of a deleterious excessive α-response by the uterus. Ephedrine (25–50 mg) i.v. is suggested as an alternative medication (Entman and Moise 1984).

The following sections and Table 12.2 summarize specific treatment plans for the more frequently occurring adverse reactions (Bush et al. 1993; Bush 1996; Harris and Bush 1996). However, these recommendations are not the only effective treatment regimens (Siegle and Lieberman 1978; Cohan and Dunnick 1988; McClennan 1994; Cohan et al. 1996). One should develop one's own protocol, and review and update it periodically.

12.4 Nausea and Vomiting

Nausea and vomiting are usually self-limited. However, these may also be early signs of a more severe reaction and Lalli (1980) found that 20% of fatal contrast reactions, occurring during urography with conventional ionic contrast media, began with nausea and vomiting. For this reason, the patient should be observed closely for systemic symptoms, while maintaining intravenous access.

Treatment: observation

12.5 Scattered Hives or Extensive Urticaria

For only a few scattered hives or pruritis, treatment is usually not necessary. Pruritis can be controlled effectively with an H_1 histamine blocker, such as diphenhydramine. For moderate urticaria, the combination of an H_1 and an H_2 antihistamine is suggested (Runge et al. 1992). However, the patient should be observed closely for other developing systemic symptoms, while maintaining intravenous access. With diffuse erythema and urticaria, "third spacing" of fluid may occur and hypotension may develop. In such situations, treatment with i.v. fluids (e.g., normal saline) and small doses of i.v. epinephrine is recommended. Intravenous epinephrine is very effective in reversing cutaneous reactions to intravascular radiocontrast and improving cardiovascular status.

Treatment:
- Pruritis: H_1 antihistamine
- Moderate urticaria: H_1 plus H_2 antihistamines
- Severe urticaria: epinephrine, either subcutaneously or i.v.

12.6 Bronchospasm

Bronchospasm, without coexisting cardiovascular problems, should be treated with oxygen and inhaled bronchodilators. Inhaled β_2-adrenergic agonists such as albuterol, metaproterenol, and terbutaline deliver large doses of bronchodilating β_2-agonist drugs directly to the airways with minimal systemic absorption and, therefore, minimal cardiovascular effects. Using a metered dose inhaler (MDI), treatment typically involves two to three deep inhalations. Aminophylline is no longer recommended as a first-line drug, having been supplanted by the β-agonist inhalers; furthermore, aminophylline may cause significant hypotension if administered too rapidly. If the initial β-agonist inhaler treatment is not fully effective, one should add nembulized β-agonist medication or inhaled mist, or administer i.v. epinephrine. Intravenous epinephrine is very effective in reversing bronchospasm.

Treatment:
- Oxygen
- β_2-agonist inhaler
- Intravenous epinephrine if the patient is not responsive to initial β-agonist inhaler

12.7 Laryngeal Edema

Laryngeal edema does not respond well to inhaled β-agonists and, in fact, these agents may actually worsen laryngeal edema. Laryngeal edema should be treated with i.v. epinephrine. Therefore, clinical evaluation and auscultation of the patient prior to beginning treatment is extremely important to differentiate laryngeal edema from bronchospasm.

Epinephrine is the primary treatment for laryngeal edema. Intravenous epinephrine, 1 ml (0.1 mg) of 1 : 10 000 solution given slowly over 2–5 min should be utilized whenever there is rapid progression of symptoms or when hypotension with possible inadequate absorption of subcutaneous medication is suspected (Bush et al. 1993; Bush and McClennan 1995a,b; Bush 1996). Using this inital low dose of i.v. epinephrine, additional small doses are given incrementally depending on response to the initial dose. Epinephrine may also be administered as an aerosolized mist, endotracheally or transtracheally.

Treatment:
- Oxygen
- Intravenous epinephrine, 1:10 000, 1 ml (0.1 mg) slowly over 2–5 min

12.8 Isolated Hypotension

Profound hypotension may occur without respiratory symptoms. Tachycardia, or possibly a normal cardiac rate, helps differentiate this reaction from the vagal reaction (hypotension plus sinus bradycardia). In patients who have been taking β-adrenergic-blocking medications (e.g., propranolol), compensatory tachycardia may not occur in response to hypotension.

Isolated hypotension is best treated initially by rapid intravenous fluid replacement, rather than by resorting to vasopressor drugs (vanSonnenberg et al. 1987). Elevation of the patient's legs is very important in that the maneuver returns about 700 ml of blood to the central circulation and is preferable to placing the patient in the Trendelenburg position (Smith and Corbascio 1970). Rapid infusion of large volumes of intravenous normal saline or Ringer's lactate may be required for adequate reversal of hypotension. Supplemental oxygen is also very important. Vasopressors (e.g., epinephrine or dopamine) are reserved for those hypotensive situations not responding to aggressive intravascular fluid therapy. An i.v. solution of epinephrine is created by mixing 1 mg of epinephrine in 250 ml of dextrose water; a beginning rate is 4 µg per minute (1 ml/min).

Treatment:
- Elevate legs
- Oxygen
- Intravenous fluids (normal saline, lactated Ringer's), rapidly infused

12.9 Vagal Reaction

Vagal reaction is characterized by sinus bradycardia and hypotension. Its exact cause is unknown. In some cases the vagal excess is elicited by just the stimulation of the procedure itself, rather than the injected contrast material or other substance. The vagal reaction results in vasodilatation and expanded vascular space. The vasodilatation is treated by elevation of the patient's legs and rapid infusion of intravenous fluids.

The excess vagal action also causes bradycardia, which is treated by intravenous administration of atropine to block the vagal stimulation of the cardiac conduction system. Since small doses of atropine can be detrimental in treating the bradycardia associated with contrast media-induced vagal reactions (Chamberlain et al. 1967; Stanley and Pfister 1976; Brown 1990), larger doses (0.6–1.0 mg) are indicated. My recommendation is 1.0 mg of atropine given intravenously (slow push) as the initial dose with additional doses of 0.6–1.0 mg every 3–5 min as needed to correct the bradycardia. The total recommended dose is 0.04 mg/kg in adults (about 3 mg) (Bush and Swanson 1991; Bush 1996). Rarely have I had to give more than two doses, i.e., 2 mg total.

Treatment:
- Elevate legs
- Oxygen
- Intravenous fluids (normal saline, lactated Ringer's), rapidly infused
- Intravenous atropine, 1 mg slow push; repeat as needed to a total of 2–3 mg

12.10 Generalized Anaphylaxis-like Reactions

Generalized anaphylaxis-like reactions are acute, rapidly progressing, systemic reactions characterized by multisystem involvement with pruritis, urticaria, angioedema, respiratory distress (bronchospasm and/or laryngeal edema), and vascular changes with hypotension. These generalized reactions require prompt and aggressive therapy. Initial treatment includes maintenance of airway, administration of supplemental oxygen, rapid infusion of intravenous fluids, and administration of adrenergic medications.

Epinephrine is the medication of choice and should be administered early and intravenously for rapid, effective action and to avoid suboptimal absorption from subcutaneous tissues because of developing hypotension (Bush and Swanson 1991; Bush et al. 1993; Sadler et al. 1995; Bush and McClennan 1995a,b). A low dose, 1.0 ml (0.1 mg) of 1:10 000 solution, is given at a relatively slow rate (over 2–5 min) and is titrated to effect (Smith and Corbascio 1970). If the reaction is not responding to this initial, slowly administered, low i.v. dose, the rate of injection should be increased. Intravenous epinephrine should be given with caution to elderly patients and in the presence of hypoxia, where there is increased risk of severe cardiac arrhythmias. Additionally, the amount of intravenous epinephrine should be limited in patients who are receiving noncardioselective β-blocking medications (e.g., propranolol) as discussed earlier.

When the use of epinephrine is inadvisable, bronchospasm can be treated with a β_2-agonist inhaler and hypotension can be treated with intravenous fluids. As discussed earlier, isoproterenol, a pure β-agonist with no α-effects, can be used in patients on noncardioselective β-blockers to "override" the β-blockade. Intravenous glucagon has also been utilized instead of epinephine in treating cardiovascular emergencies during anaphylaxis (Winbery and Lieberman 1995).

Treatment:
- Elevate legs
- Oxygen
- Intravenous fluids (normal saline, lactated Ringer's), rapidly infused
- Intravenous epinephrine, 1:10 000, 1 ml (0.1 mg) slowly over 2–5 min; repeat as necessary to total of 1 mg (10 ml)

  Secondarily add:
- β-Agonist inhaler
- H_1 antihistamine i.v.
- H_2 antihistamine i.v.
- Corticosteroids i.v.

If epinephrine is contraindicated or no response occurs to epinephrine, consider:
- Isoproterenol i.v.
- Glucagon i.v.

12.11 Angina

When angina occurs during a procedure or after contrast injection, the patient is treated symptomatically, cardiac monitoring is begun, and assistance is summoned.

Treatment:
- Oxygen
- Intravenous access (run at a slow rate to keep access open)
- Nitroglycerin: sublingual, 0.4 mg tablet, or topically, 2% ointment, 1- to 2-inch strip applied and rubbed
- Morphine sulfate i.v.

12.12 Hypertension

Hypertension is an uncommon reaction. It may be encountered during cystography in patients with upper spinal cord injury (autonomic dysreflexia), during selective renal angiography, or possibly during contrast studies on patients with pheochromocytoma. Phentolamine is specific for treating the hypertension secondary to pheochromocytoma.

Treatment of the hypertension associated with autonomic dysreflexia has been performed with oral (sublingual) nifedipine, a calcium-channel blocker. However, the absorption of nifedipine occurs via the gastrointestinal tract, and not sublingually. So the contents of the capsule should be swallowed, not held sublingually (Grossman et al. 1996). An alternative to nifedipine is topical nitroglycerin. A 1- to 2-inch strip of the 2% ointment is applied and rubbed into the skin. The application may be repeated as necessary.

Treatment:
- Oxygen
- Intravenous fluids very slowly, only to maintain i.v. access
- Nitroglycerin: sublingual, 0.4 mg tablet, or topically, 2% ointment, 1- to 2-inch strip applied and rubbed
- Nifedipine: capsule chewed or punctured and the contents swallowed
- For pheochromocytoma: phentolamine, 5 mg, i.v. slowly

12.13 Seizure

Seizures usually occur either from irritation of a focus in the brain (e.g., from metastasis) or from an episode of acute hypotension such as with an acute, pronounced vagal reaction. Primary treatment is to protect the patient from injury and assure maintenance of airway. For a syncopal episode, treatment aims to correct the hypotension. If an irritative brain focus is known to exist and the seizuring does not subside, an anticonvulsant medication can be utilized.

Treatment:
- Protect patient
- Airway: clear, control tongue
- Search for cause, e.g., hypotension, and treat appropriately
- If uncontrolled, use anticonvulsant, e.g., diazepam, 5 mg i.v.

12.14 Cardiovascular Collapse/Cardiac Arrest

Cardiac arrest is defined as having occurred when the patient is unconscious, unresponsive, and has no pulse or blood pressure. If a patient is found in this condition, a "Code" should be called and immediate cardiopulmonary resuscitation (CPR) should be started (Emergency Cardiac Care Committee, American Heart Association 1992; GRAUER and CAVALLARO 1993).

Acknowledgements. Material for this chapter has been extracted from the following articles (with permission): BUSH WH, SWANSON DP (1991) Acute reactions to intravascular contrast media: types, risk factors, recognition and specific treatment. AJR 157:1153–1161; BUSH WH, SWANSON DP (1995) Radiocontrast. In: VIRANT FS (ed) Systemic reactions. Immunol Allergy Clin North Am. Saunders, Philadelphia, pp 597–612; BUSH WH (1996) Risk factors, prophylaxis, and therapy of X-ray contrast media reactions. Advances in X-ray Contrast 3:44–53; HARRIS JB, BUSH WH (1996) How to treat adverse reactions to contrast media. Contemp Urol 8:33–46; BUSH WH (1999) Treatment of acute reactions. In: BUSH WH, KREEKE KN, KING BF, BETTMANN MA (eds) Radiology life support (RAD-LS). London, Arnold (in press).

References

Barach EM, Nowak RM, Tennyson GL, Tomlanovich MC (1984) Epinephrine for treatment of anaphylactic shock. JAMA 251:2118–2122
Brown JH (1990) Atropine, scopolamine, and antimuscarinic drugs. In: Gilman AG, Rall TW, Nies AS, Taylor P (eds) The pharmacological basis of therapeutics. McGraw-Hill, New York, pp 150–165
Bush WH (1996) Risk factors, prophylaxis and therapy of X-ray contrast media reactions. Adv X-ray Contrast 3:44–53
Bush WH (1999) Treatment of acute contrast reactions. In: Bush WH, Krecke KN, King BF, Bettmann (eds) Radiology life support (RAD-LS). London, Arnold (in press)
Bush WH, McClennan BL (1995a) Treatment of adverse contrast media reaction (letter). Radiology 194:289
Bush WH, McClennan BL (1995b) Epinephrine administration for severe adverse reactions to contrast agents (letter). Radiology 196:879
Bush WH, Swanson DP (1991) Acute reactions to intravascular contrast media: types, risk factors, recognition, and specific treatment. AJR 157:1153–1161
Bush WH, McClennan BL, Swanson DP (1993) Contrast media reactions: prediction, prevention, and treatment. Postgrad Radiol 13:137–147
Chamberlain DA, Turner P, Sneddon JM (1967) Effects of atropine on heart-rate in healthy man. Lancet 2:12–15
Cohan RH, Dunnick NR (1988) Treatment of reactions to radiologic contrast material. AJR 151:263–267
Cohan RH, Leder RA, Ellis JH (1996) Treatment of adverse reactions to radiographic contrast media in adults. Radiol Clin North Am 34:1055–1060
Emergency Cardiac Care Committee and Subcommittees, American Heart Association (1992) Guidelines for cardiopulmonary resuscitation and emergency cardiac care. III. Adult advanced cardiac life support. JAMA 268:2199–2241
Entman SS, Moise KJ (1984) Anaphylaxis in pregnancy. South Med J 77:402
Fischer HW, Colgan FJ (1976) Causes of contrast media reactions. Radiology 121:223
Goldberg M (1984) Systemic reactions to intravascular contrast media – a guide for the anesthesiologist. Anesthesiology 60:46–56
Grauer K, Cavallaro D (1993) ACLS: certification preparation and a comprehensive review, vols. I & II. Mosby, Lifeline, St. Louis
Grossman E, Messerli FH, Grodzicki T, Kowey P (1996) Should a moratorium be placed on sublingual nifedipine capsules given for hypertensive emergencies and pseudoemergencies? JAMA 276:1328–1331
Harris JB, Bush WH (1996) How to treat adverse reactions to contrast media. Contemp Urol 8:33–46
Ignarro L, Colombo C (1973) Enzyme release from polymorphonuclear leukocyte lysosomes: regulation by autonomic drugs and cyclic nucleotides. Science 180:1181–1183
Lalli AF (1980) Contrast media reactions: data analysis and hypothesis. Radiology 134:1–12
Lasser EC, Lang J, Sovak M, Kolb W, Lyon S, Hamlin AE (1977) Steroids: theoretical and experimental basis for utilization in prevention of contrast media reactions. Radiology 125:1–9
Lasser EC, Berry CC, Talner LB, et al. (1987) Pretreatment with corticosteroids to alleviate reactions to intravascular contrast media. N Engl J Med 317:845–849
Lvoff R, Wilchken DEL (1972) Glucagon in heart failure and cardiogenic shock. Circulation 45:534–539
McClennan BL (1994) Adverse reactions to iodinated contrast media. Recognition and response. Invest Radiol 29(Suppl 1):S46–S50
Morris HG (1985) Mechanisms of action and therapeutic role of corticosteroids in asthma. J Allergy Clin Immunol 75:1–13
Obeid A, Johnson L, Potts J, et al. (1975) Fluid therapy in severe systemic reaction to radiopaque dye. Ann Intern Med 83:317–321

Powers RD, Donowitz LG (1984) Endotracheal administration of emergency medications. South Med J 77:340–341
Roberts JR, Greenberg ME, Baskin SI (1979) Endotracheal epinephrine in cardiorespiratory collapse. JACEP 8:515
Runge JW, Martinez JC, Caravati EM, Williamson SG, Hartsell SC (1992) Histamine antagonists in the treatment of acute allergic reactions. Ann Emerg Med 21:237–242
Sadler DJ, Parrish F, Coulthard A (1995) Contrast media reactions (letter). Clin Radiol 50:506
Siegle RL, Lieberman P (1978) A review of untoward reactions to iodinated contrast material. J Urol 119:581–587
Smith NT, Corbascio A (1970) The use and misuse of pressor agents. Anesthesiology 33:58–101
Stanley RJ, Pfister RC (1976) Bradycardia and hypotension following use of intravenous contrast media. Radiology 121:5–7
vanSonnenberg E, Neff CC, Pfister RC (1987) Life-threatening hypotensive reactions to contrast media administration: comparison of pharmacologic and fluid therapy. Radiology 162:15–19
Winbery SI, Lieberman PL (1995) Anaphylaxis. Immunol Allergy Clin North Am 15:447–476
Zurier R, Weissmann G, Hoffstein S, et al. (1974) Mechanisms of lysosomal enzyme release from human leukocytes. II. Effects of cAMP and cGMP, autonomic agonists, and agents which affect microtubule function. J Clin Invest 53:297–309

13 Hepatic Agents

P. Leander

CONTENTS

13.1 Introduction

There is a need for accurate diagnosis of the liver as this organ is commonly involved in malignant disease. Even if such disease is currently often fatal regardless of treatment, early and accurate diagnosis is a necessary first step in the development of new therapies.

Computed tomography (CT) is at present used routinely in the workup of patients with malignant disease in the liver, but the future role of CT in abdominal workup is less clear as abdominal magnetic resonance imaging (MRI) is evolving rapidly as a modality with high sensitivity and specificity. Hepatic agents for use with MRI have already been approved for clinical use; however, to date CT systems remain more widely available and are associated with lower costs.

In order to enhance the attenuation difference between normal liver tissue and focal lesions, nonspecific extracellular contrast agents are used. Many schemes for administration of these agents have been proposed, providing indirect evidence that nonspecific extracellular contrast agents are not optimal for CT of the liver. CT arterial portography (CTAP) is considered to be the most accurate method. This method requires that the patient first undergoes an angiographic procedure to place a catheter in the superior mesenteric or splenic artery. CT scans are exposed in the portal phase so as to enhance normal liver tissue rather than tumorous tissue. Good results have been reported with CTAP (Nelson et al. 1990). However, areas of low attenuation in the liver representing perfusion abnormalities rather than tumor deposits may be produced, yielding false-positive results (Nelson et al. 1992). The method is also invasive and cumbersome and is therefore only used as a preoperative investigation in highly selected patients.

P. Leander, MD, PhD, Department of Diagnostic Radiology, Malmö University Hospital, SE-205 02 Malmö, Sweden

13.2 Hepatic Agents

The search for clinically acceptable hepatic agents has been ongoing for many years, and the best-known agent to date is probably the colloidal thorium dioxide preparation Thorotrast. It was used for many years until it was realized that its indefinite retention in the liver could induce the otherwise rare angiosarcoma. Radiographically, however, it was satisfactory and had few acute side-effects (Thomas et al. 1951).

In conventional X-ray studies the doses required for hepatic agents are high, and frequently the side-effects have precluded these agents from entering, or remaining in, the clinical armamentarium (Olsson 1941; Thomas et al. 1951). With the advent of CT the search for hepatic agents was revitalized owing to the lower doses required. Clinical studies have shown that the use of hepatic agents in CT is one way of obtaining both higher contrast between normal liver tissue and focal lesions and higher sensitivity (Ivancev et al. 1989c; Vermess et al. 1980). However, so far no hepatic agent for CT has been approved for clinical use.

A hepatic agent should be easy to use as regards intravenous administration and have a long imaging window, i.e., the time during which the contrast between normal liver tissue and focal lesions is high, to permit thorough scanning. Compared with nonspecific extracellular contrast agents, hepatic agents require lower doses as they accumulate in the liver and functional information about the liver parenchyma may be obtained if contrast uptake is related to liver function. Also, if the administration of the hepatic agent is by bolus injection, information may be obtained in the distribution phase, thereby yielding a higher specificity in the diagnosis of focal lesions in the liver.

Hepatic agents may be divided into three categories according to the mechanism of uptake for targeting to normal liver tissue: reticuloendothelial system (RES)-directed agents, hepatocyte agents, and a combination of RES-directed and hepatocyte agents.

13.2.1
RES-Directed Agents

The sinusoids of the liver are lined by Kupffer cells belonging to the RES system. Ten percent of the cells in the liver are Kupffer cells, but compared with hepatocytes they are small and their volume is only a few percent of the total liver volume. Kupffer cells constitute about 80%–90% of the fixed macrophages of the RES. Phagocytosis is responsible for the internalization of particulate material, e.g., bacteria, virus particles, and diagnostic substances such as particulate contrast agents (Jones and Summerfield 1982). Phagocytized material may be reutilized or excreted, while undigestable components may be stored indefinitely.

For a particle to be phagocytized, it must be recognized as having a foreign surface. Besides being essential for the uptake of the foreign material in the RES, this recognition of a foreign surface may cause side-effects (Violante and Fischer 1987).

13.2.1.1
Solid Particles

Besides Thorotrast, other inorganic compounds with indefinite retention have been experimentally studied as particulate contrast agents for radiography, e.g., stannic oxide (Fischer 1957), but the retention of the agents has precluded their further development. In contrast to inorganic compounds, organic compounds are cleared from the organism and contrast agents based on them have, in experimental studies, demonstrated hepatic opacification in plain film radiography (Violante and Fischer 1984). In CT, suspensions of particles formed of organic esters of water-soluble contrast agents have been experimentally studied (Gjöen et al. 1990; Violante and Dean 1980; Leander et al. 1993). These agents have been found to be efficacious in experimental settings, a dose of approximately 100 mg I/kg increasing the x-ray attenuation in normal liver tissue by more than 40 HU. Despite their ability to be excreted, these contrast agents have been abandoned due to their acute toxicity.

13.2.1.2
Emulsions

Another type of particle is emulsions (Fig. 13.1). Emulsions mainly consisting of iodinated ethyl esters of poppy-seed oil fatty acids were developed to be used as hepatic agents for CT (AG 52-315 and AG 60-99) (Alfidi and Laval-Jeantet 1976; Laval-Jeantet et al. 1982; Vermess et al. 1977). The emulsion AG 60-99 became unavailable to one research group, forcing them to develop (Vermess et al. 1979) and test (Vermess et al. 1980) a similar emulsion based on the same original idea (EOE 13). In clinical imaging studies the efficacy of these emulsions was promising, but there were serious concerns about their long-term stability and their toxicity in terms of the side-effects associated with the uptake of the emulsions in the RES. Such side-effects could be reduced significantly by steroid premedication (Vermess et al. 1982).

Perfluorchemicals are a family of organic compounds in which hydrogen has been replaced by fluorine. These chemicals are inert and have a low toxicity. Research has shown that some perfluorchemicals demonstrate potential as contrast agents

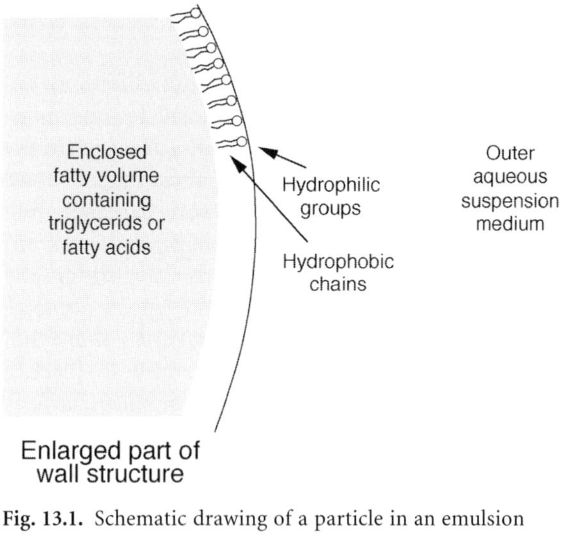

Fig. 13.1. Schematic drawing of a particle in an emulsion

for CT if the radiopaque atom bromine is incorporated (MATTREY 1989). As perfluorchemicals accumulate within Kupffer cells, specific enhancement of normal liver tissue is achieved, providing higher contrast against focal lesions in CT in both experimental and clinical settings (BEHAN et al. 1993; MATTREY 1989).

13.2.1.3
Liposomes

Liposomes were first described during the 1960s (BANGHAM et al. 1965) and are composed of lipid bilayers enclosing an aqueous volume (Fig. 13.2). They can be formed from different kinds of lipids, phospholipids being the most commonly used. Liposomes can be vehicles for water-soluble substances encapsulated in the aqueous compartment such as nonspecific extracellular contrast agents. Liposomes have been studied in several experimental investigations as hepatic agents for CT (ADZAMLI et al. 1990; KRAUSE et al. 1991; LEANDER 1996; RYAN et al. 1984; SACHSE et al. 1993; SELTZER et al. 1988).

So far liposomes have mainly been produced on a laboratory scale and authors have expressed their concerns about the possibility of large-scale production of pharmaceutically and pharmacologically acceptable liposomes (SACHSE et al. 1993; SELTZER et al. 1988). The difficulties to be mastered include encapsulation of the contrast agent and long-term stability of the liposomes (shelf-life). Encapsulation of contrast agents in liposomes is often expressed as the iodine-to-lipid ratio (I/L) on a weight basis (g/g). Older liposome technology obtained at best ratios of 1:1. However, advances in this field have now led to reports of ratios up to 5:1 for usable liposomes (JANOFF et al. 1991; PASSARIELLO et al. 1990). If the ratio is low, lipids phagocytized by the Kupffer cells in the liver lead to saturation of the cells. Although reversible, RES saturation may result in less than optimal hepatic liposome uptake and increases in the fractions delivered to other organs (JANOFF et al. 1991). A massive uptake of liposomes in the RES will also elicit side-effects, e.g., fever and malaise, showing similarities to the human response when bacteria and virus particles are phagocytized. As has been demonstrated for emulsions, such side-effects may be reduced by steroid premedication (ROZENBERG et al. 1993).

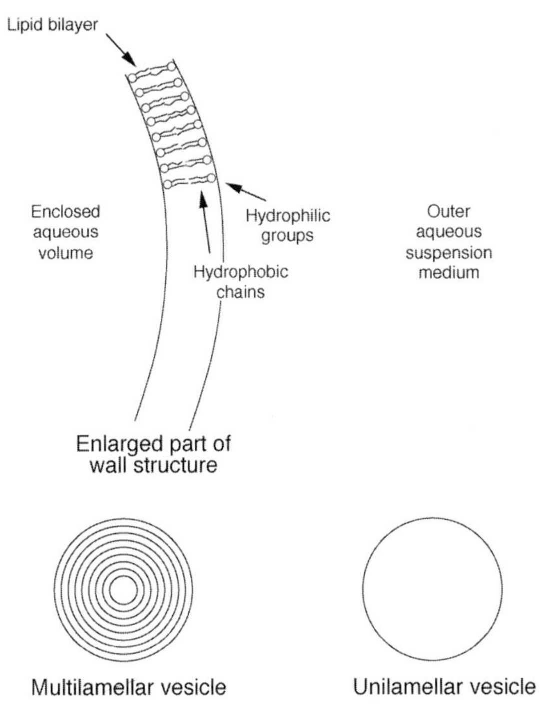

Fig. 13.2. Schematic drawing of liposomes

The lipid bilayer building up a liposomal wall is not completely tight for small water-soluble molecules such as extracellular contrast agents. Thus encapsulated contrast will inevitably leak out from the liposomes over a period of time. As has been shown, the speed is dependent on, among other factors, the osmotic pressure over the lipid wall (CHENG et al. 1987). The condition of a high encapsulation ratio and blood isotonicity may be met by a ratio 6 radiographic contrast agent (LEANDER 1996). Also, when there is a concentration gradient of the contrast agent over the lipid wall, leakage is always present. This has led to preparations where the nonencapsulated contrast agent is not removed from the final liposomal preparation, giving the same concentration of the nonencapsulated and the encapsulated contrast agent (LEANDER 1996; SACHSE et al. 1993). This ensures that there is no net exchange of the contrast agent over the liposomal wall and may result in acceptable shelf-lives. However, the presence of nonencapsulated contrast agent raises the question of unwanted imaging effects. The nonencapsulated contrast agent may accumulate in tumorous tissue in a way similar to certain situations in contrast-enhanced CT, thereby diminishing the desired increase in contrast of normal liver tissue against focal lesions. In one experimental study using a liposomal contrast agent with partly nonencapsulated iopromide at a total dose of 200 mg I/kg, high x-ray attenuation in a focal lesion compared with normal liver tissue was seen, indicating such an unwanted effect (SACHSE et al. 1993).

CTP (CT-particles) is a preparation of iodixanol-containing liposomes (Holtz et al. 1995; Leander 1996). In an experimental setting a dose of 100 mg I/kg encapsulated iodixanol gave a contrast of liver to focal lesions of 68 HU, 10 min after administration of the liposomes (Leander 1996). The first human study (phase I) of CTP showed a clear dose-response, the dose of 100 mg I/kg encapsulated iodixanol giving an increase in attenuation in the liver of 45 HU, 12.5 min after administration of the liposomes (Leander et al. 1997). The doses were given as bolus injections (2 ml/s) with a power injector and in early images there was a clinically useful increase in attenuation in the aorta, making the liposomes useful both as an agent for general abdominal CT and, after 12.5 min, as a hepatic agent (Fig. 13.3). No acute side-effects were encountered; however, particle-related side-effects commenced 1–3 h after administration. None of these side-effects were serious and all volunteers recovered spontaneously without any action having to be taken. The side-effects of CTP have stopped further development of the specific formulation used.

Another group has conducted a phase I study with their liposomal formulation without encountering any side-effects (Zaccarini et al. 1997). Their study did not include imaging but their pharmacokinetic data indicate that this liposomal formulation may be both efficacious and well tolerated.

13.2.2
Hepatocyte Agents

Hepatocytes constitute about 70% of all the cells in the liver, but represent about 80% of its volume. They are responsible for uptake of substances from blood and excretion into the bile canaliculi. Factors influencing this process include molecular weight, lipophilicity, polarity, and specific receptors (Smith 1973). A carrier-mediated uptake is believed to be involved when substances, in spite of concentration gradients between the blood and the hepatocyte or between the hepatocyte and the bile canaliculi, are excreted in the bile. These carriers, which are normally engaged in human metabolism, e.g., the uptake and excretion of bile acids and bilirubin, are relatively unspecific and may also facilitate the uptake and excretion of diagnostic substances. All iodinated bile contrast agents seem to use organic anion carrier systems (Schuhmann-Giampieri 1993). These substances may be more or less inhibited by the co-administration of other substances using the same carrier.

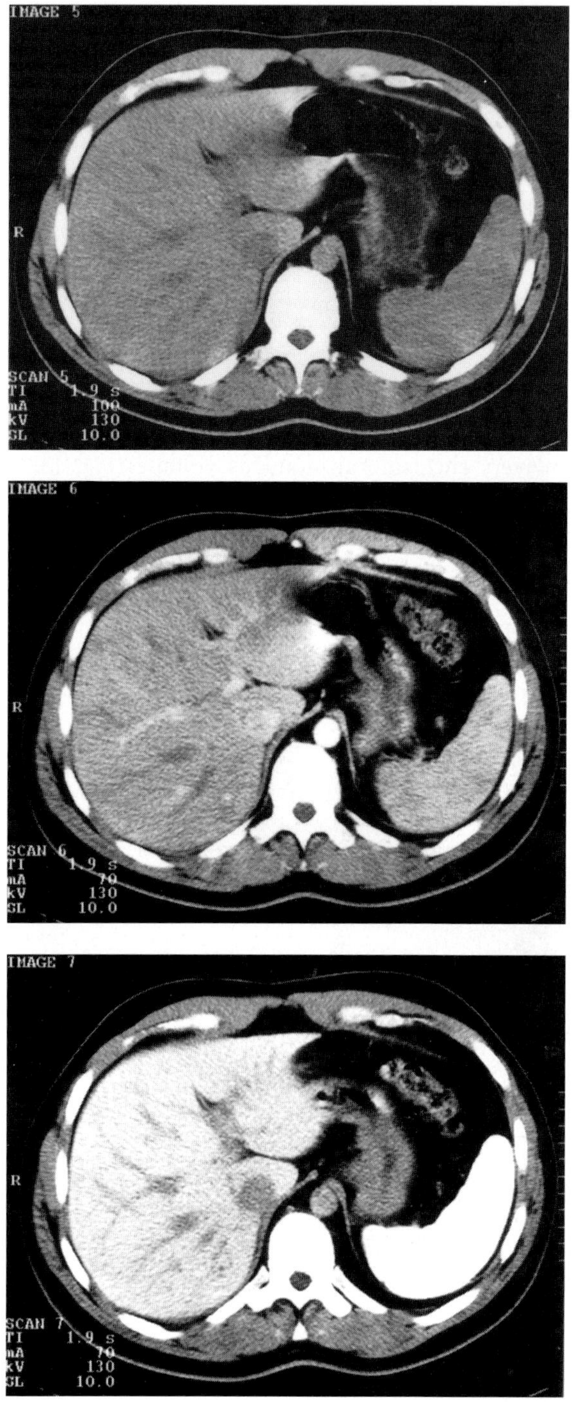

a

b

c

Fig. 13.3 a–c. Use of CTP (iodixanol-containing liposomes) in a volunteer at a dose of 100 mg encapsulated I/kg body wt. **a** Precontrast; **b** 45 s after start of administration, showing contrast enhancement in aorta; **c** 12.5 min after start of CTP administration, showing enhancement in normal liver tissue and spleen

Cholangiographic contrast agents for use in CT of the liver were studied early in the history of CT. In relation to their toxicity, the small increases in x-ray attenuation achieved with these compounds did not justify their use (Moss and Brito 1981). Experimental studies with new hepatobiliary substances are continuing and one group has shown that a hydrophobic modification of diatrizoic acid will result in a sufficiently long residence time in the liver for a significant increase in attenuation to be achieved (Arunachalam et al. 1997). However, the results show a strong species dependence, and results in man have not been presented so far. Also, recently a group has shown that an agent first intended for hepatic MRI, i.e., Gd-EOB-DTPA (Clement et al. 1992; Schuhmann-Giampieri et al. 1992) can be used in CT (Schuhmann-Giampieri et al. 1997). To obtain a higher attenuation per molar unit dysprosium was substituted for gadolinium. Their results are promising, with an enhancement in man of about 30 HU at a dose of 0.5 mmol/kg body wt.

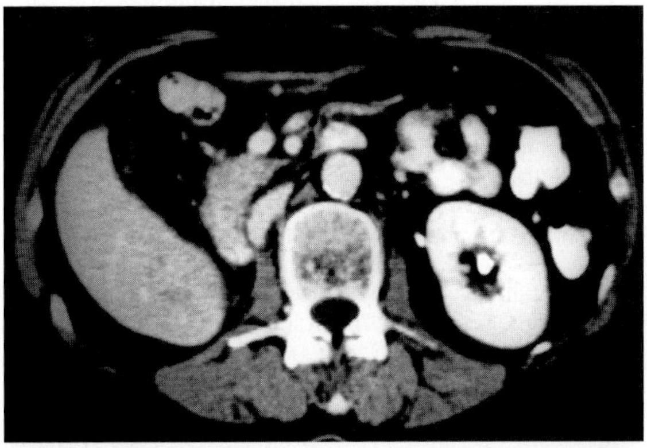

a

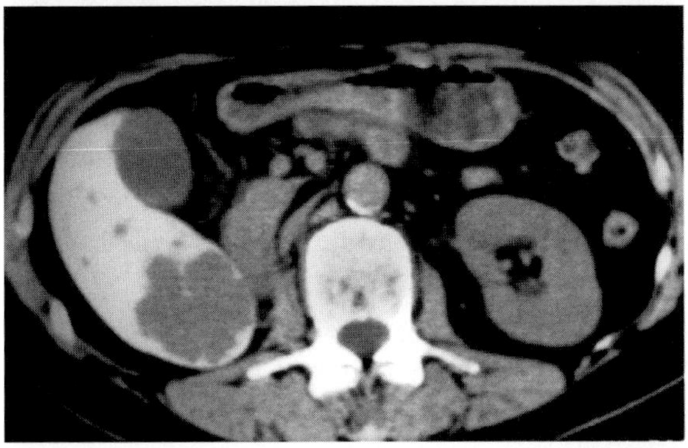

b

Fig. 13.4 a,b. Iodinated lipid emulsion. A case showing a hypervascular metastasis in the liver. **a** Contrast-enhanced CT using a nonspecific extracellular contrast agent in the equilibrium phase. **b** After iodinated lipid emulsion administration a large metastasis is clearly demonstrated which was not depicted precontrast. (Courtesy of Dr. Ivancev, Malmö, Sweden)

As mentioned above, RES-directed agents may elicit side-effects in conjunction with their uptake in Kupffer cells. Two groups have focused on this problem and found that similar reactions were seen in the early stages of the research to find parenteral lipid emulsions (Ivancev et al. 1989b). These problems were solved and parenteral lipid solutions resembling chylomicrons, which occur naturally in the metabolism of the liver, were formulated. Chylomicron remnants are phagocytized preferentially by the hepatocytes rather than by the Kupffer cells. This solution was mimicked by substituting iodine-containing triglycerides for the triglycerides normally occurring in the chylomicron core (Ivancev et al. 1989a; Lee et al. 1997). Experimental (Bergman et al. 1997; Sundin et al. 1994; Lee et al. 1997) and clinical (Ivancev et al. 1989c; Magnusson et al. 1997) results in CT are promising (Fig. 13.4). In the clinical studies only minor side-effects were seen that may be related to free iodine, i.e., iodism. A relatively slow uptake in the hepatocytes gives a blood pool effect but the attenuation values in the abdominal vessels are lower than required for abdominal CT. As yet no contrast agent approved for human use has been developed from this concept.

13.2.3 Combination of RES-Directed and Hepatocyte Agents

Only a few reports exist on combinations of RES-directed and hepatocyte agents. In one CT study a particulate contrast agent was synthesized using the biliary contrast agent iodipamide, but it was not observed that the liver enhancement of this particulate contrast was more pronounced than that of another particulate contrast agent synthesized using the nonspecific extracellular iothalamate (Violante et al. 1980). In another CT study, the biliary contrast agent iosefamate was incorporated in liposomes. Compared with free iosefamate this led to only slightly higher enhancement in the liver (Seltzer et al. 1984). Probably due to the higher toxicity of these agents, neither group pursued research into biliary contrast agents.

References

Adzamli IK, Seltzer SE, Slifkin M, et al. (1990) Production and characterization of improved liposomes containing radiographic contrast media. Invest Radiol 25:1217–1223

Alfidi RJ, Laval-Jeantet M (1976) AG 60.99: a promising contrast agent for computed tomography of the liver and spleen. Radiology 121:491
Arunachalam A, Song B, Sukumaran K, et al. (1997) Synthesis and evaluation of *N,N*-dimethydiatrizoic acid analogs as liver imaging agents (abstract). Contrast Media Research (CMR-97), Kyoto, Japan, May 18–22, 1997
Bangham AD, Standish MM, Watkins JC (1965) Diffusion of univalent ions across the lamellae of swollen phospholipids. J Mol Biol 13:238–252
Behan M, O'Connell D, Mattrey RF, et al. (1993) Perfluorooctylbromide as a contrast agent for CT and sonography: preliminary clinical results. Am J Roentgenol 160:399–405
Bergman A, Sundin A, Magnusson A (1997) An iodinated lipid emulsion for CT of the liver. Comparison with iohexol in the detection of experimental hepatic metastases. Acta Radiol 38:55–60
Cheng KT, Seltzer SE, Adams DF, et al. (1987) The production and evaluation of contrast-carrying liposomes made with an automatic high-pressure system. Invest Radiol 22:47–55
Clement O, Mühler A, Vexler V, et al. (1992) Gadolinium-ethoxybenzyl-DTPA, a new liver-specific magnetic resonance contrast agent. Kinetic and enhancement patterns in normal and cholestatic rats. Invest Radiol 27:612–619
Fischer HW (1957) Colloidal stannic oxide: animal studies on a new hepatolienographic agent. Radiology 68:488–498
Gjöen T, Holtz E, Strande P, et al. (1990) Particulate biodegradable contrast medium for computerised tomography of the liver. In: Ferrucci JT, Stark DD (eds) Liver imaging – current trends and new techniques. Andover Medical Publishers, Boston, pp 394–402
Holtz E, Heglund IF, Dyvik K, et al. (1995) Iodixanol liposomes – preclinical characteristics and imaging properties (abstract). Contrast Media Research (CMR-95), Naantali, Finland, June 17–22, 1995
Ivancev K, Lunderquist A, McCuskey R, et al. (1989a) Experimental investigation of a new iodinated lipid emulsion for computed tomography of the liver. Acta Radiol 30:407–413
Ivancev K, Lunderquist A, McCuskey R, et al. (1989b) Effect of intravenously injected iodinated lipid emulsions on the liver – an experimental study correlating computed tomography findings with in vivo microscopy and electron microscopy findings. Acta Radiol 30:291–298
Ivancev K, Lunderquist A, Isaksson A, et al. (1989c) Clinical trials with a new iodinated lipid emulsions for computed tomography of the liver. Acta Radiol 30:449–457
Janoff AS, Minchey SR, Perkins WR, et al. (1991) Interdigitation-fusion vesicles: a new approach for selective opacification of the RES. Invest Radiol 26:S167–S168
Jones EA, Summerfield JA (1982) Kupffer cells. In: Arias IM, Popper H, Schachter D, et al. (eds) The liver: biology and pathobiology. Raven Press, New York, pp 507–523
Krause W, Sachse A, Wagner U, et al. (1991) Preclinical characterization of iopromide-carrying liposomes. Invest Radiol 26:S172–S174
Laval-Jeantet AM, Laval-Jeantet M, Bergot C (1982) Effect of particle size on the tissue distribution of iodized emulsified fat following intravenous administration. Invest Radiol 17:617–620
Lee FT Jr, Chosy SG, Naidu SG, et al. (1997) CT depiction of experimental liver tumors: contrast enhancement with hepatocyte-selective iodinated triglyceride versus conventional techniques. Radiology 203:465–470
Leander P (1996) A new liposomal contrast medium for computed tomography of the liver: an imaging study in a rabbit tumour model. Acta Radiol 37:63–68
Leander P, Golman K, Strande P, et al. (1993) A comparison between IEEC, a new biodegradable particulate X-ray contrast medium and iohexol in a tumour model of computed tomography imaging of the liver. Invest Radiol 28:513–519
Leander P, Höglund P, Kloster Y, et al. New liposomal liver-specific contrast agent for CT: First human phase I clinical trail assessing efficacy and safety. Acad Radiol 1998;5:S6–8
Magnusson A, Bergman A, Carneheim C, et al. Contrast enhancement of the liver in healthy male volunteers following intravenous administration of FP 736-04. Acad Radiol 1998;5:S9–12
Mattrey RF (1989) Potential role of perfluorooctylbromide in the detection and characterization of liver lesions with CT. Radiology 170:18–20
Moss AA, Brito AC (1981) Computed tomography of the liver in rhesus monkeys following iosefamate meglumine administration. Radiology 141:123–127
Nelson RC, Chezmar JL, Sugarbaker PH, et al. (1990) Preoperative localization of focal liver lesions to specific liver segments: utility of CT during arterial portography. Radiology 176:89–94
Nelson RC, Thompson GH, Chezmar JL, et al. (1992) CT during arterial portography: diagnostic pitfalls. Radiographics 12:705–718
Olsson O (1941) On hepatosplenography with "jodsol". Acta Radiol 22:749–761
Passariello R, Pavone P, Patrizio G, et al. (1990) Liposomes loaded with nonionic contrast media. Hepatosplenic computed tomographic enhancement. Invest Radiol 25:S92–S94
Rozenberg OA, Loshakova LV, Mikhailova N, et al. (1993) Radiologic detection of triombrast in liposomes of liver and spleen (first phase of clinical trial) (in Russian). Vestn Rentgenol Radiol 5:35–38
Ryan PJ, Davis MA, DeGaeta LR, et al. (1984) Liposomes loaded with contrast material for image enhancement in computed tomography. Radiology 152:759–762
Sachse A, Leike JU, Rößling GL, et al. (1993) Preparation and evaluation of lyophilzed iopromide-carrying liposomes for liver tumor detection. Invest Radiol 28:838–844
Schuhmann-Giampieri G (1993) Liver contrast media for magnetic resonance imaging: interrelations between pharmacokinetics and imaging. Invest Radiol 28:753–761
Schuhmann-Giampieri G, Schmitt-Willich H, Press WR, et al. (1992) Preclinical evaluation of Gd-EOB-DTPA as a contrast agent in MR imaging of the hepatobiliary system. Radiology 183:59–64
Schuhmann-Giampieri G, Rupp K, Handreke K, et al. (1997) Dysprosium EOB DTPA. A new liver-specific contrast agent for computed tomography. Acad Radiol 1998;5:S90-92
Seltzer SE, Shulkin PM, Adams DF, et al. (1984) Usefulness of liposomes carrying iosefamate for CT: opacification of liver and spleen. AJR 143:575–579
Seltzer SE, Gregoriadis G, Dick R (1988) Evaluation of the dehydration-rehydration method for production of contrast-carrying liposomes. Invest Radiol 23:131–138
Smith RL (1973) The excretory function of the bile. Chapman and Hall, London
Sundin A, Ahlstrom H, Graf W, et al. (1994) Computed tomography of experimental liver metastases using an iodinated hepatocyte-specific lipid emulsion. A correlative study in the nude rat. Invest Radiol 29:963–969
Thomas SF, Henry GW, Kaplan HS (1951) Hepatolienography: past, present, and future. Radiology 57:669–683
Vermess M, Adamson RH, Doppman JL, et al. (1977) Computed tomographic demonstration of hepatic

tumor with the aid of intravenous iodinated fat emulsion. An experimental study. Radiology 125:711–715

Vermess M, Chatterji DC, Doppman JL, et al. (1979) Development and experimental evaluation of a contrast medium for computed tomographic examination of the liver and spleen. J Comput Assist Tomogr 3:25–31

Vermess M, Doppman JL, Sugarbaker P, et al. (1980) Clinical trials with a new intravenous liposoluble contrast material for computed tomography of the liver and spleen. Radiology 137:217–222

Vermess M, Doppman JL, Sugarbaker PH, et al. (1982) Computed tomography of the liver and spleen with intravenous lipoid contrast material: review of 60 examinations. AJR 138:1063–1071

Violante MR, Dean PB (1980) Improved detectability of VX2 carcinoma in the rabbit liver with contrast enhancement in computed tomography. Radiology 134:237–239

Violante MR, Fischer HW (1984) Particulate suspensions of contrast media. In: Sovak M (ed) Radiocontrast agents. Springer, Berlin Heidelberg New York, pp 543–576

Violante MR, Fischer HW (1987) Efficacy and safety of IDE particulate suspensions for liver CT enhancement. In: Parvez Z, Moncanda R, Sovak M (eds) Contrast media: biologic effects and clinical application. CRC Press, Boca Raton, Fl., pp 89–103

Violante MR, Fischer HW, Mahoney JA (1980) Particulate contrast media. Invest Radiol 15:S329–S334

Zaccarini P, Spinazzi A, Lorusso V, et al. (1997) Safety and pharmacokinetics of BR21, a liver-specific CT agent, in healthy volunteers. Acad Radiol 1998;5:S20–22

14 Lymphatic Agents

E.R. WISNER and R.W. KATZBERG

CONTENTS

14.1 Introduction

Accurate cancer staging is important for selecting initial management strategies and for monitoring response to therapy. Determination of regional lymph node involvement is crucial for establishing an accurate prognosis, selecting the most appropriate treatment modality, and surgical or radiation treatment planning. After physical examination, computed tomography (CT) is currently the non-operative modality most frequently used for evaluation of lymph node status for cancer staging. Although magnetic resonance imaging (MRI), ultrasonography and scintigraphy may also be used for this purpose, they provide lower spatial resolution and, in the case of ultrasound, may also provide less contrast resolution. Conventional direct lymphography, previously a mainstay in cancer staging, has declined in popularity since it requires a time-consuming delivery technique and its usefulness is limited to pelvic and lumbar nodal chains. Novel lymphotropic radiographic contrast media that obviate these drawbacks are under active development and are discussed in this review.

E.R. WISNER, DVM, Associate Professor and Head of Radiology, Department of Veterinary Clinical Sciences, College of Veterinary Medicine, Ohio State University, Columbus, OH 43210-1089, USA
R.W. KATZBERG, MD, Professor, Department of Radiology, School of Medicine, University of California, Davis, Sacramento, CA 95817, USA

14.2 Historical Perspective

14.2.1 Indirect Lymphography

In the 1930s, initial attempts at enhancing lymphatic vessels and lymph nodes consisted of interstitial (FUNAOKA et al. 1930; MENVILLE and ANÉ 1932; ZOLOTUKHIN 1934), intranodal (CARVALHO et al. 1931), or intraperitoneal (MENVILLE and ANÉ 1934) injection of particulate radiographic contrast materials such as Thorotrast, oily iodinated solutions, and a variety of water-soluble agents. These materials dispersed into surrounding tissues, accumulated in regional afferent lymphatics, and produced varying degrees of contrast enhancement of the regional lymphatic vessels and lymph nodes. This "indirect" technique soon lost favor since it was inefficient for concentrating contrast material into lymphatics and often did not accumulate within lymph nodes in concentrations adequate to produce sufficient tissue contrast for radiographic examination. In addition, significant concerns were raised about local tissue damage from injection of soluble iodinated agents and from the carcinogenic effects resulting from the ionizing radiation of thorium (FISCHER 1959).

14.2.2 Direct Lymphography Using Ethiodol

In the early 1950s KINMONTH described the intraoperative visualization of lymphatics by interstitial injection of vital dyes (KINMONTH 1952) and subsequently the technique for direct lymphography using water-soluble contrast agents (Kinmonth 1954). A number of investigators shortly thereafter described the current method of direct lymphography, which entailed injection of oily contrast media into a cannulated peripheral lymphatic vessel to enhance draining lymphatic vessels and regional lymph nodes (Hreschyshyn et al. 1961; Wallace et al. 1961).

Iodized poppy seed oil (Ethiodol, Savage Laboratories, Melville, N.Y.) containing 37% iodine (475 mg I/ml) organically bound to esters of fatty acids, and formulated to minimize viscosity to facilitate injection, is the contrast agent currently used for direct lymphography. After injection and transport through the afferent lymphatics, distribution of Ethiodol within lymph nodes is fairly uniform within the lymph node sinuses. On microscopic examination of contrast-containing nodes, the material appears as spherical fat globules distributed in the distended sinuses (Viamonte et al. 1963). In general, cancerous nodes resulting from regional metastasis of solid tumors are identified by characteristic contrast filling defects within the affected nodes. Lymphomatous nodes generally take on a more diffuse foamy appearance (Viamonte et al. 1963). One important advantage of lymphography in comparison to other imaging modalities is that the characteristic distribution of contrast material within enhanced nodes can allow one to discern malignant involvement in nonenlarged lymph nodes (Viamonte et al. 1963).

Conventional lymphography has been limited primarily to an assessment of the retroperitoneal lymph nodes caudal to the renal pedicles and accessible via pedal lymphatics. Thus, the value of this procedure is limited since the nodes superior to the renal pedicles, the abdominal lymph nodes, and some of the deep pelvic node groups are not accessible by the pedal approach. Although techniques have been described for visualizing other lymph node groups (Fisch and Sigel 1964), these procedures have never received widespread acceptance due to their technically difficult nature.

14.3 Staging Using Computed Tomography

With the advent and refinement of CT, conventional lymphography has gradually lost favor as a method of cancer staging (Castellino and Marglin 1982; North et al. 1982; Moskovic et al. 1991). This is in spite of the fact that lymphography is often more accurate for staging than CT or can provide significant additional diagnostic information in certain types of cancer (Sombeck et al. 1993; Baker et al. 1990; Mansfield et al. 1990; Fernando et al. 1994; Bussar-Maatz and Weissbach 1993; Horenblas et al. 1991; Marks et al. 1991; Dooms and Hricak 1986). Several factors are responsible for the decline of direct lymphography, including the technical difficulty, the time required to perform the examination, and the limited nodal region that can be effectively depicted. In addition, administration of oily contrast can occasionally lead to morbidity associated with pulmonary or parenchymal organ oil embolism, systemic chemotoxicity, allergy, and local tissue reaction (Bruna and Brunova 1994; Lossef 1994; Fuchs 1962).

Because the attenuation or signal intensity of unenhanced lymph nodes is similar to that of surrounding tissues in CT and MRI, respectively, visualization of individual lymph nodes is poor. Identification of lymph nodes usually requires that the node be surrounded by fat to provide some degree of tissue contrast. In lean patients or in anatomical regions where little fat is deposited, lymph nodes, whether normal or abnormal, may therefore be difficult to recognize. The addition of intravascular contrast provides some help in differentiating vessels and nodes. In addition, enhancement of metastatic lymph nodes has also been reported in patients with urinary bladder cancer using fast dynamic MRI techniques (MP-RAGE) after intravenous gadolinium administration (Bareentsz 1996). However, nodal enhancement in these instances is variable and appears to be dependent on neovascularity within the affected nodes. Although a few papers also report characteristics of nodal rim enhancement after intravenous contrast administration using CT, nodal architecture typically cannot be defined (Arnold et al. 1991). While characteristics such as central nodal necrosis and extracapsular spread have been suggested for differentiating cancerous from noncancerous lymph nodes (Yousem et al. 1992), size is by far the most important criterion, with 1.0–1.5 cm often defined as the maximal diameter for normal nodes on cross-sectional images depending on the anatomical location. Lymph node shape has not been shown to be particularly useful in differentiating cancerous and normal nodes (van den Brekel et al. 1990).

14.4 Rediscovery of Indirect Lymphography

Because of the excellent contrast resolution of CT and MRI as compared with conventional radiographic images, indirect methods for lymph node contrast enhancement have once again gained some attention as a means of lymphographic examination. The opportunity for smaller amounts of contrast material to adequately enhance lymph nodes and the ability to target virtually any lymph node group make interstitial contrast administration attractive with current imaging technology.

Current strategy for lymph node targeting employs particulate agents capable of being phagocytized by cells of the reticuloendothelial system after interstitial delivery. Indeed, most of the currently proposed agents have been initially or subsequently proposed as hepatosplenic contrast agents. Although none of these agents are currently available for clinical use, two agents, iodinated nanoparticles and perflubron (perfluorooctyl bromide, PFOB), have shown promise in preclinical studies.

Intravenously injected lymphotropic contrast media have been proposed for MR lymphography and these investigational agents have shown some promise in terms of lymph node enhancement (Weissleder et al. 1990, 1994). Advantages of intravenous administration are ease of administration and the potential for simultaneous enhancement of all lymph nodes. Disadvantages are the need to administer larger doses of contrast material because of the inability to target specific anatomical regions and the risk of serious systemic toxicity. Because the amount of active material required to adequately enhance lymph nodes for MR examination is orders of magnitude smaller than that required for radiographic enhancement, intravenous routes of administration appear more feasible for MRI than for CT. We are not aware of any lymphotropic intravenous agents under development for radiographic lymphography.

14.5 Lymphatic System Anatomy and Physiology

The tissue interstitium comprises a loose cross-linked gel-like matrix of collagen fibers and proteoglycan filaments. Fluid within the interstitium is an ultrafiltrate of blood whose formation is governed by Starling forces, and more than 99% is trapped within the proteoglycan gel. Because of the gel-like character of the interstitial fluid volume, movement of interstitially injected particulates may be impeded and distribution of the volume may be reduced (Guyton 1991). An interstitial macrophage population also exists within the interstitial matrix. These macrophages may be either sessile or mobile and may be recruited from the circulating blood monocyte population. Interstitial macrophages can phagocytize injected particles and either retain them at the injection site or transport them intracellularly to regional lymph nodes by traversing the lymphatic walls.

The plexus of initial microlymphatics are formed by an endothelial lining without an associated smooth muscle component. Endothelial junctions at this level lack tight junctions and macroscopic openings can be visualized when the lymphatics are distended. The initial lymphatics are therefore a leaky system and provide a network of microvalves formed by loosely overlapping endothelial cells that provide a mechanism for fluid uptake. In addition, fenestrations up to a few micrometers in width can provide both uninhibited fluid flow but also an avenue for particle uptake (Schmid-Schönbein 1990). It has been postulated that deformation of these loose junctions or fenestrations by massage may be an important factor in increasing the rate of particulate contrast uptake after interstitial contrast injections (Hanna et al. 1994). In addition, the cytoplasm of the endothelial cells has numerous vesicles which could also potentially serve as a mechanism of particle transit across the endothelial lining.

Lymph nodes are surrounded by a thick fibrous capsule. The node parenchyma is divided into poorly defined cortical (paracortical and follicular) and medullary regions (Fig. 14.1). The cortical region is made up of follicles and germinal centers containing B lymphocytes and surrounding paracortex populated by T lymphocytes. A lymph node hilus is present on the inferior surface of the node through which the efferent lymphatic and the nodal artery and vein enter or exit, respectively. Immediately deep to the capsule is a subcapsular sinus into which lymph fluid from the afferent lymphatic vessels drains. Lymph percolates through a complex cortical and medullary sinus system, exiting through the efferent lymphatic. The majority of metastatic foci are found in the subcapsular sinus of affected lymph nodes with the remainder usually occurring in the medullary sinus region. Nodal macrophages line the sinus system and are in greatest abundance in the medullary cords.

14.6 Pharmacokinetics of Interstitially Delivered Lymphatic Agents

While the ultimate fate of interstitially injected particulate agents is to accumulate within targeted

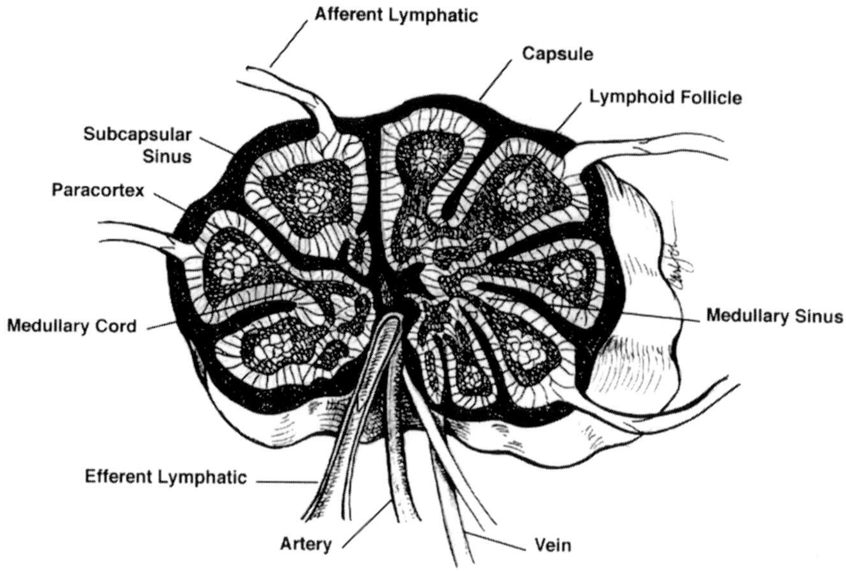

Fig. 14.1. Schematic depiction of a normal lymph node showing afferent and efferent lymphatic vessels, cortical and medullary regions, and the complex nodal sinus system

lymph nodes by macrophage phagocytosis, the initial fate of the particles after interstitial injection is less clear.

Particles of less than a few nanometers in diameter are largely removed by blood capillaries at the injection site. Particles of up to a few tens of nanometers in diameter are absorbed rapidly into the lymph capillaries. Larger particles may remain trapped within the interstitium at the injection site for a much longer time (Bergqvist et al. 1983) and at least some of the particles may be phagocytized by mobile macrophages before entering the lymphatics (Ikomi et al. 1995). Optimal colloid particle size for scintigraphic agents has been reported to be between 1–10 nm (Strand and Persson 1979) although a particle size range of 10–1000 nm has been suggested as suitable for efficient transit across the interendothelial gaps (Wolf 1995). While particle diameter is the major characteristic affecting the tendency to cross through the initial lymphatic capillary plexus, factors such as shape, chemical composition, surface charge, and other particle characteristics may also influence uptake. Muscular activity, passive limb movement, and hyperthermia have also been demonstrated to significantly increase the transport of iodinated nanoparticles (Wolf et al. 1994a; Ikomi et al. 1995) and superparamagnetic iron oxide particles (SPIO) (Elste et al. 1996). Contrast media in nanoparticulate or emulsion suspensions currently being investigated for interstitial lymphography have average particle diameters of 200–350 nm. Seaman and Powers (1955) demonstrated that interstitially injected radioactive colloidal gold administered perilesionally to breast cancer patients concentrated within cancerous nodes in amounts approximately proportional to the volume of residual normal node tissue. In addition, particles accumulate specifically within the normal tissue and not in the tumor. This also appears to be true for small particulate contrast agents which accumulate to the greatest extent within nodal macrophages in the medullary sinuses but not in follicular regions, which are devoid of macrophages (Weissleder et al. 1994). These findings have important implications regarding the expected distribution of radiographic particulate contrast agents since detection of altered nodal architecture is fundamental to the ability of the agent to detect node metastasis.

14.7 Lymphatic Agents

14.7.1 Iodinated Nanoparticles

Iodinated nanoparticles currently being investigated for indirect lymphographic applications (NC 67722 Sterile Suspension, Nycomed Inc., Wayne, Pa.) are prepared from a white crystalline material containing approximately 50% iodine by weight. The empirical formula is $C_{19}H_{23}I_3N_2O_6$.

The active compound is stabilized with polyethylene glycol and a proprietary excipient in a buffered suspension. Milling results in a final particle size of under 350 nm as determined by laser light scattering and scanning electron microscope methods. The injectable formulation is a milky white suspension containing 76 mg iodine/ml that has been formulated for subcutaneous or submucosal interstitial injection (ANONYMOUS 1996). The clinical efficacy and safety of this agent is currently under investigation with FDA phase 1 and phase 2 trials being performed in the United States and Europe.

Safety studies in animals have shown a low-grade and self-limiting foreign body reaction, typical of deposited particulate materials, at the injection site and within targeted lymph nodes. Regional lymph node enlargement occurs after contrast administration associated with physical accumulation of contrast material within the targeted nodes and due to cellular response including neutrophil infiltration, macrophage hyperplasia, and lymphoid hyperplasia. This reaction does not appear to be dose related and lymph node reactivity does not affect the overall lymph node architecture. Thus, histological diagnosis of excised nodes can be performed (ANONYMOUS 1996).

We have administered iodinated nanoparticles (NC 67722 Sterile Suspension) subcutaneously in the distal extremities of normal dogs to opacify popliteal and superficial cervical nodes or in the buccal submucosa to opacify submandibular lymph nodes in doses from 0.1 to 6.0 ml (76 mg I/ml) (Fig. 14.2). Significant enhancement occurred within 4 h of injection and peak enhancement of targeted first-order nodes on CT images was seen between 12 and 24 h after contrast administration. The dose response appeared to be roughly linear within the contrast volume ranges studied, with maximal mean attenuation of opacified nodes being between 400 and 600 HU at the highest administered volume as compared with precontrast attenuation values of approximately 35 HU. Contrast enhancement of more distal nodes in the chain was also noted in this study but not quantified (WISNER et al. 1995a).

High-resolution radiographic studies of excised contrast-enhanced normal canine lymph nodes demonstrate a fairly uniform distribution of the contrast material in the nodal sinuses, lending credence to the hypothesis that particles accumulate and concentrate in macrophages within the targeted nodes (WISNER et al. 1995a) (Fig. 14.3).

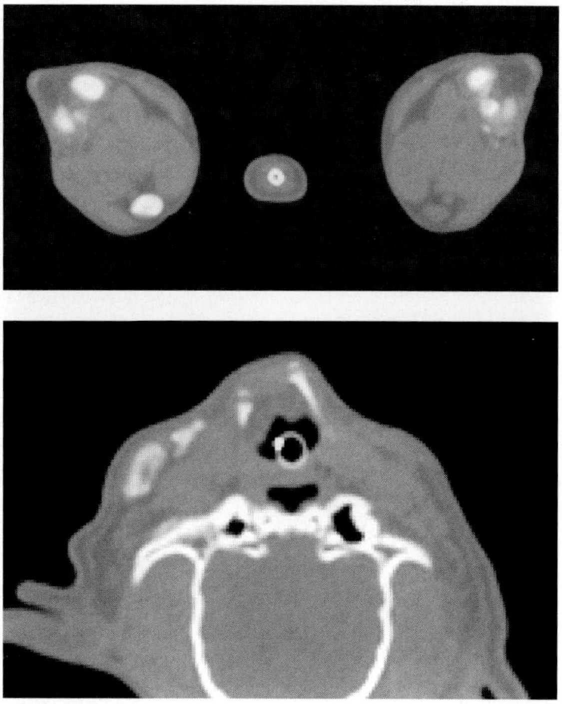

a

b

Fig. 14.2. a CT image of a normal dog at the level of the popliteal lymph nodes. This image was acquired 24 h after unilateral subcutaneous injection of an iodinated nanoparticle suspension at the level of the metatarsus. **b** CT image of a normal dog at the level of the mandibular lymph nodes. This image was acquired 24 h after unilateral submucosal injection of an iodinated nanoparticle suspension into the buccal wall of the oral cavity

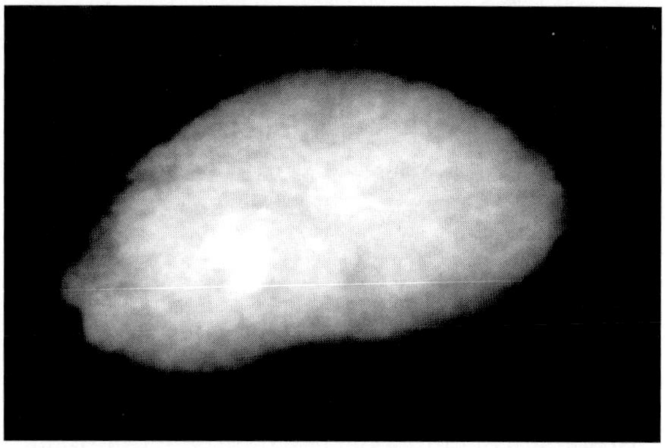

Fig. 14.3. High-resolution radiograph of an excised popliteal lymph node from a normal dog. An iodinated nanoparticle suspension was injected subcutaneously at the level of the ipsilateral metatarsus 24 h prior to excision. Contrast material is distributed throughout the lymph node parenchyma

Efficacy studies using a naturally occurring swine model of metastatic malignant melanoma have also demonstrated excellent opacification of regional lymph nodes 24 h after perilesional subcutaneous injections of contrast material. Conspicuity of normal lymph nodes after contrast-enhancement was

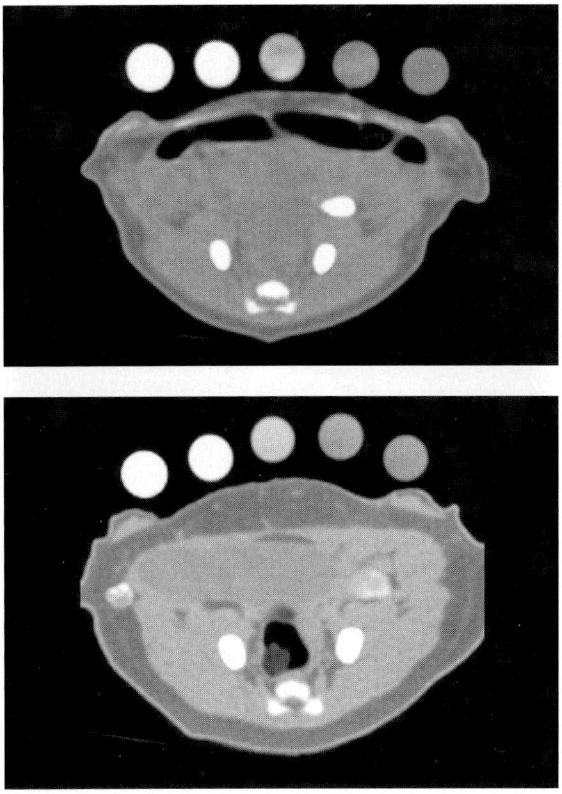

a

b

Fig. 14.4. **a** CT image of an iliac lymph node from a normal pig after contrast enhancement of the node with an interstitially delivered iodinated nanoparticle suspension. The contralateral iliac node is not enhanced and cannot be visualized. **b** CT image of a contrast-enhanced iliac lymph node from an age-matched melanoma-positive pig with regional node metastasis. An iodinated nanoparticle suspension was injected subcutaneously in a perilesional ring pattern around a cutaneous melanoma lesion on the ipsilateral flank. There is less contrast enhancement than in the normal iliac node and the pattern of contrast distribution is nonuniform, with an obvious central filling defect indicative of node metastasis. A second, smaller, cancerous node is seen in the subcutaneous fat of the opposite flank

excellent and nodal internal architecture was portrayed with medullary regions appearing to accumulate more contrast than cortex, consistent with the distribution of intranodal macrophages. Conspicuity of cancerous nodes was similarly increased, the affected nodes demonstrating obvious architectural abnormalities (Wisner et al. 1996) (Fig. 14.4).

Characteristic filling defects could be identified in regions of tumor replacement of nodal tissue and criteria such as size, shape, disruption of the corticomedullary junction, and uniformity of opacification were also suggested as potential characteristics to differentiate normal from cancerous nodes. Quantitatively, a more than 25% replacement of the node by tumor also had lower average attenuation and average iodine concentration, although total iodine uptake in these nodes was greater than in normal nodes due to an increase in total volume (Wisner et al. 1996).

Wolf et al. (1994b) have used a precursor iodinated nanoparticle formulation (WIN 8883, Nycomed, Inc., Wayne, Pa.) to quantitatively compare uptake of subcutaneously administered particles in normal and reactive popliteal lymph nodes in rabbits. In these studies, lymph nodes responding to regional septic inflammation were significantly larger than normal nodes and the average contrast enhancement was significantly less (mean attenuation 114 HU versus 84 HU) after injection of up to 2.0 ml of contrast material subcutaneously in the metacarpus.

This precursor agent has also been used to evaluate serial uptake of contrast material in popliteal, presacral, and para-aortic lymph nodes after subcutaneous metatarsal injection in normal rabbits. After injection of 0.5 ml, attenuation of these node groups was increased to at least 100 HU by 12, 30, and 45 min respectively. An increase in attenuation to 200 HU required approximately twice as long. Gentle massage at the site of injection was also found to increase both the rate of uptake and the maximal attenuation in enhanced nodes (Wolf et al. 1994a).

We have used the same agent to opacify most major lymph node groups in the normal dog model using a combination of subcutaneous, oral submucosal, and endoscopically guided injection methods. These studies have demonstrated the ability to target virtually any lymph node group through appropriate injection techniques including previously inaccessible groups such as the mediastinal, tracheobronchial, and abdominal nodes (Wisner et al. 1994, 1995b).

14.7.2 Perflubron (Perfluorooctyl Bromide, PFOB)

Perflubron is a colorless, inert liquid with the empirical formula $C_8F_{17}Br$ (Fig. 14.5). Perflubron-containing agents are prepared as 30% or 60% wt/vol emulsions (Alliance Pharmaceutical, San Diego, Calif.). Emulsions are formulated with egg yolk phospholipid (2%–9%) as an emulsifying agent along with small quantities of buffer, heavy metal chelator, and antioxidant. Mean particle diameter is 200–300 nm with 4–8 $\times$ 10^{13} particles per milliliter. Sixty percent emulsions have been used in preclini-

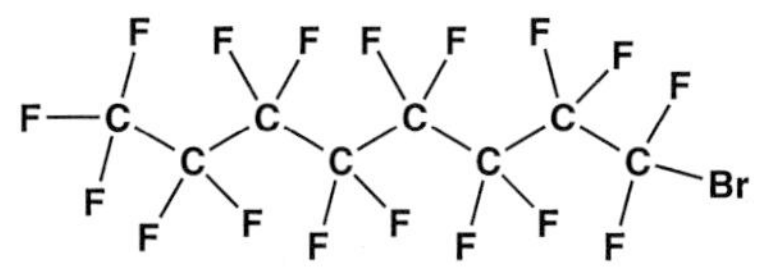

Fig. 14.5. Chemical structure of perflubron (perfluorooctyl bromide, PFOB)

cal trials (Wolf et al. 1994c). The presence of the bromine atom renders this agent radiopaque but because the atomic number of bromine is 35, these agents produce somewhat less attenuation at typical clinical imaging energies than iodinated agents (atomic number of iodine = 53) at the same concentration.

Studies performed with perflubron emulsions when used as an intravenously injected reticuloendothelial-specific agent have demonstrated localization and concentration of perflubron within cytoplasmic vacuoles of Kupffer cells (Mattrey et al. 1982). This localization within macrophages also presumably occurs after lymphatic transport to lymph nodes after interstitial injection.

Initial safety studies in healthy volunteers receiving subcutaneous injections of 1–4 ml of the emulsion injected in divided doses dorsally in the metacarpal region included monitoring hematology, coagulation, blood chemistry, urinalysis, and vital signs before and up to 28 days after contrast agent administration. Adverse events were monitored immediately after injection and at all follow-up visits. No clinically significant adverse systemic effects were reported, although transient, mild injection site discomfort associated with erythema and swelling was described, resolving in most volunteers within 2 h after contrast injection (Hanna et al. 1994).

In studies performed in normal rabbits and monkeys by Wolf et al., perflubron administered subcutaneously as either a 30% or a 60% suspension, using injection volumes of from 0.1–0.5 ml in the subcutaneous tissues of the metacarpus, produced excellent regional node enhancement, the quality of which was linearly related to the administered dose. In rabbits receiving a 0.25 ml injection volume, contrast enhancement of axillary nodes occurred by 4 h postinjection and maximal bromine accumulation within targeted nodes occurred approximately 48 h postinjection. The rate of lymph node contrast enhancement was increased by massage of the injection site. The maximal value at this dose was approximately 10 mg/ml, which translates to 170 HU at 80 kV, with more than 8 mg/ml still being present at 21 days. The estimated half-life of residence time

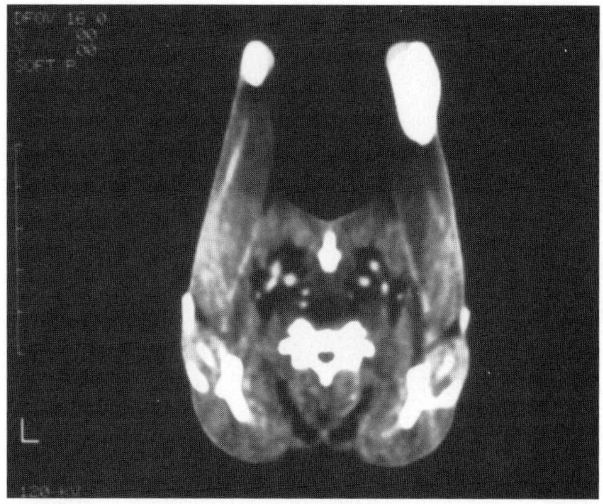

Fig. 14.6. CT image of contrast-enhanced lymph nodes of the neck of a normal rabbit. This image was acquired 1 week after injection of a perflubron suspension into the muscles of the cheek. (Courtesy of Dr. Gerald L. Wolf)

within the nodes was 63 days. In this same investigation, normal monkeys receiving 1.0 ml subcutaneous injections of 60% perflubron in the web spaces of the foot had CT-assessed contrast enhancement of the inguinal nodes that was sustained from 3 to 17 days (Wolf et al. 1994c) (Fig. 14.6).

Hanna et al., using the same animal model, concluded that volumes of at least 0.15 ml were necessary to consistently and adequately enhance the axillary nodes. In a related study that assessed extracellular versus intracellular transport and where lymphatic uptake of a 30% fluorescent labeled perflubron emulsion was measured in the lymphatic fluid from afferent lymphatic vessels draining the injection sites, the authors concluded that the extracellular component predominated. Massage of the injection site increased lymphatic uptake and also increased the intracellular uptake component. It was postulated that massage produced some degree of tissue deformation which may have facilitated movement of the agent through the interendothelial gaps of the initial lymphatic vessels (Hanna et al. 1994). In 18 normal volunteers receiving 1, 2, or 4 ml of perflubron administered subcutaneously between the dorsal metacarpals of one limb, CT scans in the axillary region obtained between 1 and 28 days postinjection showed initial contrast uptake in axillary lymph nodes on the third day which reached peak enhancement at 14 days and then decreased only slightly by 28 days postinjection. Both the extent of contrast enhancement and the number of lymph nodes opacified increased with increasing dose. The average peak enhancement for the 1-, 2-,

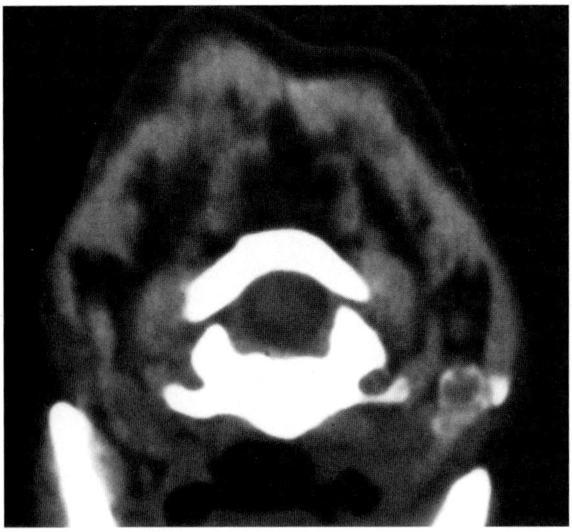

Fig. 14.7. CT image of the cervical region of a dog depicting regional metastasis of a caudal superficial cervical lymph node. Interstitial injection of a perflubron suspension produced nonuniform contrast enhancement and an obvious filling defect. (Courtesy of Dr. Deborah L. Darien, University of Wisconsin-Madison School of Veterinary Medicine)

and 4-ml groups was approximately 130, 190, and 270 HU, respectively (Hanna et al. 1994).

Subcutaneously administered perflubron has also been used to contrast enhance normal canine lymph nodes (Darien et al. 1993) and cancerous nodes in dogs with spontaneously arising metastatic cancer. Qualitative findings from lymphographic CT examinations of these animals demonstrate improved lymph node conspicuity and alterations in architecture of affected nodes (Fig. 14.7).

14.7.3 Other Agents

Water-soluble, iodinated, molecular contrast agents have also been proposed as lymphographic (Siefert et al. 1980) or lymphangiographic agents (Weissleder and Weissleder 1989) for interstitial administration. Because of their small size and solubility, these agents disperse quickly through interstitial and lymphatic fluid and across lymphatic vessel walls. In addition these small, molecular agents do not concentrate within regional lymph nodes since they are not phagocytosed. As a result, they are probably not suitable for indirect lymphography.

Iodine-carrying liposomes have been formulated as reticuloendothelial agents for hepatosplenic imaging after intravascular injection and concentrate in the targeted organs by phagocytosis by Kupffer cells of the liver and reticuloendothelial cells of the spleen (Seltzer et al. 1995). Although iodinated liposome agents could potentially be developed for lymphatic imaging applications, there are few reports characterizing these agents for this purpose.

14.8 Summary

New contrast agents for indirect lymphography permit the assessment of regional nodal groups with a technical ease not previously available. The previous severe limitations of direct lymphography, namely the tedious and time-consuming technique and the fact that its usefulness was limited to the pelvis and lower abdomen, are eliminated by the indirect methodology. Direct assessment of nodal architecture and pharmacokinetics in addition to size criteria by CT and MR-assisted modalities is advantageous in cancer staging accuracy. The capability of enhancing nodal groups in virtually any human anatomical region appears to be a realistic clinical opportunity.

References

Anonymous (1996) Sterile WIN 67722 suspension 150 mg/mL. Clinical Investigator Brochure. Nycomed Inc., Wayne, Pa

Arnold MM, Tsao SY, Kreel LK (1991) Computed tomography contrast enhancement of cervical lymphadenopathy. Ear Nose Throat J 70:355–360

Baker LL, Parker BR, Donaldson SS, Castellino RA (1990) Staging of Hodgkin disease in children: comparison of CT and lymphography with laparotomy. AJR 154:1251–1255

Barentsz JO, Jager GJ, van Vierzen PB, et al. (1996) Staging urinary bladder cancer after transurethral biopsy: value of fast dynamic contrast-enhanced MR imaging. Radiology 201:185–193

Bergqvist L, Strand S-E, Persson BRR (1983) Particle sizing and biokinetics of interstitial lymphoscintigraphic agents. Semin Nucl Med 13:9–19

Bruna J, Brunova J (1994) Complications and side-effects after lymphography. Lymphology 27(Suppl):321–324

Bussar-Maatz R, Weissbach L (1993) Retroperitoneal lymph node staging of testicular tumours. TNM Study Group. Br J Urol 72:234–240

Carvalho R, Rodriguez A, Pereina S (1931) Lamise en evidence por la radiographie du system lymphatique chez la vivant. Ann Anat Pathol (Paris) 8:193

Castellino RA, Marglin SI (1982) Imaging of the abdominal and pelvic lymph nodes. Lymphography or computed tomography? Invest Radiol 17:433–443

Darien DL, Adams WC, Duielzig RR, MacEwen EG (1993) Computed tomography evaluation of the canine and feline lymph nodes using perflubron emulsion (Imagent LN) as a contrast agent. Proceedings of the American College of

Veterinary Radiology Annual Scientific Meeting, Chicago, Ill.
Dooms GC, Hricak H (1986) Radiologic imaging modalities, including magnetic resonance, for evaluating lymph nodes. West J Med 144:49–57
Elste V, Wagner S, Taupitz M, et al. (1996) Magnetic resonance lymphography in rats: effects of muscular activity and hyperthermia on the lymph node uptake of intravenously injected superparamagnetic iron oxide particles. Acad Radiol 3:660–666
Fernando IN, Moskovic E, Fryatt I, Glaholm J, Blake PR (1994) Is there still a role for lymphography in the management of early stage carcinoma of the cervix? Br J Radiol 67: 1052–1056
Fisch UP, Sigel ME (1964) Cervical lymphatic system as visualized by lymphography. Ann Otol Rhinol Laryngol 73:869–882
Fischer HW (1959) A critique of experimental lymphography. Acta Radiol 52:448–454
Fuchs WA (1962) Complications in lymphography with oily contrast media. Acta Radiol 57:427–441
Funaoka S, Tachikawa R, Yamaguchi O, Fijita S (1930) Kurz Mitteilung über den Mechanismes der symphstromung. Ab dritten Abstr Inst Kaiserlich Univ Kyoto 1:11
Guyton AC (1991) The microcirculation and lymphatic system: capillary fluid exchange, interstitial fluid and lymph flow. In: Guyton AC (ed) Textbook of medical physiology, 8th edn. Saunders, Philadelphia, pp 173–184
Hanna G, Hopkins R, Flaim K, et al. (1994) Indirect lymphography with perflubron emulsion – preclinical and clinical results. Invest Radiol 29(Suppl 2):S33–S35
Horenblas S, van Tinteren H, Delamarre JFM, Moonen LCF, Lustig V, Kröger R (1991) Squamous cell carcinoma of the penis: accuracy of tumor, nodes and metastasis classification system, and role of lymphangiography, computerized tomography scan and fine needle aspiration cytology. J Urol 146:1279–1283
Hreschyshyn MM, Sheehan F, Holland JF (1961) Visualization of retroperitoneal lymph nodes. Lymphangiography as an aid in the measurement of tumor growth. Cancer 14: 205
Ikomi F, Hanna GK, Schmid-Schönbein GW (1995) Mechanism of colloidal particle uptake into the lymphatic system: basic study with percutaneous lymphography. Radiology 196:107–113
Kinmonth JB (1952) Lymphography in man: a method for outlining lymphatic trunks at operation. Clin Sci 11:13–21
Kinmonth JB (1954) Lymphangiography in clinical surgery and particularly in the treatment of lymphedema. Ann R Coll Surg Engl 15:300
Lossef SV (1994) Complications of lymphography. Semin Intervent Radiol 11:107–112
Mansfield CM, Fabian C, Jones S, et al. (1990) Comparison of lymphangiography and computed tomography scanning in evaluating abdominal disease in stages III and IV Hodgkin's disease. Cancer 66:2295–2299
Marks LB, Shipley WU, Walker TG, Waltman AC (1991) Role of lymphangiography in staging testicular seminoma. Urology 38:264–266
Mattrey RF, Long DM, Multer FK, Mitten R, Higgins CB (1982) Perfluoroctylbromide: a reticuloendothelial-specific and tumor-imaging agent for computed tomography. Radiology 145:755–758
Menville LJ, Ané JN (1932) Roentgen visualization of lymph nodes in animals. J Am Med Assoc 98:1796–1798
Menville LJ, Ané JN (1934) Roentgen-ray visualization of part of lymphatic system. Radiology 23:327–330
Moskovic E, Fernando I, Blake P, Parsons C (1991) Lymphography – current role in oncology. Br J Radiol 64:422–427
North LB, Lindell MM, Jing B-S, Wallace S (1982) Current use of lymphography for staging lymphomas and genital tumors. AJR 158:725–728
Schmid-Schönbein GW (1990) Microlymphatics and lymph flow. Physiol Rev 70:987–1028
Seaman WG, Powers WE (1955) Studies on distribution of radioactive colloidal gold in regional lymph nodes containing cancer. Cancer 8:1044–1046
Seltzer SE, Blau M, Herman LW, et al. (1995) Contrast material-carrying liposomes: biodistribution, clearance, and imaging characteristics. Radiology 194:775–781
Siefert HM, Mutzel W, Schobel C, Weinmann H-J, Wenzel-Hora BI, Speck U (1980) Iotasul, a water-soluble contrast agent for direct and indirect lymphography. Lymphology 13:150
Sombeck MD, Mendenhall NP, Kaude JV, Torres GM, Million RR (1993) Correlation of lymphangiography, computed tomography, and laparotomy in the staging of Hodgkin's disease. Int J Radiat Oncol Biol Phys 25:425–429
Strand S-E, Persson BRR (1979) Quantitative lymphoscintigraphy. I. Basic concepts for optimal uptake of radiocolloids in the parasternal lymph nodes of rabbits. J Nucl Med 20:1038–1046
van den Brekel MWM, Stel HV, Castelijns JA, et al. (1990) Cervical lymph node metastasis: assessment of radiologic criteria. Radiology 177:379–384
Viamonte M, Altman D, Parks R, Blum E, Bevilacqua M, Recher L (1963) Radiographic-pathologic correlation in the interpretation of lymphangioadenograms. Radiology 80:903–916
Wallace S, Jackson L, Schaffer B (1961) Lymphangiograms: their diagnostic and therapeutic potential. Radiology 76:179
Weissleder H, Weissleder R (1989) Interstitial lymphography: initial clinical experience with a dimeric nonionic contrast agent. Radiology 170:371
Weissleder R, Elizondo G, Wittenberg J, Lee AS, Josephson L, Brady T (1990) Ultrasmall superparamagnetic iron oxide: an intravenous contrast agent for assessing lymph nodes with MR imaging. Radiology 175:494–498
Weissleder R, Heautot JF, Schaffer BK, Nossiff N, Papisov MI, Bogdanov A, Brady TJ (1994) MR lymphography: study of a high-efficiency lymphotropic agent. Radiology 191:225–230
Wisner ER, Katzberg RW, Koblik PD, et al. (1994) Iodinated nanoparticles for indirect computed tomography lymphography of the craniocervical and thoracic lymph nodes in normal dogs. Acad Radiol 1:377–384
Wisner ER, Katzberg RW, Griffey SM, Drake CM, Haley PJ, Vessey AR (1995a) Indirect computed tomography lymphography using iodinated nanoparticles: time and dose response in normal canine lymph nodes. Acad Radiol 2:497–506
Wisner ER, Katzberg RW, Koblik PD, et al. (1995b) Indirect computed tomography lymphography of subdiaphragmatic lymph nodes using iodinated nanoparticles in a normal canine model. Acad Radiol 2:405–412
Wisner ER, Katzberg RW, Link DP, et al. (1996) Indirect computed tomography lymphography using iodinated nanoparticulates to detect cancerous lymph nodes in a cutaneous melanoma model. Acad Radiol 3:40–48
Wolf GL (1995) Specific imaging agents for lymph nodes. In: Torchilin VP (ed) Handbook of targeted delivery of imaging agents. CRC Press, Boca Raton, Fl., pp 365–384

Wolf GL, Na GC, Gazelle GS, McIntire GL, Cannillo J, Bacon ER, Helpern E (1994a) Time lapse quantitative computed tomography lymphography: assessing lymphatic function in vivo. Acad Radiol 1:358–363
Wolf GL, Gazelle GS, McIntire GL, Bacon ER, Toner JL, Cooper ER, Haley PJ (1994b) Percutaneous computed tomography lymphography in the rabbit by subcutaneously injected nanoparticulates. Acad Radiol 1:352–357
Wolf GL, Rogowska J, Hanna GK, Halpern EF (1994c) Percutaneous CT lymphography with perflubron – imaging efficacy in rabbits and monkeys. Radiology 191:501–505
Yousem DM, Som PM, Hackney DB, Schwaibold F, Hendrix RA (1992) Central nodal necrosis and extracapsular neoplastic spread in cervical lymph nodes: MR imaging versus CT. Radiology 182:753–759
Zolotukhin A (1934) Roentgenologic method of examination of lymphatic system in man and animals. Radiology 23:455–462

II
Magnetic Resonance Contrast Media

15 Chemical Synthesis of Paramagnetic Complexes

J.F. Desreux and D. Gilsoul

CONTENTS

15.1 Introduction

Despite the remarkable quality of the unenhanced magnetic resonance (MR) images, it rapidly became obvious that contrast agents were necessary if better morphologic and functional information was needed. Metal ions such as Gd^{3+}, Dy^{3+}, Mn^{2+}, and Fe^{3+} very effectively reduce the relaxation times T1 and T2 of water because of their magnetic properties and their high hydration numbers but they are too toxic to be injected as such. Rapid excretion from the body and very low toxicity are achieved provided the metal ions are encapsulated by an organic ligand that forms thermodynamically stable and kinetically inert chelates. Many new metal chelates can now be safely injected intravenously and bring about notable improvements in image contrast even if they are not as effective as the uncomplexed ions because of their lower hydration numbers.

The synthesis of MRI contrast agents (Brasch 1994) is a most interesting challenge for the chemists since they have to recourse to all aspects of chemistry (Desreux and Jacques 1995). Indeed, preparing new contrast agents requires the expertise of specialists in organic, coordination, physical, and analytical chemistry. For example, high-yield procedures must be devised for the synthesis of new chelating agents forming stable metal complexes. Moreover, high stability is achieved only if the coordination properties of the metal ions are taken into account when designing a new ligand, and reaching a high relaxivity requires thorough physical analyses of the dynamic properties of the complexes in aqueous solution. Finally, measurements and testings should be carried out on pure compounds of known composition. The synthesis of new MRI contrast agents is thus a field of great interest for chemists not only because of the successful applications of these compounds in medical imaging but also because of the opportunity to contribute to the fundamental understanding of the properties of paramagnetic metal complexes. The aim of the present chapter is to give an overview of synthetic methods leading to the preparation of a variety of MRI contrast agents with the hope that the nonspecialist will be better able to interact with chemists working in different fields. The emphasis will be essentially on the gadolinium complexes, Gd^{3+} being the choice ion because of its high magnetic moment and its relatively slow electronic relaxation time. Moreover, although other ligands will be mentioned, the present review will be mostly restricted to polyamino polycarboxylic complexing agents as they form the most stable gadolinium chelates. Ligands are divided below into linear and macrocyclic structures and the aim of the chemical modifications brought to each structure will be stressed, though without full details on the significance of physical parameters such as correlation times as this topic is dealt with in the preceding chapter. After reading the present chapter and going through the papers mentioned as references, the reader who is not familiar with chemistry might become convinced that a new chelate should be prepared, but he or she should always remember

J.F. Desreux, PhD, Professor, Coordination and Radiochemistry, University of Liège, Sart Tilman (B6), B-4000 Liège, Belgium
D. Gilsoul, PhD, Coordination and Radiochemistry, University of Liège, Sart Tilman (B6), B-4000 Liège, Belgium

that chemical syntheses and analyses are long and painstaking processes!

15.2 Synthesis of Linear Polyamino Polycarboxylic Ligands

DTPA, **1** (Fig. 15.1, Gd^{3+} complex: Magnevist, Schering), was the first ligand to come to mind when it became obvious that MRI contrast agents would be needed as this ligand was known to form the most stable lanthanide complexes known at the time. The gadolinium chelate of this commercially available ligand (Acros, Aldrich) is readily excreted via the renal route and its LD_{50} is quite low (8–10 mmol/kg). $GdDTPA^{2-}$ is an extracellular agent now routinely used in hospitals.

Electrically neutral chelates have been obtained with DTPA derivatives featuring two amide groups instead of two carboxylic groups. DTPA-BMA, **2** (Gd^{3+} complex: Omniscan, Nycomed), is commercially available (Strem) and its analogs can be prepared by a classical mixed anhydride approach followed by isolation by chromatography on an ion-exchanger (Sherry et al. 1988). Introducing the less strongly coordinating amide group in the DTPA structure comes at a price since the stability of the gadolinium complexes is lowered. For instance, the stability constant $\log K_{ML}$,

$$K_{\Phi\upsilon} = \frac{[ML]}{[M][L]},$$

where $[M]$, $[L]$, and $[ML]$ designate the concentrations of the metal, the ligand, and the complex at equilibrium, decreases from 22.2 for $GdDTPA^{2-}$ to 16.8 for GdDTPA-BMA. However, it should be noted that conditional constants $\log K'_{ML}$ are more indicative of the complexing ability of a ligand since they are calculated by taking the protonation processes into account. The $\log K'_{ML}$ at pH 7.4 decreases from 17.7 to 14.9 on going from $GdDTPA^{2-}$ to GdDTPA-BMA and the latter complex is not more stable than $GdEDTA^{-}$ ($\log K'_{ML} = 14.7$), a complex that is known to be toxic. Despite this low stability, GdDTPA-BMA is rapidly excreted via the renal route with little decomposition, a clear indication that thermodynamic stability is not necessarily the most important parameter and that biodistributions must be systematically evaluated (Wedeking et al. 1992).

The hydrophobicity of DTPA-like chelates has been increased by the addition of aromatic substituents so as to reach a high degree of excretion in the bile. Hepatocytes take up these chelates through their anion transporter system. An aromatic substituting group has been added either on an acetate arm, as in the case of BOPTA, **3** (Bracco), or on the polyamine chain, as in the case of EOB-DTPA, **4** (Schering). Ligands with an aromatic substituent on one of the ethylenic moieties can be prepared by the condensation of ethylene diamine with a substituted amino acid. The resulting amide is reduced with $BH_3 \cdot THF$ and acetate groups are added by reaction with a halo acid (Brechbiel et al. 1986). Ligands substituted on an acetate arm such as BOPTA are obtained by reaction between a large excess of a polyamine and an aromatic acid halogenated in the α position (Uggeri et al. 1995). Additional acetate functions are added on the remaining free amino groups by reaction with a halo acetic acid in basic medium. It should be stressed here that the addition of acetate groups to a polyamine is less straight-

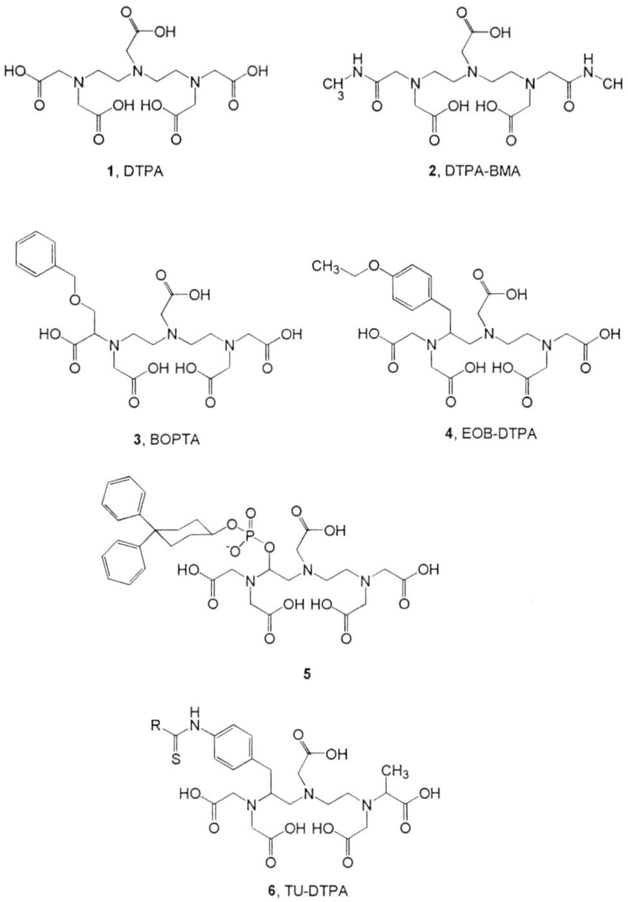

Fig. 15.1. Structure of linear polyamino polycarboxylic ligands suitable for preparing gadolinium-containing MRI contrast agents

forward than expected: yields are often low and the desired compounds must be isolated by chromatography. A synthesis via a *t*-butyl ester followed by an acid hydrolysis is sometimes advantageous (Carvalho et al. 1992; Keana and Mann 1990). It should also be noted that aromatic substituents increase the interaction of the chelates with biological macromolecules, which in turn leads to an increase in their rotation correlation times τ_r. Ligand **5**, featuring a rigid diphenylmethyl unit, has recently been synthesized to ensure that the correlation times τ_r of its gadolinium complex and of albumin are sufficiently close.

The synthetic procedures briefly described above also allow the preparation of metal complexes that can be covalently linked to macromolecules. A nitrophenyl substituent is generally preferred as the nitro group is easily transformed into an isothiocyanato function. Coupling with an amino function is then easily carried out through a thiourea unit (ligand **6**) (Keana and Mann 1990). If possible, the older method consisting in reacting DTPA anhydride (available from Aldrich) with polylysine (Manabe et al. 1986) or albumin (Lauffer and Brady 1985) should be avoided despite its simplicity as one or several acetate arms are used for the binding with the macromolecule and are no longer available for coordinating the metal ions. The stability of the complexes is then drastically reduced, as already mentioned.

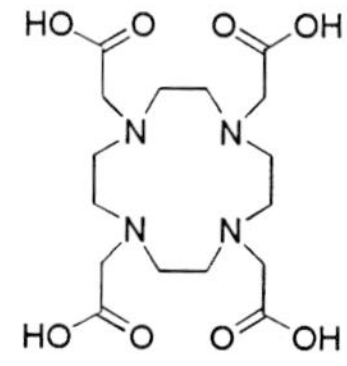

7, DOTA

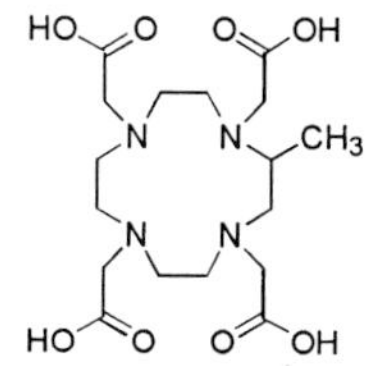

8, MDOTA

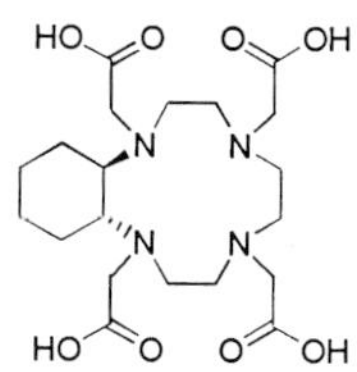

9(CY)DOTA

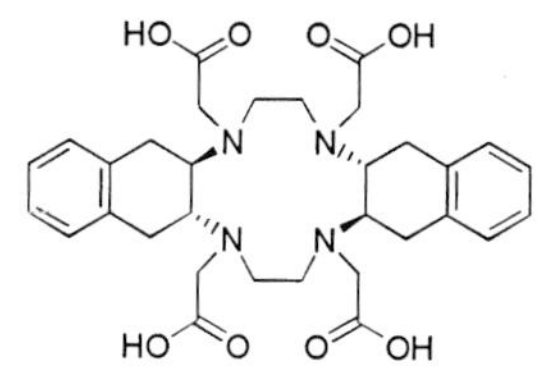

10, $(TE)_2$DOTA

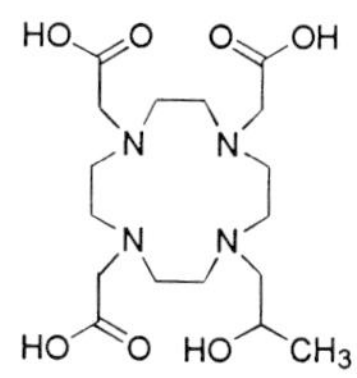

11, HPDO3A

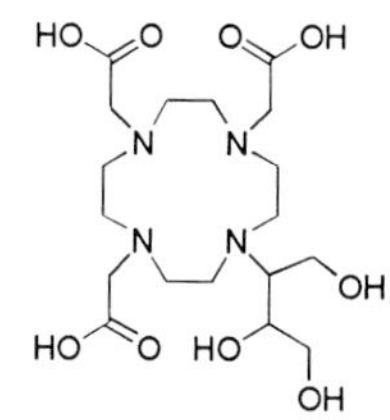

12, DOA-B

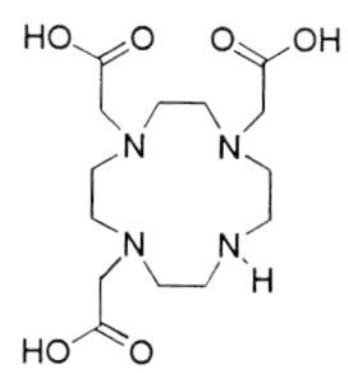

13, DO3A

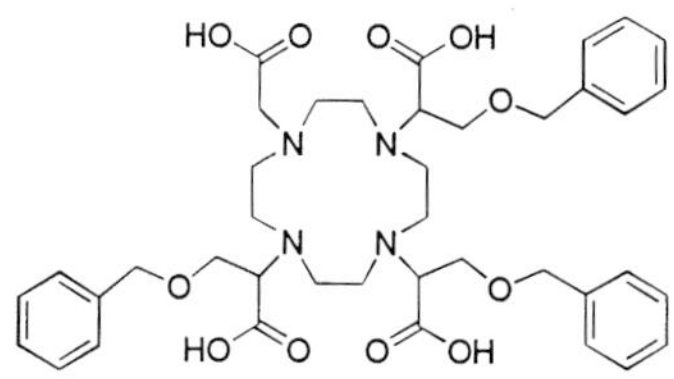

14, $DOTA(BOM)_3$

Fig. 15.2. Structure of macrocyclic polyamino polyacetic ligands suitable for preparing gadolinium-containing MRI contrast agents

15.3 Synthesis of Macrocyclic Polyamino Polycarboxylic Ligands

Most macrocyclic ligands used as MRI contrast agents are derived from DOTA, **7** (Dotarem, Guerbet; Fig. 15.2). DOTA and its derivatives are particularly interesting ligands because of the steric preferences of their 12-membered cycle. The preferred arrangement of the tetraaza ring of DOTA is a square conformation called [3333] because each side of the square is composed of three collinear bonds. This arrangement favors the formation of a square antiprismatic structure with two parallel square faces, one N_4 face with the lone pairs of the nitrogen atoms directed towards the center of the structure and one O_4 face made of the four charged carboxylic oxygen atoms. This spider-like conformation (Desreux 1980; Spirlet et al. 1984) is very stable ($\log K_{ML}$ = 25.6, $\log K'_{ML}$ = 19.0 at pH 7.4), as expected, since a square antiprism and a [3333] conformation are the sterically least demanding geometries for a 12-membered cycle and for eight coordinating atoms around a central metal ion (Kepert 1982). The DOTA lanthanide chelates are unusually rigid as observed by nuclear magnetic resonance (Desreux 1980; Jacques and Desreux 1994) and are kinetically inert (Wang et al. 1992). Kinetic inertness is the most desirable feature for an MRI contrast agent as it ensures low toxicity. The dissociation of $GdDOTA^-$ is acid catalyzed and exceedingly slow ($t_{1/2}$ = 85 days at pH 2) (Wang et al. 1992), probably because the entry of a proton in the rigid cage and the subsequent protonation of a nitrogen atom are very difficult.

It is thus not surprising that the DOTA ligand has been chemically modified in a number of ways in order to obtain some desirable property while keeping its interesting complexation features. The unsubstituted macrocycle itself, 1,4,7,10-tetraazacyclododecane, is available from Aldrich or Acros but at a hefty price. It can be synthesized in large quantities by a now classical procedure (Richman and Atkins 1974) from diethylenetriamine via the sodium salt of its tritosylated derivative or by a recent and more direct approach (Athey and Kiefer 1996) from pure triethylenetetramine (Fluka) via a bis-imidazoline. Increased rigidity and hydrophobicity can be expected for ligands featuring aliphatic or aromatic substituents. However, the synthesis of substituted tetraaza macrocycles is often more difficult because of the bulkiness of the groups added to diethylenetriamine. For instance, bases such as Cs_2CO_3 instead of Na_2CO_3 have to be used in the cyclization step yielding monomethylated DOTA, **8** (Schaeffer et al. 1991), from a ditosylamide and a ditosylate. In a different procedure, macrocycles with groups directly grafted onto the tetraaza ring are obtained by condensation between a substituted diamine and a dichlorodiamide. Ligands such as (CY)DOTA, **9**, or $(TE)_2$DOTA, **10**, are obtained after reduction with $BH_3 \cdot THF$ and reaction with a halo acid (Runge et al. 1995; Desreux et al. 1994).

Also of relevance are the various approaches devised for the synthesis of ligands with different substituents on the nitrogen atoms. The synthesis of DOTA derivatives with different combinations of acetate, acetamide, alcohol, and/or phosphonate arms requires discrimination between identical reaction sites in the tetraaza ring. The preparation of mono- (Dischino et al. 1991), di- (Dumont et al. 1994; Kovacs and Sherry 1995), and triprotected (Prasad et al. 1991) tetraaza rings has been reported. The synthesis of ligands such as HPDO3A, **11** (Proance, Bracco) (Dischino et al. 1991), or DO3A-B, **12** (Gadobutrol, Schering) (Toth et al. 1996a), can thus be carried out and electrically neutral gadolinium chelates can be used in order to avoid osmotic shocks during intravenous injections. These chelates remain kinetically inert and sufficiently stable despite the replacement of one carboxylic function by a less strongly coordinating group (Kumar et al. 1993). The ligand DO3A, **13**, is also a very good starting material for the synthesis of a variety of derivatives substituted with different coordinating functions (Dischino et al. 1991). Likewise, GdDOTA complexes with different carboxylic arms featuring pendant hydrophobic groups have been prepared to increase the interactions with albumin and reach a high relaxivity, presumably because of the formation of clathrate-type species (Aime et al. 1996).

As in the case of the linear polyamine polycarboxylic ligands, bifunctional DOTA derivatives have been synthesized for binding with biological or synthetic macromolecules. The *p*-nitrobenzyl group is again the preferred linkage unit and has been added either to the tetraaza ring or to one acetate arm (see ligands **15** and **16** in Fig. 15.3). Ring substitution has been performed by internal cyclization of a polytosylated polyamine (Moi et al. 1988), by reaction of an activated diacid with a substituted diamine (McMurry et al. 1992), by condensation of tosylated derivatives in the presence of Cs_2CO_3 (Ansari et al. 1993) or via a cyclic bis-amide (Mishra et al. 1996b). On the other hand, DOTA ligands with a nitro group grafted onto one acetate function have been obtained either directly from the unsubstituted tetraaza ring by reaction with *p*-nitrobenzyl bromide in appropri-

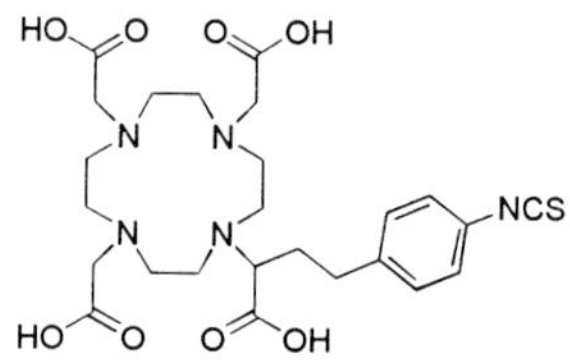

15

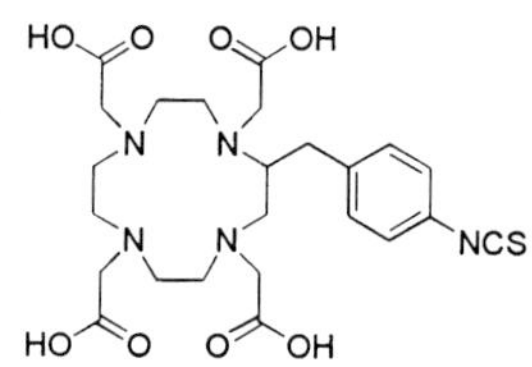

16

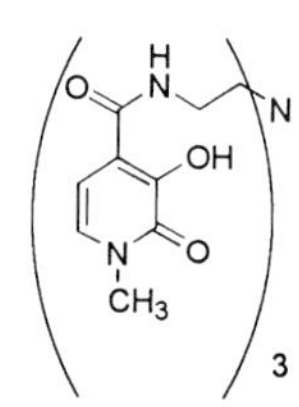

17
TREN-Me-3,2-HOPO

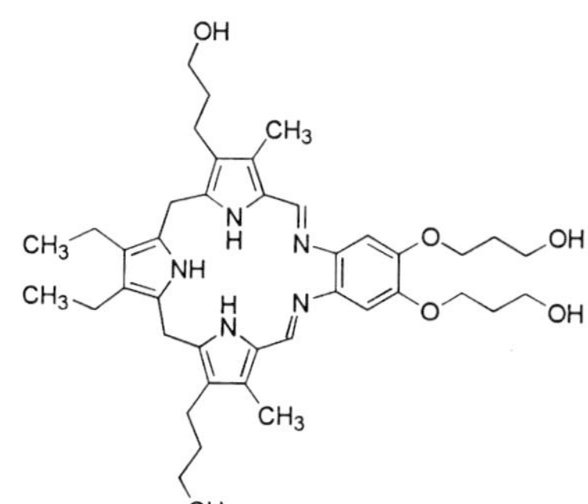

18, Texaphyrin

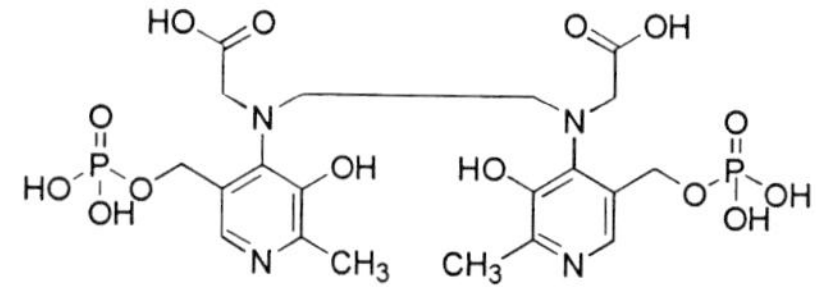

19, DPDP

Fig. 15.3. Structure of various linear and macrocyclic ligands suitable for preparing gadolinium- or manganese-containing MRI contrast agents ate concentration conditions (KRUPER et al. 1993) or from the triacetate tetraaza cycle by reaction with a substituted α-halo acid (MISHRA et al. 1996a).

15.4 Synthesis of Multimeric Polyamino Polycarboxylic Ligands

Increasing the rotational correlation time τ_r and thus the relaxivity, can be achieved by tying together several gadolinium chelates. As illustrated in Fig. 15.4, a reasonably good linear correlation is found between the molecular weight of gadolinium complexes, whether monomeric or polymeric, and their relaxivity per Gd^{3+} ion. One should not expect anything better than an approximate linear relationship in Fig. 15.4 as small differences in temperature, in degree of hydration, and in shape and rigidity could not be taken into account. In order to increase τ_r, two DO3A units have been linked together by reaction with bis-epoxides (SHUKLA et al. 1996). The relaxivity is doubled provided the bridge between the two GdDO3A units is sufficiently rigid. Two to fourfold relaxivity increases have been measured in the case of poly-DTPA (MARTIN et al. 1995) and poly-DOTA (RANGANATHAN et al. 1995) ligands featuring two to eight complexing units and possibly a tethering function for anchoring to a macromolecule. Sizeable relaxivity increases have also been achieved by covalently linking up to 192 benzyl-DTPA isocyanate moieties to polyamine dendrimers (WIENER et al. 1994). The dendrimers of interest here are nearly perfectly monodisperse polymers

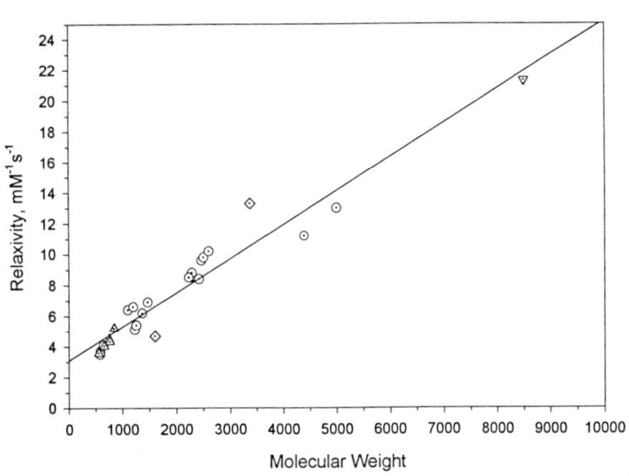

Fig. 15.4. Molecular weight dependence of the relaxivity of various gadolinium chelates at 20 MHz. Data between 25° and 37°C. *Symbols*: ⊙, RANGANATHAN et al. (1994); △, AIME et al. (1992b); ▽, WIENER et al. (1994); ◇, MARTIN et al. (1995)

whose molecular weight can be increased stepwise by adding new generations of ethylene diamine groups on the outer surface. These well-characterized polymeric materials are particularly suited for preparing high molecular weight MRI contrast agents and relaxivity of 35 $mM^{-1}s^{-1}$ per Gd^{3+} ion have been obtained. It should be noted that the relaxivity per metal ion measured for a dendrimeric DTPA polymer of generation six has not been included in Fig. 15.4 as its relaxivity, although high, is lower than predicted for a molecular weight of 139000. This phenomenon is under investigation (WIENER et al. 1994) but it remains obvious that dendrimers are not subjected to segmental motions as are linear polymers and that their overall reorientation motions are the main contribution to the τ_r correlation times of the attached gadolinium chelates. High molecular weight DTPA-dendrimers are intravascular MRI agents and bring about a prolonged vascular enhancement of the relaxivity that should prove useful in angiography.

Multimeric complexes of less well-defined stoichiometry form spontaneously by interaction between a hydrophobic chelate and biological macromolecules (MARTIN et al. 1995). Aggregates stabilized by noncovalent interactions display high relaxivities because of their long τ_r times and could also be useful blood pool agents provided they show no immunologic reactivity, a problem that could also be encountered with dendrimers. A twofold increase in relaxivity is often observed in the presence of albumin and a relaxivity of 53 $mM^{-1}s^{-1}$ has been reported for an adduct between human serum albumin and a GdDOTA chelate substituted by three benzyloxy groups, DOTA(BOM)$_3$, **14** (AIME et al. 1996). This is the highest relaxivity mentioned so far in the literature. As already mentioned, this high relaxivity could be due to an increase in the outer sphere contribution caused by the formation of a water pocket around the metal complex interacting with albumin.

The reticuloendothelial system can be targeted with liposome-based MRI agents and several procedures have been reported for substituting DTPA with long aliphatic chains usually at the cost of a loss in stability of the metal complexes because of the replacement of two or more carboxylic groups by amide functions (KABALKA et al. 1991; KIM et al. 1992). Liposomes are not only useful for imaging the liver but could also be interesting blood pool agents provided they are sufficiently stable and they are not cleared too rapidly from the circulation. To that end, methods have been developed for the synthesis of DTPA ligands with two acetamide arms substituted with long aliphatic chains featuring two polymerizable alkyne groups that are cross-linked by irradiation with ultraviolet light. Polymerizable chains comprising a biotin moiety can be included in the liposomes for coupling with proteins (STORRS et al. 1995).

Two other facts are pertinent at the end of this chapter. Firstly, the bridge covalently linking metal chelates to a synthetic macromolecule should be short and rigid to ensure that all the parts of the structure are rigidly locked with one another and exhibit τ_r values as close as possible. However, very few systematic studies of the influence of the length and rigidity of the bridge have yet been reported (TOTH et al. 1996b). A benzyl thiourea unit has been used by many authors but other entities are probably needed. Secondly, the water exchange time τ_m should be short so as to allow an efficient transfer of relaxivity to the bulk water. Of little or no importance for small rapidly tumbling chelates, τ_m becomes of paramount importance for high molecular weight compounds for which a long τ_m does not allow achievement of the large increase in relaxivity predicted by the Solomon-Bloembergen theory (POWELL et al. 1996). Amide groups instead of the more coordinating carboxylate functions appear to lengthen τ_m and ligands such as DTPA-BMA, **2**, could be less suitable for tethering to macromolecules (AIME et al. 1994; PUBANZ et al. 1995).

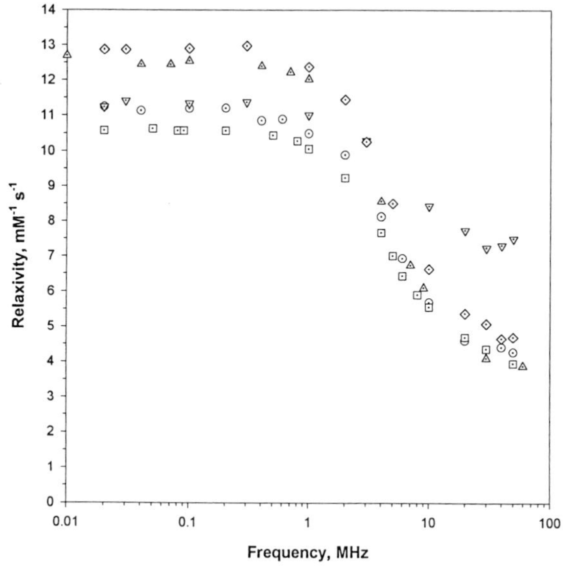

Fig. 15.5. NMR dispersion curves reported in the literature for GdDOTA at 25°C. *Symbols*: ▽, GERALDES et al. (1986); ⊙, MATON (1993); □, AIME et al. (1992a); △, HERNANDEZ et al. (1990); ◇, SHERRY et al. (1989)

15.5 Preparation and Analysis of Gadolinium Complexes

Contrast agents for MRI must be of the utmost purity to avoid toxicity problems. From a more fundamental standpoint, purity is also absolutely mandatory for correct physical measurements. This problem is illustrated in Fig. 15.5, which shows the relaxivity curves published for $GdDOTA^-$ in the literature. The discrepancies between these curves clearly show that appropriate care must be taken when preparing ligands and their metal chelates. Macrocyclic and linear polyamino polyacetic ligands are purified either by ion-exchange chromatography or, in the most difficult cases, by preparative high-pressure liquid chromatography (HPLC) on a reversed-phase support (RENN and MEARES 1992). The isolation of a pure ligand on an ion-exchanger is often performed by a two-step procedure. The ligand in the acid form is added to a sulfonated ion-exchanger and eluted with a diluted NH_4OH aqueous solution. The basic eluate is added to a quaternary ammonium ion-exchanger in the formate form and the sought compound is isolated pure by gradient elution with formic acid solutions. Finally, formic acid is eliminated as an azeotrope. The purity of the ligand can be checked by HPLC (KANG et al. 1993) using a chromophoric group, if the molecule contains such a group, or after addition of copper ions to the eluent.

Gadolinium polyamino polycarboxylic complexes are prepared by reaction of a boiling solution of the ligand in the protonated form with an equimolecular amount of either the metal oxide Gd_2O_3, chloride, $GdCl_3$ or hydroxide, $Gd(OH)_3$. Gadolinium oxide calcined at 1200°C is a standard that can be weighted and used as such for synthesizing complexes although the oxide dissolution by the ligand is often slow. A faster formation of complexes is achieved by adjusting the pH of an equimolecular ligand – $GdCl_3$ mixture with NaOH but then, the final complex solution also contains inorganic salts. A faster complexation reaction also takes place if the protonated ligand is reacted with $Gd(OH)_3$. This hydroxide must be freshly prepared by quantitative precipitation with NaOH of the required amount of $GdCl_3$, itself prepared by dissolution of the calcined oxide in HCl. After filtration, the gelatinous hydroxide precipitate is thoroughly washed with water, transferred with the filter paper into a flask, and reacted with a boiling solution of the ligand. Adding an excess of metal oxide or of hydroxide and filtering the insoluble material after several days of heating is easy but not always safe as tetra- or pentaacids such as DOTA or DTPA contain more protons than are needed for forming 1:1 chelates and dissolve an excess of oxide.

The purity of the chelates must be checked by reversed-phase HPLC using a fluorescence detector to analyze the free Gd^{3+} that might be present as well as other gadolinium-containing species (Kumar et al. 1994b). Should impurities be detected and if crystallization proves ineffective, preparative HPLC or column chromatography on divinylstyrene-based polymeric materials such as Dianion CHP (Mitsubishi) allows the isolation of the purified chelates in large quantities (Dischino et al. 1991).

15.6 Synthesis of Other Linear and Macrocyclic Gadolinium Complexes

The search for more efficient gadolinium-containing MRI contrast agents has not been restricted to polyamino polycarboxylic ligands. Several groups have explored totally different routes while still achieving the high stability and the kinetic inertness that are needed for gadolinium chelates. For instance, TREN-Me-3,2-HOPO, **17** (see Fig. 15.3), complexes Gd^{3+} better than DTPA-BMA, **2**, ($\log K_{ML}$ = 20.3) despite an open structure that allows two water molecules to be directly coordinated to the metal ion. Accordingly, the relaxivity is about 2.5 times that of $GdDTPA^{2-}$ at 20 MHz. Dihydrated Gd^{3+} chelates with similar stabilities and relaxivities have also been obtained with DO3A, **13**, and its analogs (Spirlet et al. 1997; Kumar et al. 1994a) but have not been used for practical purposes as other more stable derivatives are readily available.

Texaphyrins, **18**, are another very interesting class of ligands as they encapsulate lanthanide ions in an array of nearly coplanar nitrogen atoms leaving ample space for water molecules. The relaxivity of the Gd^{3+} complex is very high (19.0 $mM^{-1}s^{-1}$ at 20 MHz and 25°C) and its kinetics of dissociation is slow. Full experimental details on the synthesis of these ligands and their metal complexes have been reported (Sessler et al. 1993).

15.7 Complexes with Transition Metal Ions

Although gadolinium chelates are by far the most used and most extensively investigated contrast agents in MRI, transition metal complexes should not be overlooked. Divalent manganese and trivalent iron have been chosen for MRI as they exhibit a high magnetic moment and a relatively long electronic relaxation time τ_s, as does gadolinium. However, it is pertinent to note here that the coordination chemistry of the lanthanides is quite different from that of the transition metals. Lanthanides have little or no steric requirements and the geometry of their complexes is essentially governed by the conformational preferences of the ligands; hence the synthesis of so many different complexing agents. By contrast, transition metal ions with their *d* orbitals available for bonding have a strong preference for octahedral or tetrahedral arrangements. When complexed by multidentate ligands, these ions are usually nonhydrated and their relaxivity is thus entirely outer sphere in origin and much lower than in the case of the gadolinium chelates. This deficiency is no longer as significant if transition metal complexes are selectively taken up by a specific organ. This is so in the case of the Mn(II) chelate of DPDP, **19**, a vitamin $\mathbf{B_6}$ analog that is recognized by the membrane transport system of hepatocytes. The stability of this complex is not very high and it dissociates partially in the liver (Gallez et al. 1996), but the release of free Mn(II) seems to have only minor side-effects. The synthesis of ligands akin to DPDP has been reported (Rocklage et al. 1989) and the preparation of its Mn(II) derivatives poses no particular problem. The classical techniques of analytical chemistry can be relied upon for checking the purity of the complexes. Paramagnetic metalloporphyrins are also potential MRI contrast agents and their synthesis and properties have been described (Hernandez and Bryant 1991).

References

Aime S, Botta M, Ermondi G, Fedeli F, Uggeri F (1992a) Synthesis and NMRD studies of Gd complexes of macrocyclic polyamino polycarboxylic ligands bearing β-benzyloxy-α-propionic residues. Inorg Chem 31:1100–1103

Aime S, Anelli PL, Botta M, Fedeli F, Grandi M, Paoli P, Uggeri F (1992b) Synthesis, characterization, and 1/T1 NMRD profiles of gadolinium(III) complexes of monoamide derivatives of DOTA-like ligands. X-ray structure of the 10-[2-[[2-hydroxy-1-(hydroxymethyl)ethyl]amino]-1[(phenylmethoxy)methyl]-2-oxo-ethyl]-1,4,7,10,tetra-azacyclododecane-1,4,7-triacetic acid gadolinium(III) complex. Inorg Chem 31:2422–2428

Aime S, Botta M, Fasano M, Paoletti S, Anelli PL, Uggeri F, Virtuani M (1994) NMR evidence of a long exchange lifetime for the coordinated water in Ln(III)-bis(methyl amide)-DTPA complexes (Ln = Gd, Dy). Inorg Chem 33:4707–4711

Aime S, Botta M, Fasano M, Crich SG, Terreno E (1996) Gd(III) complexes as contrast agents for magnetic resonance imaging: a proton relaxation enhancement study of the interaction with human serum albumin. J Biol Inorg Chem 1:312–319

Ansari MH, Ahmad M, Dicke KA (1993) Synthesis of 2-(p-aminobenzyl) derivatives of 1,4,7-triazacyclononane-*N,N′,N″*-triacetic acid (NOTA) and 1,4,7,10-tetraazacyclododecane- *N,N′,N″,N‴*-tetraacetic acid (DOTA): macro-cyclic bifunctional chelating agents useful for antibodies labeling. Bioorgan Med Chem Lett 3:1067–1070

Athey PS, Kiefer GE (1996) Process for preparing polyazamacrocycles. Patent Application WO 95/14726:1–53

Brasch RC (1994) New developments in MRI contrast enhancement. Magma 2:161–168

Brechbiel MW, Gansow OA, Atcher RW, Schlom J, Esteban J, Simpson DE, Colcher D (1986) Synthsis of 1-(*p*-isothiocyanatobenzyl) derivatives of DTPA and EDTA. Antibody labeling and tumor-imaging studies. Inorg Chem 25:2772–2781

Carvalho JF, Kim SH, Chang CA (1992) Synthesis and Metal Complex Selectivity of Macrocyclic DTPA and EDTA bis(amide) ligands. Inorg Chem 31:4065–4068

Desreux JF (1980) Nuclear magnetic resonance spectroscopy of lanthanide complexes with a tetraacetic tetraaza macrocycle. Unusual conformation properties. Inorg Chem 19:1319–1324

Desreux JF, Jacques V (1995) Role of metal-ligand interactions in the design of MRI contrast agents. In: Berthon G (ed) Handbook of metal-ligand interactions in biological fluids. Dekker, New York, p 1109

Desreux JF, Tweedle MF, Ratsep PC, Wagler TR, Marinelli ER (1994) Hepatobiliary tetraaza macrocyclic magnetic resonance contrast agents. US Pat. 5,358,704:1–22

Dischino DD, Delaney EJ, Enswiler JE, Gaughan GT, Prasad JS, Srivastava SK, Tweedle MF (1991) Synthesis of nonionic chelates useful as contrast agents for magnetic resonance imaging. 1,4,7-tris(carboxymethyl)-10-substituted-1,4,7,10- tetraazacyclododecanes and their corresponding gadolinium chelates. Inorg Chem 30:1265–1269

Dumont A, Jacques V, Qixiu P, Desreux JF (1994) Regioselective synthesis of 1,7-diprotected 1,4,7,10-tetraazacyclododecane and preparation of a dialcohol dicarboxylic macrocyclic ligand. Tetrahedron Lett 35:3707–3710

Gallez B, Bacic G, Swartz HM (1996) Evidence for the dissociation of the hepatobiliary MRI contrast agent Mn-DPDP. Magn Reson Med 35:14–19

Geraldes CFGC, Sherry AD, Brown RD III, Koenig SH (1986) Magnetic field dependence of solvent proton relaxation rates induced by Gd^{3+} and Mn^{2+} complexes of various polyaza macrocyclic ligands: implications for NMR imaging. Magn Reson Med 3:242–250

Hernandez G, Bryant RG (1991) Proton magnetic relaxation of Mn(II) tetra(4-sulphophenyl)porphine ion in water. Bioconjugate Chem 2:394–397

Hernandez G, Tweedle MF, Bryant RG (1990) Proton magnetic relaxation dispersion in aqueous glycerol solutions of Gd(DTPA)2- and Gd(DOTA)-. Inorg Chem 29:5109–5113

Jacques V, Desreux JF (1994) Quantitative two-dimensional EXSY spectroscopy and dynamic behavior of a paramagnetic lanthanide macrocyclic chelate: YbDOTA (DOTA = 1,4,7,10-tetraazacyclododecane-*N,N′,N″,N‴*-tetraacetic acid). Inorg Chem 33:4048–4053

Kabalka GW, Davis MA, Moss TH, et al. (1991) Gadolinium-labeled liposomes containing various amphiphilic GdDTPA derivatives: targeted MRI contrast enhancement agents for the liver. Magn Reson Med 19:406–415

Kang SI, Ranganathan RS, Emswiler JE, Kumar K, Gougoutas JZ, Malley MF, Tweedle MF (1993) Synthesis, characterization, and crystal structure of the gadolinium(III) chelate of (1*R*,4*R*,7*R*)-α, α′, α″-trimethyl-1,4,7,10- tetraazacyclododecane- 1,4,7- triacetic acid (DO3MA). Inorg Chem 32:2912–2918

Keana JF, Mann JS (1990) Chelating ligands functionalized for facile attachment to biomolecules - a convenient route to 4-isothiocyanatobenzyl derivatives of diethylenetriaminepentaacetic acid and ethylenediaminetetraacetic acid. J Org Chem 55:2868–2871

Kepert DL (1982) Inorganic stereochemistry. Springer, Berlin Heidelberg New York, pp 1–227

Kim SK, Pohost GM, Elgavish GA (1992) Gadolinium complexes of [(myristoyloxy)propyl]diethylenediaminetetraacetate: new lipophilic, fatty acyl conjugated NMR contrast agents. Bioconjugate Chem 3:20–26

Kovacs Z, Sherry AD (1995) A general synthesis of 1,7-disubstituted 1,4,7,10-tetraazacyclododecanes. J Chem Soc Chem Commun 185–186

Kruper WJ, Rudolf PR, Langhoff CA (1993) Unexpected selectivity in the alkylation of polyazamacrocycles. J Org Chem 58:3869–3876

Kumar K, Chang CA, Tweedle MF (1993) Equilibrium and kinetic studies of some lanthanide complexes of macrocyclic polyaminopolycarboxylates. Inorg Chem 32:587–593

Kumar K, Chang CA, Francesconi LC, Dischino DD, Malley MF, Gougoutas JZ, Tweedle MF (1994a) Synthesis, stability, and structure of gadolinium(III) and yttrium(III) macrocyclic poly(amino carboxylates). Inorg Chem 33:3567–3575

Kumar K, Sukumaran KV, Tweedle MF (1994b) Determination of free Gd^{3+} as a cyclohexanediaminetetraacetic acid complex by reversed-phase HPLC in ionic gadolinium(III) chelates. Anal Chem 66:295–299

Lauffer RB, Brady TJ (1985) Preparation and water relaxation properties of proteins labeled with paramagnetic metal chelates. Magn Reson Imaging 3:11–16

Manabe Y, Longley C, Furmanski P (1986) High-level conjugation of chelating agents onto immunoglobulins: use of an intermediary poly(L-lysine)-diethylenetriaminepentaacetic acid carrier. Biochim Biophys Acta 883:460–467

Martin VV, Ralston WH, Hynes MR, Keana JF (1995) Gadolinium(III) di- and tetrachelates designed for in vivo noncovalent complexation with plasma proteins: a novel molecular design for blood pool MRI contrast enhancing agents. Bioconjugate Chem 6:616–623

Maton F (1993) Etude de complexes paramagnétiques en solution aqueuse. Caractérisation physico-chimique par relaxométrie protonique a champ variable (PhD Thesis). University of Mons-Hainaut, Belgium

McMurry TJ, Brechbiel MW, Kumar K, Gansow OA (1992) Convenient synthesis of bifunctional tetraaza macrocycles. Bioconjugate Chem 3:108–117

Mishra AK, Draillard K, Faivre-Cahuvet A, Gestin JF, Curtet C, Chatal J-F (1996a) A convenient, novel approach for the synthesis of polyaza macrocyclic bifunctional chelating agents. Tetrahedron Lett 37:7515–7518

Mishra AK, Gestin JF, Benoist E, Faivre-Chauvet A, Chatal JF (1996b) Simplified synthesis of the bifunctional chelating agent 2-(4-aminobenzyl)-1,4,7,10-tetraazacyclodecane-*N,N′,N″,N‴*-tetraacetic acid. New J Chem 20:585–588

Moi MK, Meares CF, DeNardo SJ (1988) The peptide way to macrocyclic bifunctional chelating agents: synthesis of 2-(*p*-nitrobenzyl)-1,4,7,10-tetraazacyclododecane-*N,N',N'',N'''*-tetraacetic acid and study of its yttrium(III) complex. J Am Chem Soc 110:6266–6267

Powell DH, Ni Dhubhghaill ON, Pubanz D, Helm L, Lebedev YS, Schlaepfer W, Merbach AE (1996) Structural and dynamic parameters obtained from 17O NMR, EPR, and NMR studies of monomeric and dimeric Gd^{3+} complexes of interest in magnetic resonance imaging: an integrated and theoretically self-consistent approach. J Am Chem Soc 118:9333–9346

Prasad JS, Okuniewicz FJ, Delaney EJ, Dischino DD (1991) Synthesis of gadolinium (+/–)-10-(1-hydroxypropan-2-yl)-1,4,7,10-tetraazacyclododecane-1,4,7-triyltriacetate via tribenzyl 1,4, 7,10-tetraazacyclododecane-1,4,7-tricarboxylate. J Chem Soc Perkin Trans I:3329–3332

Pubanz D, Gonzalez G, Powell DH, Merbach AE (1995) Unexpectedly large change of water exchange rate and mechanism on [Ln(DTPA-BMA)(H_2O)] complexes along the lanthanide(III) series. Inorg Chem 34:4447–4453

Ranganathan RS, Pillai R, Ratsep PC, Shukla R, Tweedle MF, Zhang X (1995) Enhanced relaxivity monomeric and multimeric compounds. Patent Application WO 95/31444:1–77

Ranganathan RS, Kang SI, Ratsep PC, Pillai KMR, Shukla R, Zhang X, Tweedle M (1994) New multimeric MRI contrast agents. Proceedings of the 4th Special Topic Seminar of the European Magnetic Resonance Forum, Santiago de Compostela, Spain, 28–30 September 1994, European Magnetic Resonance Forum, Mons, Belgium, pp 17–28

Renn O, Meares CF (1992) Large-scale synthesis of the bifunctional chelating agent 2-(*p*-nitrobenzyl)-1,4,7,10-tetraazacyclododecane-*N,N',N'',N'''*-tetraacetic acid, and the determination of its enantiomeric purity by chiral chromatography. Bioconj Chem 3:563–569

Richman JE, Atkins TJ (1974) Nitrogen analogs of crown ethers. J Am Chem Soc 96:2268–2271

Rocklage SM, Cacheris WP, Quay SC, Hahn FE, Raymond KN (1989) Manganese (II) *N,N'*-dipyridoxylthylenediamine-*N,N'*-diacetate 5,5'-bis(phosphate). Synthesis and characterization of a paramagnetic chelate for magnetic resonance imaging enhancement. Inorg Chem 28:477–485

Runge VM, Wells JW, Williams NM (1995) Comparison of gadolinium Cy(2)DOTA, a new hepatobiliary agent, and gadolinium HP-DO3A, an extracellular agent, in healthy liver and metastatic disease. Invest Radiol 30:123–130

Schaeffer M, Meyer D, Beaute S, Doucet D (1991) A new macrocyclic MRI contrast agent: Gd MCTA complex. Magn Reson Med 22:238–241

Sessler JL, Mody TD, Hemmi GW, Lynch V (1993) Synthesis and structural characterization of lanthanide(III) texaphyrins. Inorg Chem 32:3175–3187

Sherry AD, Cacheris WP, Kuan K-T (1988) Stability constants for Gd^{3+} binding to model DTPA-conjugates and DTPA-proteins: implications for their use as magnetic resonance contrast agents. Magn Reson Med 8:180–190

Sherry AD, Brown RD, III, Geraldes CFGC, Koenig SH, Kuan K-T, Spiller M (1989) Synthesis and characterization of the gadolinium(3+) complex of DOTA-propylamide: a model DOTA-protein. Inorg Chem 28:620–622

Shukla R, Fernandez M, Pillai RK, Raganathan R, Ratsep PC, Zhang X, Tweedle MF (1996) Design of conformationally rigid dimeric MRI agents. Magn Reson Med 35:928–931

Spirlet M-R, Rebizant J, Desreux JF, Loncin MF (1984) Crystal and molecular structure of sodium aquo(1,4,7,10-tetraazacyclododecane-1,4,7,10-tetraacetato) europate(III) tetrahydrate, NAEuDOTA.H_2O).4H_2O, and its relevance to NMR studies of the conformational behavior of the lanthanide complexes formed by the macrocyclic ligand DOTA. Inorg Chem 23:359–363

Spirlet M-R, Rebizant J, Wang XY, et al. (1997) The gadolinium(III) chelate of 1-oxa-4,7,10-triazacyclododecane-4,7,10-triacetic acid. Formation of polymeric chains in the solid state and relaxivity properties. J Chem Soc, Dalton Trans 497–500

Storrs RW, Troper FD, Li HY, et al. (1995) Paramagnetic polymerized liposomes as new recirculating MR agents. J Magn Reson Imaging 5:719–724

Toth E, Kiraly R, Platzek J, Raduchel BE, Brucher E (1996a) Equilibrium and kinetic studies on complexes of 10-[2,3-dihydroxy-(1-hydroxymethyl)-propyl]-1,4,7,10-tetraazacyclododecane-1,4,7-triacetate. Inorg Chim Acta 249:191–199

Toth E, Pubanz D, Vauthey S, Helm L, Merbach AE (1996b) The role of water exchange in attaining maximum relaxivities for dendrimeric MRI contrast agents. Chem Eur J 2:1607–1615

Uggeri F, Aime S, Anelli PL, et al. (1995) Novel contrast agents for magnetic resonance. Synthesis, and characterization of the ligand BOPTA and its Ln(III)-complexes [Ln = Gd, La, and Lu]. X-ray structure of disodium TPS-9-145337286-c-s-[4-carboxy-5,8,11- tris(carboxymethyl)-1-phenyl-2-oxa-5,8,11-triaazatridecan-13-oato(5'')]gadolinate(2'') in mixture with its enantiomer. Inorg Chem 34:633–642

Wang XY, Jin TZ, Comblin V, Lopez-Mut A, Merciny E, Desreux JF (1992) A kinetic investigation of the lanthanide DOTA chelates. Stability and rates of formation and of dissociation of a macrocyclic gadolinium(III) polyaza polycarboxylic MRI contrast agent. Inorg Chem 31:1095–1098

Wedeking P, Kumar K, Tweedle MF (1992) Dissociation of gadolinium chelates in mice: relationship to chemical characteristics. Magn Reson Imaging 10:641–648

Wiener EC, Brechbiel MW, Brothers H, Magin RL, Gansow OA, Tomalia DA, Lauterbur PC (1994) Dendrimer-based metal chelates: a new class of magnetic resonance imaging contrast agents. Magn Reson Med 31:1–8

16 Preparation and Structure-Activity Relationships of Particulate Magnetic Agents

A. Nævestad, S.L. Fossheim, and A.K. Fahlvik

CONTENTS

16.1 Introduction

Contrast agents administered systemically will distribute in the body as a function of the intrinsic properties of the substances. Conventional low molecular weight, hydrophilic agents are normally distributed throughout the extracellular compartment of the body. A possible way of achieving site-specific contrast agent delivery is by means of particulate contrast materials or particulate carrier systems for water-soluble contrast agents. The distribution of particulate agents to specific tissue sites can be considered in terms of their physicochemical properties as well as the various biological processes involved. The purpose of this chapter is to present an overview of preparation methods and to highlight important structure-activity relationships for selected parenterally applied particulate MRI contrast agents, paramagnetic liposomes, and superparamagnetic iron oxides (SPIOs).

The "structure" of a particulate agent is given by its physicochemical features such as particle size, surface charge, and surface composition. The "activity" of the particulate agent is determined by its biodistribution, diagnostic potential, and tolerability. All these factors can be optimized (for a given particulate agent) by selecting the appropriate particle design and preparation methods. The most striking feature of the particulates is their ability to, actively or passively, distribute to specific sites, thereby creating a high local concentration of the agent. In addition to allowing significant variation and flexibility in composition and size, the surface of a particulate agent will to a large extent determine its biocompatibility and general safety profile. To date, several types of particulate paramagnetic and superparamagnetic compounds have been investigated as potential MRI contrast agents, mainly for hepatosplenic imaging.

Manganese (Mn) sulfide and gadolinium (Gd) phytate were the first studied paramagnetic particulates (Chilton et al. 1984; Engelstad et al. 1984), followed by Gd oxide particles (Burnett et al. 1985) and GdDTPA-labeled starch microspheres (Rongved et al. 1991). Mn carbonate particles (Wisner et al. 1995), polyethyleneglycol (PEG)-coated Mn hydroxyapatite particles (Adzamli et al. 1997), and dysprosium-DTPA starch microspheres (Fossheim et al. 1999) have recently been investigated. However, the most widely used particulate carrier for paramagnetic substances has been the liposome (Unger et al. 1994; Schwendener 1994). Most of the research on paramagnetic particles has focused on their efficacy as a positive liver agent. However, due to confinement within the liver macrophages, no positive contrast enhancement has been observed for GdDTPA starch microspheres and liposomal GdHPDO3A (Fahlvik et al. 1990a; Fossheim et al. 1995). Such particles have shown their potential as liver susceptibility (negative) agents. Recently, new applications have arisen for PEG-coated paramagnetic liposomes such as MR angiography and lymph node imaging (Trubetskoy et al. 1995; Schwendener 1994). Traditionally, SPIO particles have been used in MRI as negative contrast agents for the gastrointestinal and hepatosplenic ar-

A. Nævestad, MSc, Department of Medicinal Chemistry, School of Pharmacy, P.O.Box 1177, Blindern, N-0316 Oslo, Norway
S.L. Fossheim, PhD, Nycomed Imaging AS, P.O.Box 4220 Torshow, N-0401 Oslo, Norway
A.K. Fahlvik, PhD, Nycomed Imaging AS, P.O.Box 4220 Torshov, N-0401 Oslo, Norway

eas. Their applications are being extended into new areas such as lymph node, bone marrow, heart, kidney, and brain imaging. Ultrasmall SPIOs with a surface structure giving extended circulation time and exhibiting a low r_2/r_1 relaxivity ratio as well as a high r_1 value, have also shown the ability to act as positive blood pool contrast agents (Chambon et al. 1993).

16.2 Preparation Methods

16.2.1 Paramagnetic Particles

Particles can be classified into nonliposomal solid particles and liposomes. As this chapter focuses on liposomes as carriers for paramagnetic agents, the synthesis of nonliposomal paramagnetic particles will be described only briefly.

16.2.1.1 Nonliposomal Particles

Solid particles are often prepared by precipitation of the paramagnetic ions in alkaline solution or by complexation with a suitable ligand, forming water-insoluble particles. For instance, Gd oxide particles were prepared by titrating a $GdCl_3$ solution with a sodium hydroxide solution to pH 7 followed by sonication (Burnett et al. 1985). Mn carbonate particles were prepared by controlled precipitation of Mn chloride and sodium carbonate (Wisner et al. 1995). In the synthesis of Mn hydroxyapatite particles, ammonium hydroxide was added to an alkaline solution containing Mn and calcium nitrate, ammonium dihydrogen phosphate, and phosphoric acid. The resulting slurry was size stabilized by addition of modified PEG and particles were obtained by high-pressure microfluidization (Adzamli et al. 1997). Alternatively, particulate attachment of the paramagnetic ions is accomplished by complexation to a ligand which is covalently linked to the particle surface. Such a synthetic strategy has been employed in the preparation of cross-linked GdDTPA starch microspheres (Rongved et al. 1991). In essence, the bis-anhydride of DTPA was reacted in anhydrous dimethylsulfoxide with cross-linked starch particles in various ratios of DTPA to glucose units. The suspension was agitated for 24 h and cooled in an ice-water bath followed by addition of water. The particles were washed several times by alternate suspension in water and centrifugation. A slight molar deficit of Gd chloride was added at pH 6, and the particulate suspension was agitated for several hours followed by dialysis. A similar synthetic route has been employed for the preparation of GdDTPA-dextran particles (Gibby et al. 1989).

16.2.1.2 Liposomes

Liposomes are versatile systems, where, for example, the size and surface properties can be easily varied by selection of a suitable preparation procedure and an appropriate combination of phospholipids (PLs) and other components. However, there are some inherent disadvantages associated with liposomes such as poor stability, safety issues, and scale-up problems. Five basic methods can be employed for liposome preparation (Lichtenberg and Barenholz 1988), based on: (a) mechanical action, (b) replacement of organic solvents by aqueous media, (c) detergent removal, (d) size transformation and fusion, and (e) pH adjustment. The key step for most methods is the hydration of the PLs, the membrane constituents of the liposome. Liposomes are first formed when PLs are dispersed in excess water above the gel-to-liquid crystal phase transition temperature (T_m) of the PLs. The resulting liposome dispersions are often heterogeneous with respect to size, number of bilayers (lamella), and morphology. Liposomes are generally classified into three general classes: multivesicular vesicles (MVVs), multilamellar vesicles (MLVs), and unilamellar vesicles. The last-mentioned are further divided on the basis of size: liposomes under 100 nm are considered small unilamellar vesicles (SUVs), while those larger than 100 nm are classified as large unilamellar vesicles (LUVs) (Talsma and Crommelin 1992).

Multilamellar vesicles are easily prepared by the thin film hydration method. Briefly, PLs are dissolved in a volatile organic solvent or a solvent mixture. To achieve high biological and chemical stability, saturated PLs with a T_m above 37°C are employed. The predominant PL is often a neutral species such as phosphatidylcholine (PC), but negatively charged PLs, like phosphatidylserine (PS) or phosphatidylglycerol (PG), may be added in small amounts to prevent liposome aggregation. The organic solvents are removed under reduced pressure, depositing a thin lipid film on the glass wall. The lipid film is hydrated under mechanical agitation with an appropriate aqueous phase containing dissolved solutes. If high T_m PLs are used, the aqueous phase should be prewarmed and the vortexing and subsequent swelling should be performed at a temperature above T_m. The MLVs are usually subjected to several freeze-thaw cycles, a process which increases the trapping volume (ml of intraliposomal volume/mol PL) (LICHTENBERG and BARENHOLZ 1988). The hydration time, agitation rate, and thickness of the lipid film (surface area) are parameters of importance for the liposome quality and influence the type of liposome formed (size, lamellarity, and trapping volume). Although thin film hydration is easily carried out on a small scale, problems relating to limitations of surface area are encountered at a manufacturing scale. An alternative is the use of spray-dried or lyophilized PLs and lipid hydration is accomplished by adding the PLs to the aqueous phase under stirring.

The resulting MLVs are large with a broad size distribution and require size reduction by mechanical treatment such as extrusion or sonication. Extrusion consists in forcing under pressure the MLV dispersion through membrane filters with a well-defined pore size by an inert gas in high-pressure cells (extruders). The MLVs must be extruded at temperatures of at least 10°C above T_m (NAYAR et al. 1989). The extrusion technique is simple and produces liposomes with a narrow size distribution, but is also time consuming when SUVs composed of saturated PLs at high lipid concentration (>100 mg/ml) are desired. Extrusion is the method of choice for the production of well-defined LUVs on a small scale. Sonication of MLVs is performed either in a bath sonicator or with a probe immersed in the sample. Probe sonication is the most widely used method for the preparation of SUVs on a small scale.

From a pharmaceutical point of view, an optimal liposomal preparation route gives high trapping efficiency (ratio between the concentration of liposome-associated material and lipid concentration), produces well-defined liposomes, and is amenable to scale-up. Other factors to be considered when selecting a preparation method are the type of liposome desired and the properties of the active ingredient.

For liposomal paramagnetic agents, the contrast material can, depending upon its properties, be (a) encapsulated into the aqueous phase of the liposome if hydrophilic, (b) incorporated into the liposome membrane through hydrophobic interactions if lipophilic, (c) intercalated within the membrane if amphiphatic, or (d) attached by a chemical bond to the surface of the PL membrane (TALSMA and CROMMELIN 1992). Table 16.1 lists some preparation and formulation methods of paramagnetic liposomes.

Table 16.1. Preparation methods and physicochemical properties of selected paramagnetic liposomes

Preparation method	Liposome formulation	Paramagnetic substance	Liposome size (nm)	Relaxivities $(s^{-1}\ mM^{-1})$[c]		References
				r_1	r_2	
Thin film hydration sonication	PC/Chol/PE-PEG (2%)[a]	GdDTPA-PE, membrane attached	205	10.1[d]		TRUBETSKOY et al. (1995)
	PC/Chol/PE-PEG (5%)[a]	GdDTPA-PE, membrane attached	205	16.0[d]		TRUBETSKOY et al. (1995)
Thin film hydration extrusion	EPC/Chol	GdDTPA, encapsulated	70	2.60	2.70	UNGER et al. (1994)
	HPC/HPS	GdHPDO3A, encapsulated	274	0.10	0.30	FOSSHEIM et al. (1995)
	DPPC/DPPG	GdHPDO3A, encapsulated	242	0.30	0.70	FOSSHEIM et al. (1995)
	EPC/DOPE	GdDTPA-SE, membrane intercalated	50	22.5		TILCOCK et al. (1992)
	EPC/DOPE	GdDTPA-SE, membrane intercalated	400	21.0		TILCOCK et al. (1992)
	EPC/DTPA-PE (12.5%)[b]	GdDTPA-PE[e], membrane attached	<200	21.0[d]		GRANT et al. (1989)
	EPC/DTPA-PE (25%)[b]	GdDTPA-PE[e], membrane attached	<200	15.0[d]		GRANT et al. (1989)
	SPC/Chol	GdBOPTA, membrane incorporated	104	4.2		SCHWENDENER (1994)
	SPC/PE-PEG/Chol	GdBOPTA, membrane incorporated	132	3.9		SCHWENDENER (1994)
	EPC/Chol	$MnCl_2$, encapsulated	≈100	30.3	65.1	UNGER et al. (1994)
	EPC/Chol	MnEDTA-DDP, membrane intercalated	≈100	30.3	36.7	UNGER et al. (1994)
	EPC/Chol	MnEDTA-DDP, membrane intercalated	≈400	5.70	7.2	UNGER et al. (1994)
	EPC	MnHSA, encapsulated	309	69.70		NAVON et al. (1986)

Chol, cholesterol; DPPC, dipalmitoylphosphatidylcholine; DPPG, dipalmitoylphospatidylglycerol; DOPE, dioleoyl phosphatidylethanolamine; EPC, egg phosphatidylcholine; HPC, hydrogenated phosphatidylcholine; HPS, hydrogenated phosphatidylserine; HSA, human serum albumin; SPC, soy phosphatidylcholine.

[a] Mole %. [b] Weight %. [c] 20 MHz unless otherwise stated. [d] 10 MHz. [e] Obtained in situ by Gd complexation to DTPA-PE.

For water-soluble agents, the trapping efficiency depends on the trapping volume and thereby the liposome size, PL composition, and lamellarity. Studies report a linear relationship between liposome diameter and trapping volume for unilamellar liposomes (Talsma and Crommelin 1992). The preparation of liposome-encapsulated paramagnetic chelates has been extensively described (Unger et al. 1994). Liposome encapsulation of paramagnetic macromolecules, such as Mn bound to human serum albumin, has also been reported (Navon et al. 1986). For liposome membrane-incorporated material, the trapping efficiency depends on the lipophilicity of the material, the PL concentration, and the phase behavior of the membrane (e.g., gel or fluid state). Lipophilic metal chelates such as GdBOPTA have been successfully incorporated into liposomes (Schwendener 1994). Amphiphatic metal chelates such as GdDTPA-stearylester (SE) and MnEDTA-decycloaminodihydroxypropyl (DDP) have been intercalated into the liposome with high efficiency (Kabalka et al. 1988; Unger et al. 1994). For compounds that are covalently bound to the liposome membrane, the availability of binding sites limits the trapping efficiency. The binding of GdDTPA to PLs has been described (Grant et al. 1989). Preformed liposomes containing DTPA-phosphatidylethanolamine (PE) were prepared and $GdCl_3$ was added to the liposome suspension, the complexation of the outer DTPA ligand molecules with Gd being complete. A new class of paramagnetic polymerized liposomes with surface-exposed lanthanide chelates has recently been introduced (Storrs et al. 1995). The liposomes were prepared from a polymerizable lipid molecule derivatized with DTPA chelates and diacetylene moieties in the hydrophobic acyl chains, which cross-linked upon ultraviolet irradiation. Frequently, liposome encapsulation or incorporation is incomplete and extraliposomal contrast material is removed by gel filtration, ultracentrifugation, ultrafiltration, or dialysis (Lichtenberg and Barenholz 1988).

16.2.2 Superparamagnetic Iron Oxide Particles

Pharmaceutically applied SPIOs are composed of iron oxide crystals coated with or embedded in polymeric materials to avoid uncontrollable aggregation of the magnetic crystals. The active ingredient of the SPIO particles is iron oxide crystals of magnetite (Fe_3O_4), maghemite (γ-Fe_2O_3), or their intermediates. Magnetite and maghemite have the same basic crystal structure, where cubic close packed oxygen ions make a lattice of tetrahedral and octahedral sites with iron ions distributed in the lattice (Schwertmann and Cornell 1991). Each SPIO particle may comprise one or more iron oxide crystals. A superparamagnetic behavior is present for iron oxide crystals of single domain size, which is below about 30 nm (Dunlop 1973). The lower threshold size for superparamagnetic behavior of the crystals has not been fully explored. The preparation method used for the SPIO determines the size of each individual iron oxide crystal, the number of crystals per particle, and the dispersity of the crystals within the carrier particle. As all these factors influence the magnetic properties of the SPIOs, the selection of synthetic route is crucial for the outcome. The degree of dispersity describes the crystal appearance as either several crystals dispersed within the coating material or a core composed of agglomerated crystals. Classically, SPIOs used in MRI are prepared by co-precipitation of magnetite in the presence of a coating material. Magnetite may also be precipitated directly without the presence of a coating material. Independently of the precipitation method, magnetite is formed in two steps:

Step 1

$$FeCl_2 + 2FeCl_3 \xrightarrow{\text{Base}} Fe(OH)_2 + Fe_2O_3{\cdot}xH_2O$$

Step 2

$$Fe(OH)_2 + Fe_2O_3{\cdot}xH_2O \longrightarrow Fe_3O_4$$

The precipitate formed in step 1 does not exhibit superparamagnetic behavior as the iron oxide/hydroxides formed are of paramagnetic nature. The amount and rate of ammonia or other bases added influence both the reaction rate of step 2 and the size of the magnetite crystal (Ronay 1982). A sufficient amount of base is important in order to maintain pH above 8 and ensure a complete transformation of iron oxide/hydroxide to magnetite (Schwertmann and Cornell 1991). An overview of preparation methods and physicochemical properties of various SPIO formulations is presented in Table 16.2. The saturation magnetization (M_{sat}), relaxivities (r_1, r_2), and the r_2/r_1 ratio are important factors describing the SPIO properties. For dextran-coated SPIOs it has been shown that a decreased dextran-to-iron ratio increases the iron oxide core size and thereby also the r_2 and r_2/r_1 ratio (Chouly et al. 1996).

Table 16.2. Preparation methods and physicochemical properties of selected SPIO formulations

Preparation method and SPIO structure	SPIO formulation	Coating material	Crystal size (nm)	Particle size (nm)	Relaxivities (s^{-1} mM^{-1}) r_1	r_2	r_2/r_1	M_{sat} (emu/g FeOx)	References
Direct precipitation; iron oxide cores of agglomerated multi-crystals (polycrystalline)	AMI-121	Siloxane	7.9–8.8[a]	300	3.2	72	22.5		JUNG and JACOBS (1995)
	HEP-SPIO	Heparin	9.3[a]	66[b] and 75[c]	35.5	270	7.6	70	SJØGREN et al. (1997)
	Anti-CEA SMP	Poly (Glu, Lys, Tyr 6 : 3 : 1) with anti-CEA mAb conjug.	9.6 ± 0.8	50		300			TIEFENAUER et al. (1993)
Co-precipitation; individual crystals dispersed in a polymer matrix (polycrystalline)	MSM	Starch	10	400	17	218	13		FAHLVIK et al. (1990b)
	AMI-25	Dextran T-10	4.8–5.6[a]	36.1 ± 15.6[b] 58.5 ± 185.8[c]	23.9	98	4.1		JUNG and JACOBS (1995)
	SHU 555A	Carboxydextran	4.2	61	24	190	8		HAMM et al. (1994), REIMER et al. (1995)
	MD	Dextran T-40	5–20	49	44	368	8.4		POULIQUEN et al. (1991)
	PEG-magnetite	Difunctionalized PEG	5	147	2.6	466	177		SUZUKI et al. (1996)
	HS	Arabinogalactan		54	21	52	2.5		JOSEPHSON et al. (1990)
Fractionation (monocrystalline)	AMI-227	Dextran T-10	5.8–6.2[a]	21[b] or 30[c]	22.7	53	2.3		JUNG and JACOBS (1995)
	USPIO	Dextran		11.4 ± 6.3	21.6	44.1	2.0	42	WEISSLEDER et al. (1990)
	AG-USPIO	Arabinogalactan		12 ± 6.5	23	49	2		REIMER et al. (1990)
	MION-37	Dextran T-10	4.6	22 ± 6	16	35	2.1		PAPISOV et al. (1993), WEISSLEDER et al. (1995)
	MION-46	Dextran T-10	4.6	21 ± 3	15	35	2.1	48	WEISSLEDER et al. (1995)

Anti-CEA SMP, Anti-carcinoembryonic antigen superparamagnetic particles; MSM, magnetic starch microspheres; HS, hepatic selective; MION, monocrystalline iron oxide nanopreparation.
[a] Determined by x-ray diffraction.
[b] Determined by dynamic light scattering, number-weighted distribution.
[c] Determined by dynamic light scattering, volume-weighted distribution.

16.2.2.1
SPIOs Prepared by Direct Precipitation

SPIO crystals can be prepared by direct precipitation when ammonia or other bases are added to an aqueous solution of ferric and ferrous iron without the presence of a stabilizer or polymer (MÜLLER et al. 1996; SJØGREN et al. 1997). The immediately formed crystals appear as µm-to-mm sized aggregates and are easily collected by use of a magnet. The excess of iron salts, ammonia, and sodium chloride is removed by washing with purified water until pH reaches 6–7. The dispersion is further homogenized by sonication in the presence of a coating material to disperse the aggregates into stable coated and nm-sized particles containing multiple crystals. The iron oxide crystals can be stabilized either by charge or sterically or by a combination of both. Polyelectrolytes such as heparinoid polymers and polyamino acids of a wide molecular weight range are well suited as coating materials (FAHLVIK et al. 1996). A high content of positively or negatively charged groups is important to ensure adsorption and multiple bond attachment of the polymer to the iron oxide crystal surface. Bonding is believed to be mainly of an electrostatic nature by interactions between charged functional groups on the polymer and the oxide and hydroxide groups of the iron oxide surface. Alternatively, pH adjustment can also be used to electrostatically stabilize the particles above or below their isoelectrical point (SONTUM et al. 1996). Iron oxide crystals may also be stabilized by coating materials with only one attachment point to the iron oxide surface (Pilgrimm 1994). In this case the binding group of the coating material has to be carefully chosen based on the affinity of the functional group for the iron oxide surface. Neutral polymers such as unmodified starch or dextran are unsuitable as stabilizers and coating materials when added to already formed iron oxide crystals. The advantage of the direct precipitation is the high flexibility in the selection of coating material. A high number of polymers and low molecular weight substances can be applied to tailor-make the SPIO formulation.

16.2.2.2 SPIOs Prepared by Co-Precipitation

Conventional SPIO formulations are prepared by modifications of the so-called Molday method, which implies co-precipitation of iron oxide and a coating material from an aqueous solution of iron salts and polymer by addition of an alkaline solution (Molday and Mackenzie 1982). The formed crystals are stabilized in the process by the coating material, which may also increase the viscosity of the reaction medium. Due to incomplete crystal formation (step 1) additional energy, e.g., in form of heating, is needed to form superparamagnetic crystals (step 2). The crystal size of the dispersion is generally homogeneous while the overall particle size distribution is relatively broad. This is due to the different numbers of iron oxide crystals and amount of polymer per particle. To achieve an optimal product, the co-precipitation method must be optimized with respect to the stoichiometric quantities of iron salts, pH, temperature, and type and amount of polymer. Hydrophilic polysaccharides such as starch and dextran are commonly used for co-precipitation. However, materials such as difunctionalized PEGs are also useful for co-precipitation (Suzuki et al. 1995). A special case of co-precipitation is the preparation of magnetoferritin. Magnetoferritin is composed of maghemite cores, oxidized from the initially precipitated magnetite cores, within an apoferritin shell. Apoferritin is an endogeneous iron storage protein and can be considered as a rigid matrix or stabilizer molecule during precipitation of magnetite. The product is, unlike the other co-precipitated SPIOs, homogeneous in size and entirely monocrystalline (Meldrum et al. 1992).

Irrespective of the synthetic route, the particle size distribution of SPIOs is relatively inhomogeneous and further purification is needed. The SPIO dispersions can be refined and purified by dialysis, ultrafiltration, or gel filtration chromatography (Pouliquen et al. 1991). Sedimentation or centrifugation can also be valuable methods to separate different fractions of the particles, at least on a limited scale (Sjøgren et al.1997).

16.3 Formulation

A pharmaceutical particulate product for parenteral administration demands high colloidal stability during both storage and use. Additionally, it must be compatible with the biological milieu, e.g., isotonic and isohydric. The design of the formulation depends upon the properties and applications of the product.

All SPIOs are coated with polymeric materials that provide electrostatic and/or steric stabilization. Charge stabilization of liposomes is achieved by imparting a surface charge to the liposome membrane, which is accomplished by employing negatively charged PLs. Polymeric coating materials, such as PEG, are also used to prevent liposome fusion or aggregation by steric hindrance.

Uncharged particles are normally formulated in saline or in other osmotic active electrolytes. Particles stabilized by charge cannot be formulated in electrolyte solution as salts induce particle aggregation. Uncharged excipients such as glucose or sucrose are employed for such particles. Sterically stabilized SPIOs are more robust and may be formulated using electrolytes or sugars. They can also be lyophilized, in contrast to electrostatically stabilized SPIOs.

Liposomes of high chemical and physical stability are normally obtained by using cholesterol and saturated PLs with a T_m above 37°C; in practice PLs with a carbon chain length of 16 or more are used. This is a crucial feature for liposome-encapsulated material as the risk of leakage during storage and also in vivo is minimized. Lyophilized formulations to be reconstituted before use may also be prepared to improve the shelf-life stability (Talsma and Crommelin 1993). Ready-to-use particulate formulations are, however, always considered advantageous. The concentration of the particles is important for the intended clinical applications. As an example, a small volume of highly concentrated SPIOs can be bolus injected while relatively diluted SPIOs are limited to infusion.

16.4 Surface Modification and Targeting Perspectives

From biomaterial science it is well known that the biological responses to foreign surfaces are related to the nature of the introduced surface. After intravascular administration, the surface of the particles, corresponding to the dosage of up to several m^2/kg body weight, will interact with blood proteins (opsonins) and other blood components. The interaction pattern will affect both the biokinetics and the biocompatability of the particle. Therefore, particles have to be carefully designed dependent upon their target application and to ensure safety. The biocompatibility of the particles needs to be evaluated to avoid adverse effects in humans. Conventional particles, when administered intravascularly, are readily opsonized and phagocytosed by the macrophages of liver and spleen, thereby having a short blood residence time. The clearance profile and kinetics can, however, be varied by surface and size modification of the particles. The macrophage uptake is faster and more efficient for large and charged particles.

The structure of negatively charged PLs also influences the liver uptake, e.g., PS promotes a higher uptake than PG (Senior 1987). Uptake of liposomes by hepatocytes requires a particle size less than the pore diameter of the endothelial fenestrations in liver sinusoids. Small liposomes (≤70 nm) have shown uptake into hepatocytes (Vion-Dury et al. 1989). For dextran-coated SPIOs, synthesized by slightly different co-precipitation conditions, various surface structures have been obtained (Weissleder et al. 1995). The MION-37 preparation, having partly exposed iron hydroxide moieties as well as dextran, adsorbed all blood proteins. MION-46 with a more dense coat of dextran, mainly adsorbed the third component of complement and had a significantly longer circulation time in blood even though the two preparations had similar particle and core size as well as dextran content. A total change of blood clearance rate and biodistribution was achieved by immobilization of poly-lysine (10 kDa) on the particle surface of MION-46 (Papisov et al. 1993). The liver uptake increased threefold when dextran-coated SPIOs, with a neutral surface charge, were chemically modified to charged SPIOs, having a surface charge between −30 and +20 mV (Chouly et al. 1996).

Coating with hydrophilic polymers such as PEG, which prevents blood protein interactions and particle recognition by macrophages, prolongs the blood residence time (Couvreur et al. 1995). The use of PEG or similar coating materials has widened the horizon of liposome applications and opened the way for passive or active targeting to other tissues. Modification of the particulate surface, such as coupling of ligands with high affinity for cell surface receptors, may result in active targeting to selected tissues (Lasic 1993; Weissleder et al. 1995). Paramagnetic polymerized liposomes labeled with antibodies against the endothelin integrin receptor, an established angiogenesis marker, have recently shown ability to detect tumor growth in vivo (Sipkins et al. 1997). Arabinogalactan-coated SPIOs were the first formulation for active targeting to hepatocytes (Josephson et al. 1990; Reimer et al. 1990). Alternatively, liver targeting has been achieved by using nonspecific IgG (Weissleder et al. 1991). SPIOs for other targets within the body can be prepared by covalent or noncovalent attachment of vectors such as antibodies and cell adhesion molecules to the particle surface provided the activity of the vector is preserved. A number of possible coupling methods are available. A common technique for SPIOs stabilized by saccharides is to perform a periodate-oxidation of the polymer which reacts with amino groups on the vector to form Schiff's base. The product is subsequently stabilized by reduction (Molday and Mackenzie 1982). Antimyosin Fab attached to MION has been used for targeting to infarcted rabbit myocardium (Weissleder et al. 1992). Also the pancreas has been targeted by MIONs with a noncovalent attached vector, cholecystokinin (Reimer et al. 1994).

16.5 Structure-Activity Relationships

16.5.1 Paramagnetic Particles

Generally, the structure of the paramagnetic particle has a profound impact on its in vitro relaxivity. When designing a liposomal contrast agent, several approaches can be used, depending on the type of agent and application desired. Table 16.1 summarizes certain physicochemical and relaxometric properties of some paramagnetic liposome preparations.

16.5.1.1
Liposome-Encapsulated Contrast Agents

For efficient relaxation enhancement to occur, water molecules have to exchange rapidly between the bulk and the liposome interior which contains the paramagnetic agent. If water diffusion through the membrane were the rate-determining step in this exchange process, it would be expected that, for a given liposome composition, the relaxivity would scale linearly with the surface-area to volume (s/v) ratio (Barsky et al. 1992). Since this ratio is inversely proportional to the radius of the liposome, the water flux across the membrane is greater for smaller liposomes. Consequently, the lifetime of a water molecule inside the liposome (τ) decreases, increasing the in vitro relaxivity. Studies have shown a linear relationship between the r_1 of liposomal GdDTPA and the s/v ratio (Tilcock et al. 1989). However, the value of r_1 will at most be equal to that of nonliposomal metal chelate, which only occurs when fast exchange (short τ) conditions are present. In order to maximize the r_1 of encapsulated agents, the liposome should be composed of PLs in the liquid state rather than in the gel state at physiological temperature. However, leakage of the paramagnetic agent during storage and in vivo is a serious liability for such formulations. To achieve high stability, saturated PLs or sterols are normally used, but the transmembrane water permeability is reduced, which impedes water exchange and decreases the relaxivity. In fact, a 95% reduction in r_1 has been observed upon encapsulation of GdHPDO3A in hydrogenated PC/PS liposomes with a T_m of 50°C (Fossheim et al. 1995). The optimal formulation is obtained when the minimum number of liposomes is used to yield a given contrast enhancement. This is generally accomplished by increasing the internal concentration of the paramagnetic agent within the liposome. However, the internal concentration can only be increased so much before the relaxivity becomes limited by slow water exchange, and the procedure becomes self-defeating (Bačič et al. 1988; Tilcock 1994).

16.5.1.2
Liposome-Intercalated or -Attached Contrast Agents

Improved relaxivities are generally obtained when the paramagnetic agent is intercalated within the membrane or attached covalently to the liposome surface. The main advantage is a lengthened rotational correlation time of the agent that increases the relaxivity at relevant MRI field strengths, if rapid water exchange conditions prevail. Relaxivities in the range of 12–21 $s^{-1} mM^{-1}$ have been reported for surface attached GdDTPA-PE (Grant et al. 1989). However, if the association of the agent to the membrane is not rigid, the agent will exhibit an anisotropic motion which is rapid compared with the rotational correlation time of the liposome itself; the relaxivity increase will then be lower than expected. In such cases, the relaxivity of surface-attached Gd-chelates, under conditions of fast water exchange, has been shown to be invariant with liposome size over a wide range (Tilcock et al. 1992). However, if the relaxivity were exchange limited by use of saturated PLs, the size would affect the relaxation contribution of Gd-chelates associated to the inner leaflet of the liposome membrane.

16.5.2
Superparamagnetic Particles

The M_{sat}, r_1, r_2, and the r_2/r_1 ratio are important factors for predicting the imaging efficacy of SPIOs. M_{sat} is determined by the iron oxide composition described by the stoichiometric amount of iron and oxygen and the crystal structure. The maximum M_{sat} for iron oxides is 92 emu/g iron oxide for Fe_3O_4 while γ-Fe_2O_3 has an M_{sat} of about 70 emu/g iron oxide. An efficient SPIO contrast agent should have high M_{sat}, preferably higher than about 40 emu/g iron oxide (Fahlvik and Briley-Sæbø 1993). Iron oxides of non-ferrite structures have a low M_{sat} while the r_1 and r_2 values and the r_2/r_1 ratio may be acceptable. However, these iron oxides are not efficacious as contrast agents. The r_1 and r_2 and the r_2/r_1 ratio are determined by the size of the iron oxide crystal as well as the iron oxide composition. Large SPIO crystals have high r_2 values while smaller crystals have lower r_2 values and r_2 is more strongly influenced by the crystal size than is r_1. Thus the r_2/r_1 ratio increases with increasing crystal size or with clustering of individual iron oxide crystals. A positive SPIO agent must exhibit a low r_2/r_1 ratio and a high r_1 value. This is only achieved with small SPIO crystals having a high M_{sat}. A negative SPIO agent, on the other hand, should have a high r_2/r_1 ratio.

16.5.3 In Vitro – In Vivo Correlation

A high relaxivity in vitro is not always synonymous with high contrast effect in vivo due to particle degradation or compartmentalization. Generally speaking, particles are internalized into intracellular lysosomes after cellular uptake, where they eventually degrade. A lack of correlation between in vitro and liver contrast effect has been shown for liposomal GdHPDO3A and dysprosium-DTPA labeled starch particles, the agents being efficient negative contrast enhancers in liver despite a low in vitro r_2 (Fossheim et al. 1995, 1999). Compartmentalization of the contrast agent within the liver macrophages promotes what is called susceptibility effects. These effects are invariant with relaxivity and depend only on the magnetization of the compartment containing the agent, which is given by the field strength, magnetic susceptibility, and concentration of the agent within the compartment. A similar compartmentalization of a positive SPIO in liver will also result in a pronounced increase in r_2 as well as in the r_2/r_1 ratio, rendering it an efficient negative SPIO.

16.6 Concluding Remarks

Particulate formulations of diagnostic agents serve to improve site-specific delivery of the contrast-enhancing material where the targeted site can be a tissue/organ, a compartment, and/or a disease. Recent developments in cell and molecular biology in combination with the increasing knowledge of physicochemical and biological foreign surface interplays are providing exciting opportunities for optimal design of particulate agents. These opportunities can only be turned into clinical success through strategies which ensure a relatively site-specific delivery of a low-toxic contrast agent which is cost-effective to produce and convenient to use. The fact that this can only be achieved with a multidisciplinary and integrated effort makes particulate contrast agent research and development both attractive and challenging.

References

Adzamli K, Dorshow RB, Hynes MR, Li D, Nosco DL, Adams MD (1997) Preliminary evaluation of a polyethyleneglycol stabilized manganese-substituted hydroxylapatite as an intravascular contrast agent for MR angiography. J Magn Reson Imaging 7:204–208

Bačič G, Niesman MR, Bennett HF, Magin RL, Swartz HM (1988) Modulation of water proton relaxation rates by liposomes containing paramagnetic materials. Magn Reson Med 6:445–458

Barsky D, Pütz B, Schulten K, Magin RL (1992) Theory of paramagnetic contrast agents in liposome systems. Magn Reson Med 24:1–13

Burnett KR, Wolf GL, Schumacher Jr HR, Goldstein EJ (1985) Gadolinium oxide: a prototype agent for contrast enhanced imaging of the liver and spleen with magnetic resonance. Magn Reson Imaging 3:65–71

Chambon C, Clement O, Le Blanche A, Schouman-Claeys E, Frija G (1993) Superparamagnetic iron oxides as positive MR contrast agents: in vitro and in vivo evidence. Magn Reson Imaging 11:509–519

Chilton HM, Jackels SC, Hinson WH, Ekstrand KE (1984) Use of a paramagnetic substance, colloidal manganese sulfide, as an NMR contrast material in rats. J Nucl Med 25:604–607

Chouly C, Pouliquen D, Lucet I, Jeune JJ, Jallet P (1996) Development of superparamagnetic nanoparticles for MRI: effect of particle size, charge and surface nature on biodistribution. J Microencapsulation 13:245–255

Couvreur P, Dubernet C, Puisieux F (1995) Controlled drug delivery with nanoparticles: current possibilities and future trends. Eur J Pharm Biopharm 41:2–13

Dunlop DJ (1973) Superparamagnetic and single-domain threshold sizes in magnetite. J Geophys Res 78:1780–1793

Engelstad BL, Wesbey GE, Huberty JP et al. (1984) *In vitro* and *in vivo* testing of metal-ion complexes used as nuclear magnetic resonance contrast media. Invest Radiol 19:S149–150

Fahlvik AK, Holtz E, Klaveness J (1990a) Relaxation efficacy of paramagnetic and superparamagnetic microspheres in liver and spleen. Magn Reson Imaging 8:363–369

Fahlvik AK, Holtz E, Leander P, Schrøder U, Klaveness J (1990b) Magnetic starch microspheres, efficacy and elimination: a new organ-specific contrast agent for magnetic resonance imaging. Invest Radiol 25:113–120

Fahlvik AK, Briley-Sæbø K (1993) Superparamagnetic iron oxide particles for liver imaging: importance of transverse relaxivity and magnetic moment. Proceedings of the European Society for Magnetic Resonance in Medicine and Biology, Rome, p 107

Fahlvik AK, Nævestad A, Gundersen H, Strande P, Klaveness J, Jacobsen A (1996). WO 96/09840

Fossheim S, Fahlvik AK, Klaveness J (1995) Paramagnetic liposomes as liver contrast agents: evaluation of in vitro relaxivity and in vivo contrast efficacy. Proceedings of the Joint Meeting of the Society of Magnetic Resonance and the European Society for Magnetic Resonance in Medicine and Biology, Nice, p 49

Fossheim SL, Kellar KE, Månsson S, Colet JM, Rongved P, Fahlvik AK, Klaveness J (1999) Investigation of lanthanide-based starch particles as a model system for liver contrast agents. J Magn Reson Imaging (in press)

Gibby WA, Bogdan A, Ovitt TW (1989) Cross-linked DTPA polysaccharides for magnetic resonance imaging: synthesis and relaxation properties. Invest Radiol 24:302–309

Grant CWM, Karlik S, Florio E (1989) A liposomal MRI contrast agent: phosphatidylethanolamine-DTPA. Magn Reson Med 11:236–243

Hamm B, Staks T, Taupitz M (1994) A new superparamagnetic iron oxide contrast agent for magnetic resonance imaging. Invest Radiol 29:S87–S89

Harashima H, Kiwada H (1996) Liposomal targeting and drug delivery: kinetic consideration. Adv Drug Deliv Rev 19:425–444

Josephson L, Groman EV, Menz E, Lewis JM, Bengele H (1990) A functionalized superparamagnetic iron oxide colloid as a receptor directed MR contrast agent. Magn Reson Imaging 8:637–646

Jung CW, Jacobs P (1995) Physical and chemical properties of superparamagnetic iron oxide MR contrast agents: ferumoxides, ferumoxtran, ferumoxsil. Magn Reson Imaging 13:661–674

Kabalka GW, Buonocore E, Hubner K, Davis M, Huang L (1988) Gadolinium-labeled liposomes containing paramagnetic amphipathic agents: targeted MRI contrast agents for the liver. Magn Reson Med 8:89–95

Lasic DD (1993) Site-specific drug delivery. In: Lasic DD (ed) Liposomes from physics to applications. Elsevier Science Publishers, Amsterdam, The Netherlands, pp 441–458

Lichtenberg D, Barenholz Y (1988) Liposomes: preparation, characterization, and preservation. Methods Biochem Anal 33:337–462

Meldrum FC, Heywood BR, Mann S (1992) Magnetoferritin: in vitro synthesis of a novel magnetic protein. Science 257:522–523

Molday RS, Mackenzie D (1982) Immunospecific ferromagnetic iron-dextran reagents for the labeling and magnetic separation of cells. J Immunol Methods 52:353–367

Müller RH, Maassen S, Weyhers H, Specht F, Lucks JS (1996) Cytotoxicity of magnetite-loaded polylactide, polylactide/glycolide particles and solid lipid nanoparticles. Int J Pharm 138:85–94

Navon G, Panigel R, Valensin G (1986) Liposomes containing paramagnetic macromolecules as MRI contrast agents. Magn Reson Med 3:876–880

Nayar R, Hope MJ, Cullis PR (1989) Generation of large unilamellar vesicles from long-chain saturated phosphatidylcholines by extrusion technique. Biochim Biophys Acta 986:200–206

Papisov MI, Bogdanov A, Schaffer B, Nossiff N, Shen T, Weissleder R, Brady TJ (1993) Colloidal magnetic resonance contrast agents: effect of particle surface on biodistribution. J Magn Magn Mater 122:383–386

Pilgrimm H (1994) Superparamagnetic particles, process for producing the same and their use. WO 94/21240

Pouliquen D, Le Jeune JJ, Perdrisot R, Ermias A, Jallet P (1991) Iron oxide nanoparticles for use as an MRI contrast agent: pharmacokinetics and metabolism. Magn Reson Imaging 9:275–283

Reimer P, Weissleder R, Lee AS, Wittenberg J, Brady TJ (1990) Receptor imaging: application to MR imaging of liver cancer. Radiology 177:729–734

Reimer P, Weissleder R, Shen T, Knoefel WT, Brady TJ (1994) Pancreatic receptors: initial feasibility studies with a targeted contrast agent for MR imaging. Radiology 193:527–531

Reimer P, Schuierer G, Balzer T, Peters PE (1995) Application of a superparamagnetic iron oxide (Resovist) for MR imaging of human cerebral blood volume. Magn Reson Med 34:694–697

Ronay M (1982) Kinetics of formation, magnetic moment, and stability of colloidal magnetite. In: Hair M, Croucher D (eds) ACS Symposium Series No. 200: Colloids and surfaces in reprographic technology, pp 553–575

Rongved P, Lindberg B, Klaveness J (1991) Cross-linked, degradable starch microspheres as carriers of paramagnetic contrast agents for magnetic resonance imaging: synthesis, degradation, and relaxation properties. Carbohydr Res 214:325–330

Schwendener RA (1994) Liposomes as carriers for paramagnetic gadolinium chelates as organ specific contrast agents for magnetic resonance imaging (MRI). J Liposome Res 4:837–855

Schwertmann U, Cornell RM (1991) Iron oxides in the laboratory. VCH, Weinheim, pp 6–12

Senior JH (1987) Fate and behavior of liposomes in vivo: a review of controlling factors. CRC Crit Rev Ther Drug Carrier Syst 3:123–193

Sipkins DA, Kazemi M, Cheresh D, Bednarski MD, Li KCP (1997) Detection of tumor angiogenesis in vivo by $\alpha_v\beta_3$-targeted magnetic resonance imaging. Proceedings of the International Society of Magnetic Resonance in Medicine, Vancouver, p 334

Sjøgren CE, Johansson C, Nævestad A, Sontum PC, Briley-Sæbø K, Fahlvik AK (1997) Crystal size and properties of superparamagnetic iron oxide (SPIO) particles. Magn Reson Imaging 15:55–67

Sontum PC, Nævestad A, Fahlvik AK, Gundersen HG (1996) Adsorption of poly(sodium(4)styrenesulfonate) on colloidal iron oxide particles. Int J Pharm 128:269–275

Storrs RW, Tropper FD, Li HY, et al. (1995) Paramagnetic polymerized liposomes: synthesis, characterization, and applications for magnetic resonance imaging. J Am Chem Soc 117:7301–7306

Suzuki M, Shinkai M, Kamihira M, Kobayashi T (1995) Preparation and characteristics of magnetite-labelled antibody with the use of poly(ethylene glycol) derivatives. Biotechnol Appl Biochem 21:335–345

Suzuki M, Shimizu W, Kosugi Y, Honda H, Kobayashi T (1996) Magnetic characterization of magnetite particles for MR contrast agents. Bull Chem Soc Jpn. 69:1143–1148

Talsma H, Crommelin DJA (1992) Liposomes as drug delivery systems. Part I. Preparation. Pharm Technol October:96–106

Talsma H, Crommelin DJA (1993) Liposomes as drug delivery systems. Part III. Stabilization. Pharm Technol January:48–59

Tiefenauer LX, Kühne G, Andres RY (1993) Antibody-magnetite nanoparticles: in vitro characterization of a potential tumor-specific contrast agent for magnetic resonance imaging. Bioconj Chem 4:347–352

Tilcock C, Unger E, Cullis P, MacDougall P (1989) Liposomal Gd-DTPA: preparation and characterization of relaxivity. Radiology 171:77–80

Tilcock C, Ahkong QF, Koenig SH, Brown RD III, Davis M, Kabalka G (1992) The design of liposomal paramagnetic MR agents: effect of vesicle size upon the relaxivity of surface-incorporated lipophilic chelates. Magn Res Med 27:44–51

Tilcock C (1994) Liposomal blood pool agents for nuclear medicine and magnetic resonance imaging. J Liposome Res 4:909–936

Trubetskoy VS, Cannilo JA, Milshtein A, Wolf GL, Torchilin VP (1995) Controlled delivery of Gd-containing liposomes to lymph nodes: surface modification may enhance MRI contrast properties. Magn Reson Imaging 13:31–37

Unger E, Fritz T, Wu G, et al. (1994) Liposomal MR contrast agents. J Liposome Res 4:811–834

Vion-Dury J, Masson S, Devoisselle JM, et al. (1989) Liposome-mediated delivery of gadolinium-diethylenetriaminopentaacetic acid to hepatic cells: a P-31 NMR study. J Pharmacol Exp Ther 250:1113–1118

Weissleder R, Elizondo G, Wittenberg J, Rabito CA, Bengele HH, Josephson L (1990) Ultrasmall superparamagnetic iron oxide: characterization of a new class of contrast agents for MR imaging. Radiology 175:489–493

Weissleder R, Lee AS, Fischman AJ, Reimer P, Shen T, Wilkinson R, Callahan RJ, Brady TJ (1991) Polyclonal human immunoglobulin G labeled with polymeric iron oxide: antibody MR imaging. Radiology 181:245–249

Weissleder R, Lee AS, Khaw BA, Shen T, Brady TJ (1992) Antimyosin-labeled monocrystalline iron oxide allows detection of myocardial infarct: MR antibody imaging. Radiology 182:381–385

Weissleder R, Bogdanov A, Neuwelt EA, Papisov M (1995) Long-circulating iron oxides for MR imaging. Adv Drug Deliv Rev 16:321–334

Wisner ER, Merisko-Liversidge E, Kellar KE, et al. (1995) Preclinical evaluation of manganese carbonate particles for magnetic resonance imaging of the liver. Acad Radiol 2:140–147

17 Magnetic Resonance Contrast Agents of Increased Specificity

H.-J. Weinmann

CONTENTS

17.1 Introduction

At the end of the 1970s and beginning of the 1980s, the first reports were published on the use of paramagnetic ions as contrast modifiers in magnetic resonance imaging (MRI) (Lauterbur et al. 1978). The intolerance of these metallic ions was, however, mentioned as a critical factor. It was therefore unclear whether administering paramagnetic substances, such as ions of the transitional elements (e.g., $MnCl_2$) and lanthanides or nitroxyl compounds, would be a feasible approach in clinical diagnosis. However, chelation of the metal ions led to a dramatic improvement of their pharmacological and toxicological properties (Weinmann et al. 1984). The chelation allows rapid renal excretion after intravenous administration, as well as elimination of the undesired toxic effects of the free metal ions. Less than 10 years after the first marketing authorization in Europe, Japan, and the United States, paramagnetic metal chelates became important tools for routine clinical MRI. Depending on factors such as indications and clinical experience, approximately 30% of all MRI studies worldwide are performed with the use of a paramagnetic complexes. Among them, gadolinium-diethylene triamine penta-acetic acid (GdDTPA) (Magnevist, Schering AG, Berlin, Germany) is the most widely used contrast agent in MRI, with more than 50% of the market share.

These agents are considered to be unspecific contrast molecules, although their distribution in the body is far from homogeneous. For example, the compounds cannot pass through the plasma membrane of cells, thus limiting their distribution to the extracellular space and precluding passage of the blood-brain barrier. Because of their almost exclusively renal elimination, much higher concentrations occur in the kidneys than in other organs. This specific accumulation allows superb visualization of the kidneys and functional studies of this excretory organ (Schad et al. 1993). Special formulations have been developed for contrasting the gastrointestinal tract after oral administration or the joint fluid after intra-articular administration (Laniado et al. 1988; Kramer et al. 1992; Schwizer et al. 1994).

Nevertheless, there is a need for materials with more specific distribution. Such compounds should highlight otherwise isointense lesions or tissues, thus permitting more specific and sensitive diagnoses. However, the new agents can no longer be biologically inert; they must bind or interact with specific molecules, proteins, receptors, or specific structures of the areas of interest.

17.2 Blood Pool Agents

Contrast materials that selectively enhance the blood vessels have been the subject of research since the early days of angiography. Most attempts to develop such materials failed because of both the low sensi-

H.-J. Weinmann, PhD, Research Laboratories of Schering AG, Fo KM für KST, D-13342 Berlin, Germany tivity of the imaging procedure and the large amount of the agent to be injected. MRI can highlight at low concentrations the contrast effect of either T1 or T2 agents given in a small dose, which is the essential prerequisite of an acceptable blood pool agent. Paramagnetic and superparamagnetic agents are now in preclinical and clinical development; each agent has interesting features, but none is ideal. Clinical studies are needed to establish the real potential of such agents. It is too early to state whether one or the other product will fulfil the high expectations of an ideal blood pool agent.

17.2.1 Low Molecular Weight Protein-Binding Gadolinium Complexes

Lauffer (EPIX Medical) has developed a low molecular weight gadolinium chelate with strong protein-binding potential (Fig. 17.1). After intravenous injection, the agent binds predominantly to albumin and therefore highlights the vascular space (Lauffer et al. 1996). Because of this strong protein binding and the increase of the rotational corre-lation time, τ_r, the agent exhibits an extremely high relaxivity (≥than $40\,l\,mmol^{-1}\,s^{-1}$). Because of its high relaxivity, a low dose exhibits excellent blood tissue contrast enhancement. Animal studies prove that doses as low as 2.5 or 5 µmol/kg are effective.

Detailed pharmacodynamic data, including toxicity statements, are still needed to evaluate the compound's properties. Initial studies in rats and monkeys showed that the compound is safe and subject to complete elimination (mostly renal) within 24 h. As with other long-circulating blood pool agents, it is not possible to differentiate between venous and arterial blood after the first passage through the capillaries.

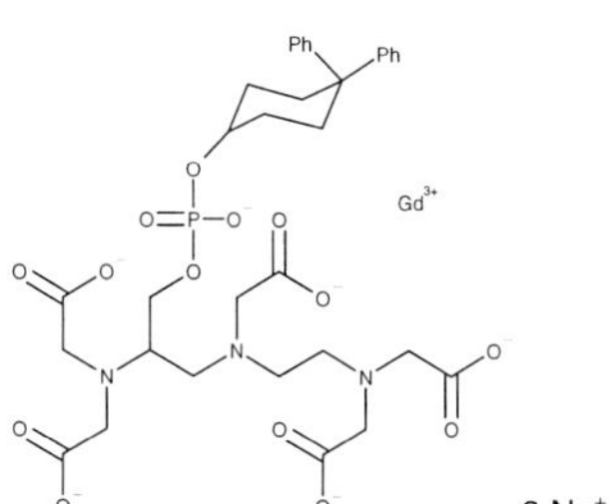

Fig. 17.1. Chemical structure of the blood pool agent, MS-325

17.2.2 Polymeric Gadolinium Complexes

Albumin covalently bound to GdDTPA as an intravascular, blood pool-enhancing agent for MRI is the polymeric agent most widely used in experimental studies in animals (Schmiedl et al. 1986, 1987; Shames et al. 1993). According to the literature, up to 40 Gd DTPA residues are attached to the protein. The studies indicate that labeled albumin distributing in the intravascular space may be effective for MRI of the blood vessels and evaluation of tissue blood volume. Because of the hyperpermeability inherent to tumor microvessels, the macromolecule permits quantitative estimates of capillary permeability in tumors (Cohen et al. 1994; Schwickert et al. 1996). Brasch and colleagues demonstrated that MRI allows estimates of plasma volume, microvascular permeability, and capillary density (Su et al. 1995; van Dijke et al. 1996).

Although the agents elicit favorable imaging characteristics, they are not suitable for clinical use. Problems include inadequate in vivo stability, low elimination, problematic synthesis, low water solubility, and large injection volume.

Dextrans, polyaspartate, polyethylene glycol, and polylysine derivatives with molecular weights ranging from 15 000 to several million daltons have been synthesized and studied by various groups (Gibby et al. 1990; Kornguth et al. 1990; Schuhmann-Giampieri et al. 1991; Bogdanov et al. 1993; Cavagna et al. 1994; Desser et al. 1994; Frank et al. 1994a; Grandin et al. 1995).

The agents exhibit a high degree of polydispersity, making it difficult to yield batches of well-defined molecular weight. Because of their large molecular size, their rotational correlation time, τ_r, is increased, and consequently all polymeric agents show an increased relaxivity per gadolinium atom of up to $20\,l\,mmol^{-1}\,s^{-1}$ at 20 MHz.

Such large molecules circulate longer in the vascular space and are interesting substances for experimental studies in animals. The agents are excellent magnetic resonance angiography (MRA) enhancers and may also be beneficial for mapping permeability surface area product. However, problematic elimination and retention in the body inhibit the agent's commercial development.

New classes of high molecular weight blood pool agents are fully synthetic cascade polymers, also known as dendrimers. These substances are spheroidal polycations that can be synthesized with a well-defined diameter and a precise number of terminal amines per dendrimer (Tomalia et al. 1990; Wiener et al. 1994). Various subtypes of the agent have been considered; for example, the paramagnetic atom was bound to the backbone by means of DTPA or macrocyclic ligands, producing polymers of anionic or neutral charge. Due to their good water solubility, highly concentrated solutions can be formulated. Nevertheless, the synthesis of compounds with consistent charge, gadolinium content, and molecular size is cumbersome.

One of the most advanced compounds is a dendrimer from Schering's research laboratories with the code number ZK 181 040 and the laboratory name Gadomer-17. The agent is characterized by a defined molecular weight of 17.5 kDa, 24 gadolinium complexes at the surface of the dendrimer, and a large hydrodynamic radius with an apparent molecular weight of about 35 kDa.

Like other polymeric gadolinium chelates, Gadomer-17 exhibits a higher T1 relaxivity ($17 l mmol^{-1} s^{-1}$) than low molecular weight contrast agents. This effect is most pronounced at 0.5–1.0 T. The agent is small enough to guarantee glomerular filtration and large enough to reduce the diffusion through the endothelial wall of intact blood vessels. The agent is eliminated by glomerular filtration within 24 h in unmetabolized form. Due to the longer extravasation and elimination time in humans, Gadomer-17 should allow contrast-enhanced MRA for at least 15 min post bolus injection in the clinical situation. Studies in dogs have shown that an improved differential diagnosis between benign and malignant neoplasms may be possible using contrast agents of this kind (Adam et al. 1996).

Little is known about the clinical safety of exobiotic polymers. Generally, large compounds that stay longer in the organism will have an increased potential for antibody cross-reactions and could therefore cause allergy-like side-effects. However, in vitro studies revealed promising results suggesting that the immunogenic potential may not be a limiting factor (Baxter et al. 1991). Medium-sized polymers, such as Gadomer-17, are useful contrast agents for MRA due to their increased relaxivity and low extravasation. In addition, the agents are eliminated quickly and completely by glomerular filtration. Medium-sized polymeric gadolinium complexes are promising new candidates for angiography and differential diagnosis in MRI.

17.2.3 Superparamagnetic Iron Oxides

Superparamagnetic iron oxides (SPIOs) are nanoparticles made of iron oxides with very high T1 and T2 relaxivities. In contrast to paramagnetic ions, the spin-spin relaxation effect is much more pronounced than the T1 effect. Because of the strong T2 effect, such compounds are of special interest in T2-weighted studies. In the first minutes after injection, before significant uptake in macrophages, SPIOs distribute in the blood space without any extravasation.

Large SPIO (Feridex, Endorem, Resovist) particles have a very strong impact on the T2 effect. But even though their T1 effect is high, it is almost insignificant because of the overwhelming spin-spin relaxation rate. The decrease in signal intensity in the vascular space may be of minor benefit for classical diagnosis of vascular abnormalities. The strong T2 effect and the rapid accumulation in macrophages disfavor the use of this class of SPIO for fast MRA.

Small-sized particles (also called ultra-small superparamagnetic iron oxides, USPIOs) such as AMI 7227 (Sinerem, Combidex) exhibit lower relaxivities, but a much more favorable T1/T2 ratio that facilitates MRA or other T1-weighted sequences (Frank et al. 1994b; McLachlan et al. 1994; Mayo-Smith et al. 1996). The compounds circulate longer in the blood pool before accumulating in the liver, spleen, and lymph nodes. During the first few minutes, or even hours, after intravenous injection a distinct T1 effect is detected in the blood or tissue. A dose of 25–50 µmol Fe/kg may be needed to obtain adequate MRA images.

In contrast to gadolinium polymers, USPIOs may be less useful for differential diagnosis and permeability-surface area product studies, since the capillary walls of carcinomas are not permeable to particles. However, detailed studies are needed to fully understand the properties of USPIOs. Results suggest that iron oxide preparations are alternatives to compounds containing macromolecular gadolinium complexes and could be useful for clinical MRA.

17.3 Liver-Specific Agents

The differential diagnosis of focal hepatic lesions continues to be a problem, even though many diagnostic methods are available. Despite the high contrast resolution of T2-weighted MRI techniques, many pathological conditions are difficult to detect or differentiate without contrast agents.

Paramagnetic extracellular contrast agents (e.g., Magnevist) improve the differential diagnosis, but not the detection rate. Using a bolus injection of 0.1–0.3 mmol/kg (~10–40 ml per patient) and fast-gradient echo sequences (dynamic imaging) results in findings similar to those obtained using contrast-enhanced spiral computed tomography (CT) (HAMM et al. 1994b; SAINI and NELSON 1995). As with contrast media-enhanced CT, gadolinium enhancement patterns reflect the degree of vascularity, flow dynamics, and vascular perfusion.

Magnevist and other extracellular contrast agents rapidly distribute in the vascular and interstitial space but do not pass cellular plasma membranes. Their hepatocellular uptake and biliary excretion are negligible. Targeting the hepatocytes and entrapping substances in macrophages of the reticuloendothelial system (RES) are both effective approaches for liver-specific agents, since both pathways have a high capacity for handling relatively unspecific bulk amounts of materials.

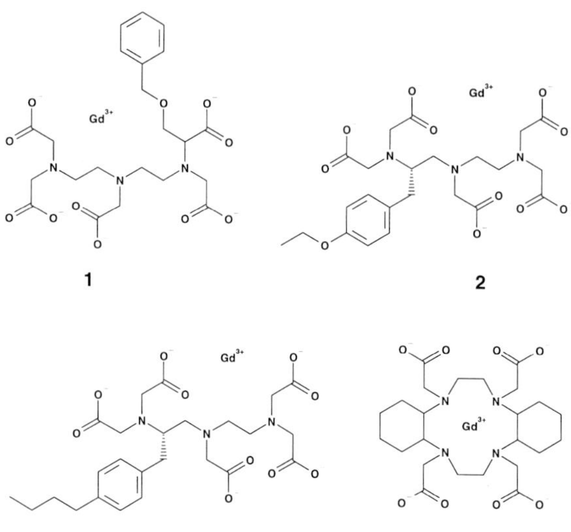

1 2 3 4

Fig. 17.2. Chemical structure of hepatobiliary gadolinium chelates. *1* (GdBOPTA = gadobenate = MultiHance; *2* (Gd-EOB-DTPA = gadoxetate = Eovist; *3* (MS 264 = Gd(1*RS*)-1-(*p*-butylbenzyl)-DTPA); *4* ($GdCy_2DOTA$)

agents will significantly improve the diagnostic accuracy of routine MRI of the liver.

17.3.1 Hepatocyte-Specific Compounds

Several compounds with different magnetic properties are currently in clinical trials. These agents include water-soluble paramagnetic chelates with hepatobiliary uptake, such as mangafodipir (MnDPDP) (Teslascan, Nycomed), Gd-benzyloxypropionictetraacetate (BOPTA) (MultiHance, gadobenate, Bracco), and Gd-ethoxybenzyl (EOB)-DTPA (Eovist, gadoxetate, Schering), as well as SPIO particles accumulating in the RES, such as AMI-25 (Feridex Berlex, Endorem Guerbet) and SHU555A (Resovist Schering) (Fig. 17.2). Special SPIO preparations with hepatocyte uptake have been studied. Arabinogalactan- and asialofetuin-coated USPIOs were developed to target the asialoglycoprotein (ASGP) receptor; these coatings direct the contrast agents exclusively to hepatocytes (WEISSLEDER et al. 1990b; SCHAFFER et al. 1993; LEVEILLE-WEBSTER et al. 1996). A dose of less than 5 μmol/kg monocrystalline iron oxide nanoparticle (MION) coated with these carbohydrates is effective in decreasing the signal intensity of the liver.

It is very likely that both paramagnetic and superparamagnetic hepatobiliary or RES-specific

17.3.1.1 Manganese Compounds

Teslascan (Mangafodipir, Nycomed) is the first manganese complex to be used as a contrast agent in clinical trials (LIM et al. 1991). The Mn^{2+} ion is a powerful T1 relaxation agent because its five unpaired electrons exhibit optimal correlation times. The agent, which demonstrates both biliary and renal excretion, has been shown to be a positive and effective liver enhancer. Its chemical similarity to vitamin B_6 is cited as the reason for the hepatocyte uptake, but some of the liver accumulation of paramagnetic manganese is probably due to the metabolism of the parent compound. The metabolic process releases free Mn^{2+} ions, which are known to accumulate in hepatocytes. Pharmacokinetic studies verified that Mn^{2+} is released in the plasma shortly after injection, and the paramagnetic ion accumulates in the liver, pancreas, and cardiac muscle (GALLEZ et al. 1996).

Peak liver enhancement occurs at 15 min after injection and persists for several hours. Since manganese is a powerful relaxation enhancer, a very small amount (5 μmol/kg) significantly enhances the contrast between the liver parenchyma and focal liver lesions (HAMM et al. 1992b; MURAKAMI et al. 1996;

ROFSKY and EARLS 1996). The level of enhancement depends upon the physiological status of the liver parenchyma. For instance, cirrhotic livers cause a heterogeneous enhancement. Patients with fibrosis and siderotic regenerating nodules exhibit decreased enhancement. Increased enhancement occurs with benign regenerating nodules. Although Teslascan is generally tolerated, transient facial flushing has been observed. European marketing authorization was granted in May 1997.

17.3.1.2
Hepatobiliary Gadolinium Chelates

Chelates with lipophilic components were investigated as potentially liver-specific compounds (VITTADINI et al. 1988; WEINMANN et al. 1991; SCHUHMANN-GIAMPIERI et al. 1992; PETRÉ et al. 1995; RUNGE and WELLS 1995). All hepatocyte-specific agents are ionic metal chelates and, unlike many other hepatotropic compounds, display a relatively pronounced hydrophilicity. These compounds enter the intracellular space of the most common liver cell, the hepatocytes. For two gadolinium compounds, gadobenate and gadoxetate, studies proved that there was carrier-mediated accumulation in the hepatocyte.

Transport is mediated by two membrane-bound transporters localized in the sinusoidal and canalicular side of the hepatocytes (WEINMANN et al. 1996). Despite a pronounced hydrophilic character, chelates accumulate quickly in the hepatocyte. No accumulation has been reported with other highly hydrophilic substances. The uptake is not mediated by cytosolic binding proteins but by a complex interplay of various carrier systems that are at least partly energy dependent. After entering the intracellular space, the gadolinium chelate is sequestered in the bile in an unaltered form.

In rats receiving up to 100 µmol/kg of Eovist, about two-thirds of the agent is eliminated in feces and one-third in urine. Because of its hepatocellular accumulation and high relaxivity, as little as 10 µmol/kg of Eovist is sufficient for improved detection of liver tumors.

The tolerability and pharmacokinetics of Gd-EOB-DTPA were studied in healthy volunteers after intravenous bolus injection (HAMM et al. 1995). A dose of 10–25 µmol/kg was sufficient to selectively enhance the signal intensity of healthy liver parenchyma. The highest dose of 100 µmol/kg tested in this series produced a distinct dip in the enhancement curve at about 30 min indicating a T2 effect because of too high a Gd concentration in the hepatocytes. Eovist was completely eliminated from the body via urine and feces. No adverse reactions or meaningful changes of biological parameters were observed after intravenous injection of up to 100 µmol/kg.

Use of the early perfusion pattern in combination with delayed images improves the characterization and detection of even small liver lesions (REIMER et al. 1996; VOGL et al. 1996).

Other hepatobiliary gadolinium chelates are being tested in animal models (RUNGE et al. 1996). These electrically neutral macrocyclic compounds exhibit excellent efficacy in animal studies and may accumulate in the liver using a different transporter than gadobenate or gadoxetate.

17.3.2
RES-Specific Compounds

17.3.2.1
Superparamagnetic Iron Oxides

Special iron oxide aggregates are extremely effective T2 relaxation agents. When placed in a magnetic field, they behave like ferromagnetic substances. Outside the magnetic field, SPIO particles do not exhibit the magnetic memory of ferromagnetic materials. The diameter of such particles is in the nanometer range, as large as proteins such as ferritin. The iron core itself has a diameter of just 3–5 nm. The apparent size of the particles in blood is larger, within 30–100 nm, because of hydration of the coating material and potential association with each other or biological substances. These iron particles are coated with polysaccharides (e.g., dextranes) and form a mahogany-colored aqueous solution. The coating of the iron core, the size of the particles, and their electrical charge influence their pharmacodynamic properties significantly. Smaller particles generally circulate longer in the blood space, finally accumulating in the macrophages of the lymph nodes, liver, spleen, and lung. The larger species-target the Kupffer cells of the RES system very effectively, especially those in the liver.

SPIO particles produce a dramatic long-range disturbance in magnetic field homogeneity. The strong T2 effect is especially apparent when the agents distribute nonhomogeneously. T2 relaxivities of more than 150 $l\,mmol^{-1}\,s^{-1}$ are common with liver-specific SPIOs.

After intravenous administration, SPIO particles are sequestered within minutes by normal RES phagocytic Kupffer cells, but they are not retained in metastases and no uptake has been observed in hepatocytes. Instead they distribute in a relatively small volume of the target: in the case of the liver, only about 2%–3% of its total cell population. Inside these Kupffer cells, the particles are clustered in lysosomal vacuoles. The strong susceptibility effect effectively influences the signal intensity, especially when T2-weighted sequences are used. Just 3 µg Fe/g liver will cause a signal decrease of 50% in a standard T2-weighted sequence.

SPIOs are metabolized into a soluble, nonsuperparamagnetic form of iron. This iron is incorporated into the normal iron pool (e.g., ferritin, hemosiderin, and hemoglobin) within a few days.

Two different preparations are currently under clinical investigation: Advanced Magnetic's AMI-25 (Feridex, Endorem) and Schering's Resovist. Using T2-weighted imaging techniques, a dose of about 10 µmol Fe/kg produced excellent clinical results (Hamm et al. 1994a; Chachuat and Bonnemain 1995; Reimer et al. 1995; Petersein et al. 1996). Doses ranging from 5 to 40 µmol Fe/kg were investigated in patients suffering from focal liver lesions. A low dose of 8 µmol Fe/kg of the Resovist preparation produced a strong decrease in signal intensity that paralleled a significant increase in the contrast-to-noise ratio. SPIO-enhanced images of the liver significantly increased the number of hepatic lesions detected and reduced the threshold size for detection to less than 5 mm.

While the particles do not accumulate in metastases, some uptake has been observed in hepatocellular carcinoma and focal nodular hyperplasia. SPIO-enhanced images during the retention phases offer improved diagnostic accuracy in detecting focal liver lesions. Studies demonstrate that even without the use of SPIO, MRI has higher diagnostic accuracy and greater effect on patient management than CT arterial portography (CTAP) (Semelka et al. 1996). It is likely that SPIO-enhanced MRI will replace CTAP because of its improved diagnostic accuracy, better tolerance, and cost-effectiveness (Rummeny et al. 1995; Seneterre et al. 1996).

Special attention must be focused on patient tolerance to these materials to ensure that their diagnostic benefits are not obtained at the cost of a higher incidence of adverse reactions. Early preparations caused severe cardiovascular side-effects. No significant, clinically relevant adverse reactions or changes in laboratory parameters have been observed with the latest formulations. However, the margin of safety in some cases exceeds several hundred or even thousand. The iron oxides are not subject to classical elimination pathways (e.g., renal excretion), but their metabolism into protein-incorporated iron (hemosiderin, hemoglobin, etc.) may be a significant advantage over gadolinium-containing long-circulating molecules. The total additional iron load per single dose represents less than 2% of the total iron content of the human body.

17.3.2.2
Liposomal Encapsulated Complexes

Liposomal gadolinium contrast agents have been investigated for liver enhancement by Unger and collaborators (Unger et al. 1990, 1991, 1993). The gadolinium is encapsulated in the form of its diethylene triamine penta-acetic acid (DTPA) or 1,4,7,10-tetraazacyclododecane-*N*,*N*′,*N*″,*N*‴ (DOTA) complexes or is incorporated into the phospholipid bilayer (Kabalka et al. 1991; Kim et al. 1991, 1992; Unger et al. 1991; Tilcock et al. 1992). The vesicles are recognized by the RES, permitting passive delivery of the gadolinium label to the liver and spleen.

Depending on the preparation, the vesicles have diameters ranging between about 50 and 500 nm. Smaller liposomes circulate longer in the blood pool and function as vascular contrast enhancers.

Decomplexation with release of free gadolinium is a clinical concern. Radiotracer studies gave evidence of in vivo decomplexation for some gadolinium chelates entrapped in liposomes (Unger et al. 1991). The tolerance of such preparations, and the in vitro and in vivo stability of liposomal-encapsulated gadolinium complexes, are still critical issues.

17.4
Lymph Node-Specific Agents

17.4.1
Gadolinium Chelates

Since endolymphatic administration is an invasive and cumbersome procedure, agents that accumulate in the lymphatics after interstitial or intravenous injection were desired. Lymphotropic paramagnetically labeled substances would result in increased signal intensity of the normal tissue; this would, in turn, lead to better detection of metastasis by fast and high-quality T1-weighted imaging procedures. Special carbohydrated polymers labeled with GdDTPA accumulate in the lymph nodes of rats after intravenous injection (HARIKA et al. 1996). This polyglucose-associated macrocomplex (PGM)-based graft copolymer significantly increases signal intensity for MRI of normal (but not metastatic) lymph nodes without causing distortion artifacts. It is too early to draw conclusions from these findings, since limited data have been published on tolerance and general pharmacology.

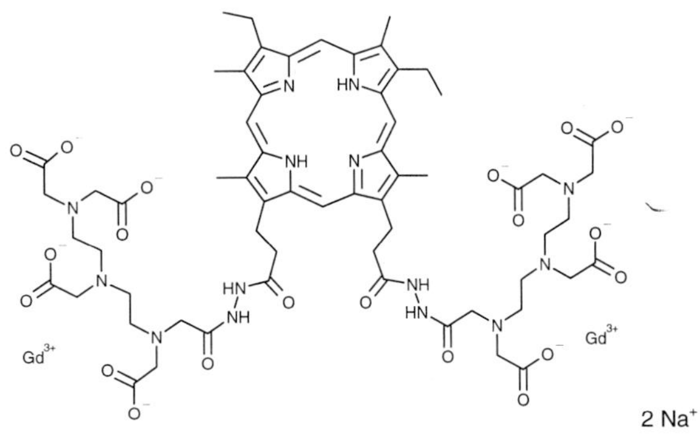

Fig. 17.3. Chemical structure of Gadophrin-2

17.4.2 SPIOs and USPIOs

SPIOs are potent contrast agents for lymphography. After endolymphatic administration, trace amounts were found to cause a darkening of the lymphatic vessels and lymph nodes (HAMM et al. 1992a; TAUPITZ et al. 1993).

Hydrophilically coated small particles circulate longer in the blood space and will not rapidly accumulate in the RES of the liver and spleen. USPIOs, also used as T1 blood pool contrast agents, are phagocytosed by the macrophages of the lymphatic system. The inhomogeneous distribution within the lymph node increases their susceptibility effect (T2*) and leads to a reduction of the signal intensity. A significant reduction of the signal intensity of the normal lymph nodes occurs 24h after intravenous injection. A dose of about 50 µmol/kg is effective in detecting metastatic involvement of lymph nodes. (WEISSLEDER et al. 1990a, 1994; BENGELE et al. 1994; GUIMARAES et al. 1994; VASSALLO et al. 1994; ELSTE et al. 1996; MCLACHLAN et al. 1996).

Screening various metalloporphyrins as tumor-specific contrast agents demonstrated that some porphyrins – e.g., bis-GdDTPA mesoporphyrin (Gadophrin-2, Schering AG, Berlin) – accumulate in necrotic tissue (SCHNEIDER et al. 1995; NI et al. 1996) (Fig. 17.3). Marchal and co-workers could identify small infarcts (induced in the myocardium or renal tissue) using 100 µmol Gd/kg 24h after dosing (MARCHAL et al. 1996). Gadophrin-2 positively stained the nonvital tissue within an infarcted area 3–24h after injection. This area matched well with the negatively stained triphenyl tetrazolium chloride area. The porphyrins induce a strong and persistent enhancement, which remains visible for several days. No such contrast effect occurs in scar tissue. The mechanism that drives the agent specifically to necrotic tissue has not been identified. The metalloporphyrins are a promising new class of contrast agents for detecting and quantifying necrosis, especially within acute myocardial infarct. An early evaluation of the physiological status of jeopardized myocardium is most important for beneficial therapy.

17.5 Cardiac-Specific Agents

Magnetic resonance imaging is a promising imaging modality for diagnosing cardiac morphology, function, and pathology. Contrast media may help position MRI as the ultimate diagnostic tool for cardiology. Pathology-specific compounds based on T1 or T2 materials are needed for more precise diagnoses, which can lead to faster and more effective treatment. Weissleder showed that superparamagnetic particles (MION) attached to antimyosin Fab accumulated in the infarcted area of the heart, but not in the healthy myocardium of rats (WEISSLEDER et al. 1992).

17.6 Adrenal Gland-Specific Agents

Coupling cholesterol with a paramagnetic label resulted in an organ-specific contrast agent for MRI of the adrenal glands (MÜHLER et al. 1995). The highly protein-bound gadolinium-DO3A-cholesterol elicited high relaxivities in water and plasma. After intravenous injection, the agent accumulated in the liver and adrenal glands. A 162% enhancement was seen in the adrenal glands of rats 2h after intravenous injection. A totally different type of molecule, cationic GdDTPA-polylysine, was shown to produce a detectable uptake and MRI enhancement in the adrenal glands of rats (WEISSLEDER et al. 1993). Microscopic studies verified the targeting of this relatively large polymeric agent to the adrenal medulla. MnDPDP or the released Mn^{2+} ion also accumulated in the adrenal glands and produced significant contrast enhancement (MITCHELL et al. 1995).

17.7 Pancreas-Specific Agents

The early detection of pancreatic tumors is still a critical issue in diagnostic imaging. New specific contrast materials may provide an additional tool to achieve that goal. In the course of the clinical development of MnDPDP as a liver-specific contrast agent, it was observed that this agent also enhanced pancreatic tissue. The accumulation may be due to the release of Mn^{2+}, which is known to bind to pancreatic tissue. Additional clinical trials are needed to investigate the diagnostic and therapeutic consequences of this finding (GEHL et al. 1993; KETTRITZ et al. 1996).

Special iron particles (MION) were used to target pancreatic receptors. Particles coated with cholecystokinin or secretin (secretin-biotin-streptavidin-MION construct) accumulated in the rat pancreas and yielded a significant signal reduction of this tissue (REIMER et al. 1994; SHEN et al. 1996).

17.8 Tumor-Specific Agents

The general understanding has been that, like metal-free porphyrins, metalloporphyrins target tumor cells. Most studies have been conducted using the manganese complex of tetra (4-sulfonatophenyl)-porphine (Mn^{3+} TPPS4); in some experiments, the corresponding gadolinium complex has been evaluated (PATRONAS et al. 1986; OGAN et al. 1987; PLACE et al. 1990; NELSON and SCHMIEDL 1991; HINDRÉ et al. 1993; NI 1996). Although strong enhancement results from the intravenous injection of the colored complexes, the specificity of the increase in signal enhancement is not clear. None of the known porphyrins fulfil the characteristics of specific tumor binding (EBERT et al. 1992).

Paramagnetic chelate-labeled monoclonal antibodies are believed to be the ultimate tumor-seeking materials. Several groups have studied this approach in detail (KORNGUTH et al. 1987; GÖHR-ROSENTHAL et al. 1993; HINDRÉ et al. 1994). Indeed, experimental studies in small animals revealed that it was possible to achieve a higher and more specific concentration of the magnetic label at the target. Although detectable by standard MRI sequences, the required dose (mg/kg body weight) of the gadolinium-labeled antibody was still too high to make commercial development promising. In regard to relaxation properties and the minimal dose of agents, SPIOs are more powerful than gadolinium compounds (WEISSLEDER et al. 1991; REMSEN et al. 1996).

Studies confirmed that, when using MION, a specific enhancement is achievable after an intravenous dose of 2 mg antibody/kg. Conjugation of monoclonal antibodies with MION particles may provide a method with which to obtain specific diagnoses of tumor involvement.

17.9 Diagnostic Agents with Therapeutic Properties

A novel porphyrin-like gadolinium complex elicited interesting characteristics as an MRI agent and as a therapeutic agent (YOUNG et al. 1994, 1996). Gd^{3+} texaphyrin is representative of a new class of radiation sensitizers with paramagnetic properties detectable by MRI (Fig. 17.4). After intravenous injection, the accumulation in tumor tissue was demonstrated by means of MRI. The gadolinium complex shows a high electron affinity and forms long-lived radicals after x-ray exposure. Animal studies confirmed that the agent is an efficient radiation sensitizer. Preliminary clinical studies in patients with brain tumors are ongoing.

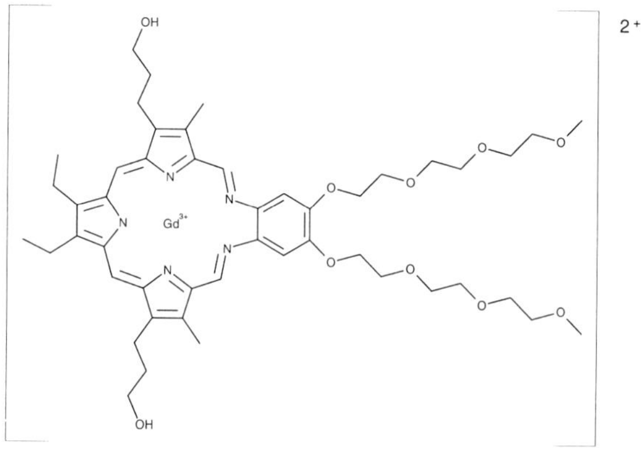

Fig. 17.4. Chemical structure of Gd^{3+} texaphyrin

17.10 Conclusion

Paramagnetic contrast agents have become an integral part of the daily practice of MRI because of both their efficacy and their excellent tolerance profile. MRI is more sensitive to the contrast-agent effect, allowing a significant reduction in dose. However, gram amounts per patient are necessary for enhancing brain tumors by means of such standard contrast materials as gadopentetate. Thus, MRI is far less sensitive than either single-photon emission tomography or positron emission tomography. New MR agents with increased selectivity and improved paramagnetic effects - either T1 or T2 - will reduce the gap between MRI and nuclear medicine in terms of dosage. The first tissue-specific agents for liver enhancement have been introduced onto the market, and lymphotropic and blood pool agents may follow soon. It is likely that within 10 years a palette of lesion- or tissue-specific agents will be standard equipment in diagnostic imaging.

Acknowledgements. I would like to express my thanks to my colleagues at Schering AG, especially Prof. Speck, Dr. Radüchel, and all members of the MR research department. Without their assistance and great support this chapter would not have been possible.

References

Adam G, Mühler A, Spuntrup E, Neuerburg JM, Kilbinger M, Bauer H, Fucezi L (1996) Differentiation of spontaneous canine breast tumors using dynamic magnetic resonance imaging with 24-gadolinium-DTPA-cascade-polymer, a new blood-pool agent. Preliminary experience. Invest Radiol 31:267–274

Baxter AB, Melnikoff S, Stites DP, Brasch RC (1991) AUR Memorial Award 1991. Immunogenicity of gadolinium-based contrast agents for magnetic resonance imaging. Induction and characterization of antibodies in animals. Invest Radiol 26:1035–1040

Bengele HH, Palmacci S, Rogers J, Jung CW, Crenshaw J, Josephson L (1994) Biodistribution of an ultrasmall superparamagnetic iron oxide colloid, BMS 180549, by different routes of administration. Magn Reson Imaging 12:433–442

Bogdanov AJ, Weissleder R, Frank HW, Bogdanova AV, Nossif N, Schaffer BK, Tsai E (1993) A new macromolecule as a contrast agent for MR angiography: preparation, properties, and animal studies. Radiology 187:701–706

Cavagna F, Luchinat C, Scozzafava A, Xia Z (1994) Polymetallic macromolecules are potential contrast agents of improved efficiency. Magn Reson Med 31:58–60

Chachuat A, Bonnemain B (1995) European clinical experience with Endorem. A new contrast agent for liver MRI in 1000 patients. Radiologe 35(11 Suppl 2):S274–S276

Cohen FM, Kuwatsuru R, Shames DM, Neuder M, Mann JS, Vexler V, Rosenau W (1994) Contrast-enhanced magnetic resonance imaging estimation of altered capillary permeability in experimental mammary carcinomas after X-irradiation. Invest Radiol 29:970–977

Desser TS, Rubin DL, Muller HH, Qing F, Khodor S, Zanazzi G, Young SW (1994) Dynamics of tumor imaging with Gd-DTPA-polyethylene glycol polymers: dependence on molecular weight. J Magn Reson Imaging 4:467–472

Ebert E, Hofmann S, Swiderski U, et al. (1992) Metallopophyrins: tumor-specific contrast agents? In: Rinck PA, Muller RN (eds) New developments in contrast agent research. European Magnetic Resonance Forum Foundation, Hamburg, pp 127–140

Elste V, Wagner S, Taupitz M, Pfefferer D, Kresse M, Hamm B, Berg R (1996) Magnetic resonance lymphography in rats: effects of muscular activity and hyperthermia on the lymph node uptake of intravenously injected superparamagnetic iron oxide particles. Acad Radiol 3:660–666.

Frank H, Weissleder R, Brady TJ (1994a) Enhancement of MR angiography with iron oxide: preliminary studies in whole-blood phantom and in animals. Am J Roentgenol 162:209–213

Frank H, Weissleder R, Bogdanov AJ, Brady TJ (1994b) Detection of pulmonary emboli by using MR angiography with MPEG-PL-GdDTPA: an experimental study in rabbits. Am J Roentgenol 162:1041–1046

Gallez B, Bacic G, Swartz HM (1996) Evidence for the dissociation of the hepatobiliary MRI contrast agent Mn-DPDP. Magn Reson Med 35:14–19

Gehl HB, Urhahn R, Bohndorf K, Klever P, Hauptmann S, Lodemann KP, Matern S (1993) Mn-DPDP in MR imaging of pancreatic adenocarcinoma: initial clinical experience. Radiology 186:795–798

Gibby WA, Billings J, Hall J, Ovitt TW (1990) Biodistribution and magnetic resonance imaging of cross-linked DTPA polysaccharides. Invest Radiol 25:164–172

Göhr-Rosenthal S, Schmitt-Willich H, Ebert W, Conrad J (1993) The demonstration of human tumors on nude mice using gadolinium-labelled monoclonal antibodies for magnetic resonance imaging. Invest Radiol 28:789–795

Grandin C, Van Beers BE, Demeure R, Goudemant JF, Mottet I, Pringot J (1995) Comparison of gadolinium-DTPA and polylysine-gadolinium-DTPA-enhanced magnetic resonance imaging of hepatocarcinoma in the rat. Invest Radiol 30:572–581

Guimaraes R, Clement O, Bittoun J, Carnot F, Frija G (1994) MR lymphography with superparamagnetic iron nanoparticles in rats: pathologic basis for contrast enhancement. Am J Roentgenol 162:201–207

Hamm B, Taupitz M, Hussmann P, Wagner S, Wolf KJ (1992a) MR lymphography with iron oxide particles: dose-response studies and pulse sequence optimization in rabbits. Am J Roentgenol 158:183–190

Hamm B, Vogl TJ, Branding G, et al. (1992b) Focal liver lesions: MR imaging with Mn-DPDP - initial clinical results in 40 patients. Radiology 182:167–174

Hamm B, Staks T, Taupitz M, Maibauer R, Speidel A, Huppertz A, Frenzel T (1994a) Contrast-enhanced MR imaging of liver and spleen: first experience in humans with a new superparamagnetic iron oxide. J Magn Reson Imaging 4:659–668

Hamm B, Thoeni RF, Gould RG, Bernardino ME, Luning M, Saini S, Mahfouz AE (1994b) Focal liver lesions: characterization with nonenhanced and dynamic contrast material-enhanced MR imaging. Radiology 190:417–423

Hamm B, Staks T, Mühler A, Bollow M, Taupitz M, Frenzel T, Wolf KJ (1995) Phase I clinical evaluation of Gd-EOB-DTPA as a hepatobiliary MR contrast agent: safety, pharmacokinetics, and MR imaging. Radiology 195:785–792

Harika L, Weissleder R, Poss K, Papisov MI (1996) Macromolecular intravenous contrast agent for MR lymphography: characterization and efficacy studies. Radiology 198:365–370

Hindré F, LePlouzennec M, de Certaines JD, Foultier MT, Patrice T, Simonneaux G (1993) Tetra-*p*-aminophenylporphyrin conjugated with Gd-DTPA: tumor-specific contrast agent for MR imaging. J Magn Reson Imaging 3:59–65

Hindré F, Curtet C, deMarco G, Pouliquen D, Chatal J-F, LeJeune JJ, Jalle P (1994) Contrast agent: magnetite-dextran labeled with anti-CEA monoclonal antibody. Society of Magnetic Resonance, 3rd Annual Scientific Meeting. Nice, France, p 1134

Kabalka GW, Davis MA, Moss TH, Buonocore E, Hubner K, Holmberg E, Maruyama K (1991) Gadolinium-labeled liposomes containing various amphiphilic Gd-DTPA derivatives: targeted MRI contrast enhancement agents for the liver. Magn Reson Med 19:406–415

Kettritz U, Warshauer DM, Brown ED, Schlund JF, Eisenberg LB, Semelka RC (1996) Enhancement of the normal pancreas: comparison of manganese-DPDP and gadolinium chelate. Eur Radiol 6:14–18

Kim SK, Pohost GM, Elgavish GA (1991) Fatty-acyl iminopolycarboxylates: lipophilic bifunctional contrast agents for NMR imaging. Magn Reson Med 22:57–67

Kim SK, Pohost GM, Elgavish GA (1992) Gadolinium complexes of [(myristoyloxy)propyl]diethylenetriaminetetraacetate: new lipophilic, fatty acyl conjugated NMR contrast agents. Bioconjug Chem 3:20–26

Kornguth SE, Turski PA, Perman WH, Schultz R, Kalinke T, Reale R, Raybaud F (1987) Magnetic resonance imaging of gadolinium-labeled monoclonal antibody polymers directed at human T lymphocytes implanted in canine brain. J Neurosurg 66:898–906

Kornguth S, Anderson M, Turski P, Sorenson J, Robins HI, Cohen J, Rappe A (1990) Glioblastoma multiforme: MR imaging at 1.5 and 9.4 T after injection of polylysine-DTPA-Gd in rats. Am J Neuroradiol 11:313–318

Kramer J, Stiglbauer R, Engel A, Prayer L, Imhof H (1992) MR contrast arthrography (MRA) in osteochondrosis dissecans. J Comput Assist Tomogr 16:254–260

Laniado M, Kornmesser W, Hamm B, Clauss W, Weinmann H-J, Felix R (1988) MR imaging of the gastrointestinal tract: value of Gd-DTPA. Am J Roentgenol 150:817–821

Lauffer RB, Parmelee DJ, Quellet HS, Dolan RP, Sajiki HS, Scott DM, Bernard PJ (1996) MS-325: a small-molecule vascular imaging agent for magnetic resonance imaging. Acad Radiol 3:S356–S358

Lauterbur PC, Mendonca-Dias MH, Rudin AM (1978) Augmentation of tissue water proton spin-lattice relaxation rates by in-vivo addition of paramagnetic ions. Front Med Biol Eng 1:752–759

Leveille-Webster CR, Rogers J, Arias IM (1996) Use of an asialoglycoprotein receptor-targeted magnetic resonance contrast agent to study changes in receptor biology during liver regeneration and endotoxemia in rats. Hepatology 23:1631–1641

Lim KO, Stark DD, Leese PT, Pfefferbaum A, Rocklage SM, Quay SC (1991) Hepatobiliary MR imaging: first human experience with MnDPDP. Radiology 178:79–82

Marchal G, Ni Y, Herijgers P, Flameng W, Petre C, Bosmans H, Yu J (1996) Paramagnetic metalloporphyrins: infarct avid contrast agents for diagnosis of acute myocardial infarction by MRI. Eur Radiol 6:2–8

Mayo-Smith WW, Saini S, Slater G, Kaufman JA, Sharma P, Hahn PF (1996) MR contrast material for vascular enhancement: value of superparamagnetic iron oxide. Am J Roentgenol 166:73–77

McLachlan SJ, Morris MR, Lucas MA, Fisco RA, Eakins MN, Fowler DR, Scheetz RB (1994) Phase I clinical evaluation of a new iron oxide MR contrast agent. J Magn Reson Imaging 4:301–307

McLachlan SJ, Morris M, Lucas MA, Baum LM (1996) Preliminary clinical experience with AMI 227. Acad Radiol 3:S295–S296

Mitchell DG, Outwater EK, Matteucci T, Rubin DL, Chezmar JL, Saini S (1995) Adrenal gland enhancement at MR imaging with Mn-DPDP. Radiology 194:783–787

Mühler A, Platzek J, Radüchel B, Frenzel T, Weinmann H-J (1995) Characterization of a gadolinium-labeled cholesterol derivative as an organ-specific contrast agent for adrenal MR imaging. J Magn Reson Imaging 5:7–10

Murakami T, Baron RL, Peterson MS, Oliver JH, Davis PL, Confer SR, Federle MP (1996) Hepatocellular carcinoma: MR imaging with mangafodipir trisodium (Mn-DPDP). Radiology 200:69–77

Nelson JA, Schmiedl U (1991) Porphyrins as contrast media. Magn Reson Med 22:366–371; discussion 378

Ni Y, Marchal G, Herijgers P, Flameng W, Petre C, Ebert W, Hilger CS (1996) Paramagnetic metalloporphyrins: from enhancers of malignant tumors to markers of myocardial infarcts. Acad Radiol 3:S395–S397

Ogan MD, Revel D, Brasch RC (1987) Metalloporphyrin contrast enhancement of tumors in magnetic resonance imaging. A study of human carcinoma, lymphoma, and fibrosarcoma in mice. Invest Radiol 22:822–828

Patronas NJ, Cohen JS, Knop RH, Dwyer AJ, Colcher D, Lundy J, Mornex F (1986) Metalloporphyrin contrast agents for magnetic resonance imaging of human tumors in mice. Cancer Treat Rep 70:391–395

Petersein J, Saini S, Weissleder R (1996) Liver. II. Iron oxide-based reticuloendothelial contrast agents for MR imaging. Clinical review. Magn Reson Imaging Clin North Am 4:53–60

Petré C, Ni Y, Marchal G, Yu J, Wevers M, Lauffer RB, Baert AL (1995) Detection and characterization of primary liver cancer in rats by MS-264-enhanced MRI. Magn Reson Med 35:532–539

Place DA, Faustino PJ, van Zijl PC, Chesnick A, Cohen JS (1990) Metalloporphyrins as contrast agents for tumors in magnetic resonance imaging. Invest Radiol 25:S69–S70

Reimer P, Weissleder R, Shen T, Knoefel WT, Brady TJ (1994) Pancreatic receptors: initial feasibility studies with a targeted contrast agent for MR imaging. Radiology 193:527–531

Reimer P, Rummeny EJ, Daldrup HE, Balzer T, Tombach B, Berns T, Peters PE (1995) Clinical results with Resovist: a phase 2 clinical trial. Radiology 195:489–496

Reimer P, Rummeny EJ, Shamsi K, Balzer T, Daldrup HE, Tombach B, Hesse T (1996) Phase II clinical evaluation of Gd-EOB-DTPA: dose, safety aspects, and pulse sequence. Radiology 199:177–183

Remsen LG, McCormick CI, Roman-Goldstein S, Nilaver G, Weissleder R, Bogdanov A, Hellstrom I (1996) MR of carcinoma-specific monoclonal antibody conjugated to monocrystalline iron oxide nanoparticles: the potential for noninvasive diagnosis. Am J Neuroradiol 17:411–418

Rofsky NM, Earls JP (1996) Mangafodipir trisodium injection (Mn-DPDP). A contrast agent for abdominal MR imaging. Magn Reson Imaging Clin North Am 4:73–85

Rummeny EJ, Reimer P, Daldrup H, Peters PE (1995) Detection of liver tumors. Radiologe 35(11 Suppl 2):S252–S258
Runge VM, Wells JW (1995) A comparison of MR hepatobiliary gadolinium chelates. Am J Roentgenol 164:122
Runge VM, Wells JW, Williams NM (1996) Evaluation of gadolinium 2,5-BPA-DO3A, a new macrocyclic hepatobiliary chelate, in normal liver and metastatic disease on high field magnetic resonance imaging. Invest Radiol 31:11–16
Saini S, Nelson RC (1995) Technique for MR imaging of the liver. Radiology 197:575–577
Schad LR, Semmler W, Knopp MV, Deimling M, Weinmann H-J, Lorenz WJ (1993) Preliminary evaluation: magnetic resonance of urography using a saturation inversion projection spin-echo sequence. Magn Reson Imaging 11:319–327
Schaffer BK, Linker C, Papisov M, Tsai E, Nossiff N, Shibata T, Bogdanov AJ (1993) MION-ASF: biokinetics of an MR receptor agent. Magn Reson Imaging 11:411–417
Schmiedl U, Ogan MD, Moseley ME, Brasch RC (1986) Comparison of the contrast-enhancing properties of albumin-(Gd-DTPA) and Gd-DTPA at 2.0 T: and experimental study in rats. Am J Roentgenol 147:1263–1270
Schmiedl U, Ogan M, Paajanen H, Marotti M, Crooks LE, Brito AC, Brasch RC (1987) Albumin labeled with Gd-DTPA as an intravascular, blood pool-enhancing agent for MR imaging: biodistribution and imaging studies. Radiology 162:205–210
Schneider G, Hayd C, Müller A, Gohl D, Urbschat K, Ebert W, Pfefferer D (1995) Contrast enhanced MRI of exp. induced brain infarctions in rabbits using Bis-Gd-MP as MR contast agent. Society of Magnetic Resonance, 3rd Annual Scientific Meeting. Nice, France, p 1144
Schuhmann-Giampieri G, Schmitt-Willich H, Frenzel T, Press W-R, Weinmann H-J (1991) In vivo and in vitro evaluation of Gd-DTPA-polylysine as a macromolecular contrast agent for magnetic resonance imaging. Invest Radiol 26:969–974
Schuhmann-Giampieri G, Schmitt-Willich H, Press W-R, Negishi C, Weinmann H-J, Speck U (1992) Preclinical evaluation of Gd-EOB-DTPA as a contrast agent in MR imaging of the hepatobiliary system. Radiology 183:59–64
Schwickert HC, Stiskal M, Roberts TP, van Dijke CF, Mann J, Mühler A, Shames DM (1996) Contrast-enhanced MR imaging assessment of tumor capillary permeability: effect of irradiation on delivery of chemotherapy. Radiology 198:893–898
Schwizer W, Fraser R, Maecke H, Siebold K, Funck R, Fried M (1994) Gd-DOTA as a gastrointestinal contrast agent for gastric emptying measurements with MRI. Magn Reson Med 31:388–393
Semelka RC, Schlund JF, Molina PL, Willms AB, Kahlenberg M, Mauro MA, Weeks SM (1996) Malignant liver lesions: comparison of spiral CT arterial portography and MR imaging for diagnostic accuracy, cost, and effect on patient management. J Magn Reson Imaging 6:39–43
Seneterre E, Taourel P, Bouvier Y, Pradel J, Van Beers B, Daures JP, Pringot J (1996) Detection of hepatic metastases: ferumoxides-enhanced MR imaging versus unenhanced MR imaging and CT during arterial portography. Radiology 200:785–792
Shames DM, Kuwatsuru R, Vexler V, Mühler A, Brasch RC (1993) Measurement of capillary permeability to macromolecules by dynamic magnetic resonance imaging: a quantitative noninvasive technique. Magn Reson Med 29:616–622
Shen TT, Bogdanov A Jr, Bogdanova A, Poss K, Brady TJ, Weissleder R (1996) Magnetically labeled secretin retains receptor affinity to pancreas acinar cells. Bioconjug Chem 7:311–316
Su MY, Najafi AA, Nalcioglu O (1995) Regional comparison of tumor vascularity and permeability parameters measured by albumin-Gd-DTPA and Gd-DTPA. Magn Reson Med 34:402–411
Taupitz M, Wagner S, Hamm B, Dienemann D, Lawaczeck R, Wolf KJ (1993) MR lymphography using iron oxide particles. Detection of lymph node metastases in the VX2 rabbit tumor model. Acta Radiol 34:10–15
Tilcock C, Ahkong QF, Koenig SH, Brown RD, Davis M, Kabalka G (1992) The design of liposomal paramagnetic MR agents: effect of vesicle size upon the relaxivity of surface-incorporated lipophilic chelates. Magn Reson Med 27:44–51
Tomalia DA, Naylor AM, Goddard IWA (1990) Starburst-Dendrimer: Kontrolle von Größe, Gestalt, Oberflächenchemie, Topologie und Flexibilität beim Übergang von Atomen zu makroskopischer Materie. Angew Chem 102:119–157
Unger E, Cardenas D, Zerella A, Fajardo LL, Tilcock C (1990) Biodistribution and clearance of liposomal gadolinium-DTPA. Invest Radiol 25:638–644
Unger E, Shen DK, Wu GL, Fritz T (1991) Liposomes as MR contrast agents: pros and cons. Magn Reson Med 22:304–308; discussion 313
Unger EC, Shen DK, Fritz TA (1993) Status of liposomes as MR contrast agents. J Magn Reson Imaging 3:195–198
van Dijke CF, Brasch RC, Roberts TP, Weidner N, Mathur A, Shames DM, Mann JS (1996) Mammary carcinoma model: correlation of macromolecular contrast-enhanced MR imaging characterizations of tumor microvasculature and histologic capillary density. Radiology 198:813–818
Vassallo P, Matei C, Heston WD, McLachlan SJ, Koutcher JA, Castellino RA (1994) AMI-227-enhanced MR lymphography: usefulness for differentiating reactive from tumor-bearing lymph nodes. Radiology 193:501–506
Vittadini G, Felder E, Tirone P, Lorusso V (1988) B-19036, a potential new hepatobiliary contrast agent for MR proton imaging. Invest Radiol 23:S246–S248
Vogl TJ, Kummel S, Hammerstingl R, Schellenbeck M, Schumacher G, Balzer T, Schwarz W (1996) Liver tumors: comparison of MR imaging with Gd-EOB-DTPA and Gd-DTPA. Radiology 200:59–67
Weinmann H-J, Brasch RC, Press W-R, Wesbey GE (1984) Characteristics of gadolinium-DTPA complex: a potential NMR contrast agent. Am J Roentgenol 142:619–624
Weinmann H-J, Schuhmann-Giampieri G, Schmitt-Willich H, Vogler H, Frenzel T, Gries H (1991) A new lipophilic gadolinium chelate as a tissue-specific contrast medium for MRI. Magn Reson Med 22:233–237; discussion 242
Weinmann H-J, Berndorf D, Mühler A, Ebert W (1996) Mechanism of hepatic uptake of Gd-EOB-DTPA. Acad Radiol 3(Suppl 2):S232–S234
Weissleder R, Elizondo G, Wittenberg J, Lee AS, Josephson L, Brady TJ (1990a) Ultrasmall superparamagnetic iron oxide: an intravenous contrast agent for assessing lymph nodes with MR imaging. Radiology 175:494–498
Weissleder R, Reimer P, Lee AS, Wittenberg J, Brady TJ (1990b) MR receptor imaging: ultrasmall iron oxide particles targeted to asialoglycoprotein receptors. Am J Roentgenol 155:1161–1167
Weissleder R, Lee AS, Fischman AJ, Reimer P, Shen T, Wilkinson R, Callahan RJ (1991) Polyclonal human immu-

noglobulin G labeled with polymeric iron oxide: antibody MR imaging. Radiology 181:245–249
Weissleder R, Lee AS, Khaw BA, Shen T, Brady TJ (1992) Antimyosin-labeled monocrystalline iron oxide allows detection of myocardial infarct: MR antibody imaging. Radiology 182:381–385
Weissleder R, Wang YM, Papisov M, Bogdanov A, Schaffer B, Brady TJ, Wittenberg J (1993) Polymeric contrast agents for MR imaging of adrenal glands. J Magn Reson Imaging 3:93–97
Weissleder R, Heautot JF, Schaffer BK, Nossiff N, Papisov MI, Bogdanov AJ, Brady TJ (1994) MR lymphography: study of a high-efficiency lymphotrophic agent. Radiology 191:225–230
Wiener EC, Brechbiel MW, Brothers H, Magin RL, Gansow OA, Tomalia DA, Lauterbur PC (1994) Dendrimer-based metal chelates: a new class of magnetic res-onance imaging contrast agents. Magn Reson Med 31:1–8
Young SW, Sidhu MK, Qing F, Muller HH, Neuder M, Zanassi G, Mody TD (1994) Preclinical evaluation of gadolinium (III) texaphyrin complex. A new paramagnetic contrast agent for magnetic resonance imaging. Invest Radiol 29:330–338
Young SW, Qing F, Harriman A, Sessler JL, Dow WC, Mody TD, Hemmi GW (1996) Gadolinium(III) texaphyrin: a tumor selective radiation sensitizer that is detectable by MRI. Proc Natl Acad Sci U S A 93:6610–6615

18 Central Nervous System

I. Berry, J.-P. Ranjeva, M. Clanet, and C. Manelfe

CONTENTS

I. Berry, MD, PhD, Department of Neuroradiology, University Hospital Purpan, and Department of Biophysics and Nuclear Medicine, University Hospital Rangueil, 1, avenue Jean-Poulhès, F-31054 Toulouse Cédex, France
J.-P. Ranjeva, PhD, Department of Neuroradiology, University Hospital Purpan, Place du Docteur Baylac, F-31059 Toulouse, France
M. Clanet, MD, Department of Neurology, University Hospital Purpan, Place du Docteur Baylac, F-31059 Toulouse, France
C. Manelfe, MD, Department of Neuroradiology, University Hospital Purpan, Place du Docteur Baylac, F-31059 Toulouse, France

18.1 Introduction

The excellent screening sensitivity of morphological magnetic resonance imaging (MRI) rapidly came to require the complementary use of paramagnetic contrast agents with interstitial diffusion. In the case of central nervous system (CNS) imaging such agents are capable of visualizing sites of breakdown of the blood-brain barrier. Dynamic observation of the kinetics of contrast enhancement is one of the issues already explored with computed tomography (CT) that has been revisited with MRI. The information thereby obtained on the permeability of the blood-brain barrier is of theoretical importance and also has limited application in the clinical setting. The dose of paramagnetic chelates to be employed is periodically subjected to renewed scrutiny. Use of the magnetization transfer technique to highlight contrast enhancement has recently offered another opportunity to reassess this question, but no clear consensus has emerged from the various series as to whether a higher or a lower dose than that originally recommended, i.e., 0.1 mmol/kg of 0.5 *M* solutions (i.e., 0.2 cm^3/kg), should be employed in clinical routine. Different routes of administration have recently been explored such as intrathecal injection.

A more functional application of the use of contrast media in the CNS has appeared achievable. Assessment of the cerebral blood volume and/or perfusion is possible using blood pool contrast agents, or on the basis of the magnetic susceptibility changes that accompany the first passage of paramagnetic bolus. Compared with other techniques used in hemodynamic studies, such as positron emission tomography (PET) and single-photon emission computed tomography, MRI offers higher spatial resolution, which appears advantageous. Currently no routine clinical applications of contrast-enhanced MRI have been established in this field, but promising approaches include evaluation of cerebrovascular pathology and use of functional MRI in brain activation studies.

18.2 The Blood-Brain Barrier and MRI Contrast Agents

18.2.1 Contrast Enhancement in the Central Nervous System

The diagnostic power of MRI relies heavily on its sensitivity to tissue water content. Most pathologies produce an increase in water content and consequently in T1 and T2 relaxation times (Brant-Zawadzki et al. 1984). Agents applicable in MRI decrease the proton relaxation times of water molecules, either because of water exchange between compartments or by migration of the agent in the interstitium. The latter is the dominant mechanism in the CNS, and its occurrence is significant only when the blood-brain barrier is ruptured (McNamara et al. 1986).

The normal blood-brain barrier is composed of endothelial cells with scarce pinocytosis, connected together by tight junctions, lying on a thick basement membrane. Permeability is limited to water, oxygen, carbon dioxide, and lipophilic substances. Contrast media, with hydrophilic molecules, cannot cross the normal blood-brain barrier (Sage 1982). Therefore in clinical routine, contrast media are employed in MRI of the CNS as a means of evaluating the blood-brain barrier status in vivo. Gadolinium chelates, which are the most widely used contrast agents, are injected intravenously in this indication in ca. one-quarter of the neurological MRI examinations in order to determine whether lesions visualized on T2-weighted sequences are macroscopically deleterious to the blood-brain barrier. This is similar to the use of contrast agents in CT of the CNS, in which iodinated contrast agents also localize blood-brain barrier breakdowns. Indeed, the molecular weights of both classes of agents are similar (in the order of 600 daltons), both are hydrophilic and neither is carried by proteins. Contrast enhancement is based on interstitial distribution of the agent, which is mandatory for the local expression of the paramagnetic effect when the imaging parameters employed are those usually used under clinical conditions. Extravascular diffusion of such agents is free throughout the body, except in the case of the structures covered by the blood-brain barrier. In the normal CNS, no physiological enhancement is noticeable in the white or the gray matter (Berry et al. 1986).

Despite the aforementioned similarities, the strategies underlying the use of contrast media in the two modalities, CT and MRI, is extremely different: contrast media increase the sensitivity of CT in the screening of intra-axial lesions, whereas in MRI of the CNS T2-weighted sequences are employed for screening (Brant-Zawadzki et al. 1984) and contrast agents are used primarily to improve the selectivity of the information. Clinical evaluation of Gd-DTPA-dimeglumine, the first molecule to reach clinical trials, confirmed its usefulness in the diagnosis and follow-up of both intra-axial (Brant-Zawadzki et al. 1986) (Fig. 18.1) and extra-axial lesions (Berry et al. 1986) (Figs. 18.2, 18.3).

18.2.2 Permeability of the Blood-Brain Barrier

A more quantitative approach to the use of gadolinium chelates entails the measurement of leakage through a defective blood-brain barrier. Various methods of measurement of blood-brain permeability have been proposed, based on compartmental analysis (Tofts and Kermode 1991; Larsson et al. 1990; see Larsson and Tofts 1992 for a comparison). Repetition of T1-weighted image acquisition allows enhancement of the signal time evolution curve and estimation of the blood-to-tissue transport coefficient.

An earlier stage of blood-brain barrier disruption was detected by Rousseau et al. (1997) using magnetite-dextran nanoparticles, which showed a decrease in T2-weighted signal intensity in the area of the disruption. Macrophages are suspected to be involved in the passage of the contrast agent across the blood-brain barrier, and this opens up a totally different field in the understanding of the uptake mechanism.

The quantity of Gd-DTPA transferred across the blood-brain barrier after intravenous injection has been studied using cerebrospinal fluid (CSF) T1 and T2 measurements at 1.5 T in order to assess integrity of the blood-brain barrier in disease states not noted for focal blood-brain barrier disruption, such as Alzheimer's disease (Ibrahim et al. 1998). The lowest Gd-DTPA concentration tested was 1.98×10^{-3} m*M*. A single measurement of the relaxation time of CSF samples performed after contrast-enhanced imaging could be used to confirm the absence of parenchymal enhancement.

Investigation of the time course of enhancement can be performed using faster techniques of initial

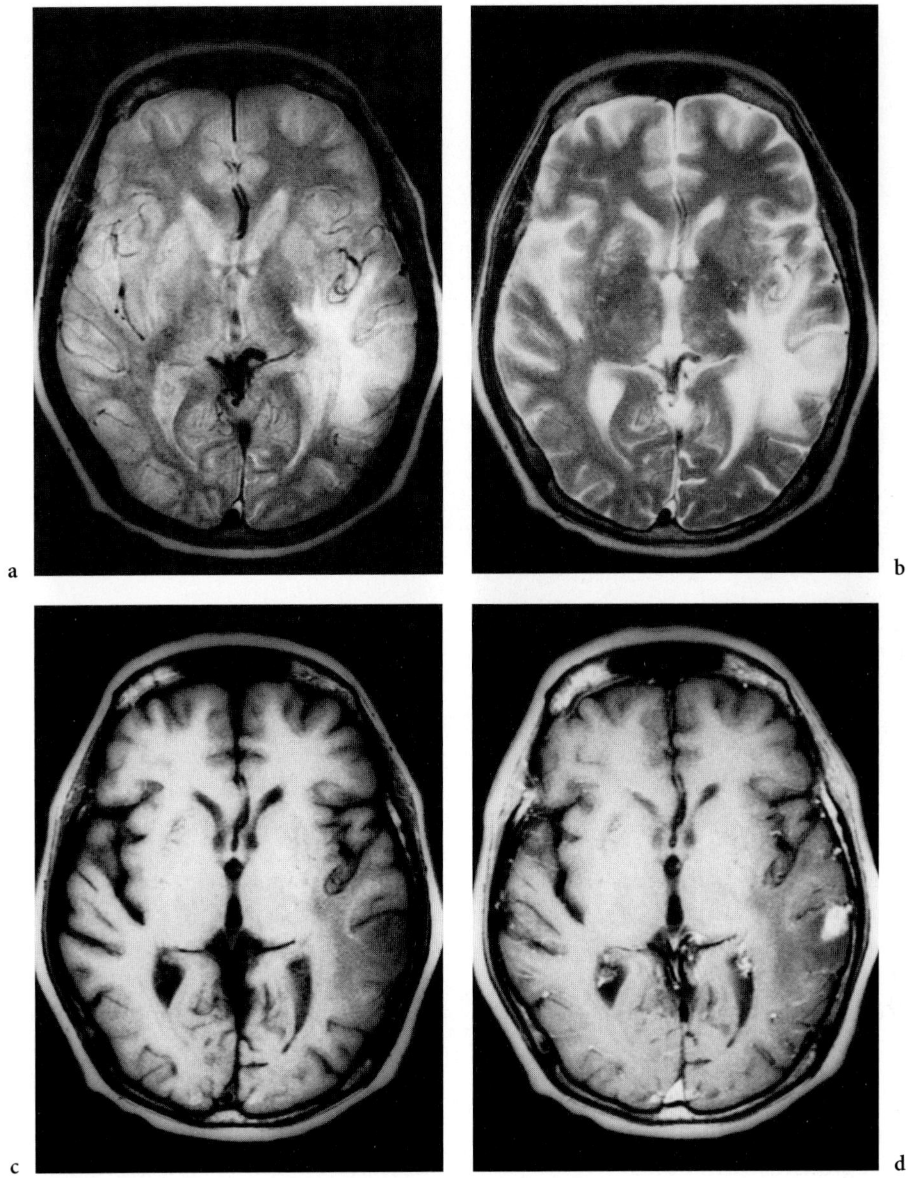

Fig. 18.1 a–d. Intra-axial lesion. T2-weighted first echo (a) and second echo (b) images show a large infiltrative hyperintense mass effect in the left temporal lobe involving both the cortex and the white matter. T1-weighted images at the same level before (c) and after (d) injection of gadolinium show enhancement restricted to a single focus in the temporal cortex representing the localization of a metastasis with neovascularization, surrounded by edema without blood-brain barrier disruption

data collection and/or by prolonged observation for several hours after the injection. This allows one to take into account the entry of the contrast agent into the cerebral capillaries, which reflects the vascularity of the tissue (BULLOCK et al. 1991; GOWLAND et al. 1992). "Dynamic MRI" is the term used to describe the acquisition of a series of T1-weighted images following a bolus injection of contrast in order to evaluate the rate of contrast uptake. Two phases occur: an early one, thought to reflect the intravascular distribution of contrast, and a late one, resulting from diffusion of contrast into the adjacent interstitial space. Most of the variability between lesions occurs in the first 100 s. Analyses of signal and concentration changes with time allow mapping of the capillary permeability-surface area product, the tissue leakage space, the enhancement onset time, the mean enhancement gradient, and the maximum enhancement level (PARKER et al. 1997). Wash-out of the contrast agent from a site of enhancement occurs

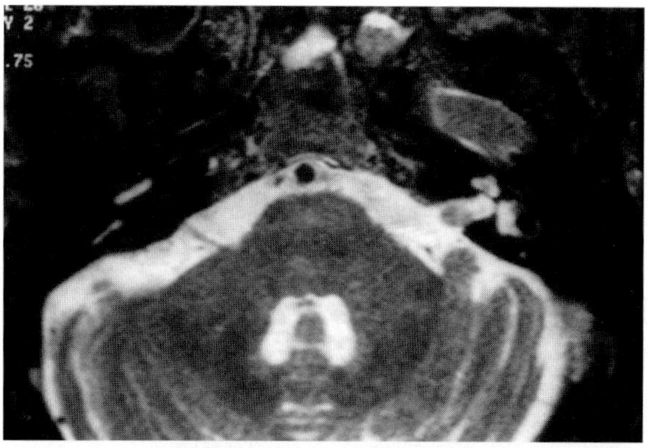

a

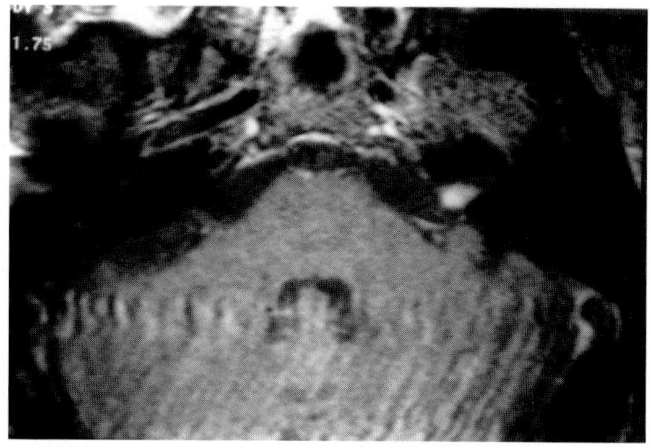

b

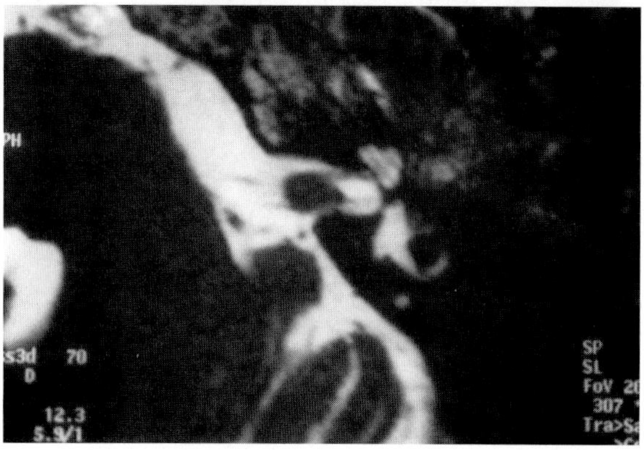

c

Fig. 18.2 a–c. Extra-axial lesion. **a** T2-weighted high-resolution 2-mm-thick slice centered on the left acoustic and facial nerves, suggesting a small mass in the internal auditory canal. **b** Post-gadolinium T1-weighted slice confirms contrast enhancement of a grade I neurinoma. **c** CISS 3D acquisition with millimetric reconstruction visualizes the neurinoma but does not replace the contrast injection test for confirmation of the extra-axial enhancing tumor

when the concentration of the agent in the blood is less than that in the tissue. This process can also be modeled (Gowland et al. 1992) and is of some interest for characterization of the size of the extracellular matrix of a lesion (Ikushima et al. 1997).

18.2.3 Optimization of Enhancement: Dose, Delay, and Magnetization Transfer Technique

Magnetic resonance signal depends upon proton density and T1 and T2 relaxation times. The timing and length of the radiofrequency pulses can be selected such that the image is weighted to depend primarily on one or other of these relaxation times, or to represent mainly proton density. Paramagnetic centers decrease each relaxation time in the same proportion. Correct combination of the effect of the contrast agent with the weighting of the image produces exploitable contrast. The relationship between the concentration of gadolinium chelates in the brain tissue and the MR signal is approximately linear for repetition time (TR) values of about 500 ms or less in spin-echo (Larsson et al. 1990). TR is therefore easily set to optimize T1 weighting of images. Decreased T1 increases signal intensity as long as the decrease in T2 is not too large. Increased signal intensity requires a low local concentration of contrast agent: excessive concentrations will promote decreased signal intensity. The dose-effect relationship is consequently complex, and determination of the optimal dose is a controversial issue. The clinically recommended dose is 0.1 mmol/kg of 0.5 M solutions. The injected volume is therefore quite small: 0.2 cm^3/kg.

Several clinical trials have compared series of patients receiving the standard dose or a triple dose of gadolinium chelates. The occurrence of adverse events was found not to increase with the triple dose. The enhancement was stronger with the triple dose, and additional lesions were discovered in a limited number of cases, particularly in patients with brain metastases and multiple sclerosis; however, this was considered to have limited implications for patient management (Runge et al. 1992; Yuh et al. 1992; Haustein et al. 1993; Haughton 1994; Van Dijk et al. 1997) (Figs. 18.4, 18.5). Flow artifacts are increased after administration of high-dose contrast agents, particularly in the posterior fossa; in addition the increase in cost is quite significant. Accordingly, such studies have not produced a major change in examination strategy, with the exception of some

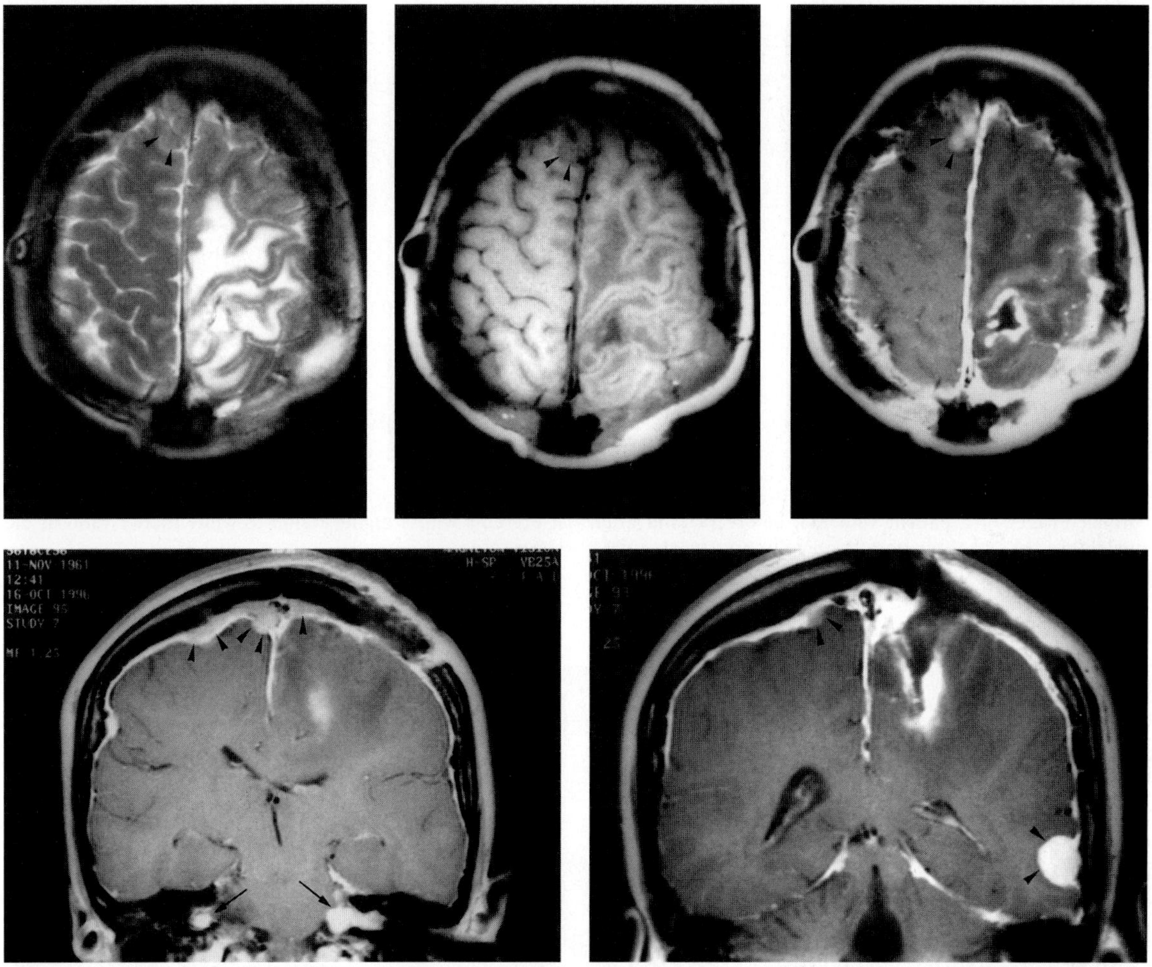

a,b c d e

Fig. 18.3 a–e. Complex examination showing both intra- and extra-axial lesion enhancement in a patient with von Recklinghausen neurofibromatosis type II with bilateral acoustic neurinomas, meningiomatosis, meningitis, and staphylococcus abscess following surgery on a parasagittal meningioma. **a** T2-weighted slice showing a left frontoparietal hyperintense mass effect of the abscess and a right anterior frontal meningioma (*arrowheads*) with the same intensity as brain parenchyma. **b, c** T1-weighted precontrast (**b**) and postcontrast (**c**) axial slices showing rim enhancement of the abscess, meningeal enhancement of the infection, and enhancement of the meningiomatosis (*arrowheads*). **d, e** Postcontrast T1-weighted coronal slices showing diffuse meningeal enhancement related to infection, additional meningioma enhancement both at the vertex and in the left temporal region (*arrowheads*), and enhancement of the abscess and bilateral acoustic neurinomas (**d**, *arrows*)

protocols in which a double dose is recommended (as in some clinical trials in patients with multiple sclerosis).

Other parameters also need to be taken into consideration with respect to enhancement. The optimal delay between injection and imaging is usually 5 min. Longer delays do not produce a significant increase in intensity according to HAUSTEIN et al. (1992) and AKESON et al. (1997), though others have found a moderate increase in sensitivity, particularly in the detection of multiple sclerosis lesions (FILIPPI et al. 1997a; SILVER et al. 1997). In fact the technique of magnetization transfer (WOLFF and BALABAN 1994) focuses to a far greater extent on increasing contrast on the basis of decreased signal intensity of nonenhancing tissue. A comparison of triple dose versus standard dose with magnetization transfer showed equally good lesion-to-white matter contrast; the triple-dose magnetization transfer technique further increased lesion-to-white matter contrast but did not show additional lesions (KNAUTH et al. 1996). On the other hand in the detection of multiple sclerosis lesions the interobserver agreement has been found to be better with triple-dose than with single-dose gadolinium when using the magnetization transfer technique (VAN

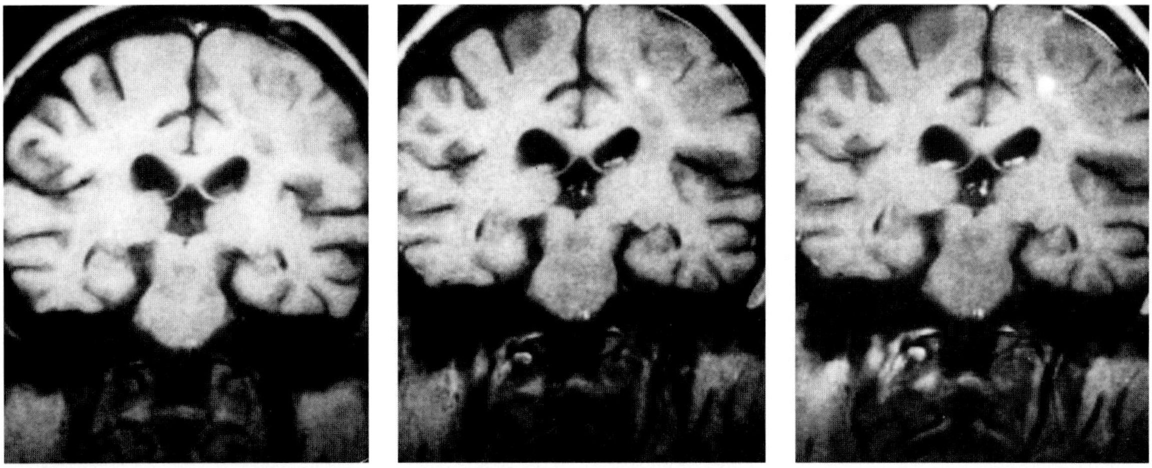

a,b c

Fig. 18.4 a–c. Triple-dose gadolinium study. T1-weighted coronal images of a patient with MS, before (**a**) and after single-dose (**b**) and triple-dose (**c**) gadolinium chelate injection. Enhancing plaque in the left parietal white matter is visible after both the single dose and the triple dose, although it presents with a higher lesion-to-white matter ratio in the latter case

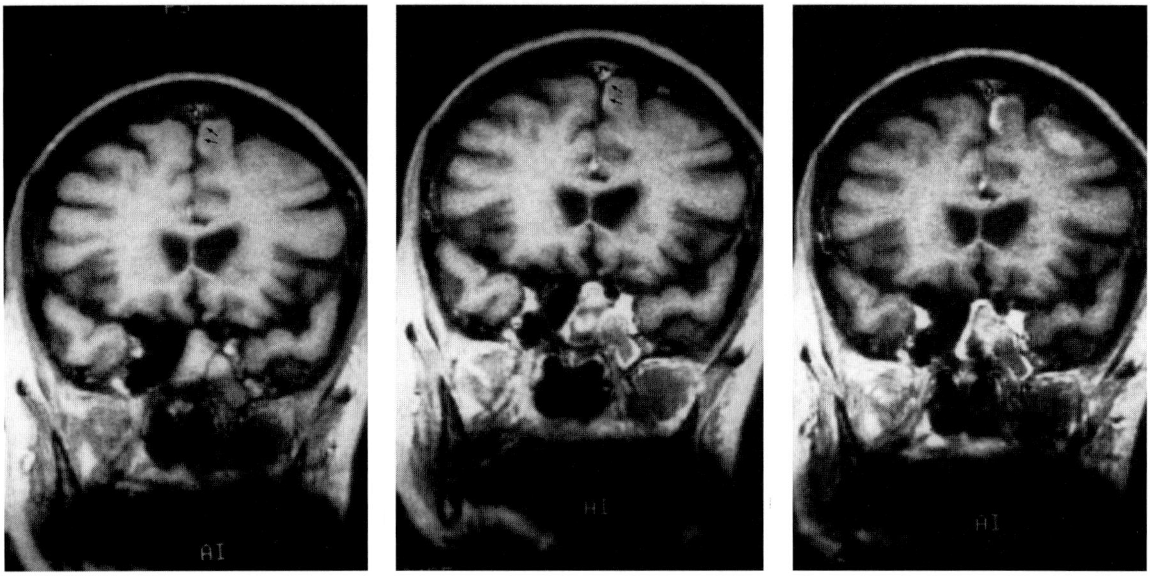

a,b c

Fig. 18.5 a–c. Triple-does gadolinium study revealing contrast enhancement. T1-weighted coronal images of a patient with a venous brain infarct, before (**a**) and after single-dose (**b**) and triple-dose (**c**) gadolinium chelate injection. A petechial left midline cortical lesion (*arrows*) enhances faintly after the single dose and markedly after the triple dose. A prefrontal cortical lesion enhances only after the triple dose

Waesberghe et al. 1997). When using magnetization transfer after contrast injection it is important also to obtain precontrast images with magnetization transfer since some high-signal lesions on T1-weighted images may be disclosed by magnetization transfer and should not be mistaken for contrast enhancement (Meyer et al. 1997). This applies for lesions less structured than normal tissue, such as are found in patients with tuberous sclerosis (Jeong et al. 1997) (Fig. 18.6) or multiple sclerosis (Bozzao et al. 1996).

18.2.4 Alternative Routes of Administration

Intraventricular administration of gadolinium chelate for MRI of the CSF was tested at a dose of

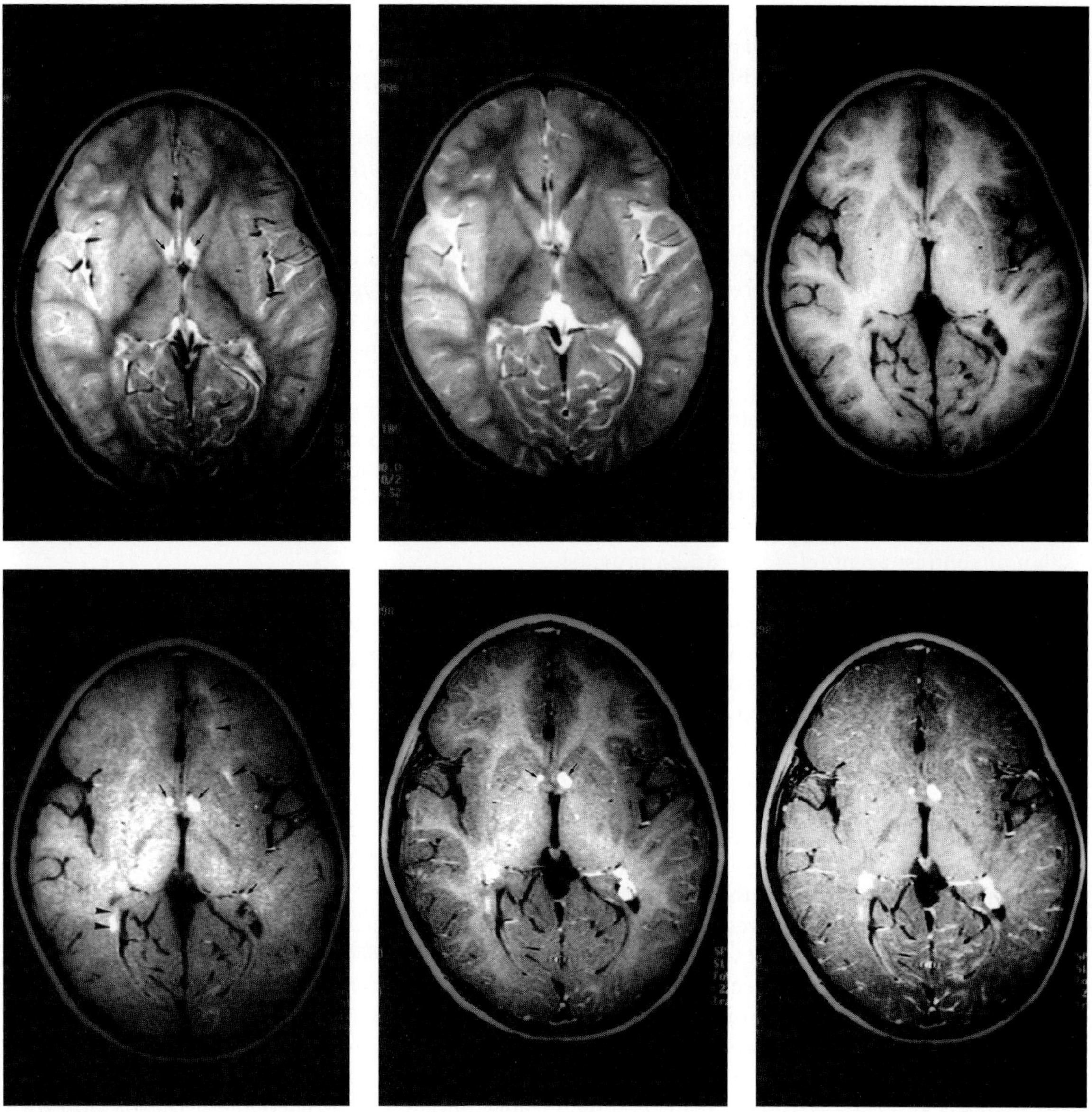

a,b c

d,e f

Fig. 18.6 a–f. Bourneville syndrome studied with magnetization transfer in a 3-year-old boy with left motor seizures. **a,b** T2-weighted first (**a**) and second echo (**b**) images show hyperintense subependymal nodules located at both foramina of Monro (*arrows*). **c** T1-weighted sequence depicts only their mass effect. **d** With the addition of magnetization transfer saturation pulse three subependymal nodules (*arrows*) present bright signal intensity as well as abnormalities in the subcortical left frontal and periventricular right temporal white matter (*arrowheads*). **e** Contrast injection reveals enhancement in the subependymal nodules but becomes ambiguous in the vicinity of the choroid plexuses, which also enhance. **f** Postgadolinium T1-weighted sequence with magnetization transfer saturation pulse achieves the best contrast-to-noise ratio for the visualization of subependymal nodules

0.01 mmol in two patients with leptomeningeal carcinomatosis (Siebner et al. 1997). Such a dose only achieved enhancement close to the site of injection. This procedure may be of interest to check the efficiency of drug administration devices, for example. The safety of the subarachnoid injection of MR contrast media has been addressed by Skalpe (1998).

18.3 Contrast Agents for Brain Perfusion Assessment

The cerebral intravascular space represents only 5% of the brain; therefore extracting its contribution from the signal of the whole brain is difficult. Three approaches allow amplification of the blood pool MR signal: perfusion techniques based on the differential velocities of water molecules (Le Bihan et al. 1988), spin labeling of water protons (Williams et al. 1992), and the use of contrast agents. The contrast agents employed are either nondiffusible agents imaged at a stable concentration in the circulation (Berry et al. 1996) or agents rapidly imaged during their first passage in the brain, which relfects cerebral blood volume and cerebral blood flow (Villringer et al. 1988).

18.3.1 First Passage

Dynamic MRI, in which a series of images are rapidly acquired over several minutes following a bolus injection of contrast agent (cf. Sect. 18.2.2), provides information on both tissue perfusion and disruption of the blood-brain barrier. Information on blood flow can be more specifically obtained if one considers the initial changes in signal as the contrast agent passes through the vessels of the brain. Perfusion imaging can be achieved by rapid acquisition of either T1- or T2*-weighted images. This is usually called "magnetic susceptibility imaging." A drop in signal in a T2*-weighted sequence is observed, lasting about 15 s. Among fast imaging techniques, echoplanar imaging (EPI) achieves the best temporal resolution for monitoring the cerebrovascular transit of magnetic susceptibility contrast media. On the other hand T2*-weighted gradient-echo produces better signal-to-noise ratios. The resulting curves of signal intensity over time are fitted and integrated to quantify cerebral blood volume (Belliveau et al. 1990; Rosen et al. 1990, 1991; Sorensen et al. 1997). Deconvolution of cerebral blood flow and mean transit time is also possible (Edelman et al. 1990) (Fig. 18.7). In magnetic susceptibility imaging, disruptions of the blood-brain barrier produce a less pronounced fall in signal intensity which underestimates the local perfusion. Hybrid imaging allows for concomitant rapid acquisition of T1- and T2*-weighted images (Miyati et al. 1997).

The mechanism of magnetic susceptibility contrast media is completely different from the T1 relaxation acceleration exploited for morphological purposes, even if the same diffusible agents can serve both goals because of the high magnetic moment of gadolinium chelates. Magnetic susceptibility (T2*) contrast agents induce microscopic magnetic field inhomogeneities, resulting in a loss of signal intensity in perfused tissue. Gadolinium chelates have been used in various clinical indications for brain hemodynamic assessment at rest (Aronen et al. 1994; Renshaw et al. 1997; Stehling et al. 1998) and for evaluation of cerebrovascular reserve using CO_2 or acetazolamide (Gückel et al. 1996; Nighoghossian et al. 1997; Berthezene et al. 1998). Superparamagnetic iron oxide (SPIO) particles, 40 nm in diameter, have also been used as first-pass contrast agents and produce a very large signal loss (Forsting et al. 1994; Reith et al. 1995). The high magnetic susceptibility and T1 and T2 relaxivities of SPIOs allow smaller injection volumes to be used than is the case with paramagnetic contrast agents (Josephson et al. 1991; Haraldseth et al. 1996), which will be advantageous when the former become available for human investigations.

18.3.2 Blood Pool Contrast Agents

The signal of the blood pool can be enhanced for longer than the first passage if the contrast agent used has a long half-life in the vascular compartment and if its relaxation properties are sufficiently strong. Paramagnetic macromolecules (such as albumin-gadolinium-DTPA and dextran-gadolinium-DTPA) have produced quite disappointing results, with minimal signal enhancement of the brain (Schmiedl et al. 1987; Moseley et al. 1992). In fact such macromolecules offer better possibilities for fine determination of capillary permeability (Van Dijke et al. 1996). Particulate compounds with a short plasma half-life, such as SPIOs, can be imaged during the first pass or during the initial minutes after injection, and reflect the perfusion through a decrease in signal intensity (Majumdar et al. 1988; Gore and Majumdar 1990; Kent et al. 1990; Forsting et al. 1994; Reith et al. 1995). Although the high magnetic susceptibility and the relaxivity of these agents mean that, as compared with paramagnetic compounds, lower doses are required in order to produce an effect, imaging time and doses are restricted by the transient action of SPIOs.

Another type of agent, ultrasmall superparamagnetic iron oxide (USPIO) particles, has been designed to remain longer in the bloodstream; these agents produce an efficient and quite prolonged magnetic susceptibility effect in the brain parenchyma, thereby allowing high-resolution imaging to be repeated (Fig. 18.8). USPIO particles are cleared from the bloodstream by the macrophage

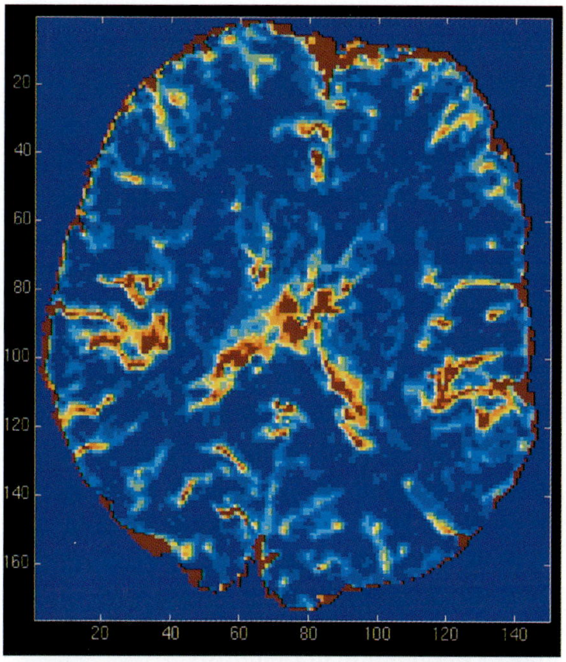
a

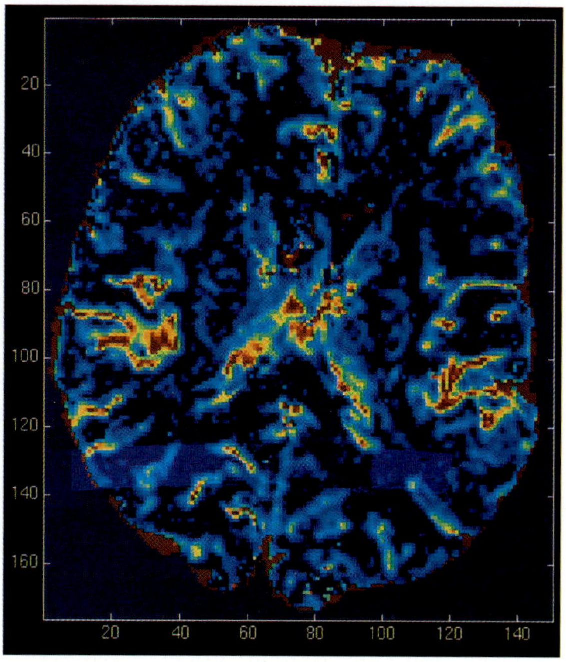
b

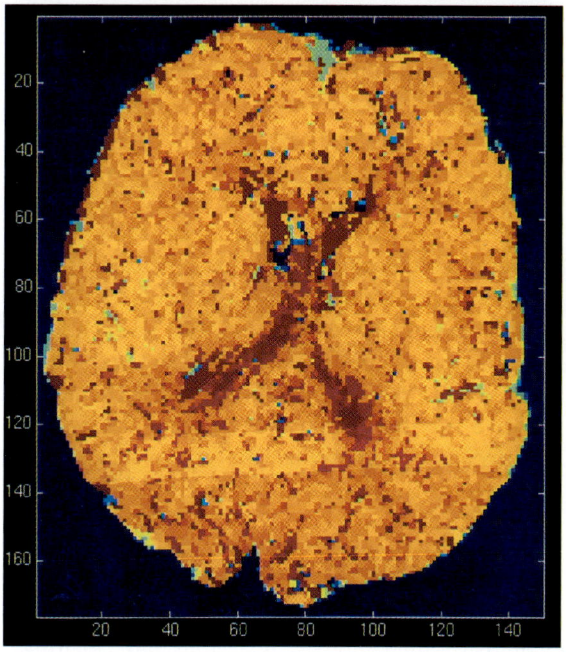
c

Fig. 18.7 a–c. Hemodynamically weighted images obtained by magnetic susceptibility echo-planar imaging during a bolus injection of gadolinium chelate. **a** Cerebral blood volume map shows higher blood volume in the gray matter (cortex and basal ganglia). **b** Relative cerebral blood flow map follows the same pattern. **c** Mean transit time map evidences the watershed areas of junctions between the territories of the middle cerebral artery and the posterior cerebral artery (red is prolonged mean transit time on the color scale)

monocyte phagocytic system (MMPS) and have a longer life span than larger particles (Weissleder et al. 1990; Mühler et al. 1995). These nanoparticles have a low charge and a hydrophilic coating. They are composed of an iron oxide crystalline core measuring 4–6 nm and coated by a dextran surfactant. The entire mean particle size is 20 nm. After intravenous administration in the rat, USPIO particles are distributed to the blood pool; they are then slowly taken up by the MMPS with a 120-min plasma half-life. They are concentrated in the spleen (35%), the lymph nodes (4%), the bone marrow (1%–2%), and the liver (20%) (Chambon et al. 1993). A single USPIO dose of 60–80 µmol iron/kg body weight combined with T2*-weighted gradient-echo or echo-planar imaging allows multislice high-resolution acquisition which is of great interest in the screening for discrete lesions. In pathological conditions of the

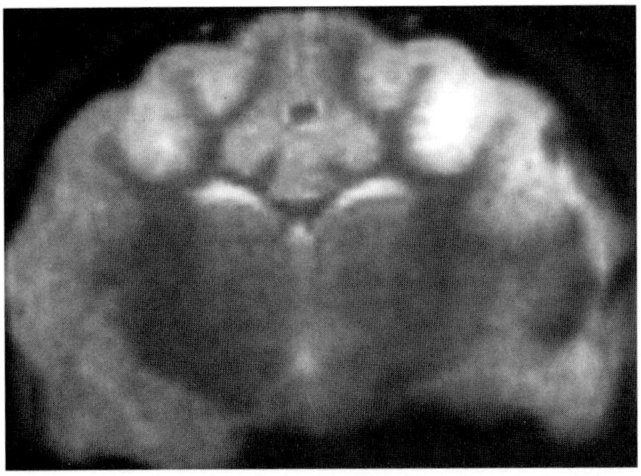

a

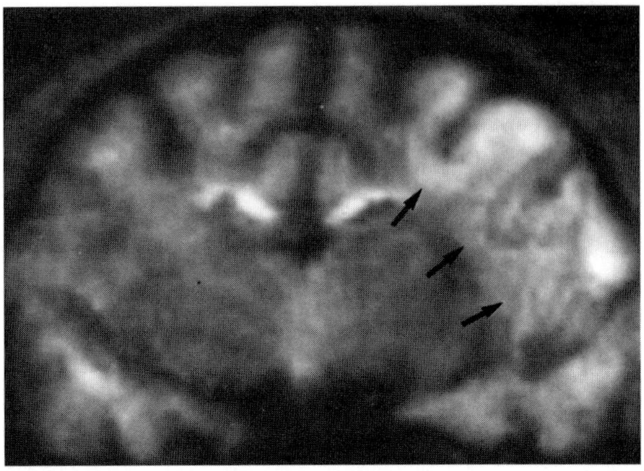

b

Fig. 18.8 a,b. Coronal T2*-weighted gradient-echo images of cat brain before (**a**) and after (**b**) injection of USPIO particles at a dose of 150 μmol iron/kg body weight 4 h after middle cerebral artery occlusion. USPIO predominantly decreases the signal of the normal territory and improves delineation of the injury (*arrows*). Note the greater signal decrease of the normal gray matter, which has a higher blood volume than the normal white matter

brain, capillary permeability is another element to be taken into consideration. Bulte et al. (1992) showed an accumulation of particles at the site of blood-brain barrier disruption in a model of freezing injury in the rat, producing a pronounced decrease in signal.

18.4 Role of Contrast Agents in MRI of Multiple Sclerosis

Magnetic resonance imaging has substantially modified our understanding of multiple sclerosis (MS). It reveals abnormalities in more than 95% of patients with definite MS and facilitates diagnosis of the disease. It is a reliable tool for objective and reproducible assessment of treatment effect and is widely used for assessment of outcome in therapeutic trials. However, the most effective way to use MRI in MS remains to be established because the relationship between the clinical symptoms, the neuropathological lesions, and their interpretation through MRI is highly complex (Miller et al. 1998). Recent MRI developments such as magnetization transfer imaging, spectroscopic imaging, diffusion imaging, and functional imaging will assist in clarifying the underlying biology of the disease by permitting better identification of the elementary pathophysiological components conditioning the reversibility of the lesions. Nevertheless, the use of paramagnetic contrast agents in this disease is of importance and deserves consideration with regard to diagnosis and prognostic assessment (Fig. 18.9).

18.4.1 Role of Gadolinium in Diagnosis

Magnetic resonance imaging can be used both to evaluate the risk of development of MS following a clinically isolated symptom (e.g., optic neuritis or a brain stem or spinal symptom) or to define the probability of the diagnosis in an individual patient. Barkhof et al. (1997) confirmed that a four-parameter dichotomized MRI model including gadolinium enhancement and juxtacortical, infratentorial, and periventricular lesions predicts the conversion to clinically definite MS with an accuracy of 80%. This model performs better than the criteria of Paty et al. (1988) or Fazekas et al. (1988), the comparative specificities being 78%, 54%, and 54%, respectively. If gadolinium were not to be used, the same level of diagnostic accuracy would require a minimum of nine lesions, a much larger number than the threshold of four considered appropriate according to the criteria of Paty et al.

Imaging of the spinal cord can contribute to the diagnosis when no brain lesions are identified (Thorpe et al. 1996). Activity in the spinal cord is approximately 10% of that in the brain, but these lesions are more likely to result in clinical relapses. The optic nerve may be imaged with thin slices and contrast enhancement can be best evaluated with the fat suppression technique (Amano et al. 1997) (Fig. 18.10).

Despite the aforementioned findings, Miller et al. (1998) concluded that the diagnosis of MS remains based on clinical criteria and that MRI findings should only be considered as offering sup-

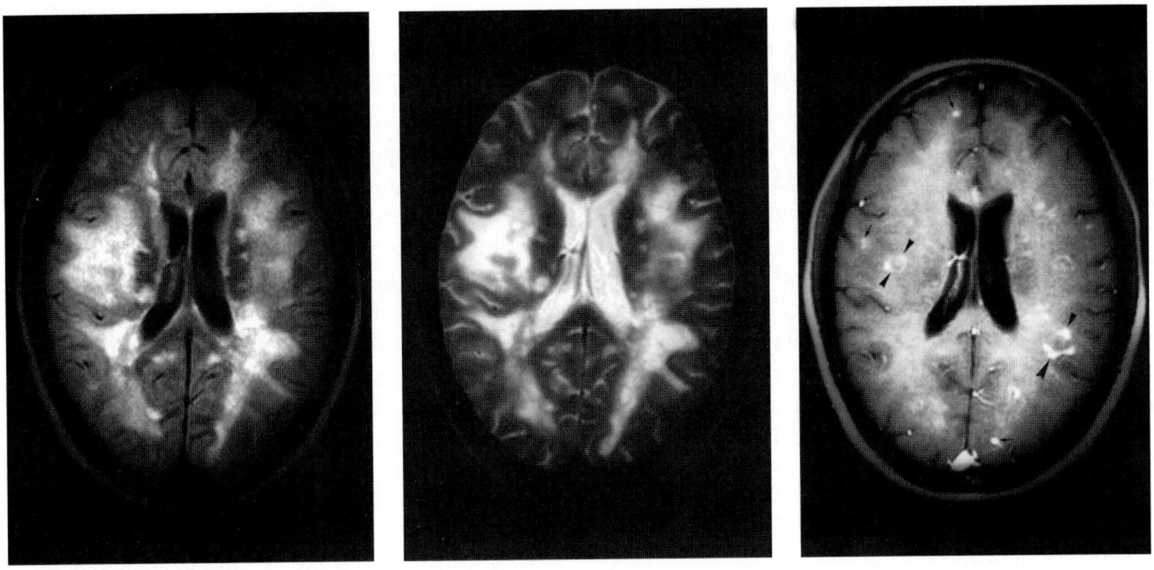

a,b c

Fig. 18.9 a–c. MS plaque enhancement. **a,b** T2-weighted first (**a**) and second echo (**b**) slices showing extensive demyelinating and edematous lesions predominantly in the white matter in a patient with relapsing MS. Periventricular lesions are better seen on the first echo image. **c** T1-weighted image obtained 5 min following gadolinium injection shows a combination of new plaqus with homogeneous enhancement (*arrows*) and reactivated plaques with rim enhancement (*arrowheads*)

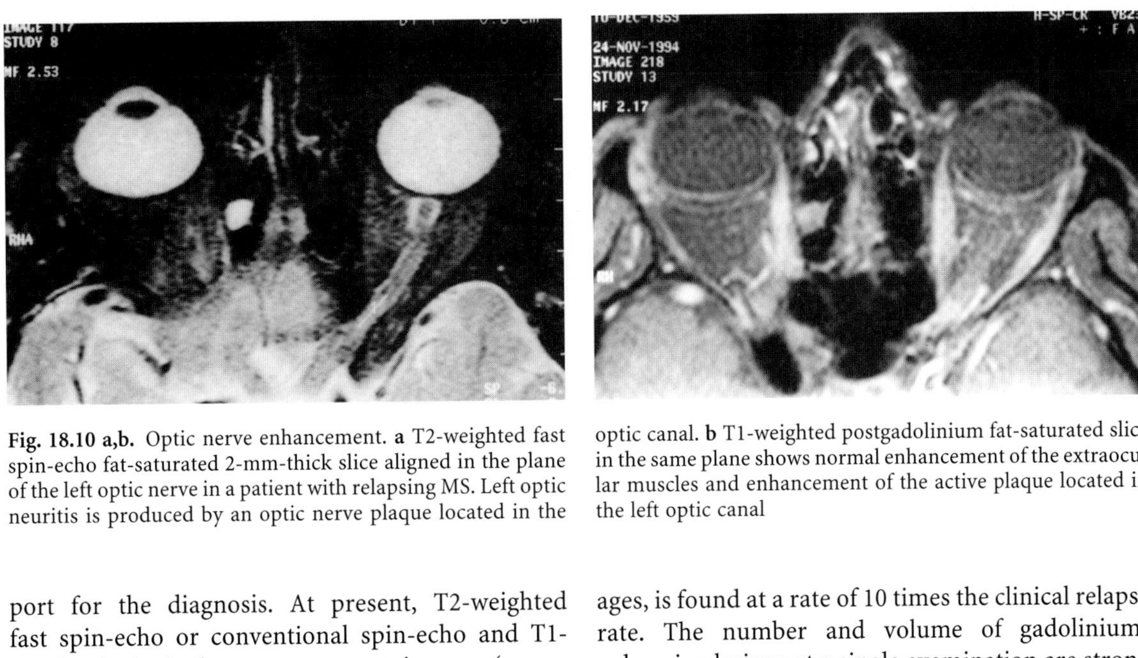

a b

Fig. 18.10 a,b. Optic nerve enhancement. **a** T2-weighted fast spin-echo fat-saturated 2-mm-thick slice aligned in the plane of the left optic nerve in a patient with relapsing MS. Left optic neuritis is produced by an optic nerve plaque located in the optic canal. **b** T1-weighted postgadolinium fat-saturated slice in the same plane shows normal enhancement of the extraocular muscles and enhancement of the active plaque located in the left optic canal

port for the diagnosis. At present, T2-weighted fast spin-echo or conventional spin-echo and T1-weighted single-dose postcontrast images (sometimes) should be the standard imaging protocols used in diagnostic tests.

18.4.2 Use of Gadolinium to Assess Disease Activity

Disease activity, as assessed by the presence of gadolinium-enhancing lesions on T1-weighted images, is found at a rate of 10 times the clinical relapse rate. The number and volume of gadolinium-enhancing lesions at a single examination are strong short-term predictors of subsequent clinical and MRI disease activity (Koudriavtseva et al. 1997). The sensitivity of MRI as a surrogate marker of short-term activity (i.e., by visualization of gadolinium-enhancing lesions on T1-weighted images and new, enlarging or recurring lesions on T2-weighted images) has led to its use in phase II clinical trials, in which it provides a primary end point that shortens the duration of the trial and limits the number of patients required to demonstrate a drug effect (MILLER et al. 1996). The clinical safety of serial monthly administrations was established in 56 patients followed up over a 4-year period (TRESLEY et al. 1997).

Various authors have addressed the questions of the most appropriate imaging technique (T1 weighting, delay between injection and imaging, and use of magnetization transfer) and the optimal dose of gadolinium in the context of MS. The initial guidelines on the use of MRI in clinical trials recommended a short delay of 5 min between injection and imaging (MILLER et al. 1991). This issue was again addressed by FILIPPI et al. (1997a), who found only a moderate increase in sensitivity (6.4%) when the interval was increased to 20–30 min. This is in keeping with the work of AKESON et al. (1997) showing that there is no advantage in waiting longer than 5 min as the effect does not change during the next 25 min. SILVER et al. (1997) reported that the sensitivity of contrast-enhanced MRI can be dramatically increased by the combination of triple-dose gadolinium and delayed (40–60 min) magnetization transfer imaging, doubling the detection of contrast-enhancing lesions. However, this technique has not yet been validated in clinical trials.

Recently SIMON et al. (1998) reported on the use of MRI in conjunction with interferon beta-1a (Avonex) in MS. In this trial, annual gadolinium-enhanced MRI studies demonstrated treatment effect. The multiple regression model used in the analysis confirmed the importance of the gadolinium enhancing status at baseline, which was predictive of the change in the T2 lesion volume after 2 years. This finding was confirmed in a study by MOLYNEUX et al. (1998), in which the number of enhancing lesions on the entry scan was predictive of subsequent relapse rate over the study duration (11 months) and also correlated with the subsequent enhancing lesion activity over the study period. A significant correlation was found between change in lesion load and disease activity on the monthly scans. This observation is in agreement with the finding that, in relapsing patients with a long-term monthly MRI follow-up, the average lesion frequency tends to show a similar rate over several years (STONE et al. 1997). Such MRI activity is not restricted to relapsing patients, as TUBRIDY et al. (1998) have very recently demonstrated that MRI activity is generally high in patients with a secondary progressive course, even when they do not have superimposed relapses.

The beta-interferons as a class induce a decline in the number of contrast-enhancing lesions in MS [cf. findings of SIMON et al. (1998) with respect to interferon beta-1a and The IFNB MS Study Group (1995) with respect to interferon beta-1b]. Histologically, extensive gadolinium enhancement has been associated with leakage of the blood-brain barrier due to massive cellular infiltration (mainly macrophages) in the acute lesions (MORRISSEY et al. 1996). It is probable that interferons act by decreasing the macrophage activation and infiltration of the white matter. Moreover an increase in soluble vascular cell adhesion molecule has been reported during treatment with interferon beta-1b, and this increase was found to correlate with the decrease in the number of contrast-enhancing lesions (CALABRESI et al. 1997). This is consistent with the hypothesis of direct interference of interferon beta-1b with the adhesion cascade, which may prevent activated T cells from trafficking into the CNS. Additionally it has been established that interferon beta-1a prolongs the beneficial effects of steroids on the blood-brain barrier, resulting in a significant reduction in the mean number and volume of enhancing lesions (GASPERINI et al. 1998). However, gadolinium enhancement was observed by BRUCK et al. (1997) also to be associated with inactive, demyelinated, or remyelinating lesions, confirming that a moderate blood-brain barrier breakdown exists in chronic lesions. This raises the question of whether the use of excessively sensitive techniques for the detection of active enhancing lesions will decrease the specificity of the correlation with the inflammatory process.

18.4.3 MRI as a Predictor of Disease Severity

The majority of reports have emphasized that the conventional MRI parameters are poorly correlated with disability as evaluated by the usual disability scoring system EDSS (MILLER et al. 1998). This suggests that the factors contributing to the disability cannot yet be recognized on MRI, i.e., it is difficult to extract the significant contributions from an abnormal T2 signal. MRI activity, including the rate of gadolinium enhancement, is well correlated with clinical exacerbations (SMITH et al. 1993) but poorly correlated with disability, and this also holds true for the total lesion load on T2-weighted images. Edema, membrane disruption, demyelination, cellular infiltration, gliosis, and axonal loss are the elementary components of the plaques and are present in different proportions according to the stage of evolution, which conditions the reversibility (STORCH and LASSMANN 1997). USPIO particles are taken up by macrophages; they have been imaged experimentally in a model of allergic encephalomyelitis and detected in immunoactive lesions (Dousset et al. 1997).

New MRI techniques are now available which allow greater pathophysiological accuracy. Some of the findings obtained with these techniques have cast new light on plaque activity. Using spectroscopic imaging, Narayana et al. (1998) have recently shown the presence of lipid peaks in active lesions, and the fact that these sometimes occurred in the absence of gadolinium enhancement in MRI-defined lesions suggests that demyelination may occur independently of perivenous inflammatory changes. Findings on magnetization transfer imaging, a method to show the transfer of molecules of water between a macromolecular environment (bound water) such as myelin and a free compartment (free water), correlate with the extent of tissue abnormalities, reflecting mainly demyelination and more generally the amount of destructuring of the underlying tissue (Gass et al. 1994; Campi et al. 1996). A follow-up study of enhancing lesions screened with single-dose and triple-dose gadolinium has evaluated the heterogeneity of the lesion population: using the magnetization transfer technique, Filippi et al. (1998a) established that the tissue damage occurring within lesions enhancing only after triple-dose injection is less severe than that in lesions enhancing after the injection of a single dose. The abnormalities in the brain, including both macroscopic and microscopic disease (Filippi et al. 1995, 1997b; Hiele et al. 1995; van Buchem et al. 1996), have been recognized to occur weeks prior to gadolinium enhancement of the lesions (Filippi et al. 1998b).

In addition to its diagnostic value, MRI provides some clues to the different pathological aspects of MS. Differentiation of these fundamental processes cannot be achieved using a single MRI technique, and all the new imaging modalities under investigation are complementary. Such intensive studies will yield more reliable prognostic parameters for prediction of potential reversibility and functional restoration, and will also permit more accurate monitoring of the natural history of MS.

18.5 Role of Contrast Agents in MRI of Tumors

18.5.1 Evaluation of the Histological Grade of Gliomas

Magnetic resonance imaging is more sensitive than CT for the detection of gliomas. Nevertheless this higher sensitivity is not associated with greater specificity in either the differential diagnosis or the grading of gliomas. T1-weighted, T2-weighted, and proton density images do not discriminate between normal tissue and the various types of tumoral tissue (Just and Thelen 1988). In fact only contrast enhancement and edema are significant for tumor grading (Tervonen et al. 1992). This was also the conclusion reached by Kelly et al, (1987), who conducted a correlative study of histology, CT, and MRI on 1242 samples from 319 gliomas.

In high-grade gliomas, contrast enhancement corresponds to the extent of the bulk tumor (i.e. the solid part of a tumor removed during debulking), in which neovascularization allows interstitial access to contrast agents because capillaries are abnormal and fenestrated, with pinocytosis in the endothelial cells. Tissues with abnormal signal but without enhancement are the site of scattered tumor cell infiltration. These cells invade larger zones than is suspected on CT, and therefore tumoral infiltration is better estimated on the basis of increased T2 signal intensity rather than by reference to CT hypodensity. It has been pointed out, however, that on MRI, too, tumor cells may be present in wider areas than the hyperintense lesion (Watanabe et al. 1992).

In low-grade gliomas, such as fibrillary astrocytomas, there may be hypodensity on CT without contrast enhancement. MRI shows hypointense T1-weighted signal and hyperintense T2-weighted signal. Histologically, isolated tumor cells are scattered in an edematous parenchyma. High signal areas on T2-weighted sequences are usually large because of the high sensitivity of this sequence to increased free water. Contrast enhancement is not the rule, but can exist. If homogeneous, it may correspond to tumoral tissue of a pilocytic astrocytoma, a low-grade well-circumscribed tumor that displays slow progression and can be well treated surgically. Otherwise, in low-grade gliomas with contrast enhancement mean survival is shortened to 4.9 years (7.9 years in cases without enhancement) and post-surgical tumor recurrence occurs 6.8 times more frequently (McCormack et al. 1992).

Comparison of histological and imaging findings generated the architectural classification of tumors proposed by Daumas-Duport et al. (1987). Type I tumors comprise those such as pilocytic astrocytoma, composed exclusively of bulk tumor tissue with sharp margins. Less frequently, type I tumors occurring in the young prove to be oligodendrogliomas, which can be surgically removed. In type III tumors, such as fibrillary astrocytomas, scattered tumor cells infiltrate normal a,b e

c,d f

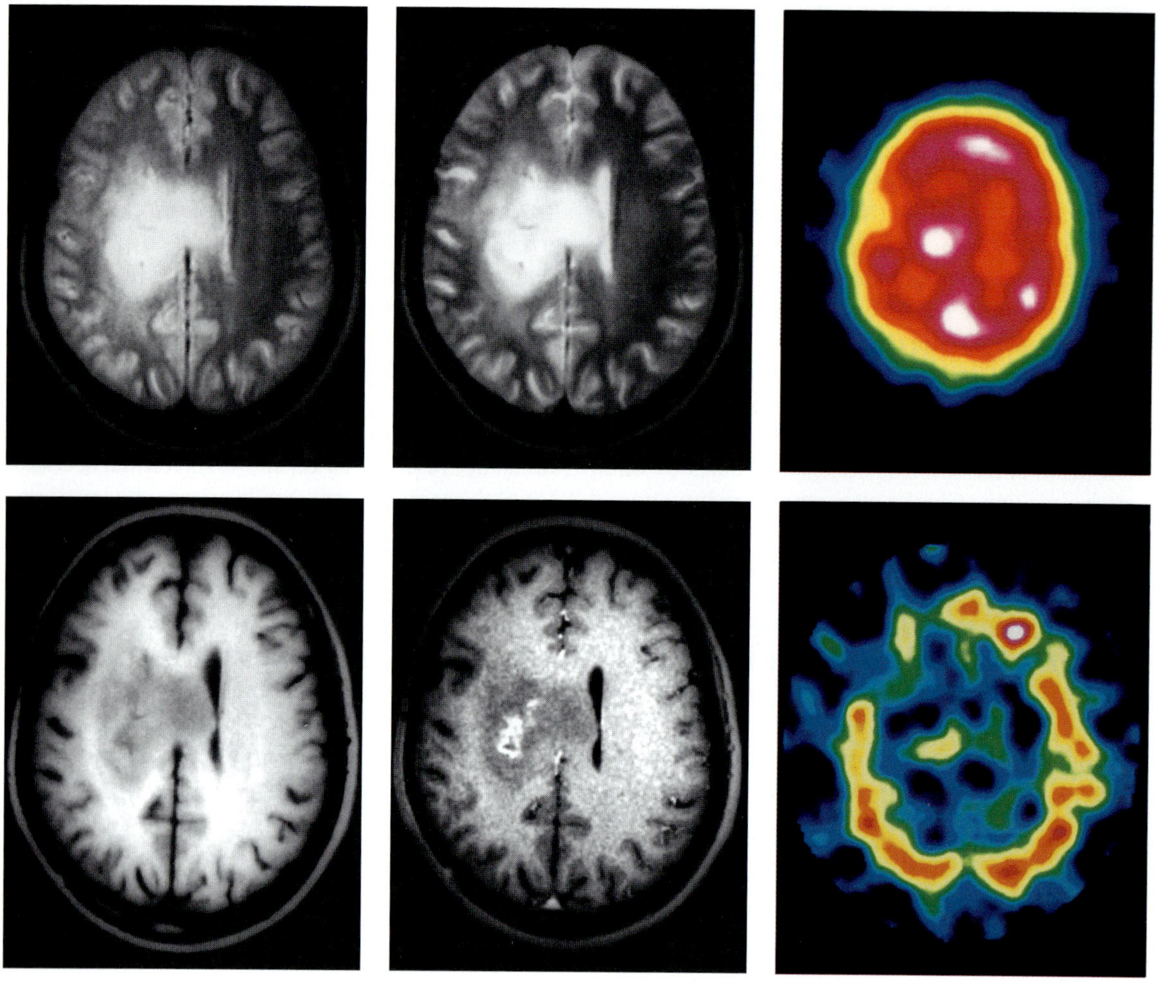

Fig. 18.11 a–f. Brain tumor enhancement. Grade 3 astrocytoma with hyperintense mass effect with fuzzy margins on T2-weighted first (**a**) and second echo (**b**) images T1-weighted precontrast hypointensity (**c**) is slightly inhomogeneous and contrast enhancement (**d**) is limited to the center of the tumor. HMPAO perfusion scintigraphy (**e**) shows increased perfusion in the tumor and decreased perfusion in the projection cortex, probably due to the deafferentation mechanism. Thallium brain scan (**f**) reveals moderately high uptake, with a lesion to scalp ratio of 4.7

tissue. In type II tumors (the most frequent) a bulk tumor is associated with peripheral infiltration; most of the high-grade glial tumors fall into this category. Exceptionally, low-grade gliomas are of type II, with the hypodense area on CT containing bulk tumor zones surrounded by scattered cells. Conversely, some high-grade tumors can exhibit a type III pattern in which many tumor cells display a high rate of mitosis but remain in a normal parenchyma without constitution of bulk tumor. This classification, based to a large extent on the contrast enhancement information, has generated a decision tree for the surgery of brain tumors (Kelly 1991).

Contrast enhancement and edema are the two main MRI features of significance for prediction of the histological grade of gliomas (Tervonen et al. 1992) (Figs. 18.11, 18.12). The intensity of contrast enhancement and the development of peritumoral edema are themselves highly correlated in high-grade glial tumors, which further confirms the relationship of these two factors with alteration of the blood-brain barrier (Pronin et al. 1997). Contrast enhancement reflects tumoral regions of highest growth potential (Yoshii et al. 1992). A combination of nine MRI parameters has been proposed to yield a morphological score that takes into account inhomogeneity, cyst or necrosis, midline shift, edema, mass effect, hemorrhage, tumor margins, flow effects, and contrast enhancement (Asari et al. 1994). Grading accuracy is 90% with this score.

Brain scintigraphy with metabolic radiotracers such as thallium-201 (Ancri et al. 1978) has been

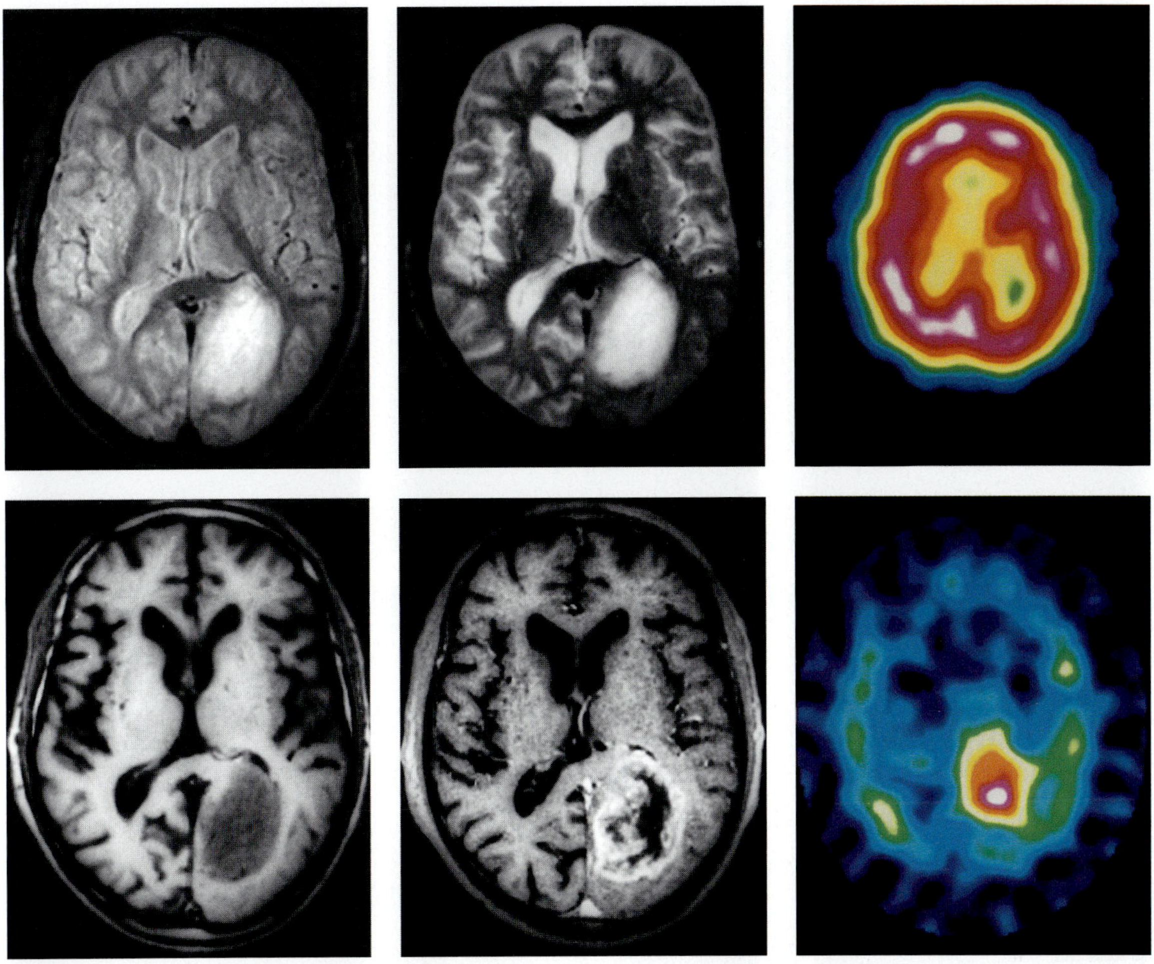

a,b e
c,d f

Fig. 18.12 a–f. Brain tumor enhancement. Grade 3 astrocytoma showing a homogeneous hyperintense mass effect with sharp margins on T2-weighted first (**a**) and second echo (**b**) images. T1-weighted precontrast hypointensity (**c**) is also surprisingly homogeneous and contrast enhancement (**d**) is markedly inhomogeneous. HMPAO perfusion scintigraphy (**e**) shows decreased perfusion and thallium brain scan (**f**) reveals high uptake with a lesion to scalp ratio of 6.2

evaluated for its ability to complement CT and MRI contrast agents in the grading of brain tumors. The behavior of thallium is analogous to that of potassium and permits the assessment of Na^+/K^+-ATPase function, increase in blood-brain barrier permeability, and preservation of local blood flow. Normally thallium dose not cross the blood-brain barrier and is not taken up by healthy brain tissue. Tumor neovascularization allows the passage of thallium, and this may help in differentiation between high- and low-grade gliomas (Black et al. 1989; Slizofski et al. 1995). The uptake index seems to have some prognostic value (Vertosick et al. 1994). This question has also been addressed with dynamic MRI and a correlation with clinical outcome has recently been demonstrated in patients with malignant gliomas (Wong et al. 1998). The vascular proliferation in malignant gliomas is expected to produce high maximum uptake rates during the first, vascular phase. Additionally the aforementioned study showed that higher maximum uptake rates are associated with shorter survival. The correlation of delayed uptake with survival is less significant.

Cerebral blood volume (CBV) maps obtained with magnetic susceptibility MRI have been found to correlate with tumor vascularity (Aronen et al. 1994) (Fig. 18.13). The range of values obtained for high-grade gliomas was larger (0.82–5.4 ml/100 g) than that found for low-grade gliomas (1.01–1.21 ml/100 g), and inhomogeneity was more pronounced in high-grade lesions. These findings concur with those of other studies regarding the perfusion of gliomas. To date such studies have mainly been performed with radiotracers; they have been regarded as con-

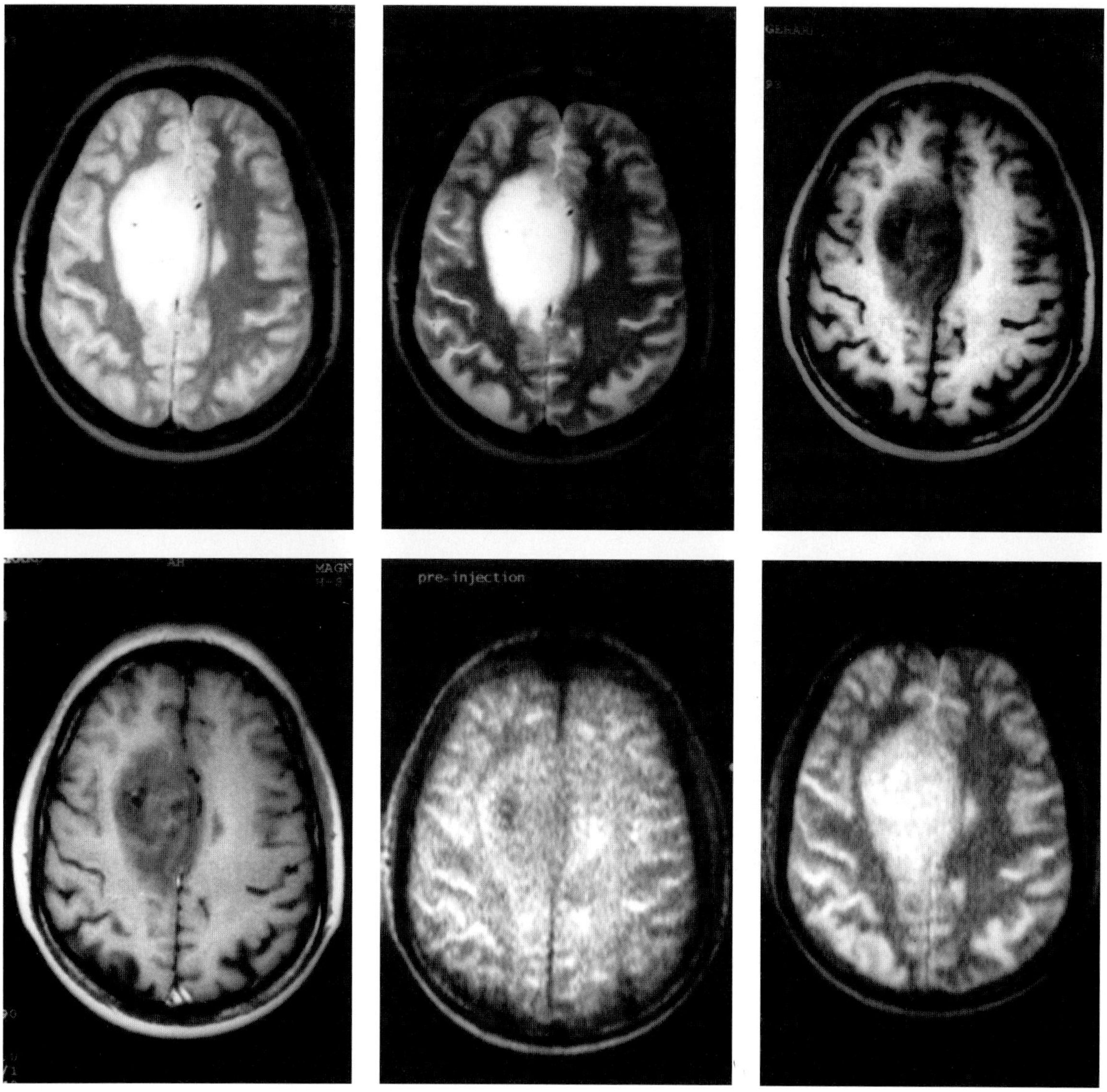

a,b c

d,e f

Fig. 18.13 a–f. Vascularity of brain tumor. **a,b** T2-weighted axial slices: first (**a**) and second echo (**b**) images of a right midline low-grade astrocytoma. **c,d** T1-weighted slices before (**c**). and after (**d**) contrast injection showing absence of tumor enhancement. **e** T2*-weighted gradient-echo image acquired before the bolus injection of gadolinium chelate. **f** Cerebral blood volume map calculated with pixel-by-pixel integration of the signal curve shows high blood volume in the tumor, suggestive of high vascularity, despite its low grade

troversial, and have not had a very significant impact on clinical practice. CBV maps may nevertheless be a useful addition to routine MRI follow-up because they seem to allow earlier detection of progression and combine the information on perfusion and early blood-brain barrier disruption (Siegal et al. 1997).

Although theoretically of interest for treatment adjustment, the quantification of blood-brain barrier permeability in brain tumors has only limited applicability in the clinical setting. The blood-to-tissue transport coefficient (see Sect. 18.2.2) could be helpful in optimizing the combination of radiation and chemotherapy. Radiation therapy changes the vascular permeability of brain tumors and the tumors themselves display great variability in vascular permeability, as shown experimentally (Schmiedl et al. 1992).

Technetium-99m sestamibi, which is tending to replace thallium for myocardial scintigraphy, has properties analogous to those of thallium at the level of the brain and the additional ability to assess the expression of P-glycoprotein, which is encoded by the MDR1 (multidrug resistance) gene. P-glycoprotein is thought to extrude the radiotracer from the tumor cells by the same mechanism by which it extrudes chemotherapic agents, thereby rendering the tumor resistant to therapy (Rao et al. 1994).

Positron emission tomography (PET) can be used to trace radioactive atoms such as ^{15}O, ^{11}C, ^{13}N, and ^{18}F, which can be incorporated in various metabolic pathways. Those pathways relevant to brain tumors are glycolysis, which is increased in malignant tumors as reflected by ^{18}F-deoxyglucose (FDG) uptake, and protein synthesis, shown by uptake of ^{11}C-L-methylmethionine. PET is a research tool which is not used at the diagnotic stage in patients with brain tumors, but which in some cases may assist in deciding which treatment to employ (Davis et al. 1993).

18.5.2 Evaluation of Residual Tumor Following Surgery

Evaluation of residual tumor volume may serve as a basis for modification of subsequent therapeutic strategy and provides the baseline for follow-up. Postoperative changes are difficult to interpret and both tumor and normal surgical reaction contribute to edema and contrast enhancement (Fig. 18.14). However, Forsting et al. (1993) have established that contrast enhancement related to surgery does not occur until the 3rd day following surgery and lasts for 6 months. Therefore CT or, more sensitively and more specifically, MRI performed within 2 days of surgery with and without contrast agent administration is the best means of detecting residual tumor. Beyond this timepoint, performance of MRI on days 3–5 following surgery minimizes the confounding effects of postsurgical enhancement and methemoglobin (Forsyth et al. 1997). Leter, however, the contrast enhancement of the surgical bed, which is smooth and peripheral, is more difficult to differentiate from that of residual tumor, which is nodular and inhomogeneous. Early postoperative MRI is also beneficial in pediatric brain tumor surgery (Oser et al. 1997). Thallium scintigraphy can help in selected cases when evidence of residual tumor is provided by uptake of radiotracer. FDG-PET uptake demonstrating increased glycolysis may only be located in residual tumor. Methionine uptake is also elevated in residual tumor, but this finding may be ambiguous after surgery because some subacute hematomas are also associated with peripheral increased metabolism.

18.5.3 Differentiation Between Tumor Recurrence and Radiation Necrosis

Most of the local radiation changes are related to demyelination and do not enhance, but radiation necrosis is more difficult to differentiate from tumor recurrence because both are associated with edema, contrast enhancement, and mass effect. Recognition of radionecrosis is important because it has a better prognosis than tumor recurrence and does not require the same treatment. Its incidence is 5%–18%. It can occur as soon as 6 months after irradiation but more usually does so from 8 to 24 months (Madison et al. 1994). In fact radiation necrosis occurs significantly only after curietherapy and radiosurgery.

Peterson et al. (1995) showed that CT or MRI follow-up is useful to differentiate tumor recurrence from radiation necrosis because high-grade gliomas usually progress on a continuous basis, in contrast to the rapid onset of radiation necrosis lesions. The combination of thallium and perfusion scintigraphy is quite specific in differentiating viable tumoral tissue from necrosis. A thallium uptake index (comparing uptake by the lesion and by the scalp) higher than 3.5 is specific for tumor, whereas a value lower than 3.5 in combination with a low perfusion index is suggestive of necrosis (Carvalho et al. 1992). On PET, radiation necrosis shows decreased glycolytic metabolism and decreased methionine uptake.

18.6 Role of Contrast Agents in Stroke

Morphological changes observed after brain vessel occlusion include edema, which modifies the appearance of the affected parenchyma on T1- and T2-weighted images. There is a correlation between the volume of the lesion and the outcome. Vascular flow-related abnormalities, including absence of normal flow void and presence of arterial enhancement, are the earliest MR findings, being detected within minutes of onset (Yuh et al. 1991). Arterial enhancement is caused by arterial slowing and indicates decreased brian perfusion (Mueller et al. 1993). Moderate and delayed contrast enhancement reflects the breakdown of the blood-brain barrier, and typically is not found in cortical infarctions during the first 24h. Only early and intense parenchymal enhancement indicates a favorable prognosis because it correlates with efficiency of leptomeningeal vascu-

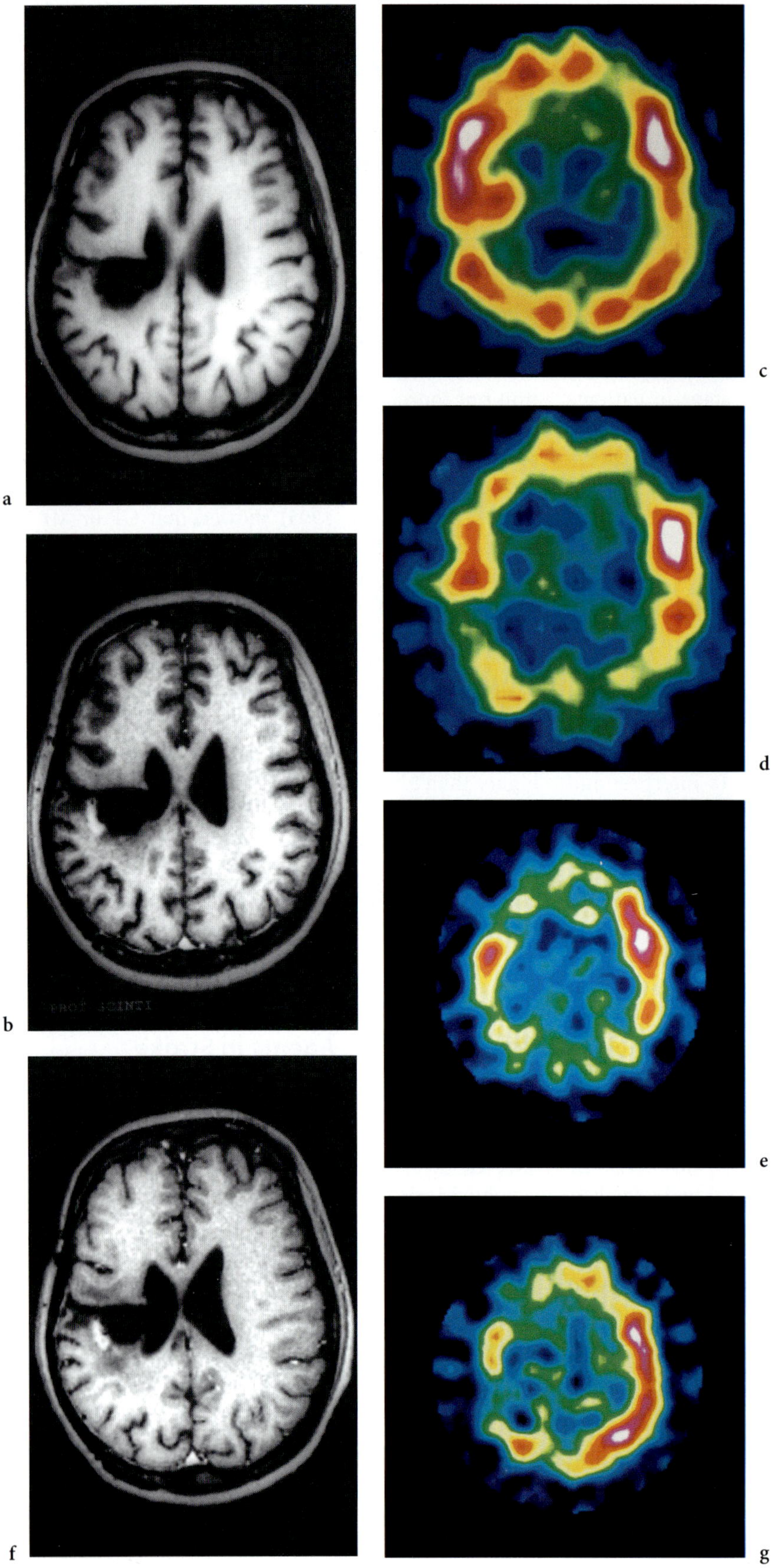
a
b
f
c
d
e
g

larization (Crain et al. 1991). Such enhancement is observed in transient occlusions, partial occlusions, and isolated watershed infarctions. Cortical vascular enhancement is the main imaging manifestation of slow flow in leptomeningeal collaterals. It does not necessarily indicate a state of impaired cerebral hemodynamics, and may be observed during the first 2 weeks and in combination with parenchymal enhancement (Essig et al. 1996).

The multiple capabilities of MRI allow the depiction of brain ischemia on the basis of not only the morphological changes but also the metabolic and functional consequences. Hemodynamic failure is the initial step in the development of ischemia. Although the initial decrease in blood flow does not influence morphological imaging, this early phase can be shown either with diffusion imaging or with cerebral blood volume imaging. Perfusion deficits may be visualized within less than 1 h after vessel occlusion in stroke, i.e., before extensive pathological changes occur and before reliable depiction is possible by standard proton MRI techniques. In comparison, standard T2-weighted MRI without contrast enhancement typically fails to demonstrate any significant signal changes before the presence of cerebral edema, which induces a relative increase in signal approximately 4 h after vessel occlusion (Warach et al. 1992; Röther et al. 1996). Perfusion deficits are well seen on dynamic susceptibility MRI, which additionally provides hemodynamic information on the status of the rest of the brain. The prolongation of mean transit time of the bolus of contrast agent in unaffected territories suggests poor collateral supply (Reith et al. 1997) (Fig. 18.15). Experimental stroke models show an early decrease in the apparent diffusion coefficient (ADC) in ischemic territories, prior to any modification of the T2-weighted sequence. This is related to the presence of cytotoxic edema, which shows a close correlation with further infarction (Moseley et al. 1990; Hoehn-Berlage 1995).

Prognostic factors are the volume of the lesion and the decrease in the ADC. The latter is correlated with the local reduction in cerebral blood flow

a 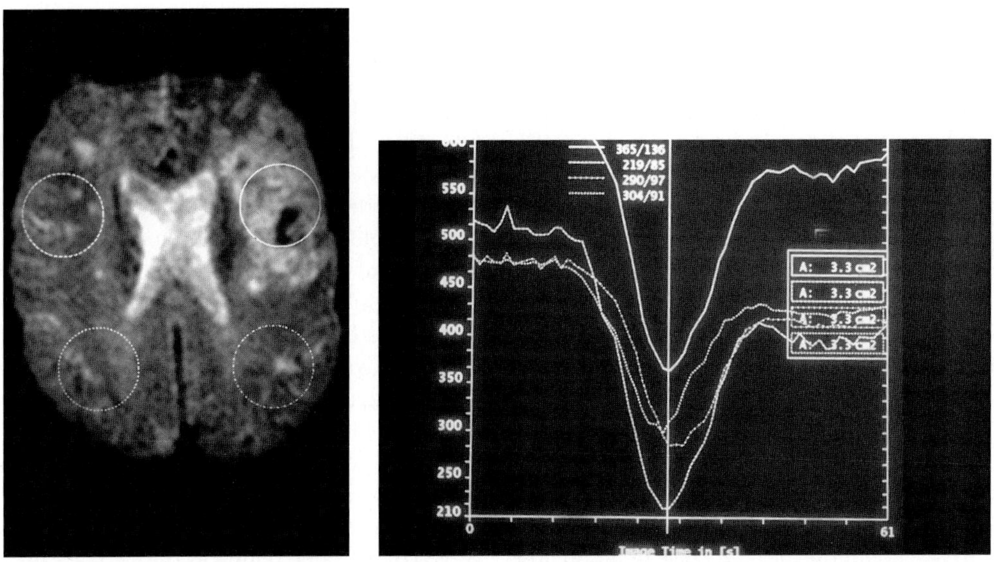 b

Fig. 18.15 a,b. Magnetic susceptibility study of stroke. **a** T2-weighted echo-planar image showing a left chronic lesion corresponding to left middle cerebral artery stroke. Regions of interest allow the temporal evolution of the signal curves to be studied (**b**). The right anterior cortical territory of the unaffected middle cerebral artery presents the largest decrease in signal, reflecting the perfusion. The left posterior region of interest shows delayed perfusion, probably because of the involvement of more collateral flow from the posterior cerebral artery due to the anterior ipsilateral lesion

Fig. 18.14 a–g. Anaplastic tumor treated by surgical removal and radiation therapy. **a–c** Follow-up examination after radiation therapy disclosed a contrast-enhancing rim of tissue at the edge of the surgical bed [T1-weighted images before (**a**) and after (**b**) contrast injection], with elevated thallium uptake (**c**). Repeat MRI at 3 months remained unchanged but thallium uptake decreased (**d**). This trend was confirmed on subsequent control examinations (**e** thallium brain scan at 10 months, **f** T1-weighted postcontrast MRI and **g** thallium brain scan almost 3 years later)

(Mancuso et al. 1995). ADC is less decreased in the penumbra than in the infarction and an ADC threshold of tissue viability will certainly be established. Additionally there is preliminary evidence that some of the functional changes seen using the combination of diffusion and perfusion MRI may be of prognostic value (Quast et al. 1993; Fisher and Garcia 1996). Dynamic susceptibility contrast MRI imaging may be used in conjunction with diffusion-weighted imaging; the former provides distinctive hemodynamic information on regions of ischemic penumbra, whereas on diffusion-weighted imaging it is difficult to distinguish normal regions from penumbra because of the small difference in ADC (Maeda et al. 1993). In many patients the initial lesion extension seen on diffusion-weighted imaging is smaller than the perfusion alteration and later the lesion visible on T2-weighted images (Fisher and Garcia 1996; Sorensen et al. 1996). A region of hypoperfusion larger than the region of diffusion abnormality may be predictive of ischemic lesion enlargement (Baird et al. 1997). On the other hand during the hyperacute phase of experimental ischemia, a decreased diffusion coefficient may be present in regions where perfusion is still preserved. This diffusion abnormality is probably reversible at this stage (Quast et al. 1993). Warach et al. (1996) showed that clinical outcome after stroke is better predicted by initial diffusion and perfusion MRI, which were more accurate than conventional MRI when performed in the first 6 h.

18.7 Role of Contrast Agents in Functional MRI of Brain Activation

Visualization of the modifications of MRI signal intensity that accompany brain activation was first achieved using contrast agents and comparing first passage of bolus at rest and during task performance in order to document the local increase in blood flow (Belliveau et al. 1991). Subsequentiy another approach to functional MRI was indentified, directly based upon blood oxygen concentration and what was termed the blood oxygen level dependent (BOLD) effect Ogawa et al. 1990). The safety, repeatability, and good spatial resolution of this technique have ensured its wide utilization both in the field of cognitive research and in clinical applications. Its main drawback is the small difference in signal (4%–6%) achieved on a clinical 1.5-T imager between rest and activation epochs.

The hemodynamic changes of the brain can be assessed by perfusion-weighted imaging. Cerebral vascular reactivity is visible with magnetic susceptibility boluses of diffusible contrast agents (Rostrup et al. 1996; Gückel et al. 1996; Nighoghossian et al. 1997; Berthezene et al. 1998) and has also been illustrated with long half-life agents in animals (Moseley et al. 1992; Lin et al. 1997), which is a more interesting approach for the repeated comparison of status.

The feasibility of amplification of the difference in signal in functional MRI by the administration of a blood pool contrast agent has been investigated. Berry et al. (1996) combined suppression of the BOLD effect by hyperoxygenation and the use of USPIO particles to visualize hemodynamic changes in the rabbit brain induced by hypercapnia and achieved a signal difference of 8%, suggesting that this approach could produce larger signal changes and thereby be a more sensitive technique for functional MRI. Nevertheless, these experiments were performed with a conventional gradient-echo sequence with a low temporal resolution (15 s) and a model quite far removed from real neuronal activation. De Crespigny et al. (1997) tested a forepaw stimulation paradigm in the rat at 4.7 T and confirmed a larger gradient-echo signal change (15%–20%) with USPIO particles than with the BOLD effect (4%–5%). The same strategy for functional MRI was further tested using echo-planar imaging (EPI) on a rabbit model under 5% CO_2 inhalation to increase cerebral blood volume (Noel et al. 1997). In the presence of nanoparticles (60 and 80 µmol iron/kg body weight), the EPI MR signal decreased by 8%. In a second step, a functional MRI experiment with a visual activation paradigm under air respiration showed significant positive changes in the occipital lobe related to the BOLD effect. When the BOLD effect was suppressed by hyperoxygenation with an IFO_2 (inspired fraction of oxygen) of 70%, a significant decrease in signal during activation was observed in the same region as the decrease observed in the presence of USPIO particles at a dose of 80 µmol iron/kg body weight. In a somatosensory experiment involving electrical forepaw stimulation in the rat, Mandeville et al. (1998) found an increase in the functional contrast-to-noise ratio relative to BOLD imaging by 5.7 at 2.0 T and by 1.5 at 4.7 T when using dynamic measurements of regional changes in cerebral blood volume after injection of USPIO (ca. 180 µmol iron/kg body weight). A loss in temporal resolution was the counterpart of this improvement in sensitivity because the cerebral blood volume responded more slowly to stimulus than did the BOLD signal.

References

Akeson P, Nordstrom CH, Holtas S (1997) Time dependency in brain lesion enhancement with gadodiamide injection. Acta Radiol 38:19–24

Amano Y, Amano M, Kumazaki T (1997) Normal contrast enhancement of extraocular muscles: fat-suppressed MR findings. AJNR Am J Neuroradiol 18:161–164

Ancri D, Basset JY, Lonchampt MF, Etavard C (1978) Diagnosis of cerebral lesions by thallium 201. Radiology 128:417–422

Aronen HJ, Gazit IE, Louis DN, et al. (1994) Cerebral blood volume maps of gliomas: comparison with tumor grade and histologic findings. Radiology 191:41–51

Asari S, Makabe T, Katayama S, Itoh T, Tsuchida S, Ohmoto T (1994) Assessment of the pathological grade of astrocytic gliomas using an MRI score. Neuroradiology 36:308–310

Baird AE, Benfield A, Schlaug G, et al. (1997) Enlargement of human cerebral ischemic lesion volumes mesasured by diffusion-weighted magnetic resonance imaging. Ann Neurol 41:581–589

Barkhof F, Filippi M, Miller DH, et al. (1997) Comparison of MRI criteria at first presentation to predict conversion to clincally definite multiple sclerosis. Brain 120:2059–2069

Belliveau JW, Rosen BR, Kantor HL, et al. (1990) Functional cerebral imaging by susceptibility-contrast NMR. Magn Reson Med 14:538–546

Belliveau JW, Kennedy DN, McKinstry RC, et al. (1991) Functional mapping of the human visual cortex by magnetic resonance imaging. Science 254:716–719

Berry I, Brant-Zawadzki M, Brasch R, Osaki L, Murovick J, Newton T (1986) Gd-DTPA in clinical MR of the brain. 2. Extraaxial lesions and normal structures. AJNR Am J Neuroradiol 7:789–793

Berry I, Benderbous S, Ranjeva JP, Gracia-Meavilla D, Manelfe C, Le Bihan D (1996) Contribution of USPIO used as blood-pool contrast agent: detection of cerebral blood volume changes during apnea in rabbit. Magn Reson Med 36:415–419

Berthezene Y, Nighoghossian N, Meyer R, et al. (1998) Can cerebrovascular reactivity be assessed by dynamic susceptibility contrast-enhanced MRI? Neuroradiology 40:1–5

Black KL, Hawkins RA, Kim KT, Becker DP, Lerner C, Marciano D (1989) Use of thallium 201 SPECT to quantitate malignancy grade of gliomas. J Neurosurg 71:342–346

Bozzao A, Bastianello S, Ferone E, Giugni E, Paolillo A, Bozzao L (1996) Enhanced and unenhanced MR with magnetization transfer in multiple sclerosis. AJNR Am J Neuroradiol 17:1837–1842

Brant-Zawaszki M, Norman D, Newton TH, et al. (1984) Magnetic resonance of the brain: the optimal screening technique. Radiology 152:71–77

Brant-Zawadzki M, Berry I, Osaki L, Brasch RC, Murovick J, Norman D (1986) Gd-DTPA in clinical MR imaging of the brain. 1. Intraaxial lesions. AJNR Am J Neuroradiol 7:781–788

Bruck W, Bitsch A, Kolenda H, Bruck Y, Stiefel M, Lassmann H (1997) Inflammatory central nervous system demyelination: correlation of magnetic resonance imaging findings with lesion pathology. Ann Neurol 42:783–793

Bullock PR, Mansfield P, Gowland P, Worthington BS, Firth JL (1991) Dynamic imaging of contrast enhancement in brain tumors. Magn Reson Med 19:293–298

Bulte JWM, DeJonge MWA, Kamman RL, et al. (1992) Dextran-magnetite particles: contrast-enhanced MRI of blood-brain barrier disruption in a rat model. Magn Reson Med 23:215–223

Calabresi PA, Tranquill LR, Dambrosia JM, et al. (1997) Increases in soluble VCAM-1 correlate with a decrease in MRI lesions in multiple sclerosis treated with interferon beta-1b. Ann Neurol 41:669–674

Campi A, Filippi M, Comi G, Scott IG, Gerevini S, Dousset V (1996) Magnetisation transfer ratios of contrast-enhancing and non-enhancing lesions in multiple sclerosis. Neuroradiology 38:115–119

Carvalho PA, Schwartz RB, Alexander E III, et al. (1992) Detection of recurrent gliomas with quantitative thallium-201/technetium-99m single photon emission computerized tomography. J Neurosurg 77:565–570

Chambon C, Clément O, LeBlanche A, Schouman-Claeys E, Frija G (1993) Superparamagnetic iron oxides as positive MR contrast agents: in vitro and in vivo evidence. Magn Reson Imaging 11:509–519

Crain MR, Yuh WTC, Greene GM, Loes DJ, Ryals TJ, Sato Y, Hart MN (1991) Cerebral ischemia: evaluation with contrast-enhance MR imaging. AJNR Am J Neuroradiol 12:631–639

Daumas-Duport C, Scheithauer BW, Kelly PJ (1987) A histologic and cytologic method for the spatial definition of gliomas. Mayo Clin Proc 62:435–449

Davis WK, Boyko OB, Hoffman JM, et al. (1993) [^{18}F]2-fluoro-2-deoxyglucose-positron emission tomography correlation of gadolinium-enhanced MR imaging of central nervous system neoplasia. AJNR Am J Neuroradiol 14:515–523

de Crespigny AJ, Busch E, Palmer JT, Williams SP, Beaulieu C, van Bruggen N (1997) High resolution functional imaging in rat brain using intravascular iron oxide contrast. Int Soc Magn Reson Med proceedings, p 628

Dousset V, Delalande C, Benderbous S, et al. (1997) Cerebral MR imaging of cells with iron burden after USPIO injection. Int Soc Magn Reson Med proceedings, p 1602

Edelman RR, Mattle HP, Atkinson DJ, et al. (1990) Cerebral blood flow: assessment with dynamic contrast-enhanced T2* weighted MR imaging at 1.5 T. Radiology 176:211–220

Essig M, Von Kummer R, Egelhof T, Winter R, Sartor K (1996) Vascular MR contrast enhancement in cerebrovascular disease. AJNR Am J Neuroradiol 17:887–894

Fazekas F, Offenbacher H, Fuchs S, Schmidt R, Niederkorn K, Horne S (1988) Criteria for an increased specificity of MRI interpretation in elderly subjects with suspected MS. Neurology 38:1822–1825

Filippi M, Campi A, Dousset V, Baratti C, Martinelli V, Canal N, Scotti G, Comi G (1995) A magnetization transfer imaging study of normal-appearing white matter in multiple sclerosis. Neurology 45:478–482

Filippi M, Yousry T, Rocca MA, Fesl G, Voltz R, Comi G (1997a) Sensitivity of delayed gadolinium-enhanced MRI in multiple sclerosis. Acta Neurol Scand 95:331–334

Filippi M, Campi A, Martino G, Colombo B, Comi GA (1997b) A magnetization transfer study of white matter in siblings of multiple sclerosis patients. J Neurol Sci 147:151–153

Filippi M, Rocca MA, Rizzo G, et al. (1998a) Magnetization transfer ratios in multiple sclerosis lesions enhancing after different doses of gadolinium. Neurology 50:1289–1293

Filippi M, Rocca MA, Martino G, Horsfield MA, Comi G (1998b) Magnetization transfer changes in the normal appearing white matter precede the appearance of enhancing lesions in patients with multiple sclerosis. Ann Neurol 43:809–814

Fisher M, Garcia JH. (1996) Evolving stroke and the ischemic penumbra. Neurology 47:884–888

Forsting M, Albert FK, Kunze S, Adams HP, Zenner D, Sartor K (1993) Extirpation of glioblastomas: MR and CT follow-up of residual tumor and regrowth. AJNR Am J Neuroradiol 14:77–87

Forsting M, Reith W, Dörfler A, von Kummer R, Hacke W, Sartor K (1994) MRI in acute cerebral ischaemia: perfusion imaging with superparamagnetic iron oxide in a rat model. Neuroradiology 36:23–26

Forsyth PA, Petrov E, Mahallati H, et al. (1997) Prospective study of postoperative magnetic resonance imaging in patients with malignant gliomas. J Clin Oncol 15:2076–2081

Gasperini C, Pozzili C, Bastianello S, et al. (1998) Effects of steroids on Gd-enhancing lesions before and during recombinant beta interferon 1 a treatment in relapsing remitting multiple sclerosis. Neurology 50:403–406

Gass A, Barker GJ, Kidd D, et al. (1994) Correlation of magnetization transfer ratio with clinical disability in multiple sclerosis. Ann Neurol 36:62–67

Gore JC, Majumdar S (1990) Measurement of tissue blood flow using intravascular relaxation agents and magnetic resonance imaging. Magn Reson Med 14:242–248

Gowland P, Mansfield P, Bullock P, Stehling M, Worthington B, Firth J (1992) Dynamic studies of gadolinium uptake in brain tumors using inversion-recovery echo-planar imaging. Magn Reson Med 26:241–258

Gückel FJ, Brix G, Schmieedek P, et al. (1996) Cerebrovascular reserve capacity in patients with occlusive cerebrovascular disease: assessment with dynamic susceptibility contrast-enhanced MR imaging and the acetazolamide stimulation test. Radiology 201:405–412

Haraldseth O, Jones RA, Müller TB, Fahlvik AK, Oksendal AN (1996) Comparison of dysprosium DTAP BMA and superparamagnetic iron oxide particles as susceptibility contrast agents for perfusion imaging of regional cerebral ischemia in the rat. JMRI 6:714–717

Haughton VM (1994) A multicenter trial of high-dose gadodiamide injection for imaging the central nervous system and spine. Acad Radiol 1:10–14

Haustein J, Laniado M, Niendorf H-P, Hilbertz T, Planitzer J, Schörner W, Louton T (1992) Administration of gadopentetate dimeglumine in MR imaging of intracranial tumors: dosage and field strength. AJNR Am J Neuroradiol 13:1199–1206

Haustein J, Laniado M, Niendorf H-P, et al. (1993) Triple-dose versus standard-does gadopentetate dimeglumine: a randomized study in 199 patients. Radiology 186:855–860

Hiele JF, Grossman RI, Ramer KN, Gonzalez-Scarano F, Cohen JA (1995) Magnetization transfer effects in MR-detected multiple sclerosis lesions: comparison with gadolinium-enhanced spin-echo images and nonenhanced T1-weighted images. Am J Neuroradiol 16:69–77

Hoehn-Berlage M (1995) Diffusion-weighted NMR imaging: applications to experimental focal cerebral ischemia. NMR Biomed 8:345–358

Ibrahim MA, Emerson JF, Cotman CW (1998) Magnetic resonance imaging relaxation times and gadolinium-DTPA relaxivity values in human cerebrospinal fluid. Invest Radiol 33:153–162

Ikushima I, Korogi Y, Kuratsu J, Hirai T, Hamatake S, Takahashi M, Ushio Y (1997) Dynamic MRI of meningiomas and schwannomas: is differential diagnosis possible? Neuroradiology 39:633–638

Jeong MG, Chung TS, Coe CJ, Jeon TJ, Kim DI, Joo AY (1997) Application of magnetization trasfer imaging for intracranial lesions of tuberous sclerosis. J Comput Assist Tomogr 21:8–14

Josephson L, Bigler J, White D (1991) The magnetic properties of some materials affecting MR images. Magn Reson Med 22:204–208

Just M, Thelen M (1988) Tissue characterization with T1, T2 and proton density values: results in 160 patients with brain tumors. Radiology 169:779–785

Kelly PJ (1991) Glial neoplasms. In: Kelly PJ (ed) Tumor stereotaxis. W.B. Saunders,Philadelphia, pp 296–357

Kelly PJ, Daumas-Duport C, Scheithauer BW, Kall BA, Kispert DB (1987) Stereotactic histologic correlations of computed tomography and magnetic resonance imaging-defined abnormalities in patients with glial neoplasms. Mayo Clin Proc 62:450–459

Kent TA, Quast MJ, Kaplan BJ, Lifsey RS, Eisenberg HM (1990) Assessment of a superparamagnetic iron oxide (AMI-25)* as a brain contrast agent. Magn Reson Med 13:434–443

Knauth M, Forsting M, Hartmann M, Heiland S, Balzer T, Sartor K (1996) MR enhancement of brain lesions: increased contrast dose compared with magnetization transfer. AJNR Am J Neuroradiol 17:1853–1859

Koudriavtseva T, Thompson AJ, Fiorelli M, et al. (1997) Gadolinium enhanced MRI predicts clinical and MRI disease activity in relapsing-remitting multiple sclerosis. J Neurol Neurosurg Psychiatry 62:285–287

Larsson HBW, Tofts PS (1992) Measurement of blood-brain barrier permeability using dynamic Gd-DTAP scanning – a comparison of methods. Magn Reson Med 24:174–176

Larsson HBW, Stubgaard M, Frederiksen JL, Jensen M, Henriksen O, Paulson OB (1990) Quantitation of blood-brain barrier defect by magnetic resonance imaging and gadolinium-DTPA in patients with multiple sclerosis and brain tumors. Magn Reson Med 16:117–131

Le Bihan D, Breton E, Lallemand D, Grenier P, Cabanis E, Laval-Jeantet M (1986) MR imaging of intravoxel incoherent motions: application to diffusion and perfusion in neurologic disorders. Radiology 161:401–407

Le Bihan D, Breton E, Lallemand D, Aubin ML, Vignaud J, Laval-Jeantet M (1988) Separation of diffusion and perfusion in intravoxel incoherent motion MR imaging. Radiology 168:497–505

Lin W, Paczynski RP, Kuppusamy K, Hsu CY, Haacke AM (1997) Quantitative measurements of regional cerebral blood volume using MRI in rats: effects of arterial carbon dioxide tension and mannitol. Magn Reson Med 38:420–428

Madison MT, Hall WA, Latchaw RE, Loes DJ (1994) Radiologic diagnosis, staging and follow-up of adult central nervous system primary malignant glioma. Radiol Clin North Am 32:183–196

Maeda M, Itoh S, Ide H, Matsuda T, Kobayashi H, Kubota T, Ishhii Y (1993) Acute stroke in cats: comparison of dynamic susceptibility-contrast MR imaging with T2- and diffusion-weighted MR imaging. Radiology 189:227–232

Majumdar S, Zoghbi SS, Gore JC (1988) Regional differences in rat brain displayed by fast MRI with superparamagnetic contrast agents. Magn Reson Imag 6:611–615

Mancuso A, Karibe H, Rooney WD, et al. (1995) Correlation of early reduction in the apparent diffusion coefficient of water with blood flow reduction during middle cerebral artery occlusion in rats. Magn Reson Med 34:368–377

Mandeville JB, Marota JJA, Kosofsky BE, Kelner JR, Weissleder R, Rosen BR, Weisskoff RM (1998) Dynamic functional imaging of relative cerebral blood volume during rat forepaw stimulation. Magn Reson Med 39:615–624

McCormack BM, Miller DC, Budzilovitch GN, Voorhees GJ, Ransohoff J (1992) Treatment and survival of low-grade astrocytoma in adults 1977–1988. Neurosurgery 31:636–642

McNamara M, Brant-Zawadzki M, Berry I, et al. (1986) Acute experimental cerebral ischemia: MRI enhancement using Gd-DTPA. Radiology 158:701–705

Meyer JR, Androux RW, Salamon N, et al. (1997) Contrast enhanced magnetization transfer MR of the brain: importance of precontrast imaging. AJNR Am J Neuroradiol 18:1515–1521

Miller DH, Barkhof F, Berry I, Kappos L, Scotti G, Thompson AJ (1991) Magnetic resonance imaging in monitoring the treatment of multiple sclerosis: concerted action guidelines. J Neurol Neurosurg Psychiatry 54:683–688

Miller DH, Albert PS, Barkhof F, et al. (1996) Guidelines for the use of MR techniques in monitoring the treatment of MS. Ann Neurol 39:6–16

Miller DH, Grossman RI, Reingold SC, McFarland HF (1998) The role of MR techniques in understanding and managing multiple sclerosis. Brain 121:3–24

Miyati T, Banno T, Mase M, Kasai H, Shundo H, Imazawa M, Ohba S (1997) Dual dynamic contrast-enhanced MR imaging. Magn Reson Imaging 7:230–235

Molyneux PD, Filippi M, Barkhof F, et al. (1998) Correlations between monthly enhanced MRI lesion rate and changes in T2 lesion volume in multiple sclerosis. Ann Neurol 43:332–339

Morrissey SP, Stodal H, Zettl U, et al. (1996) In vivo MRI and its histological correlates in acute adoptive transfer experimental allergic encephalomyelitis. Quantification of inflammation and oedema. Brain 119:239–248

Moseley ME, Cohen Y, Mintorovitch J, et al. (1990) Early detection of regional cerebral ischemia in cats: comparison of diffusion- and T_2-weighted MRI and spectroscopy. Magn Reson Med 14:330–346

Moseley ME, Chew WM, White DL, et al. (1992) Hypercarbia-induced changes in cerebral blood volume in the cat: an ^1H MRI and intravascular contrast agent study. Magn Reson Med 23:21–30

Mueller DP, Yuh WTC, Fisher DJ, Chandran KB, Crain MR, Kim Y-H (1993) Arterial enhancement in acute cerebral ischemia: clinical and angiographic correlation. AJNR Am J Neuroradiol 14:661–668

Mühler A, Zhang X, Wang H, Lawaczeck R, Weinmann H-J (1995) Investigation of mechanisms influencing the accumulation of ultrasmall superparamagnetic iron oxide particles in lymph nodes. Invest Radiol 30:98–103

Narayana PA, Doyle TJ, Lai D, Wolinsky JS (1998) Serial proton magnetic resonance spectroscopic imaging, contrast-enhanced magnetic resonance imaging, and quantitative lesion volumetry in multiple sclerosis. Ann Neurol 43:56–71

Nighoghossian N, Berthezene Y, Meyer R, et al. (1997) Assessment of cerebrovascular reactivity by dynamic susceptibility contrast-enhanced MR imaging. J Neurol Sci 149:171–176

Noel JB, Ranjeva JP, Benderbous S, Franconi JM, Maelfe C, Berry I (1997) Activation of primary visual cortex of rabbits in presence and absence of USPIO. Int Soc Magn Reson Med proceedings, p 738

Ogawa S, Lee T-M, Nayak AS, Glynn P (1990) Oxygenation-sensitive contrast in magnetic resonance image of rodent brain at high magnetic fields. Magn Reson Med 14:68–78

Oser AB, Moran CJ, Kaukman BA, Park TS (1997) Intracranial tumor in children: MR imaging findings within 24 hours of craniotomy. Radiology 205:807–812

Parker GJ, Suckling J, Tanner SF, Padhani AR, Revell PB, Husband JE, Leach MO (1997) Probing tumor microvascularity by measurement, analysis and display of contrast agent uptake kinetics. J Magn Reson Imaging 7:564–574

Paty DW, Oger JJF, Kastrukoff FF, Hashimoto SA, Hooge JP, Eisen AA (1988) MRI in the diagnosis of MS: a prospective study with comparison of clinical evaluation, evoked potentials, oligoclonal banding and CT. Neurology 38: 180–185

Peterson K, Clark HB, Hall WA, Truwit CL (1995) Multifocal enhancing magnetic resonance imaging lesions following cranial irradiation. Ann Neurol 38:237–244

Pronin IN, Holodny AI, Petraikin AV (1997) MRI of high-grade glial tumors: correlation between the degree of contrast enhancement and the volume of surrounding edema. Neuroradiology 39:348–350

Quast MJ, Huang NC, Hillman GR, Kent TA (1993) The evolution of acute stroke recorded by multimodal magnetic resonance imaging. Magn Reson Med 11:465–471

Rao VV, Chiu ML, Kronauge JF, Piwnica-Worms D (1994) Expression of recombinant human multidrug resistance P-glycoprotein in insect cells confers decreased accumulation of technetium-99m-sestamibi. J Nucl Med 35:510–515

Reith W, Forsting M, Vogler H, Heiland S, Sartor K (1995) Early detection of experimentally induced cerebral ischemia using magnetic susceptibility contrast agents: comparison between gadopentetate dimeglumine and iron oxide particles. AJNR Am J Neuroradiol 16:53–60

Reith W, Heiland S, Erb G, Benner T, Forsting M, Sartor K (1997) Dynamic contrast-enhanced T2*-weighted MRI in patients with cerebrovascular disease. Neuroradiology 39:250–257

Renshaw PF, Levin JM, Kaufman MJ, Ross MH, Lewis RF, Harris GJ (1997) Dynamic susceptibility contrast magnetic resonance imaging in neuropsychiatry: present utility and future promise. Eur Radiol 7:216–221

Rosen BR, Belliveau JW, Verea JM, Brady TJ (1990) Perfusion imaging with NMR contrast agents. Magn Reson Med 14: 249–265

Rosen BR, Belliveau JW, Aronen HJ, et al. (1991) Susceptibility contrast imaging of cerebral blood volume: human experience. Magn Reson Med 22:293–299

Rostrup E, Larsson HB, Tofts PB, Garde K, Ring PB, Henriksen O (1996) Suscepptibility contrast imaging of CO_2-induced changes in the blood volume of the human brain. Acta Radiol 37:813–822

Röther J, Gückel F, Neff W, Schwartz A, Hennerici M (1996) Assessment of regional cerebral blood volume in acute human stroke by use of single-slice dynamic susceptibility contrast-enhanced magnetic resonance imaging. Stroke 27:1088–1093

Rousseau V, Denizot B, Pouliquen D, Jallet P, LeJeune JJ (1997) Investigation of blood-brain barrier permeability to magnetite-dextran nanoparticles (MD3) after osmotic disruption in rats. MAGMA 5:213–222

Runge VM, Kirsch JE, Burke VJ, et al. (1992) High-dose gadoteridol in MR imaging of intracranial neoplasms. JMRI 2:9–18

Sage MR (1982) Blood brain barrier: phenomenon of increasing importance to the imaging clinician. AJR Am J Roeutgenol 138:887–898

Schmiedl U, Ogan M, Paajanen H, Marotti M, Crooks LE, Brito AC, Brasch RC (1987) Albumin labeled with Gd-DTPA as an intravascular, blood pool enhancing agent for MR imag-

ing: biodistribution and imaging studies. Radiology 162:205–210
Schmiedl UP, Kenney J, Maravilla KR (1992) Kinetics of pathologic blood-brain-barrier permeability in an astrocytic glioma using contrast-enhanced MR. AJNR Am J Neuroradiol 13:5–14
Siebner HR, Gräfin von Einsiedel H, Conrad B (1997) Magnetic resonance ventriculography with gadolinium-DTPA: report of two cases. Neuroradiology 39:418–422
Siegal T, Rubinstein R, Tzuk-Shina T, Gomori JM (1997) Utility of relative cerebral blood volume mapping derived from perfusion magnetic resonance imaging in the routine follow up of brain tumors. J Neurosurg 86:22–27
Silver NC, Good CD, Barker GJ, et al. (1997) Sensitivity of contrast enhanced MRI in multiple sclerosis. Effects of gadolinium dose, magnetization transfer contrast and delayed imaging. Brain 120:1749–1761
Simon JH, Jacobs LD, Campion M, et al. (1998) Magnetic resonance studies of intramuscular interferon beta-la for relapsing multiple sclerosis. The Multiple Sclerosis Collaborative Research Group. Ann Neurol 43:79–87
Skalpe IO (1998) Is it dangerous to inject magnetic resonance contrast media into the subarachnoid space (letter)? Eur Radiol 8:427
Slizofski WJ, Krishna L, Katsetos CD, et al. (1995) Thallium imaging for brain tumors with results measured by a semiquantitative index and correlated with histopathology. Cancer 74:3190–3197
Smith ME, Stone LA, Albert PS, et al. (1993) Clinical worsening in multiple sclerosis is associated with increased frequency and area of gadopentetate dimeglumine-enhancing magnetic resonance imaging lesions. Ann Neurol 33:480–489
Sorensen AG, Buonanno FS, Gonzalez RG, et al. (1996) Hyperacute stroke: evaluation with combined multisection diffusion-weighted and hemodynamically weighted echoplanar MR imaging. Radiology 199:391–401
Sorensen AG, Tievsky AL, Ostergaard L, Weisskoff RM, Rosen BR (1997) Contrast agents in functional MR imaging. Magn Reson Imaging 7:47–55
Stehling MK, Brüning R, Rosen BR (1998) Perfusion imaging with echo-planar imaging. In: Schmitt F, Stehling MK, Turner R (eds) Echo-planar imaging. Theory, technique and application. Springer, Berlin Heidelberg New York, pp 419–464
Stone LA, Frank JA, Albert PS, Bash CN, Calabresi PA, Maloni H, McFarland HF (1997) Characterization of MRI response to treatment with interferon beta-lb: contrast-enhancing MRI lesion frequency as a primary outcome measure. Neurology 49:862–869
Storch M, Lassmann H (1997) Pathology and pathogenesis of demyelinating diseases. Curr Opin Neurol 10:186–192
Tervonen O, Forbes G, Scheithauer BW, Dietz MJ (1992) Diffuse "fibrillary" astrocytomas: correlation of MRI features with histopathologic parameters and tumor grade. Neuroradiology 34:173–178
The IFNB Multiple Sclerosis Study Group: University of British Columbia MS/MRI Analysis Group (1995) Interferon beta 1b in the treatment of MS. Final outcome of the randomized controlled trial. Neurology 45:1277–1285
Thorpe JW, Kidd D, Moseley IF, Thompson AJ, MacManus DG, Compston DA (1996) Spinal MRI in patients with suspected MS and negative brain MRI. Brain 119:709–714
Tofts PS, Kermode AG (1991) Measurement of the blood-brain barrier permeability and leakage space using dynamic MR imaging. 1. Fundamental concepts. Magn Reson Med 17:357–367
Tresley RM, Stone LA, Fields N, Maloni H, McFarland H, Frank JA (1997) Clinical safety of serial monthly administrations of gadopentetate dimeglumine in patients with multiple sclerosis: implications for natural history and early-phase treatments trials. Neurology 48:832–835
Tubridy N, Coles AJ, Molyneux P, et al. (1998) Secondary progressive multiple sclerosis: the relationship between short-term MRI activity and clinical features. Brain 121: 225–231
Van Buchem MA, McGowan GC, Kolson DL, Grossman RI (1996) Quantitative volumetric magnetization transfer analysis in MS. Estimation of macroscopic and microscopic disease burden. Magn Reson Med 36:632–636
Van Dijk P, Sijens PE, Schmitz PIM, Oudkerk M (1997) Gd-enhanced MR imaging of brain metastases: contrast as a function of dose and lesion size. Magn Reson Imag 15:535–541
Van Dijke C, Brasch R, Roberts T, et al. (1996) Mammary carcinoma model: correlation of macromolecular contrast enhanced MR imaging characterizations of tumor microvasculature and histologic capillary density. Radiology 198:813–818
Van Waesberghe JH, Castelijns JA, Roser W, et al. (1997) Single dose with magnetization transfer versus triple dose gadolinium in the MR detection of multiple sclerosis lesions. AJNR Am J Neuroradiol 18:1279–1285
Vertosick FT Jr, Selker GR, Grossman SJ, Joyce JM (1994) Correlation of thallium-201 single photon emission computed tomography and survival after treatment failure in patients with glioblastoma multiforme. Neurosurgery 34:396–401
Villringer A, Rosen B, Belliveau JW, et al. (1988) Dynamic imaging with lanthanide chelates in normal brain: contrast due to magnetic susceptibility effects. Magn Reson Med 6:164–174
Warach S, Li W, Ronthal M, Edelman RR (1992) Acute cerebral ischemia: evaluation with dynamic contrast-enhanced MR imaging and MR angiography. Radiology 182:41–47
Warach S, Dashe JF, Edelman RR (1996) Clinical outcome in ischemic stroke predicted by early diffusion-weighted and perfusion magnetic resonance imaging: a preliminary analysis. J Cereb Blood Flow Metab 16:53–59
Watanabe M, Tanaka R, Takeda N (1992) Magnetic resonance imaging and histopathology of cerebral gliomas. Neuroradiology 34:463–469
Weissleder R, Elizondo G, Wittenberg J, Rabito CA, Bengele HH, Josephson L (1990) Ultrasmall superparamagnetic iron oxide: characterisation of a new class of contrast agents for MR imaging. Radiology 175:489–493
Williams DS, Detre JA, Leigh JS, Koretsky AS (1992) Magnetic resonance imaging of perfusion using spin-inversion of arterial water. Proc Natl Acad Sci USA 89:212–216
Wolff SD, Balaban RS (1994) Magnetization transfer imaging: practical aspects and clinical applications. Radiology 192:593–599
Wong ET, Jackson EF, Hess KR, et al. (1998) Correlation between dynamic MRI and outcome in patients with malignant gliomas. Neurology 50:777–781
Yoshii Y, Komatsu Y, Yamada T, Hyodo A, Nose T, Kobayashi E (1992) Malignancy and viability of intraparenchymal brain tumors: correlation between Gd-DTPA contrast MR images and proliferative potentials. Acta Neurochir (Wien) 117:187–194
Yuh WTC, Crain MR, Loes DJ, Greene GM, Ryals TJ, Sato Y (1991) MR imaging of cerebral ischemia: findings in the first 24 hours. AJNR Am J Neuroradiol 12:621–629
Yuh WTC, Engelken JD, Muhonen MG, Mayr NA, Fisher DJ, Ehrhardt JC (1992) Experience with high-does gadolinium MR imaging in the evaluation of brain metastases. AJNR Am J Neuroradiol 13:335–345

19 Liver and Pancreas

P. Pavone, A. Laghi, and C. Catalano

CONTENTS

19.1 Introduction

Magnetic resonance imaging (MRI) has been proposed as a newer technique to visualize liver or pancreatic lesions with an intrinsically high contrast. The major difference between MRI and other imaging techniques lies in the fact that image contrast may be modified by changing imaging parameters, namely TE, TR, and flip angle.

In the early years of clinical application of abdominal MRI, Stark et al. (1986) proposed that the intrinsic contrast could be improved by using a heavily T1-weighted sequence, with a very short TR (260–300 ms), and a TE of 10–15 ms. In clinical trials he was able to demonstrate that T1-weighted sequences are more sensitive than T2-weighted sequences in the detection of focal hepatic lesions (i.e., the opposite of the situation for detection of brain lesions). However, subsequent studies were never able to show a clear superiority of non-contrast-enhanced MRI over more widely available and less expensive procedures, such as ultrasonography and computed tomography (CT). Therefore, the need for a contrast agent able to improve these results was evident from the very early experiences with liver MRI.

Various authors tried to improve results in lesion detection and characterization using conventional, intravascular-extracellular contrast agents. However, the rapid diffusion through the interstitial tissue of the liver and neoplastic parenchyma obtained with these agents is often responsible for obscuring the evidence of hepatic lesions, and only the use of dynamic sequential images acquired immediately after contrast agent injection may improve the detection of lesions.

A different and more valid approach was to use contrast agents able to directly and selectively reach the liver. Two methods may be used to achieve this: either hepatobiliary secretion or reticuloendothelial deposition of the contrast agent. All major research performed by the industry has been directed towards this goal, and nowadays a number of contrast agents are already commercially available which are able to produce selective enhancement (either positive or negative) of the liver parenchyma.

As far as the pancreas is concerned, the peculiar characteristics of this organ, with very little interstitial space, requires that images must be acquired in a dynamic way following injection of contrast agents, in order to improve evidence of focal lesions. One of the hepatobiliary contrast agents (Mn-DPDP) has proven able to provide strong selective enhancement of the pancreatic parenchyma.

In this chapter we will discuss the main results obtained to date with enhanced MRI of the liver and pancreas, and some potential contrast agents still in the early experimental phase.

19.2 Contrast Agents for Clinical Use

Contrast agents used in liver imaging may be divided as follows: nonspecific paramagnetic contrast agents with an intravascular-extracellular distribution, and hepatospecific agents with either biliary excretion or affinity for the reticuloendothelial system.

P. Pavone, MD, Università Degli Studi di Roma "La Sapienza", Istituto di Radiologia Cattedra II, Policlinico Umberto I, I-00161 Roma, Italy
A. Laghi, MD, Università Degli Studi di Roma "La Sapienza", Istituto di Radiologia Cattedra II, Policlinico Umberto I, I-00161 Roma, Italy
C. Catalano, MD, Università Degli Studi di Roma "La Sapienza", Istituto di Radiologia Cattedra II, Policlinico Umberto I, I-00161 Roma, Italy

19.2.1
Intravascular-Extracellular Paramagnetic Contrast Agents

19.2.1.1
Technical Notes

The pharmacokinetics of gadolinium chelates is similar to that of iodinated contrast agents: they distribute very rapidly between intravascular and extravascular compartments. Therefore, a relatively short window before the equilibrium phase is available to obtain images of diagnostic quality. As a consequence, the combination of rapid bolus injection and rapid acquisition time is mandatory in order to avoid loss of tumor-to-liver contrast. Usually, T1-weighted gradient-echo sequences with an acquisition time of 10–30 s are acquired, and the liver is imaged during the arterial, portal venous, and delayed phases after bolus injection of gadolinium. Using an automatic injector increases the quality of contrast enhancement and a bolus test improves the exact timing of image acquisition.

19.2.1.2
Clinical Applications

19.2.1.2.1
LESION IDENTIFICATION
Clinical results are similar to those obtained with spiral CT, where hypervascular tumors [hepatocellular carcinoma (HCC), carcinoid, hypervascular metastases] are better detected in the arterial phase, whereas hypovascular metastases are better defined in the portal venous phase. Recent studies suggest that the overall accuracy of contrast-enhanced MR images is superior to that of unenhanced images in tumor detection, and that contrast-enhanced MRI is superior to spiral CT in detecting hypervascular tumors owing to the greater contrast resolution. The detection of hypervascular tumors is greatly improved by use of an optimal scanning technique (exact timing, adequate bolus injection, rapid acquisition).

19.2.1.2.2
LESION CHARACTERIZATION
After gadolinium injection, lesion characterization is based on the same diagnostic criteria as are used in contrast-enhanced CT.

Hypervascular nodules in a cirrhotic liver suggest HCC. In some cases HCC is well circumscribed and a hypervascular "capsule" may be demonstrated. Central areas of low attenuation secondary to necrosis may be observed.

Rim enhancement is seen in most metastatic lesions, which are more commonly hypovascular compared with normal hepatic parenchyma. In some cases (metastatic disease from renal cell cancer, islet cell tumor, and carcinoid tumor) a hypervascular lesion may be observed, with transient enhancement in early arteriographic phases and isointensity on delayed images.

Hemangiomas are the most common liver tumors, occurring in about 4%–7% of patients. Characterization is performed using the typical enhancement pattern, represented by peripheral nodular enhancement with progressive centripetal filling; persistence of hyperintensity on delayed images is another sign, but caution should be exercised because some metastatic lesions may be isointense to surrounding liver on delayed images.

A transient increase in signal intensity is more typical for adenoma, where the diagnosis is also suggested by intralesional hemorrhagic areas. Differential diagnosis with focal nodular hyperplasia (FNH) is sometimes necessary. FNH shows a typical enhancement pattern, with initial central hyperintensity (enhancement of the central scar), progressive centrifugal and very rapid wash-in, and, finally, persistent hyperintensity of the central scar on delayed images.

19.2.2
Hepatospecific Contrast Agents

The major categories into which hepatospecific contrast agents can be divided are: (a) contrast agents with hepatobiliary excretion; (b) contrast agents with superparamagnetic properties. Most of these agents are now in an advanced experimental phase of investigation, and they will become available for routine clinical use in the near future.

19.2.2.1
Hepatobiliary Agents

19.2.2.1.1
TECHNICAL NOTES
Hepatobiliary agents are paramagnetic contrast agents with selective biliary excretion. They are compounds of either gadolinium or manganese chelated with lipophilic molecules containing aromatic

groups. After intravenous administration they are taken up by hepatocytes and excreted through the bile ducts. The result is a strong enhancement of normal hepatic parenchyma, with filling defects represented by benign and malignant lesions. A compound of manganese (Mn-DPDP) has recently been introduced onto the European market, while compounds of gadolinium are under preclinical evaluation.

19.2.2.1.2
CLINICAL APPLICATIONS

Hepatobiliary agents significantly increase liver/nonhepatocellular tumor contrast on T1-weighted images, resulting in improved detection of metastases. It has been demonstrated that 5-mm metastases can be easily detected after contrast medium injection, and that there is also better demarcation between metastases and surrounding tissue. The further advantage of hepatobiliary agents is that they are used for T1-weighted images, where the signal-to-noise ratio is considerably higher compared with T2-weighted images.

Characterization may be facilitated by selective hepatobiliary uptake, which allows distinction between tumors of hepatocytic origin and other lesions. The enhancement pattern of HCC is quite variable and probably dependent on the contrast medium used for the study. In fact, if gadoxetate disodium is administered, most HCCs are hypointense relative to the liver because of lower enhancement, whereas strong enhancement is seen in the case of well-differentiated HCCs. If mangafodipir trisodium is used, most well-differentiated HCCs appear hyperintense after contrast injection, and distinction between well-differentiated and undifferentiated HCCs may be possible on the basis of the different enhancement pattern. A rim enhancement pattern is observed in liver metastases. Bolus injection, limited only to gadoxetate disodium for safety reasons, may provide additional information.

19.2.2.2 Reticuloendothelial Agents

19.2.2.2.1
TECHNICAL NOTES

The action of reticuloendothelial contrast agents relies upon the presence of a strong magnetic effect of aggregates of iron microparticles. After intravenous administration they are taken up by the Kupffer cells of the liver and spleen and produce a strong effect on local magnetism. The result is a marked reduction in the signal intensity of the normal parenchyma, with no influence on the MR signal of neoplastic tissues, where the Kupffer cells are not represented.

These agents are currently available for routine clinical use. Care must be taken to perform a slow injection of the contrast material in order to avoid side-effects. In fact, after rapid infusion low back pain has been described in many patients.

19.2.2.2.2
CLINICAL APPLICATIONS

The effect of superparamagnetic contrast agents is to reduce the signal intensity of liver tissue, without any effect on lesions with no reticuloendothelial cells. Therefore, an increase in tumor-to-liver contrast is obtained, allowing the detection of more lesions compared with unenhanced images. The superparamagnetic effect is better visible if T2*-weighted gradient-echo or moderately T2-weighted spin-echo sequences are employed. Initial studies demonstrated a better result if mid-field strength equipment was used, although a European multicenter trial has suggested an improvement in lesion detection with high-field strength equipment, if used with new optimized pulse sequences.

In a recent study, images obtained at 0.5 T after administration of iron oxides presented the same diagnostic accuracy as CT portography in the detection of hepatic metastases.

Even if the main role of superparamagnetic agents is in identifying secondary hepatic lesions, they can also help in characterization, in selected cases. In fact, uptake of superparamagnetic agents, with a decrease in signal intensity, is present in all lesions with reticuloendothelial cells, like FNH, adenomas, and well-differentiated HCC; these can be easily differentiated from metastatic lesions, which typically do not have Kupffer cells. Hemangiomas have peculiar features after iron oxide administration, showing hyperintense signal on T1-weighted images and decreased signal intensity on T2-weighted images.

19.3 Future Perspectives

New classes of contrast agent are under development, i.e., hepatospecific agents directed to membrane cell receptors and blood pool agents, a new class of intravascular contrast media with long persistence in the blood vessels.

Receptor agents are iron oxide particles covered with polysaccharides which interact with the specific receptors of the sinusoidal surface of the hepatocytes. Following the interaction, the receptor-ligand complex is phagocytosed and intracellular lysosomal degradation occurs. Two contrast agents are under experimental development: arabinogalactan-coated ultrasmall superparamagnetic iron oxide particles (AG-USPIO) and arabinogalactan-coated monocrystalline iron oxide nanocompound (AG-MION). Both decrease the signal intensity of liver tissue, possibly in a more homogeneous way compared with reticuloendothelial system agents because of the more widespread distribution of iron oxide particles through liver tissue. No clinical results are available, since both compounds are in the preclinical phase of development.

Blood pool agents are contrast media with a prolonged blood half-life. They may be divided into macromolecular agents and particles. The *former* are represented by a gadolinium compound linked to a macromolecular backbone, such as albumin, dextran, and polylysine, with a high molecular weight resulting in prolonged retention in blood. No human experiments have been performed with these contrast media because of the possible dissociation between gadolinium and the macromolecule with a consequent high risk of toxic effects. The *latter* are represented by small particles (20–30 nm), usually ultrasmall superparamagnetic iron oxide particles coated with dextran, with a prolonged blood half-life and lymph node and reticuloendothelial cell uptake.

References

Adam G, Neuerburg J, Spuntrup E, Muhler A, Scherer K, Gunther RW (1994) Gd-DTPA-cascade-polymer: potential blood pool contrast agent for MR imaging. J Magn Reson Imaging 4:462–466

Bartolozzi C, Colagrande S, Pellicanò G, Olmastroni M, Agostini S, Zampa V (1990) Agenti di contrasto in Risonanza Magnetica. Diagnostica con Risonanza Magnetica - Quaderno 9 di Aggiornamento Professionale Continuativo: 273–286

Bloembergen N (1957) Proton relaxations times in paramagnetic solutions. J Chem Phys 27:572–579

Cavagna F, Dapra M, Maggioni F, de Haen C, Felder E (1991) Gd-BOPTA/Dimeg: experimental disease imaging. Magn Reson Med 22:329–333

Chou CK, Liu GC, Yang LT, Chen RS, Jaw TS (1993) Abdominal MR imaging following antegrade air introduction into the intestinal loops. Abdom Imaging 18:205–210

Dawson P, Blomley M (1994) Gadolinium chelate MR contrast agents. Clin Radiol 49:439–442

Hahn PF, Stark DD, Lewis JM, et al. (1990) First clinical trial of a new superparamagnetic iron oxide for use as an oral gastrointestinal contrast agent for MR imaging. Radiology 175:695–770

Harpur ES, Worah D, Hals PA, Holtz E, Furuhama K, Nomura H (1993) Preclinical safety assessment and pharmacokinetics of gadodiamide injection, a new MRI contrast agent. Invest Radiol 28(Suppl 1):S28–S43

Laniado M, Kornmesser W, Hamm B, Clauss W, Weinmann HJ, Felix R (1988) MR imaging of the gastrointestinal tract: value of Gd-DTPA. AJR 150:817–821

Lonnemark M, Hemmingsson A, Ericsson A, Gundersen HG, Bach-Gansmo T (1990) Oral superparamagnetic particles for MRI: effect in plain and viscous aqueous suspensions. Acta Radiol 31:303–307

Mattrey RF, Hajek P, Gylys-Morin VM, et al. (1987) Perfluorochemicals as gastrointestinal contrast agents for MR imaging: preliminary studies in rats and humans. AJR 148:1259–1263

Ni Y, Marchal G, Lukito G, Yu J, Muhler A, Baert AL (1994) MR imaging evaluation of liver enhancement by Gd-EOB-DTPA in selective and total bile duct obstruction in rats: correlation with serologic, microcholangiographic and histologic findings. Radiology 190:753–758

Niendorf HP, Haustein J, Cornelius I, Alhassan A, Clauss W (1991) Safety of gadolinium-DTPA: extended clinical experience. Magn Reson Med 22:358–363

Parienty RA, Smolarski N, Pradel J, Ducellier R, Lubrano JM (1979) Computed tomography of the gastrointestinal tract – lesion recognition and pitfalls. J Comput Assist Tomogr 3:615–619

Rinck PA, Smevik O, Nilsen G, Klepp O, Onsrud M, Oksendal A, Borseth A (1991) Oral magnetic particles in MR imaging of the abdomen and pelvis. Radiology 178:775–779

Rofsky NM, Weinreb JC, Bernardino ME, Young SW, Lee JK, Noz ME (1993) Hepatocellular tumors: characterization with Mn-DPDP-enhanced MR imaging. Radiology 188:53–59

Runge VM, Gelblum DY, Pacetti ML, Carolan F, Heard G (1990) Gd-HP-DO3A in clinical MR imaging of the brain. Radiology 177:393–400

Runge VM, Kirsch JE, Thomas GS (1991) High-dose applications of gadolinium chelates in magnetic resonance imaging. Magn Reson Med 22:222–228

Schuhmann-Giampieri G (1993) Liver contrast media for magnetic resonance imaging. Interrelations between pharmacokinetics and imaging. Invest Radiol 28:753–761

Schuhmann-Giampieri G, Schmitt-Willich H, Press WR, Negishi C, Weinmann HJ, Speck U (1992) Preclinical evaluation of Gd-EOB-DTPA as a contrast agent in MR imaging of the hepatobiliary system. Radiology 183:59–64

Stark DD, Wittenberg J, Edelman RR, et al. (1986) Detection of hepatic metastases: analysis of pulse sequence performance in MR imaging. Radiology 159:365–370

Watson AD, Rocklage SM (1992) Theory and mechanisms of contrast-enhancing agents. In: Higgins CB, Hricak H, Helms CA (eds) Magnetic resonance imaging of the body. Raven Press, New York, pp 1257–1288

Weinmann HJ, Brasch RC, Press WR, Wesbey GE (1984) Characteristics of gadolinium DTPA complex: a potential NMR contrast agent. Am J Roentgenol 142:619–624

Winter TC 3rd, Freeny PC, Nghlem HV, Mack LA, Patten RM, Thomas CR Jr, Elliot S (1993) MR imaging with i.v. superparamagnetic iron oxide: efficacy in the detection of focal hepatic lesions. Am J Roentgenol 161:1191–1198

20 Heart

M. Lombardi and A. L'Abbate

CONTENTS

20.1 Introduction

In recent decades imaging techniques have contributed greatly to the impressive advances in cardiology. Among the new imaging techniques, magnetic resonance imaging (MRI) is progressively becoming more interesting for both research and clinical applications. Certain advantages make this technique unique in the technological panorama: MRI offers a natural contrast between blood, myocardium, and surrounding structures, and the fine depiction of morphology is nowadays routinely used in congenital heart disease as well as in acquired diseases (Higgins and Caputo 1992). Furthermore, MR images, by their intrinsic nature, are influenced by the chemical structure of the different tissues and their physical properties (T1, T2, proton density). Accordingly, MRI has been proposed as the reference technique in the diagnosis of right ventricular dysplasia (Blake et al. 1994), where fat or fibrous-fatty infiltration of the right ventricle free wall is present. Diagnostic changes in T1 and T2 induced by infarction have also been documented both in animals and in man (Williams et al. 1980; McNamara et al. 1985; Fisher et al. 1987).

The use of contrast agents significantly enriches the potential of MRI by facilitating the detection of signal intensity inhomogeneity due to myocardial tissue abnormalities. Among the various pathophysiological aspects of cardiac disease, researchers are devoting their energies in particular to four topics: cardiac tumors, myocardial infarction, quantitative myocardial perfusion, and coronary angiography.

M. Lombardi, MD, C.N.R. Clinical Physiology Institute, Via Paolo Savi, 8, I-56126, Pisa, Italy
A. L'Abbate, MD, C.N.R Clinical Physiology Institute, Via Paolo Savi, 8, I-56100 Pisa, Italy

20.2 Cardiac Tumors

The excellent spatial and contrast resolution of MRI allows the detection, anatomical localization, and description of the size of cardiac and paracardiac masses (Lund et al. 1989; Gomes et al. 1987). Moreover, the large field of view facilitates imaging of the mediastinum and provides information on the relationship between the tumoral mass and the surrounding structures (Amparo et al. 1984; Barakos et al. 1989). However, with MRI, as with other imaging techniques, the spatial definition of the landmarks between an infiltrating tumor and the surrounding normal myocardial tissue may be a difficult task (Lund et al. 1989). To this purpose the use of T2-weighted spin-echo (SE) images may be of some help, although the prolonged TE causes a significant degradation of images of the beating heart. The use of contrast agents together with T1-weighted images can be helpful in inducing differential contrast enhancement of tumors as compared with normal myocardium and surrounding structures (Funari et al. 1991; Weinreb et al. 1990) (Fig. 20.1).

Currently the most frequently used contrast agent is gadolinium diethylene triamine penta-acetic acid (Gd-DTPA), the distribution of which is primarily located in the extracellular space. Tumors with augmented vascularization, such as carcinoid tumors, or with significant enlargement of the interstitial space, such as myxomas, may show a substantial signal enhancement. In addition, nonvascularized, necrotic, or cystic areas inside the tumor can induce heterogeneous contrast enhancement of the neoplastic mass

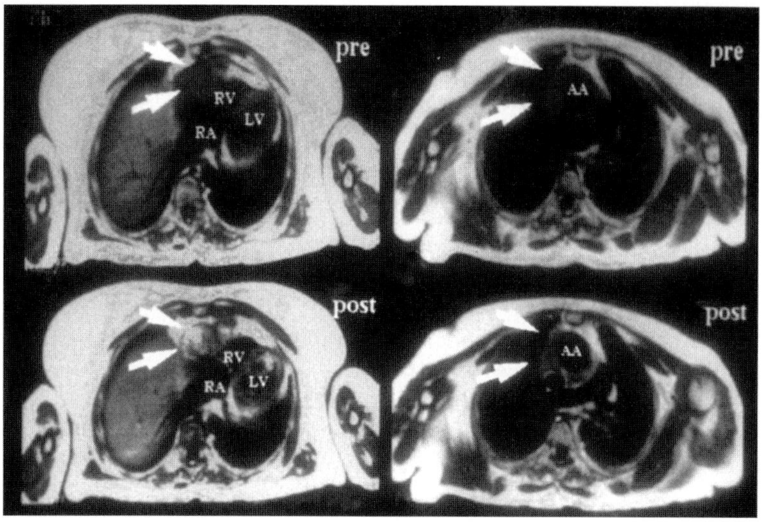

Fig. 20.1. Demonstration of a lymphoma (*arrows*) involving the free wall of the right ventricle (*left panel*) and the perivascular space around the great vessels (*right panel*), before (*upper panels*) and after (*lower panels*) injection of Gd-DTPA. With the contrast agent present, a higher and inhomogeneous enhancement of the neo-plastic mass is evident. *LV*, Left ventricle; *RA*, right atrium; *RV*, right ventricle; *AA*, aortic artery. (Courtesy of Dr. V. ZAMPA, Imaging Department, University of Pisa, Pisa, Italy)

a

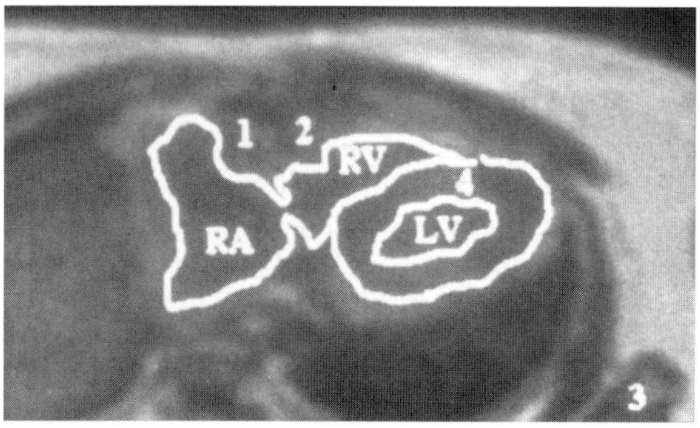

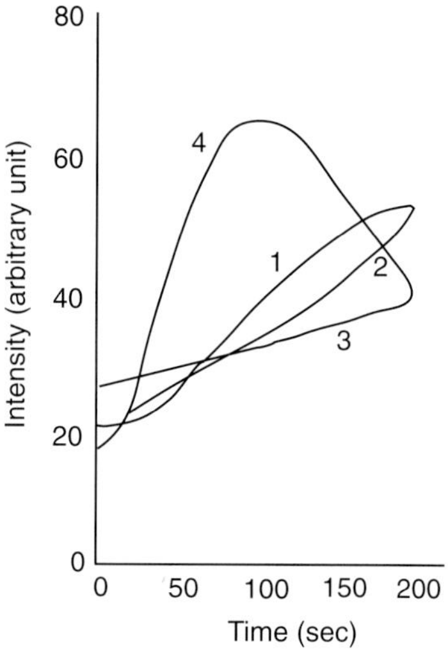

b

Fig. 20.2. Evaluation by the dynamic approach of the same tumoral mass (lymphoma) as is shown in Fig. 20.1. The signal intensity behavior after injection of a bolus of Gd-DTPA is shown in the time domain. In this case, eight SE images were obtained before and after the injection of the contrast agent. On each image, four regions of interest were drawn: the tumoral mass (identified by *1* and *2*), normal myocardium (identified by *4*), and skeletal muscle (identified by *3*). The time-intensity curves show lower signal intensity with depression of the curves in the time domain at the level of the tumor, interpreted as indicating a low-degree of vascularization of the tumoral mass. *LV*, Left ventricle; *RA*, right atrium; *RV*, right ventricle. (Courtesy of Dr. V. ZAMPA, Imaging Department, University of Pisa, Pisa, Italy)

due to the absence of contrast medium (FUNARI et al. 1991).

An empirical but widely used approach to the evaluation of cardiac tumors consists in evaluation of the dynamic behavior of the signal changes in the time domain following the intravenous injection of contrast agent (Fig. 20.2). Sequential images are acquired using SE or preferably gradient-echo (GRE) or turbo GRE sequences to obtain T1-weighted images. The behavior of the signal intensity in the time domain is influenced by several factors such as the vascularization of the mass, which is indirectly evaluated by this approach.

Despite the fact that neither large series nor systematic comparative studies on the different types of cardiac tumors have been produced, one may assert that it is likely that the use of contrast agent can be extremely helpful in differentiating between normal and infiltrating neoplastic tissue. Finally, the use of contrast agents can be proposed in order to differentiate between intracardiac tumors and acute or subacute thrombotic masses since the latter are not vascularized and therefore cannot be enhanced by contrast media. In rare cases, chronic thrombi are vascularized (CIPRIANO and GUTHANER 1978), in which case they may show signal enhancement after contrast administration.

20.3 Diagnosis and Quantitation of Myocardial Infarction

Myocardial infarction is one of most common diseases and a major cause of morbidity and mortality in Western countries. In the era of thrombolysis and coronary revascularization, it is of clinical relevance to differentiate between irreversibly damaged myocardium on the one hand and dysfunctioning though still viable tissue such as stunned and hibernating myocardium on the other. Furthermore, the presence of residual ischemia and the underlying coronary anatomy are important aspects to be addressed.

Magnetic resonance imaging has some intrinsic advantages for the detection and quantitation of infarcted myocardium. It has been shown that, from the analysis of relaxation times (T1 and T2) and proton density, it is possible to differentiate normal from ischemic damaged myocardium (HIGGINS et al. 1983). Based on these considerations, a number of studies have been performed to examine changes in signal intensity within the infarction both in animal models and in human beings (MCNAMARA et al. 1985; PFLUGFELDER et al. 1986; TSCHOLAKOFF et al. 1986; WESBEY et al. 1984a; WILLIAMS et al. 1980; WISEMBERG et al. 1988). These studies have shown that changes in T1 and T2 are precociously detected after infarction; using T2-weighted images it is possible to appreciate a signal intensity increase 60 min after coronary artery occlusion, peaking at about 4 h after occlusion. The reported magnitude of the signal increase varies according to the magnetic field and the pulse sequence used. Using T1-weighted images, an increase in signal intensity of about 66% has been reported. This alteration is detectable during the acute phase, increases progressively, and then declines.

Reperfusion of the ischemic/infarcted region can also affect the T2 relaxation time. Thirty minutes after the onset of reperfusion, reperfused myocardium shows a prolonged T2 (SLUTSKY et al. 1984; RATNER et al. 1985; JOHNSTON et al. 1985, 1987). A correlation between enhanced signal intensity and jeopardized myocardium has been reported (BUDA et al. 1985; BOUCHARD et al. 1989).

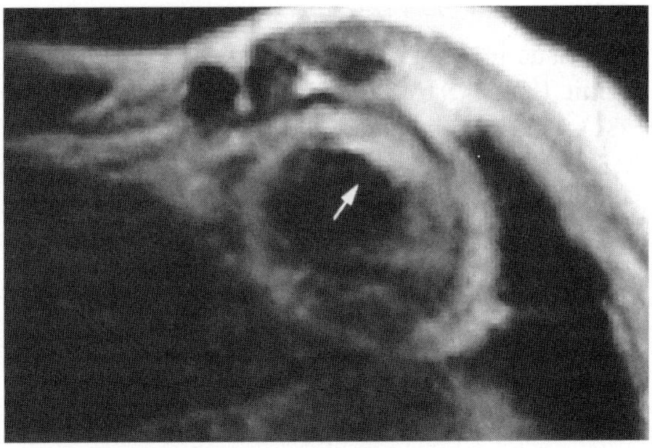

Fig. 20.3. SE image obtained in a patient 1 week after a transmural myocardial infarction. The image was obtained after injection of 0.1 mmol/kg b.w. of gadodiamide (Nycomed, Oslo, Norway). The infarcted region (*arrow*) shows an increased signal intensity compared with normal regions

It is not completely clear why T1 and T2 relaxation times are altered. The initial hypothesis that tissue edema could be responsible for such a phenomenon has been challenged by further studies showing the persistence of signal intensity alteration after several weeks in the absence of edema. In the rabbit T2 has been shown to remain enhanced for up to 3 months within the infarcted area (JOHNSTON et al. 1988). Changes of T1 and T2 are likely the consequence of many factors including changes in the myocardial water content (CANBY et al. 1987), compartmentalization of water, concentration and type of lipid present, macromolecular environment, temperature, variation in electrolyte concentrations, and presence of granulation (JOHNSTON et al. 1988).

The detection of acute infarction with unenhanced MRI does not occur until several hours after coronary occlusion (WILLIAMS et al. 1980; PFLUGFELDER et al. 1986). Furthermore, changes in T1 and T2 may not be sufficient to provide enough contrast to adequately visualize the infarcted areas. The use of contrast agents may facilitate the detection of signal intensity inhomogeneity due to the presence of necrotic as well as ischemic regions.

It has been shown that the administration of contrast agents enhances the differences between normal and infarcted tissue (WESBEY et al. 1984b) (Fig. 20.3). Five minutes after injection of a gadolinium-based contrast agent, infarcted regions showed a shortening of T1 and T2 with respect to normal tissue (PESHOCK et al. 1986; MCNAMARA et al. 1986). Furthermore, low signal intensity has been reported in non-reperfused regions generally surrounded by an area with higher signal intensity. The peri-infarction zone is commonly believed to represent tissue in which myocytes are still alive but ischemic (Helfant et al. 1978; Hearse and Yellon 1981). This inhomogeneity disappears subsequently.

The use of MRI in conjunction with contrast agents has to take into account the potential problems related to the complexity of mechanisms involved in signal changes (Wolf 1990). Factors to be considered are the indirect effect on both T1 and T2 relaxation times, their different and usually opposing effects on final image intensity, the pharmacokinetic properties of the contrast agents, blood flow and blood volume, and the presence and duration of reperfusion. Particularly for low molecular weight contrast agents, changes in the distribution volume from exclusively extracellular to extracellular and intracellular due to the loss of compartmentalization as a consequence of the cell membrane disruption play a major role in determining the local concentration. For Gd-DTPA the pharmacokinetic characteristics have been investigated in an animal model with a well-defined ischemic territory (Pereira et al. 1996). The kinetics of the contrast agent uptake can be modeled by the modified Kety model (Diesbourg et al. 1992; Pereira et al. 1996; Tong et al. 1993):

$$[\text{Gd–DTPA}]_i(t) = FE \sum_0^t [\text{Gd–DTPA}]_a(\tau)e^{-FE\lambda(t-\tau)}d\tau,$$

where F is the regional perfusion, E is the extraction fraction of Gd-DTPA, $[\text{Gd-DTPA}]_a$ and $[\text{Gd-DTPA}]_i$ are the arterial and tissue concentrations, respectively, and λ is the partition coefficient of Gd-DTPA. According to the equation, if the input arterial function $[\text{Gd-DTPA}]_a$ is maintained constant so that the tissue and blood concentrations of Gd-DTPA will eventually reach equilibrium, λ will simply be the ratio of tissue and arterial concentrations of Gd-DTPA. Under this condition, the increased distribution volume, which is the consequence of loss of integrity of ischemic myocardial cells (i.e., loss of viability), leads to an increased amount of Gd-DTPA per unit mass of tissue, which results in greater signal enhancement relative to normal tissue on T1-weighted images.

Despite the limitations inherent to the complexity of the mechanisms involved in the signal intensity changes, the extent of myocardial necrosis can be accurately estimated with Gd-DTPA-enhanced images in both animals (Nishimura et al. 1989a) and humans (De Roos et al. 1990). The differentiation between reperfused and non-reperfused infarct is made possible by the injection of a low molecular weight gadolinium-based contrast agent such as gadodiamide (gadolinium diethylene triamine penta-acetic acid bismethylamide, Gd-DTPA-BMA). Immediate enhancement of reperfused regions has been documented after the injection of the contrast agent. This enhancement may be related to several mechanisms, including vascular extravasation, postischemic hyperemia, and expansion of the extracellular space. Afterwards, delayed clearance of the contrast agent from the reperfused infarcted zone is, presumably, caused by neutrophil- and platelet-mediated obstruction of microvasculature, which is often observed during reperfusion, and by edema that results in compression of the venous bed. Similarity in the enhancement profiles of the peri-infarction zone and the reperfused infarct suggests the possibility of common mechanisms of enhancement (Masui et al. 1991).

In clinical studies the enhancement of infarcted areas has been shown in the acute and subacute phase (McNamara et al. 1985; Fisher et al. 1987) while in chronic infarction the poorly vascularized scar does not show significant enhancement (Nishimura et al. 1989b); the optimal delay prior to imaging following the acute event is about 1 week (Van Dijkman et al. 1991). Furthermore, different patterns of enhancement (diffuse, subendocardial, dark areas of hemorrhage, and doughnut pattern) have been obtained in patients with myocardial infarction with and without reperfusion as assessed by coronary angiography (De Roos et al. 1989).

By contrast, with magnetic susceptibility contrast agents such as dysprosium chelates, a decrease in signal intensity of normally perfused and alive myocardium, with preservation of compartmentalization, is obtained. In fact, these contrast agents induce local magnetic field inhomogeneities that result in signal loss on both T2- and T2*-weighted images (Saeed et al. 1989). Using dysprosium diethylene triamine penta-actetic acid bismethylamide (Dy-DTPA-BMA), a close relationship has been shown between the area demarcated by the contrast agent and the area of deficient perfusion (Yu et al. 1993).

Manganese compounds have also been used for myocardial imaging. Manganese has a marked, dose-dependent effect on the myocardial T1 relaxation time. At higher doses of manganese, T2 shortening occurs, counteracting the effect on T1 on final image intensity. Infarct size has been successfully measured by manganese (Goldman et al. 1982). Manganese is actively taken up by viable myocardium and distributes throughout the myocardium in linear relation to myocardial blood flow. The infarcted regions display a relatively low signal intensity as compared with normal myocardium.

Macromolecular blood volume contrast agents have been shown to be able to elicit regional myocardial blood volume content inhomogeneities and identify infarcted regions on the basis of capillary leakage of contrast agent (SCHMIEDL et al. 1987).

Other contrast agents have also been shown to be potential markers of myocardial necrosis. There is evidence that paramagnetic metalloporphyrins are avidly taken up by necrotic tissue, allowing discrimination between reperfused and non-reperfused infarction (NI et al. 1996).

Overall, then, several MR contrast agents have been successfully tested in experimental models and to a minor degree in humans. MRI seems to greatly benefit from the use of contrast agents for the detection and quantitation of myocardial infarction and, to some extent, for the depiction of the complex and dynamic changes occurring in the evolution of cardiac ischemic events.

20.4 Quantitative Myocardial Perfusion

Several methods have been developed in recent years to evaluate myocardial perfusion by MRI. Some of them do not require the administration of contrast agent, e.g., the intravoxel incoherent motion technique (LE BIHAN et al. 1988) or magnetization transfer techniques (PRASAD et al. 1993; TSEKOS et al. 1994; WILLIAMS et al. 1993). These approaches have the intrinsic advantage of being totally noninvasive; they allow repeated measurements and avoid the build-up of contrast agent due to repeated injections, such as during stress studies. However, they suffer from intrinsic limitations related to the complexity of the mechanisms responsible for the contrast effect, which make these techniques sensitive to heart motion and the results difficult to interpret.

As an alternative, fast MRI techniques offer a sufficiently high temporal resolution to follow the first pass through the heart of a bolus of contrast agent (Fig. 20.4). Several groups have shown the potential value of this approach (ATKINSON et al. 1990; MANNING et al. 1991; WILKE et al. 1993; SAEED et al. 1993; LOMBARDI et al. 1997).

Figure 20.5 depicts time-intensity curves obtained from different regions of interest of the left ventricular wall during the passage of the contrast agent through the myocardium. From these time-intensity curves a number of parameters can be derived, e.g., the wash-in slope, the peak intensity level, and the area under the curve etc. These derived parameters have been shown to be representative, to some extent, of the local myocardial blood flow and volume (WILKE et al. 1993; SAEED et al. 1995; LOMBARDI et al. 1997) and to correlate with tomographic technetium-99m sestamibi imaging in patients with coronary artery disease (MATHEIJSSEN et al. 1996). Furthermore, the use of ultrarapid techniques such as echo-planar imaging has been proposed to further reduce the image acquisition time to a few tenths of

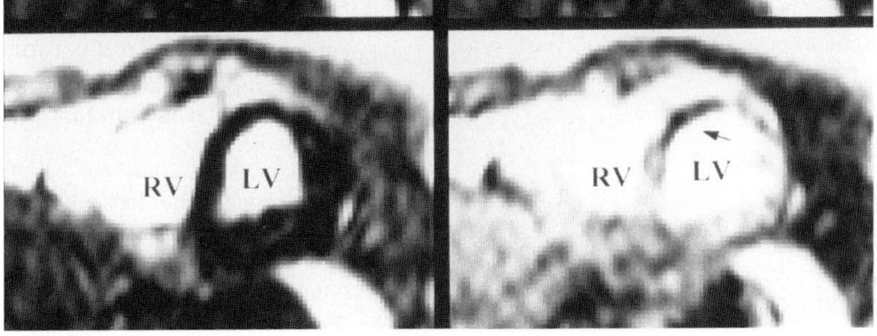

Fig. 20.4. Four out of a sequence of 64 images (one per heart beat) depicting the first pass of a bolus of Gd-DTPA (0.05 mmol/kg b.w.), intravenously injected. This sequence was obtained in a patient 1 week after a transmural myocardial infarction at the level of the anteroseptal wall. *Upper left panel*: preinjection; *upper right panel*, first pass of the contrast agent at the level of the right ventricle (*RV*); *lower left panel*, first pass of the contrast agent at the level of the left ventricle (*LV*); *lower right panel*, first pass of the contrast agent at the level of the myocardium. Within the infarcted area reduced enhancement of the signal is evident. In this patient the left anterior descending coronary artery was occluded

a millisecond (WENDLAND et al. 1993). Beside the advances in MRI equipment, a deeper knowledge of the potential and the limitations of low molecular weight contrast agents such as Gd-DTPA has been achieved. In addition to the above-mentioned Kety equation for modeling the variations of Gd-DTPA concentration with time, other mathematical models have been proposed to describe the complex behavior of this kind of contrast agent. For example, the relation between the unidirectional influx constant for Gd-DTPA, its extraction fraction, and the plasma perfusion rate has been described according to the following equation (LARSSON et al. 1994):

$$K_i = F \cdot \left(1 - e^{PS/F}\right),$$

where K_i is the unidirectional influx constant describing the unidirectional transport of Gd-DTPA across the capillary membrane, F is the plasma perfusion rate, and PS is the permeability surface-area product.

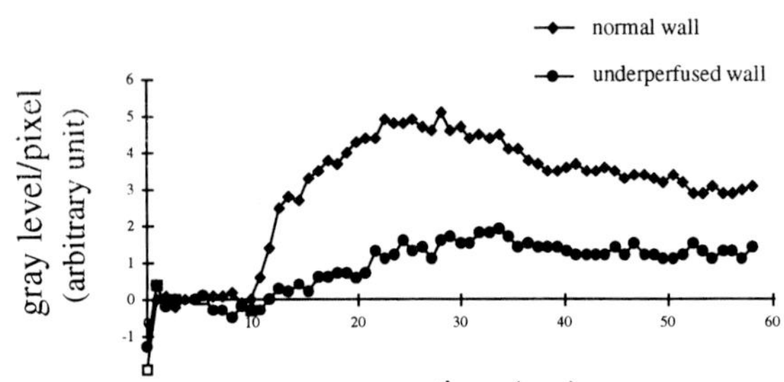

Fig. 20.5. Myocardial first pass of a bolus of Gd-DTPA (0.05 mmol/kg b.w.) intravenously injected in a living animal model with reduced perfusion within the territory of the left anterior descending coronary artery. The time-intensity curve generated from the region of interest positioned at the level of the ischemic wall shows a decreased signal intensity as compared with the normally perfused wall

To avoid the limitations inherent to multicompartmental distribution, a number of strictly intravascular compounds are under study (Gd-DTPA-polylysine, liposomes, iron oxide particles, etc.). Conjugating paramagnetic or superparamagnetic ligands to polysaccharides, polymeres, proteins, and lipids allows the distribution of such contrast agents to be confined within the intravascular space. Their use may give rise to a significant positive contrast effect with heavily T1-weighted images (CANET et al. 1993). In particular, using intra-atrial injection of polylysine-Gd-DTPA, reliable estimation of regional myocardial blood flow and vascular blood volume has been achieved (KROLL et al. 1996; WILKE et al. 1995).

An iron-based superparamagnetic contrast agent has been successfully used for relative quantitation of myocardial blood flow after injection in a peripheral vein (Fig. 20.6) (LOMBARDI et al. 1996).

While some of these agents are expected to evolve side-by-side with the traditional low molecular weight contrast agents, new imaging modalities allow the simultaneous depiction of multiple slices of the heart (WALSH et al. 1995), further increasing the potential of MRI in the evaluation of myocardial perfusion.

Although the development of these contrast agents and of ultra-fast imaging modalities may further improve the capability of MRI in the evaluation of myocardial perfusion, other factors have to be

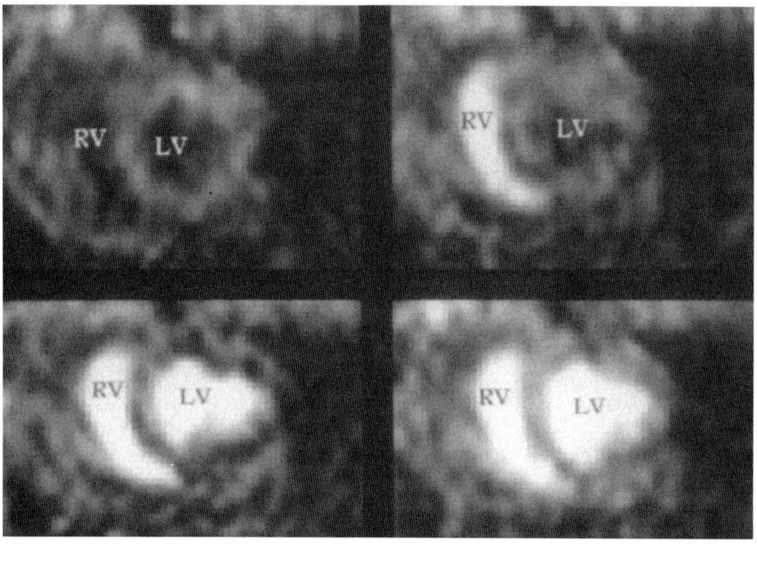

Fig. 20.6. Four images obtained with a Turbo FLASH pulse sequence during the first pass of a bolus (5 µmol/kg) of superparamagnetic iron-based contrast agent (PEG-IMP, Nycomed, Oslo, Norway), intravenously injected in a living animal. *Upper left panel*, precontrast; *upper right panel*, first pass through the right ventricle (*RV*); *lower left panel*, first pass through the left ventricle (*LV*); *lower right panel*, first pass through the myocardium. This contrast agent remains confined to the intravascular space

taken into account in order to derive absolute flow values from first-pass curves. In fact, the assumption that regional variations in contrast agent concentration produced by regional variations in blood flow lead to signal changes which are linearly related to the flow changes is not acceptable in vivo. The interlinkage of compartments (plasma, red blood cells, interstitium, tissue cells) by proton exchange propagates the effect of contrast agents into compartments without contrast agent, reducing the advantage of using intravascular contrast media (Bauer et al. 1996; Donahue et al. 1996) unless exchange-insensitive sequences are used (Donahue et al. 1996).

20.5 Visualization of the Coronary Arteries

The spatial resolution of currently available MRI equipment allows the visualization only of the major coronary artery segments (Manning et al. 1993). Several factors limit imaging of coronary arteries such as their tortuous nature and their cyclic movement. Technical advances such as the navigator-echo real-time respiratory gating may reduce the negative effect of respiration on image quality (Wang et al. 1996). The natural contrast offered by MRI can be further improved by the use of specific techniques already in use in MR angiography such as magnetization-prepared T2 contrast (Brittain et al. 1995). The feasibility of using contrast agents to improve the signal-to-noise ratio is now under investigation. The blood pool agents seem very promising for this purpose because of their favorable characteristic of remaining within the intravascular space for a long period (Frank et al. 1994; Stillman et al. 1996). However, it is too early to state whether MRI coronary angiography will have a definite role in coronary artery disease and whether the use of contrast agents will be necessary.

20.6 Conclusions

From this short overview it can be concluded that MRI, used in conjunction with adequate contrast agents, has the potential to become the only tool in cardiology, fulfilling the "one-stop shop" philosophy, i.e., comprehensive evaluation of heart morphology, coronary artery anatomy, ventricular function, and myocardial perfusion. To overcome the present limitations, the development of organ-specific contrast agents and of contrast agents with different pharmacokinetic properties is required.

References

Amparo EG, Higgins CB, Farmer D, Gasmu G, McNamara M (1984) Gated MRI of cardiac and paracardiac masses: initial experience. AJR 143:1151–1156

Atkinson D, Burstein D, Edelman RR (1990) First-pass cardiac perfusion: evaluation with ultrafast MR imaging. Radiology 174:757–762

Barakos JA, Brown JJ, Higgins CB (1989) MR imaging of secondary cardiac and paracardiac lesions. AJR 153:47–50

Bauer WR, Hiller K-H, Roder F, Rommel E, Ert G, Haase A (1996) Magnetisation effects in capillaries by microcirculation affects diffusion controlled spin relaxation: a model which describes the effect of perfusion on relaxation enhancement by intravascular contrast agents. Magn Reson Med 35:43–55

Blake LM, Scheinman MM, Higgins CB (1994) MR features of arrhythmogenic right ventricular dysplasia. AJR 162:809–812

Bouchard A, Reeves RC, Cranney G, Bishop SP, Pohost GM (1989) Assessment of myocardial infarct size by means of T2 weighted ^{1}H nuclear magnetic resonance imaging. Am Heart J 117:281–289

Brittain JH, Hu BS, Wright GA, et al. (1995) Coronary angiography with magnetization prepared T2 contrast. Magn Reson Med 33:689–696

Buda AJ, Aisen AM, Juni JE, Callagher KP, Zotz RJ (1985) Detection and sizing of myocardial ischemia and infarction by nuclear magnetic resosonance imaging in the canine heart. Am Heart J 110:1284–1290

Canby RC, Reeves RC, Evanochko WT, Elgavish GA, Pohost GM (1987) Proton nuclear magnetic resonance relaxation times in severe myocardial ischemia. J Am Coll Cardiol 10:412–420

Canet E, Revel D, Forrat R, et al. (1993) Superparamagnetic iron oxide particles and positive enhancement for myocardial perfusion studies assessed by subsecond T1-weighted MRI. Magn Reson Med 11:1139–1145

Cipriano PR, Guthaner DF (1978) Organized left atrial mural thrombus demonstrated by coronary angiography. Am Heart J 96:166–169

DeRoos A, Van Rossum AC, Van der Wall EE, et al. (1989) Reperfused and non-reperfused myocardial infarction: potential of gadolinium-DTPA enhanced MR imaging. Radiology 172:717–720

De Roos A, Matheijssen NAA, Doornbos J, et al. (1990) Myocardial infarct size after reperfusion therapy: assessment with Gd-DTPA-enhanced MR imaging. Radiology 176:517–521

Diesbourg LD, Proat FS, Wisemberg G, et al. (1992) Quantification of myocardial blood flow and extracellular volumes using a bolus injection of Gd-DTPA: kinetic modelling in canine ischemic disease. Magn Reson Med 23:239–253

Donahue KM, Weisskoff RM, Chesler DA, Kwong KK, Bogdanov AA Jr, Mandeville JB, Rosen BR (1996) Improving MR quantification of regional blood volume with intravascular T1 contrast agents: accuracy precision and water exchange. Magn Reson Med 36:858–867

Fisher MR, McNamara MT, Higgins CB (1987) Acute myocar-

dial infarction: MR evaluation in 29 patients. AJR 148:247–251
Frank H, Weissleder R, Brady TJ (1994) Enhancement of MR angiography with iron oxide: preliminary studies in whole-blood phantom and in animal. AJR 162:209–213
Funari M, Fujita N, Wallace WP, Higgins CB (1991) Cardiac tumors: assessment with Gd-DTPA enhanced MR imaging. J Comput Assist Tomogr 15:953–958
Goldman MR, Brady TJ, Pykett IL, et al. (1982) Quantification of experimental myocardial infarction using nuclear magnetic resonance imaging and paramagnetic ion contrast enhancement in excised canine hearts. Circulation 66:1012–1016
Gomes AS, Lois JF, Child JS, Bown K, Batra P (1987) Cardiac tumors and thrombus: evaluation with MR imaging. AJR 149:895–899
Hearse DJ, Yellon DM (1981) The border zone in evolving myocardial infarction: controversy or confusion? Am J Cardiol 47:1321–1334
Helfant RH, Banka VS, Bodenheimer WM (1978) Perplexities and complexities concerning the myocardial infarction, border zone and its salvage. Am J Cardiol 47:345–347
Higgins CB, Caputo GR (1992) Acquired heart disease. In: Higgins CB, Hricak H, Helms CA (eds) Magnetic resonance imaging of the body. Raven Press, New York, pp 525–566
Higgins CB, Herfkens R, Lipton MJ, et al. (1983) Nuclear magnetic resonance imaging of acute myocardial infarction in dogs: alterations in magnetic relaxation times. Am J Cardiol 52:184–188
Johnston DL, Brady TJ, Ratner AV, et al. (1985) Assessment of myocardial ischemia with proton magnetic resonance: effects of a three hour coronary occlusion with and without reperfusion. Circulation 71:595–601
Johnston DL, Liu P, Rosen BR, et al. (1987) In vivo detection of reperfused myocardium by nuclear magnetic resonance imaging. J Am Coll Cardiol 9:127–135
Johnston DL, Homma S, Liu P, et al. (1988) Serial changes in nuclear magnetic resonance relaxation times after myocardial infarction in the rabbit: relationship to water content, severity of ischemia, and histopathology over a six-month period. Magn Res Med 8:363–379
Kroll K, Wilke N, Jerosch-Herold M, et al. (1996) Modeling regional myocardial flows from residue functions of an intravascular indicator. Am J Physiol 271 (Heart Circ Physiol 40):H1643–H1655
Larsson HBW, Stubgaard M, Søndergaard L, Henriksen O (1994) In vivo quantification of the unidirectional influx constant for Gd-DTPA diffusion across the myocardial capillaries with MR imaging. J Magn Reson Imag 4:433–440
Le Bihan D, Breton E, Lallemand D, et al. (1988) Separation of diffusion and perfusion in intravoxel incoherent motion MR imaging. Radiology 168:497–505
Lombardi M, Jones RA, Westby J, et al. (1996) Relative quantitation of myocardial perfusion by MRI and intravenous iron based contrast in the open chest pig. Circulation 94;8:I-418
Lombardi M, Jones RA, Westby J, et al. (1997) Magnetic resonance imaging for the evaluation of regional myocardial perfusion in an experimental animal model. J Magn Reson Imag 7:987–995
Lund JT, Ehman RL, Julsrud PR, Sinak LJ, Tajik AJ (1989) Cardiac masses: assessment by MR imaging. AJR 152:469–473
Manning WJ, Atkinson DJ, Grossman W, Paulin S, Edelman RR (1991) First-pass nuclear magnetic resonance imaging studies using gadolinium-DTPA in patients with coronary artery disease. J Am Coll Cardiol 18:959–965
Manning WJ, Li W, Edelman RR (1993) A preliminary report comparing magnetic resonance coronary angiography with conventional angiography. N Engl J Med 328:828–832
Masui T, Saeed M, Wendland MF, Higgins CB (1991) Occlusive and reperfused myocardial infarcts: MR imaging differentiation with nonionic Gd-DTPA-BMA. Radiology 181:77–83
Matheijssen NAA, Louwerenburg HW, Van Rugge PF, et al. (1996) Comparison of ultrafast dipyridamole magnetic resonance imaging with dipyridamole sestaMIBI SPECT for detection of perfusion abnormalities in patients with one-vessel coronary artery disease: assessment by quantitative model fitting. Magn Reson Med 35:221–228
McNamara MT, Higgins CB, Schechtmann N, et al. (1985) Detection and characterisation of acute myocardial infarction in man with the use of gated magnetic resonance. Circulation 71:717–724
McNamara MT, Tscholakoff D, Revel D, et al. (1986) Differentiation of reversible and irreversible myocardial injury by MR imaging with and without gadolinium-DTPA. Radiology 158:765–769
Ni Y, Marchal G, Herijgers P, et al. (1996) Paramagnetic metalloporphyrins: from enhancers of malignant tumors to markers of myocardial infarcts. Acad Radiol 3:S395–S397
Nishimura T, Yamada Y, Hayashi M, et al. (1989a) Determination of infarct size of acute myocardial infarction in dogs by magnetic resonance imaging and gadolinium-DTPA: comparison with indium-111 antimyosin imaging. Am J Physiol Imag 4:83–88
Nishimura T, Kobayashi G, Ohara Y (1989b) Serial assessment of myocardial infarction by using gated MR imaging and Gd-DTPA. AJR 153:715–720
Pereira RS, Prato FS, Wisenberg G, Sykes J (1996) The determination of myocardial viability using Gd-DTPA in a canine model of acute myocardial ischemia and reperfusion. Magn Reson Med 36:684–693
Peshock RM, Malloy CR, Buja LM, et al. (1986) Magnetic resonance imaging of acute myocardial infarction: gadolinium diethylenetriamine-pentaacetic acid as a marker of reperfusion. Circulation 74:1434–1440
Pflugfelder PW, Wisenberg G, Prato FS, Carrol SE (1986) Serial imaging of canine myocardial infarction by in vivo nuclear magnetic resonance. J Am Coll Cardiol 7:843–849
Prasad PV, Burstein D, Edelman RR (1993) MRI evaluation of myocardial perfusion without a contrast agent using magnetisation transfer. Magn Reson Med 30:267–270
Ratner AV, Okada RD, Newell JB, Pohost GM (1985) The relationship between proton nuclear magnetic resonance relaxation parameters and myocardial perfusion with acute coronary arterial occlusion and reperfusion. Circulation 71:823–828
Saeed M, Wendland MF, Tomei E, et al. (1989) Demarcation of myocardial ischemia: magnetic susceptibility effect of contrast medium in MR imaging. Radiology 173:763–767
Saeed M, Wendland MF, Yu KK, Li HT, Higgins CB (1993) Dual effect of gadodiamide injection in depiction of the region of myocardial ischemia. J Magn Reson Imag 3:21–29
Saeed M, Wendland MF, Sakuma H, et al. (1995) Coronary artery stenosis: detection with contrast-enhanced MR imaging in dogs. Radiology 196:79–84
Schmiedl U, Moseley ME, Sievers R, et al. (1987) Magnetic resonance imaging of myocardial infarction using albumin-(Gd-DTPA), a macromolecular blood-volume contrast agent in a rat model. Invest Radiol 22:713–721
Slutsky RA, Brown JJ, Peck WW, Stritch G, Andre MP (1984)

Effects of transient coronary ischemia and reperfusion on myocardial edema formation and in vitro magnetic relaxation times. J Am Coll Cardiol 3:1454–1460
Stillman AE, Wilke N, Li D, Haacke M, McLachlan S (1996) Ultrasmall superparamagnetic iron oxide to enhance MRA of the renal and coronary arteries: studies in human patients. J Comput Assist Tomogr 20:51–55
Tong CY, Prato FS, Wisenberg G, et al. (1993) Measurement of the extraction efficiency and distribution volume for Gd-DTPA in normal and diseased canine myocardium. Magn Reson Med 30:337–346
Tscholakoff D, Higgins CB, McNamara MT, Derugin N (1986) Early-phase myocardial infarction by MR imaging. Radiology 159:667–672
Tsekos NV, Zhang Y, Merkle H, Wilke N, Urgubil K (1994) Assessment of myocardial perfusion state with magnetization transfer during coronary artery occlusion and adenosine vasodilation. In: Proc. of SMR San Francisco, USA 3:1480
Van Dijkman PRM, Van der Wall EE, De Roos A, et al. (1991) Acute, subacute and chronic myocardial infarction: quantitative analysis of gadolinium-enhanced MR images. Radiology 180:147–151
Walsh EG, Doyle M, Lawson MA, Blackwell GG, Pohost GM (1995) Multislice first-pass myocardial perfusion imaging on a conventional clinical scanner. Magn Reson Med 34:39–47
Wang Y, Rossman PJ, Grimm RC, Riederer SJ, Ehman RL (1996) Navigator-ECHO-based real-time respiratory gating and triggering for reduction of respiratory effects in three-dimensional coronary MR angiography. Radiology 198:55–60
Weinreb JC, Davis SD, Berkmen YM, Isom W, Naidich DP (1990) Pulmonary artery sarcoma: evaluation using Gd-DTPA. J Comput Assist Tomogr 14:647–649
Wendland MF, Saeed M, Masui T, et al. (1993) Echo-planar MR imaging of normal and ischemic myocardium with gadodiamide injection. Radiology 186:535–542
Wesbey G, Higgins CB, Lanzer P, Botvinick E, Lipton MJ (1984a) Imaging and characterisation of acute myocardial infarction in vivo by gated nuclear magnetic resonance. Circulation 69:125–130
Wesbey GE, Higgins CB, McNamara MT, et al. (1984b) Effects of gadolinium-DTPA on the magnetic relaxation times of normal and infarcted myocardium. Radiology 153:165–169
Wilke N, Simm C, Zhang J, et al. (1993) Contrast-enhanced first pass myocardial perfusion imaging: correlation between myocardial blood flow in dogs at rest and during hyperemia. Magn Reson Med 29:485–497
Wilke N, Kroll K, Merkle H, et al. (1995) Regional myocardial blood volume and flow: first pass MR imaging with polylysine-Gd-DTPA. J Magn Reson Med 5:227–237
Williams ES, Kaplan JI, Thatcher F, Zimmerman G, Knoebel SB (1980) Prolongation of proton spin lattice relaxation times in regionally ischemic tissue from dog hearts. J Nucl Med 21:449–453
Williams DS, Grandis DJ, Zhang W, Koretsky AP (1993) Magnetic resonance imaging of perfusion in the isolated rat heart using spin inversion of arterial water. Magn Reson Med 30:361–365
Wisemberg G, Prato FS, Carroll SE, Turner KL, Marshall MT (1988) Serial nuclear magnetic resonance imaging of acute myocardial infarction with and without reperfusion. Am Heart J 115:510–518
Wolf GL (1990) Role of magnetic contrast agents in cardiac imaging. Am J Cardiol 66:59F–62F
Yu KK, Saeed M, Wendland MF, et al. (1993) Comparison of T1-enhancing and magnetic susceptibility magnetic resonance contrast agents for demarcation of the jeopardy area in experimental myocardial infarction. Invest Radiol 28:1015–1023

21 Kidneys and Adrenal Glands

G.P. Krestin

CONTENTS

21.1 Introduction

Magnetic resonance (MR) examination of the kidneys and adrenal glands is rendered difficult by artifacts due to respiratory motion and the proximity of the abdominal vessels. On the other hand, the kidneys are the most important organs for maintaining homeostasis in the human body; consequently, the diagnosis of renal diseases must cover not only possible morphological changes but also, and in particular, any functional disturbances. The use of a contrast material permits the assessment of different states of perfusion, with better delineation and better differentiation of pathological processes. Moreover, visualization of the passage of a renally eliminated contrast agent also provides information on the excretory function of the kidneys. Therefore, contrast-enhanced MRI of the kidneys differs fundamentally from other imaging techniques, since for the first time one single method permits simultaneous assessment of macroscopic changes and evaluation of functional derangements (Krestin 1990; von Schulthess 1989).

In the imaging diagnosis of adrenal disorders two major patient groups can be differentiated: a smaller group with clinical and laboratory findings of an adrenal endocrinopathy, and a second, much larger group with an incidentally found enlargement of the adrenal glands. The diagnostic approach in these two groups is totally different, since in the first category imaging methods are used for localization of an adrenal pathology while in the second group the lesion is found during the course of a routine imaging examination or a staging workup for a malignant primary tumor. In the first group, computed tomography (CT) remains the imaging method of choice, while in the second MRI is probably more accurate (Krestin 1990).

21.2 MR Imaging Strategies

In order to provide morphological information that may compete with the results of CT and ultrasound (US), special techniques like artifact compensation and fast imaging have to be employed. The additional use of a renally eliminated paramagnetic contrast agent like gadolinium-DTPA (Gd-DTPA) or Gd-DOTA permits the assessment of different states of perfusion and the visualization of the passage of the contrast medium, providing information on hyper- or hypoperfused lesions and on the excretory function of the kidneys. The recent development of fat suppression techniques, fast spin-echo sequences, and ultrafast imaging have further expanded the list of potential applications of MRI in the kidneys and adrenal glands.

G.P. Krestin, MD, Professor and Chairman, Department of Radiology, Academic Hospital, Erasmus University Rotterdam, Molewaterplein 40, 3015 GD Rotterdam, The Netherlands

Examination of retroperitoneal organs should be tailored considering the main clinical questions. However, a partial standardization is possible, as discussed below.

21.2.1 Examination of the Kidneys

21.2.1.1 Standard Sequence for Orientation

Between 10 and 16 transversal T1-weighted sections of the upper abdomen are acquired with a slice thickness of 10 mm. T1-weighting can be achieved using either spin-echo sequences with motion compensation techniques (ROPE, flow compensated) or gradient-echo sequences during suspended respiration (FLASH, SPGR, FFE) using a short TR (20–30 ms) and TE (10–15 ms) in combination with large flip angles (40–70°).

21.2.1.2 Tissue Characterization

T2-weighted sequences may help to better delineate the extrarenal extent of malignant renal masses. Fast spin-echo sequences (RARE) with motion compensation (TR = 3000–4000 ms; TE = 90–120 ms) or T2-weighted gradient-echo sequences (FISP, GRASS, FFE) with small flip angles (10–15°) are best suited for this purpose. For renal masses an additional fat suppression technique may help to visualize the peri- and pararenal extension of disease.

21.2.1.3 Delineation of Pathological Lesions

The extent of the lesion may be visualized in an additional plane. A coronal section is best suited for delineation of most tumors of the kidneys and adrenal glands. Breath-hold, fat-suppressed T1-weighted gradient-echo sequences (SPGR, FLASH, FFE with flip angles >40° and a slice thickness of 10 mm) can be used for this purpose and later compared with contrast-enhanced scans obtained with the same imaging parameters.

21.2.1.4 Vascular Diagnosis

For better delineation of the renal arteries and, in particular, veins in patients with perivascular malignant tumors, transversal gradient-echo images with flow compensation are mandatory. The best image quality can be achieved using a short TR (<30 ms), a short TE (<15 ms), and small flip angles (<20°).

21.2.1.5 Dynamic Contrast-Enhanced Perfusion Studies

Five to six repeated single or multiple slices in the same position before and 20, 40, 60, 120, and 240 s after bolus injection of 0.1 mmol/kg of a paramagnetic contrast agent (Gd-DTPA or Gd-DOTA) allows estimation of the early perfusion of a renal or adrenal mass. The use of fast imaging (T1-weighted gradient-echo sequences like SPGR, FLASH or FFE) in the plane of maximal tumor extent offers the possibility of rapid image repetition during suspended respiration.

21.2.1.6 Dynamic Functional Studies

In patients with renal parenchymal diseases, dynamic functional studies may be performed using a gradient-echo sequence with simultaneous T1 and T2 influence (GRASS, FFE, FLASH without spoiling gradients). Rapid repetition of 16–32 single scans in the same position with TR = 30 ms, TE = 16 ms, and flip angle = 70° using a reduced (190 × 256) matrix allows a reduction of acquisition times to 5–6 s/slice; these are followed by breathing periods of 4–5 s, resulting in a temporal resolution of 10 s. Gd-DTPA or Gd-DOTA is administered after the first scan as a bolus at a concentration of 0.1 mmol/kg body weight.

21.2.1.7 Delayed Contrast-Enhanced Images

For evaluation of late perfusion effects and of the perirenal extent of renal masses, T1-weighted fat-suppressed images may be acquired in the same plane and with the same parameters as the plain images obtained for lesion delineation. In this way one can compare the pre- and postcontrast examination for evaluation of pathologically enhancing regions.

21.2.2 Examination of the Adrenal Glands

21.2.2.1 Standard Sequence for Orientation

The standard sequence for orientation is usually an axial T1-weighted and/or T2-weighted spin-echo sequence with 5–7 mm section thickness. The use of a T2-weighted fast spin-echo sequence instead of the conventional technique reduces acquisition time and thus motion artifacts, resulting in better image quality. As an alternative to T2-weighted spin-echo sequences, a fast GRE sequence with relative T2-weighting (TR = 60 ms, TE = 30 ms, flip angle = 15°) may be used. This technique has the advantage of a shortened acquisition time, which allows for imaging during suspended respiration, resulting in improved image quality.

On T1- and T2-weighted pulse sequences, the normal adrenal glands appear iso- or hypointense compared with the liver. If fat suppression is applied, the glands become isointense to the liver on T1-weighted and hyperintense on T2-weighted images. Advantages of fat suppression are reduced noise and sharper depiction of organ architecture, reduced respiratory motion-induced artifacts, elimination of chemical shift artifacts, and expanded gray scale to accentuate small differences in tissue contrast. Disadvantages include fewer sections per acquisition and possible inhomogeneity of fat suppression throughout the image.

21.2.2.2 Lesion Characterization

Adrenal adenomas and nodular hyperplasia contain large amounts of fat, whereas metastases and pheochromocytomas contain no, or very little, lipid. Thus *chemical shift imaging* with in-phase and opposed-phase gradient-echo images has been advocated to distinguish adenomas, i.e., fatty, from nonadenomatous, i.e., nonfatty, lesions. On a 1.5-T MR system (64 MHz), lipid and water protons have a frequency difference of about 224 Hz. Thus, a phase cycling of water and lipid spins occurs every 2.24 ms after the excitation pulse. At this interval, lipid and water spins are alternatively in- and out-of-phase. The signal intensity of opposed-phase images depends on the proportion of lipid and water content within the tissue. Compared with non-lipid-containing tissue, fat-containing tissue will thus present low signal intensity on opposed-phase images. Tsushima et al. (1992, 1993) propose FLASH (fast low-angle shot) images obtained breath-held with a TR of 100 ms and a TE of 11 ms for the opposed-phase images and a TE of 13 ms for the in-phase images with a flip angle of 20°. Mitchell et al. (1992) used a gradient recalled echo sequence (GRE) with a 90° flip angle, TR = 59–142 ms, and TE = 2.3–2.5 ms for the opposed-phase images.

21.2.2.3 Dynamic Multiplanar Fast Gradient-Echo MRI

Dynamic multiplanar fast gradient-echo MRI with bolus injection during suspended respiration allows for high image quality as well as visualization of functional processes after administration of contrast material. It is reliable for demonstration and characterization of adrenal masses, providing a statistically significant differentiation of adenomas, metastases, and pheochromocytomas, although some overlap is still seen between these pathologies. Dynamic MRI can be achieved by using a GRE sequence with a TR of 30 ms, a TE of 15 ms, and a flip angle of 70°. Orientation in the coronal section allows simultaneous imaging of the adrenal glands, liver, and kidneys. Repeated imaging up to 15 min after intravenous administration of 0.1 mmol/kg body weight of a gadolinium compound should be performed.

21.3 Evaluation of Renal Excretory Function

The paramagnetic chelate Gd-DTPA is completely filtered in the glomerulus. The distinct concentration-dependent change of the tissue relaxation times brought about by Gd-DTPA allows an insight into the excretory kinetics (Choyke et al. 1989).

21.3.1 Patterns of Contrast Enhancement in Normally Functioning Kidneys

An increase in the signal intensity in the renal cortex can be observed just 10–20 s after injection of the contrast agent. A maximum value is reached about 20–50 s after the first signs of perfusion, followed by a slow, constant fall in the signal intensity. This finding is due to the pronounced arterial perfusion of the renal cortex that leads to an early appearance of Gd-DTPA in this region. The T1 shortening effects of gadolinium produce a visible increase in the signal intensity; the onset of glomerular filtration and the dilution in the extravascular space manifest themselves as a subsequent slow decrease in signal intensity (Fig. 21.1).

Signal intensity changes are different in the medulla: an increase can be observed about 10–20 s later than in the cortex. The maximum signal intensity values are the same as in the cortex or even slightly higher. Between 30 and 40 s after the first visible signs of perfusion, the signal intensity

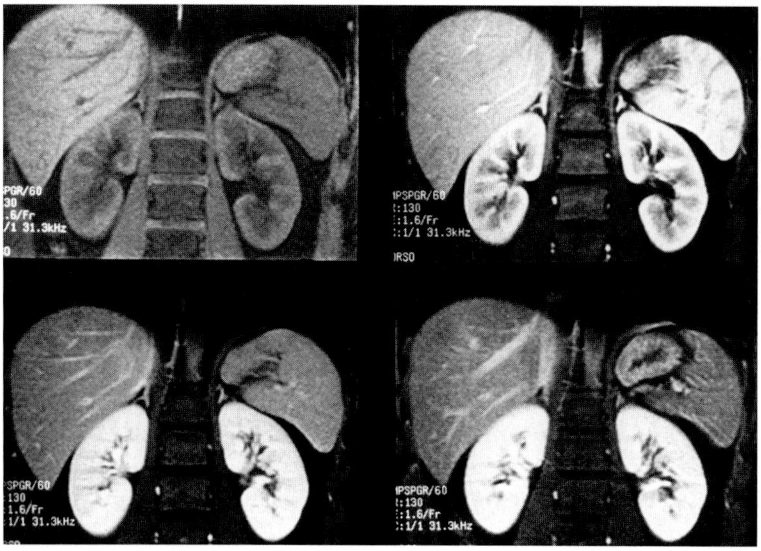

Fig. 21.1. Normal enhancement pattern of the kidneys and adrenal glands. Dynamic examination before (*top left*) and 30 (*top right*), 60 (*bottom left*) s and 120 (*bottom right*) s following injection of 0.1 mmol/kg Gd-DTPA. Note the good corticomedullary differentiation on the early postcontrast image and homogeneous parenchymal enhancement on later images, as well as the early enhancement of the adrenal tissue with rapid wash-out

decreases steeply to a minimum value which is comparable to the initial value of the precontrast image. Only when the contrast agent passes into the calyces and is diluted with noncontrasted glomerular filtrate does the signal intensity increase again to values approximately equal to those in the cortex. Excretion into the calyces usually may be demonstrated at this point: it is characterized by a decrease in signal intensity in the region of the renal pelvis, which is also followed by susceptibility artifacts (KRESTIN et al. 1990).

These changes in the signal intensity must be interpreted with reference to the effects of Gd-DTPA on the relaxation times of tissues. Since medulla accounts for only about 1%–6.5% of the entire blood supply to the kidneys, it is understandable that Gd-DTPA perfusion of the medullary structures is delayed in comparison with that of the cortex. The onset of glomerular filtration of the contrast agent and the reabsorption of water in the proximal convoluted tubule, in the loop of Henle, and particularly in the collecting duct result in a marked concentration of Gd-DTPA (50- to 100-fold concentration). Depending on the sequence used, however, contrast reversal occurs because of the now predominant T2 shortening effects of gadolinium. Therefore a reduction in signal intensity in the medullary pyramids is an effect of the high concentration of the paramagnetic contrast agent (KRESTIN et al. 1990).

The described alterations of signal intensity in renal cortex, medulla, and calyces are characteristic of undisturbed renal function and can be evaluated using signal versus time plots. On the other hand, excellent delineation of the corticomedullary junction is possible in the early perfusion phase (10–20 s after injection) and in the early excretory phase (50–90 s after injection), allowing accurate detection of the internal structural derangements of the kidney (Fig. 21.2).

21.3.2 Renal Functional Disorders

Due to the almost complete (>98%) elimination of Gd-DTPA by glomerular ultrafiltration, a correlation between enhancement patterns in the renal parenchyma and glomerular filtration rate can be expected. Dynamic examinations can be quantitatively evaluated by plotting the signal intensity values in the renal cortex and medulla as a function of time. In this way time intervals between the first signs of cortical perfusion and maximal or minimal signal intensity in the medullary pyramids can be calculated.

In the majority of cases with acute obstruction of the urinary tract, no signal intensity alterations are demonstrable with MRI. The signal intensity plots display the same pattern as in patients without functional impairment. The preserved signal intensity decrease in renal medulla proves the preserved ability of the kidney to concentrate the contrast agent. Delayed excretion can be observed in the case of already affected renal function. In these patients a normal perfusion of the renal cortex

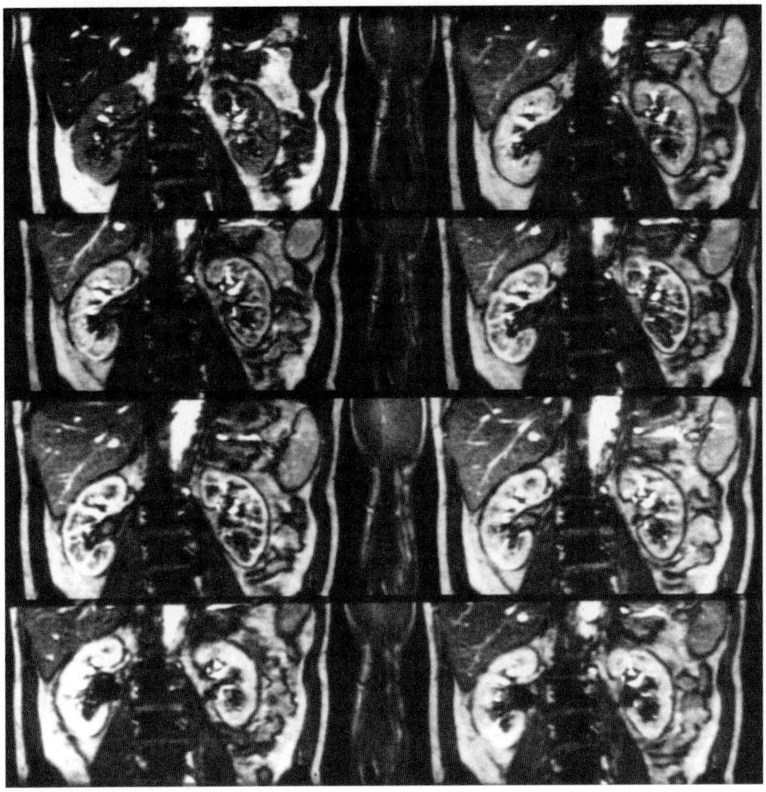

Fig. 21.2. Functional examination of the kidneys in a healthy subject with normal concentration of the contrast agent and consecutive signal decrease in the medulla commencing 30 s after injection. Repeated breath-held unspoiled gradient-echo images in the coronal plane before and 20, 30, 40, 50, 60, 70, and 120 s (*from left to right and top to bottom*) after administration of 0.1 mmol/kg Gd-DTPA

is followed by a delayed increase in the signal intensity in the medulla. Maximal signal intensity is reached here only after 40–70 s; the drop in signal intensity is less pronounced and the minimal value is seen after 60–100 s (Choyke et al. 1989).

In chronically obstructed, nonfunctioning kidneys, signal intensity alterations are more evident. A normal enhancement in the renal cortex is followed by a delayed increase in signal intensity in the medulla that reaches a plateau without demonstrable concentration of the contrast agent in the collecting ducts. Thus there is no reduction in signal intensity in the medulla and no time intervals can be measured on the signal intensity plots (Kikinis et al. 1987) (Fig. 21.3).

In patients with bilateral functional damage the bilaterally delayed concentration of Gd-DTPA in the collecting ducts or complete loss of the ability to concentrate the contrast agent in the renal medulla correlates well with the creatinine clearance ($r = 0.78$). However, the temporal resolution of 10 s/single slice allows only a rough splitting of the results. Using dynamic MRI, patients with a creatinine clearance between 50 and 80 ml/min display a 10- to 20-s delay in the reduction of signal intensity in the medulla compared with patients who have a normal excretory function. A delay of more than 20 s can be expected in patients with creatinine clearance values of about 30–50 ml/min, while time intervals are not measurable because of a complete loss of the Gd-DTPA concentration in patients with clearance values under 30 ml/min (Krestin et al. 1992, 1993) (Fig. 21.4).

In summary, semiquantitative evaluation of renal excretory function is possible using dynamic MR studies. If patients with acute urinary obstruction do not display any delay in the decrease in signal intensity in the medulla, as a sign of an adequate T2 shortening due to high Gd-DTPA concentration in the collecting ducts, a normal excretory function of the kidney can be assumed. Damage to the tubular function, leading to reduced tubular secretion and water reabsorption, occurs when intraluminal pressure exceeds a certain level. Consequently, the contrast agent that has already been filtered is not concentrated in the tubules and ducts, the result of which is a delayed and flattened decrease in the signal intensity in the medulla. When excretory function is completely lost, only signs of perfusion without sufficient concentration are visible.

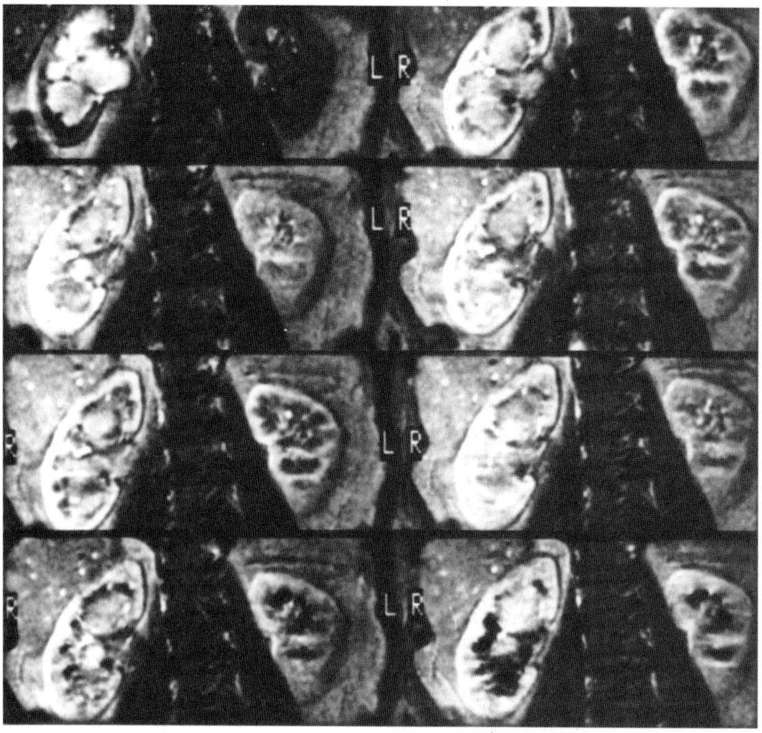

Fig. 21.3. Functional examination of the kidneys in a patient with chronic obstruction of the right kidney and thus delayed concentration of the contrast agent compared with the normally functioning right side. Repeated breath-held gradient-echo images in the coronal plane before and 20, 30, 40, 50, 60, 70, and 120 s (*from left to right and top to bottom*) after administration of 0.1 mmol/kg Gd-DTPA

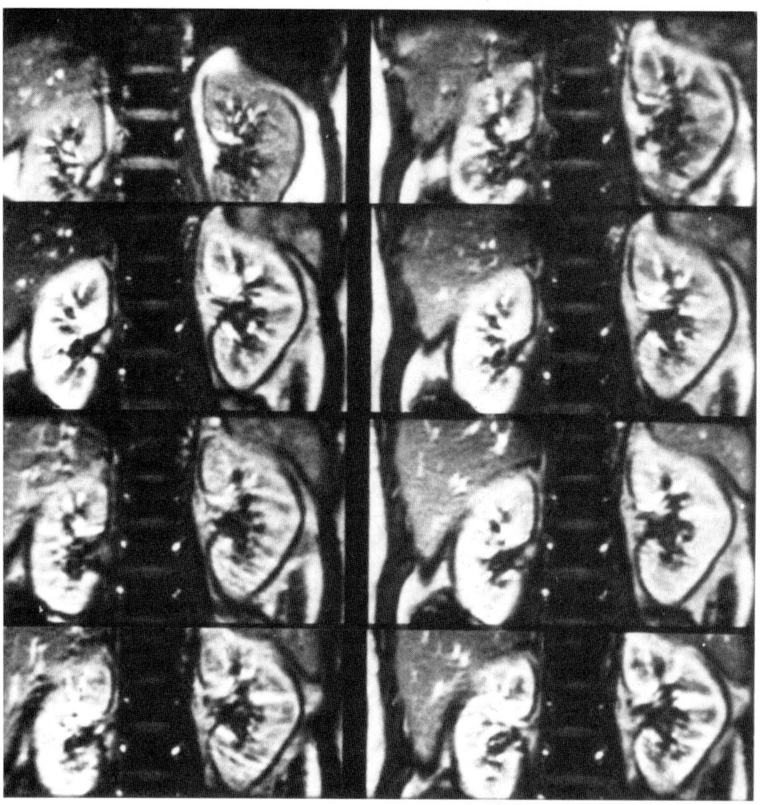

Fig. 21.4. Functional examination of the kidneys in a patient with nephrosclerosis and creatinine clearance of 40 ml/min with bilaterally delayed concentration ability in the medulla. Repeated breath-held gradient-echo images in the coronal plane before and 20, 30, 40, 50, 60, 70, and 120 s (*from left to right and top to bottom*) after administration of 0.1 mmol/kg Gd-DTPA

21.4 Renal Mass Lesions

21.4.1 Detection

On plain MR images, solid as well as cystic renal and pararenal masses often present the same signal intensities as the adjacent renal tissue. Therefore detection of such tumors is based only on the visible displacement or alteration of organ contours. Delineation from the surrounding renal parenchyma is successful with the aid of contrast-enhanced examinations. Hyperperfused masses are clearly distinguishable on early dynamic scans, while hypo- or unperfused lesions may be detected better on late postcontrast images. State-of-the-art MRI with optimal technical skills allows delineation of even very small lesions with a diameter of approximately 1 cm. Additional techniques, like fat suppression, provide a further improvement of lesion detection, allowing demonstration of small cysts or hypoperfused solid masses with diameters of less than 1 cm. However, only in a very restricted number of cases have the lesions visible on MRI not been detected previously using CT or US (EILENBERG et al. 1990; HRICAK et al. 1988; KRESTIN 1994).

21.4.2 Differentiation

Plain and especially contrast-enhanced MRI can help to differentiate renal and pararenal lesions. A nonenhancing mass with low signal intensities on T1-weighted images and a marked signal increase on T2-weighted scans represents a simple cyst in the majority of cases. But MRI is needed for this classification only if the patient has a contraindication for the use of iodinated contrast agents. Other cystic lesions may display similar signal intensities and, although MRI is highly sensitive in demonstrating hemorrhage, one cannot differentiate between hemorrhagic cysts and cystic tumors with hemorrhage. Even complicated cysts with a high content of protein can mimic solid avascular or hypovascular lesions (MAROTTI et al. 1987; KRESTIN 1994; SEMELKA et al. 1992) (Figs. 21.5, 21.6).

Among solid tumors of the kidney, MRI allows accurate detection only of fat-containing angiomyolipomas (Fig. 21.7). Other solid lesions like oncocytoma, adenoma, or renal cell carcinoma show very similar signal intensities and enhancement patterns (Fig. 21.8). However, dynamic MR after administration of Gd-DTPA, performed by repeated imaging in the same position at short time intervals,

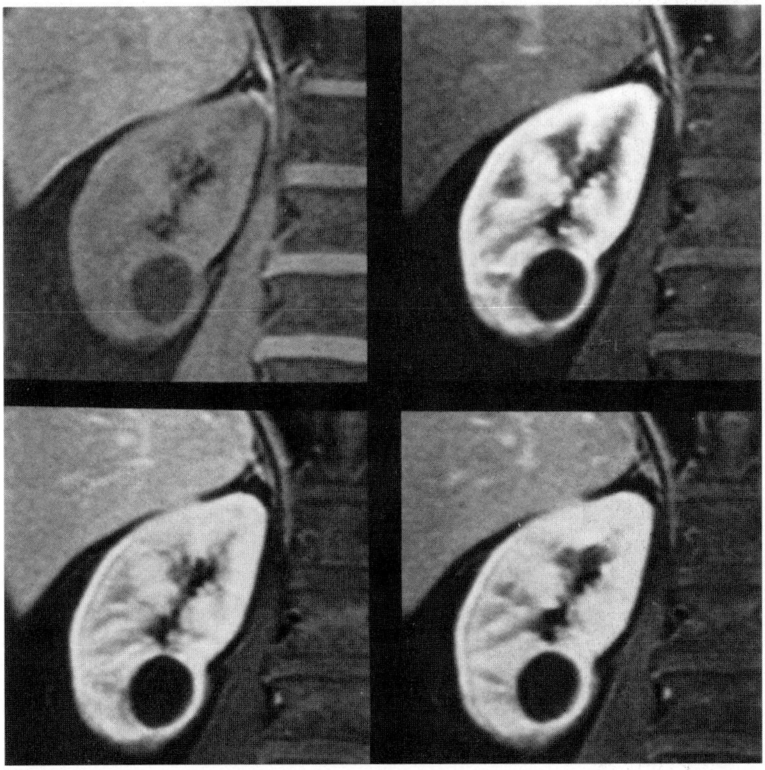

Fig. 21.5. Dynamic contrast-enhanced examination of the right kidney depicting a simple cortical cyst. Coronal images before (*top left*) and 30 (*top right*), 60 (*bottom left*), and 120 (*bottom right*) s following injection of 0.1 mmol/kg Gd-DOTA

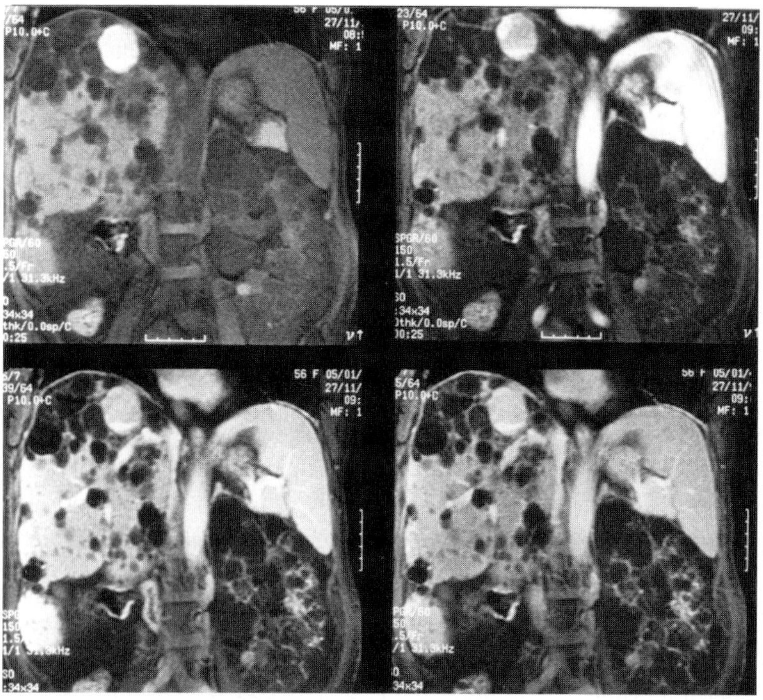

Fig. 21.6. Polycystic kidney disease with bilaterally enlarged kidneys demonstrating multiple cysts of different signal intensities without evidence of contrast uptake. Note also the presence of multiple liver cysts. Coronal dynamic contrast-enhanced examination with images before (*top left*) and 30 (*top right*), 60 (*bottom left*), and 120 (*bottom right*) s following injection of 0.1 mmol/kg Gd-DOTA

a

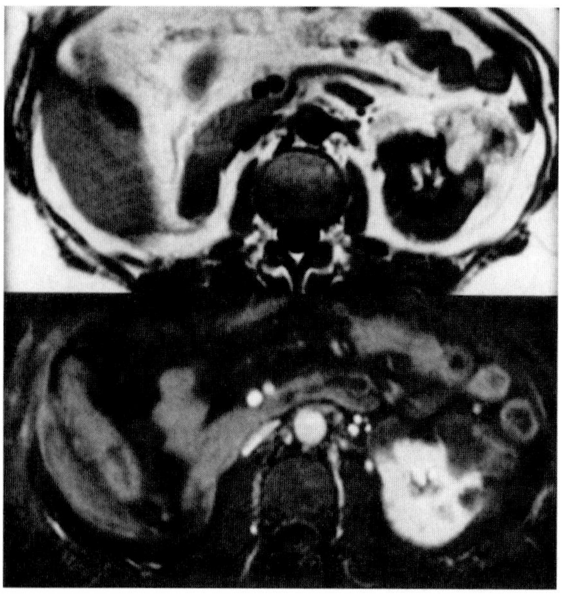

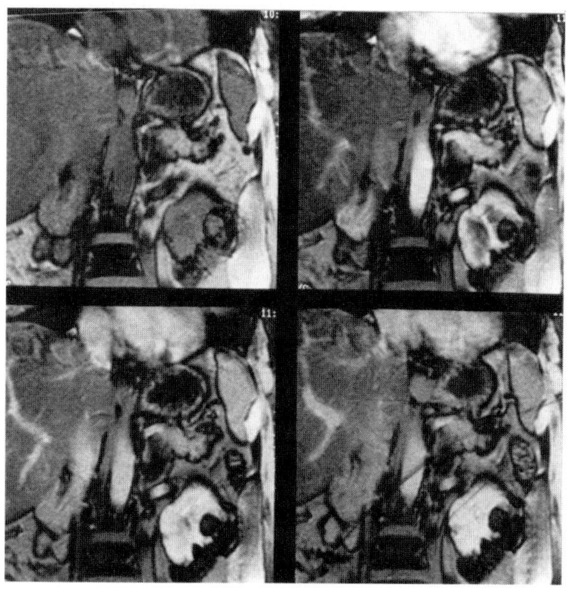

b

Fig. 21.7. a,b. Multiple angiomyolipomas of the left kidney. **a** T1-weighted (*top*) and fat-suppressed T2-weighted (*bottom*) axial images showing fat-containing regions in the left kidney with high signal intensity on the T1-weighted image and decreased signal intensity on the fat-suppressed image. **b** Coronal dynamic contrast-enhanced gradient-echo images, showing low signal intensities of the angiomyolipomas (chemical shift effect) without evidence of a pathological enhancement before (*top left*) and 30 (*top right*), 60 (*bottom left*), and 120 (bottom right) s following injection of 0.1 mmol/kg Gd-DTPA

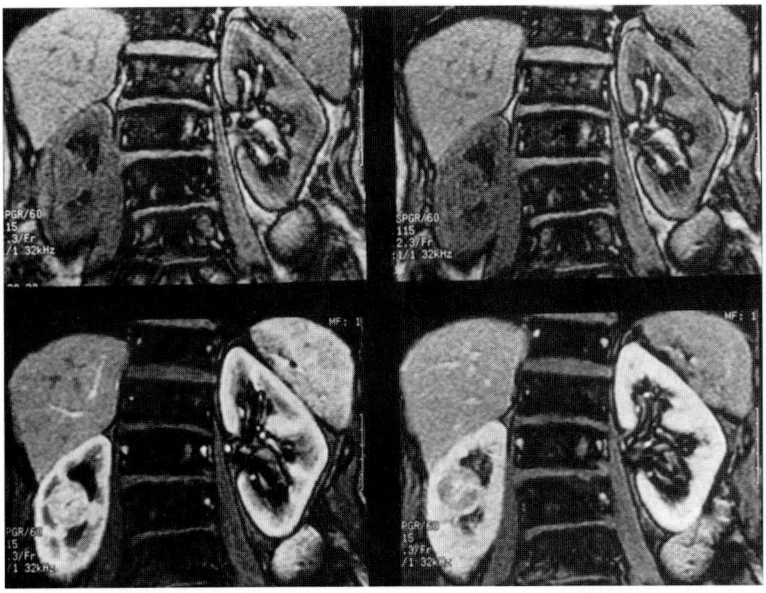

Fig. 21.8. Oncocytoma of the right kidney with strong early enhancement and small central scar. Coronal dynamic contrast-enhanced examination with images before (*top left*) and 30 (*top right*), 60 (*bottom left*), and 120 (*bottom right*) s following injection of 0.1 mmol/kg Gd-DOTA

allows optimal delineation of the normally functioning renal parenchyma and good visualization of the cortico-medullary junction. Using such sequences, renal and extrarenal masses can be differentiated accurately. Additional imaging planes may help to differentiate retroperitoneal masses which are only displacing and compressing the renal parenchyma (Rofsky et al. 1991).

21.4.3 Staging of Renal Cell Carcinoma

The most important tasks during preoperative staging of renal cell carcinoma are evaluation of the intra- and extrarenal extent of tumor and assessment of involvement of perirenal fat, of renal veins and the inferior vena cava (IVC), and of regional lymph nodes. Most of these problems can be solved using CT, but MRI seems to provide better results in the evaluation of perirenal and vascular involvement (Hricak et al. 1988; Krestin 1990).

Dynamic MR studies are useful for delineation of the intrarenal extent of primary renal malignancies as well. Although this does not help in terms of correct staging of the tumor, it may allow planning of a partial resection, if indicated (Figs. 21.9, 21.10). Differentiation between stages T2 and T3A is very important since tumors that are not confined to the kidney lead to a decrease in the 5-year survival rate of more than 50%. Invasion of perinephric fat may be well visualized with gradient-echo MRI using adequate echo times. When fat and water protons are out of phase a signal loss marks the presence of tumor cells in perirenal fat. However, similar alterations can be observed simply due to lymphatic or venous edema around the kidneys. In such cases detection of perirenal invasion can be improved using fat-suppressed contrast-enhanced images. Enhancement of previously dark areas in perirenal tissue is indicative of extrarenal tumor invasion.

Magnetic resonance imaging is the best noninvasive method for the assessment of tumor thrombi in the renal veins or the IVC. MRI provides the same information as venography. Gradient-echo images even allow delineation of thrombi in nondilated veins due to a lack of high signal intensity of flowing blood (Figs. 21.11, 21.12). Using gradient-echo images, retroperitoneal lymphadenopathy may be detected as accurately as with CT or US. However, as with those methods, the only criterion for diagnosis of malignant involvement remains the measurement of lymph node size (Hricak et al. 1988; Roubidoux et al. 1992; Semelka et al. 1992).

21.5 Adrenal Endocrinopathies

21.5.1 Cushing's Syndrome

In patients with Cushing's syndrome the role of imaging is to distinguish between adrenal hyperplasia a 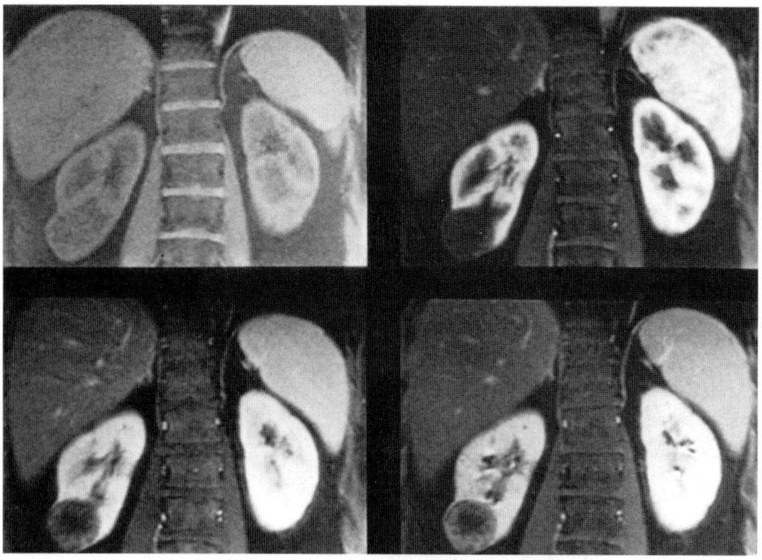

b 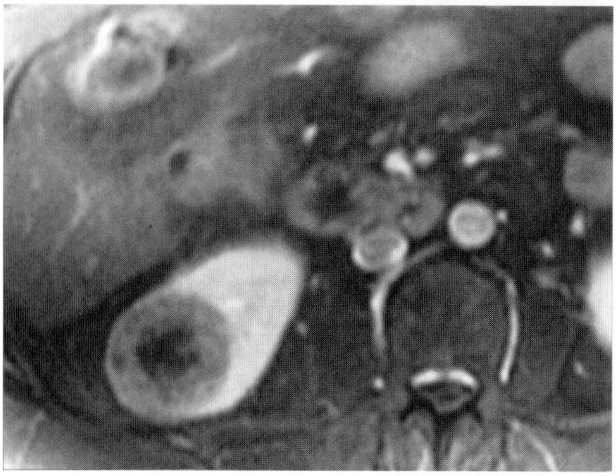

Fig. 21.9 a,b. Stage T2 renal cell carcinoma of the right kidney. **a** Dynamic contrast-enhanced examination demonstrating a rounded, well-defined mass with peripheral enhancement. Images obtained before (*top left*) and 30 (*top right*), 60 (*bottom left*), and 120 (*bottom right*) s following injection of 0.1 mmol/kg Gd-DOTA. **b** Axial delayed postcontrast T1-weighted fat-suppressed image. No evidence of perirenal enhancement

and an adrenal tumor. Most patients (85%) with Cushing's syndrome will have bilateral more or less visible adrenal hyperplasia, whereas only 10% have benign adrenal adenoma and 5% an adrenocortical carcinoma. Differentiation between hyperplasia and adenoma is usually easy since hyperplastic adrenals usually look normal or only slightly enlarged with a preserved triangular shape on CT or MRI, while Cushing adenomas are quite large, with a diameter of 2–5 cm (Fig. 21.13). Due to the higher spatial resolution and the possibility of visualizing even glands which are not enlarged, CT is the imaging method of choice in Cushing's syndrome. The only problem remains the distinction between nodular hyperplasia with a single dominant nodule and a true adenoma. However, plasma ACTH levels are generally high in patients with nodular hyperplasia whereas they are suppressed or low in patients with adenomas.

One-third of cortisol-producing adrenal tumors are malignant and most hyperfunctioning adrenal carcinomas manifest themselves as Cushing's syndrome. Only in such cases may imaging diagnosis stop after performing percutaneous US, since in a patient with Cushing's syndrome an adrenal mass larger than 6 cm in diameter is practically always malignant. MRI may show the exact location, extent, and relationships of the mass with a characteristic strong contrast enhancement and slow wash-out, but should be used only as a secondary diagnostic method following US or CT (van Erkel et al. 1994).

21.5.2 Conn's Syndrome

Primary hyperaldosteronism is due to unilateral adrenal adenoma in most patients, and only 20%–

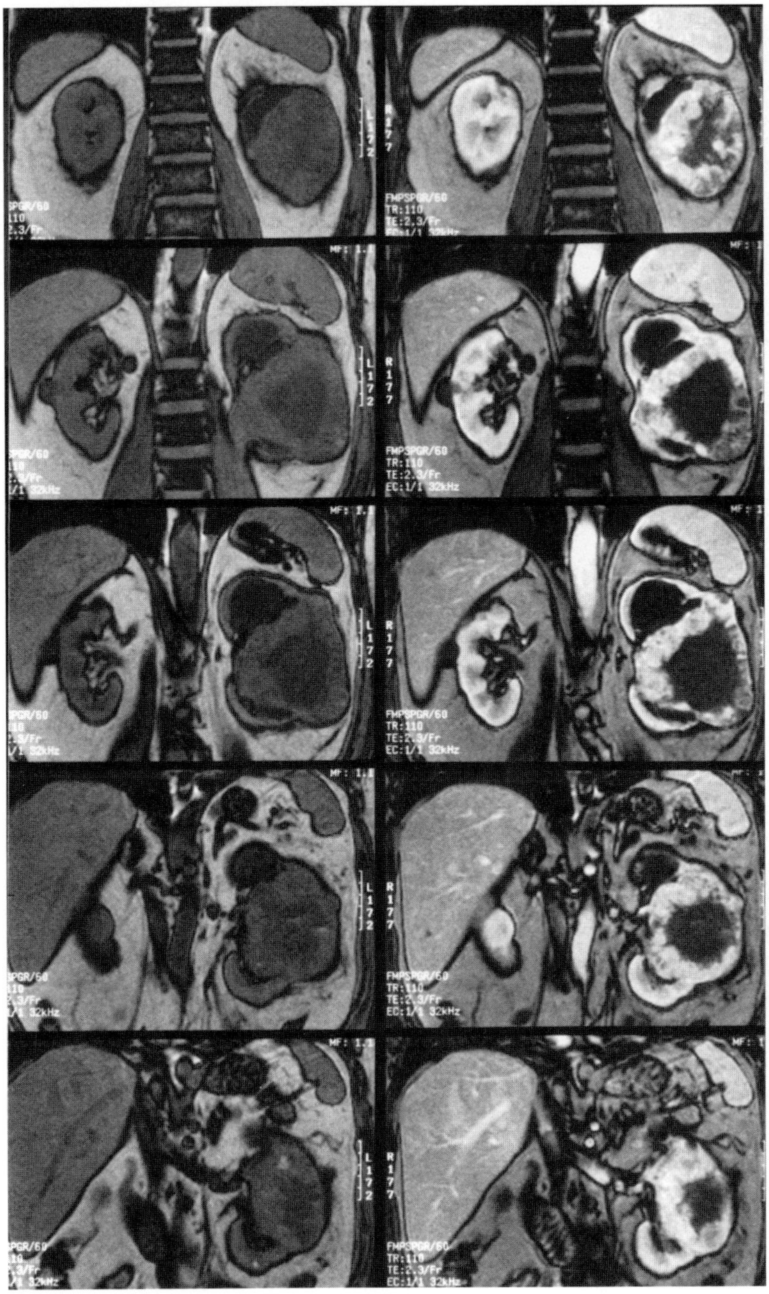

Fig. 21.10. Large, centrally necrotic stage T2 renal cell carcinoma of the left kidney. Dynamic contrast-enhanced ultrafast multiple slice images before (*left*) and 60 s (*right*) following injection of 0.1 mmol/kg Gd-DTPA

30% will present with bilateral hyperplasia or, in rare cases, with a carcinoma. Distinction between adenoma and cortical hyperplasia is, however, very important because the treatment for adenoma is adrenalectomy, whereas medical therapy is indicated in hyperplasia. Adenomas in Conn's syndrome are typically small and therefore best visualized using CT. The accuracy of CT in detecting adenomas depends on their size. A sensitivity of 100% has been reported in the literature in respect of adenomas larger than 15 mm, but this falls to only 50% for adenomas with a diameter between 10 and 15 mm and to less than 30% for lesions with a diameter of less than 10 mm. An adequate imaging technique with thin sections is therefore mandatory. Distinction between nodular hyperplasia and adenoma is equally difficult. Single nodules are more likely to be adenomas, whereas detection of multiple nodules requires further investigation with scintigraphy.

The detection of unilateral uptake of radiolabeled nor-cholesterol without or preferentially under dexamethasone suppression proves the presence of an

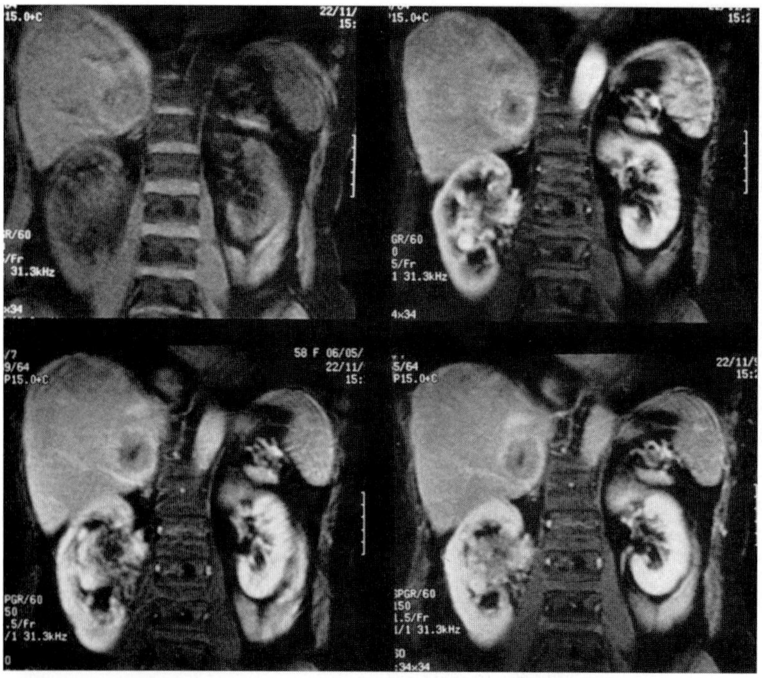

a

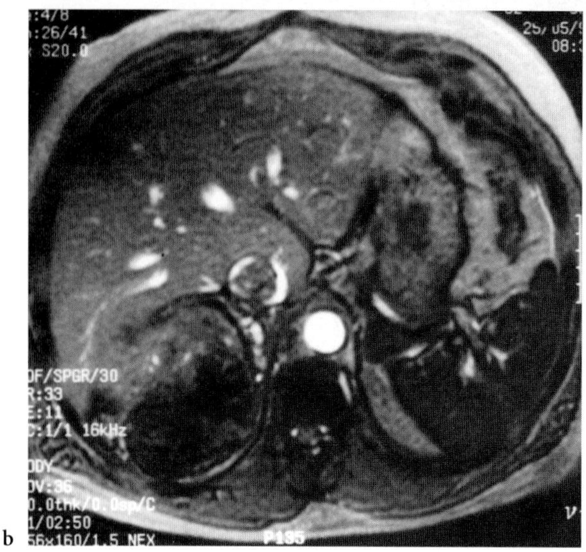

b

Fig. 21.11 a,b. Stage T3B renal cell carcinoma of the right kidney. **a** Centrally located tumor invading the renal vessels. Coronal dynamic contrast-enhanced examination with images before (*top left*) and 30 (*top right*), 60 (*bottom left*), and 120 (*bottom right*) s following injection of 0.1 mmol/kg Gd-DOTA. **b** Axial gradient-echo sequence (TOF) showing tumor thrombus in the inferior vena cava surrounded by high signal intensity flowing blood

adenoma. Only in still equivocal cases should one consider selective venous sampling for final evaluation. This method has lost its importance due to the relatively high number of technical failures of selective sampling of the right adrenal vein, which drains directly into the IVC (VAN ERKEL et al. 1994).

21.5.3 Pheochromocytoma

Pheochromocytoma and neuroblastoma are the most common hyperfunctioning tumors of the adrenal medulla. Neuroblastoma is mainly seen in the pediatric population and will thus not be addressed in this overview. Pheochromocytomas may arise anywhere in the autonomic nervous system, but 90% originate in the adrenal medulla. About 10% are inherited and they can be associated with systemic disease complexes such as neurofibromatosis, von Hippel-Lindau syndrome, or multiple endocrine neoplastic syndrome. Most adrenal pheochromocytomas are hormonally active, secreting parathyroid hormone, calcitonin, gastrin, serotonin, ACTH, and/or catecholamines.

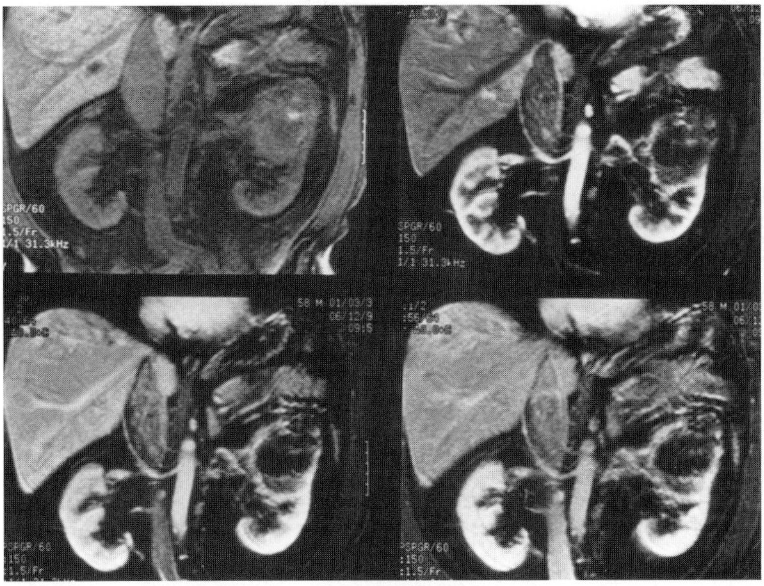

Fig. 21.12. Stage T3B renal cell carcinoma of the left kidney, with large tumor thrombus visible in the left renal vein and the infrahepatic as well as intrahepatic portions of the inferior vena cava. Coronal dynamic contrast-enhanced examination with images before (*top left*) and 30 (*top right*), 60 (*bottom left*), and 120 (*bottom right*) s following injection of 0.1 mmol/kg Gd-DOTA

a

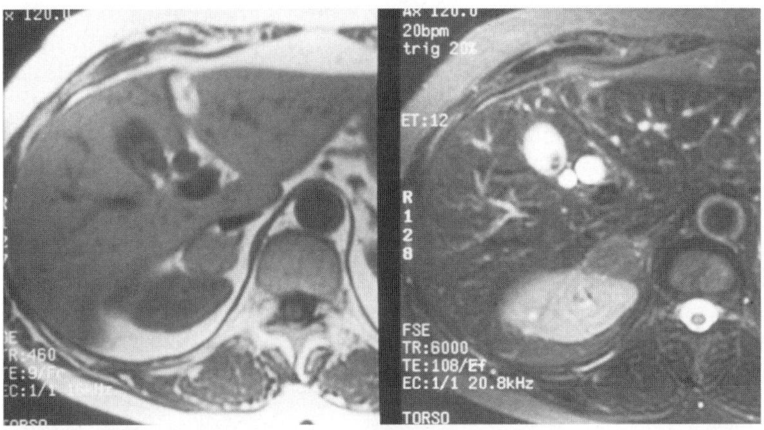

b

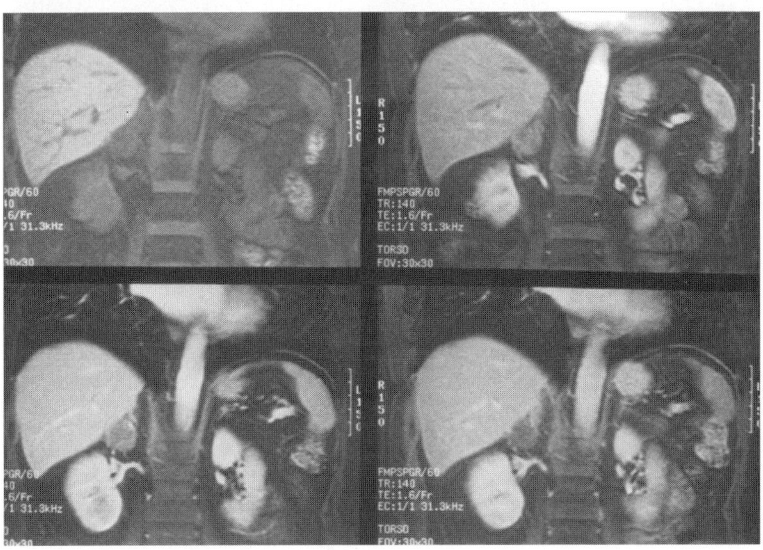

Fig. 21.13. a,b. Cushing adenoma of the right adrenal gland. **a** T1-weighted (*left*) and fat-suppressed T2-weighted (*right*) images of the enlarged right adrenal gland, showing low signal intensities on both images. **b** Coronal dynamic contrast-enhanced images, before (*top left*) and 30 (*top right*), 60 (*bottom left*), and 300 (*bottom right*) s following injection of 0.1 mmol/kg Gd-DTPA, demonstrating enhancement of the adrenal mass with rapid wash-out

Adrenal medullary hyperfunction due to pheochromocytoma can be evaluated using either CT or MRI scanning or with metaiodobenzylguanidine (MIBG) scintigraphy. On T1-weighted precontrast MR images, pheochromocytomas present with a signal intensity similar to or lower than that of the liver, but they are markedly hyperintense on T2-weighted images. Following administration of contrast material, an avid, rapid enhancement and a slow washout similar to those seen in primary or secondary malignancies are observed. On chemical shift imaging, pheochromocytomas can usually be distinguished from adenomas by virtue of their lack of signal reduction. However, they may occasionally contain normal lipid-rich adrenocortical cells or even undergo lipid degeneration and can then mimic adrenal adenomas on opposed-phase images. Pheochromocytomas cannot be differentiated from metastases or primary adrenal malignancies with any of the currently used MRI techniques; rather, diagnosis is usually made on clinical grounds.

Due to the very high signal intensity on T2-weighted images and to the marked enhancement following administration of a paramagnetic contrast agent, MRI has a high sensitivity for the detection of extra-adrenal pheochromocytoma. However, while sensitivity for detection of an adrenal pheochromocytoma is nearly 100% by CT or MRI and above 90% by iodine-MIBG scintigraphy, for the detection of an extra-adrenal lesion scintigraphy has the better overall accuracy(van Gils et al. 1991) (Fig. 21.14).

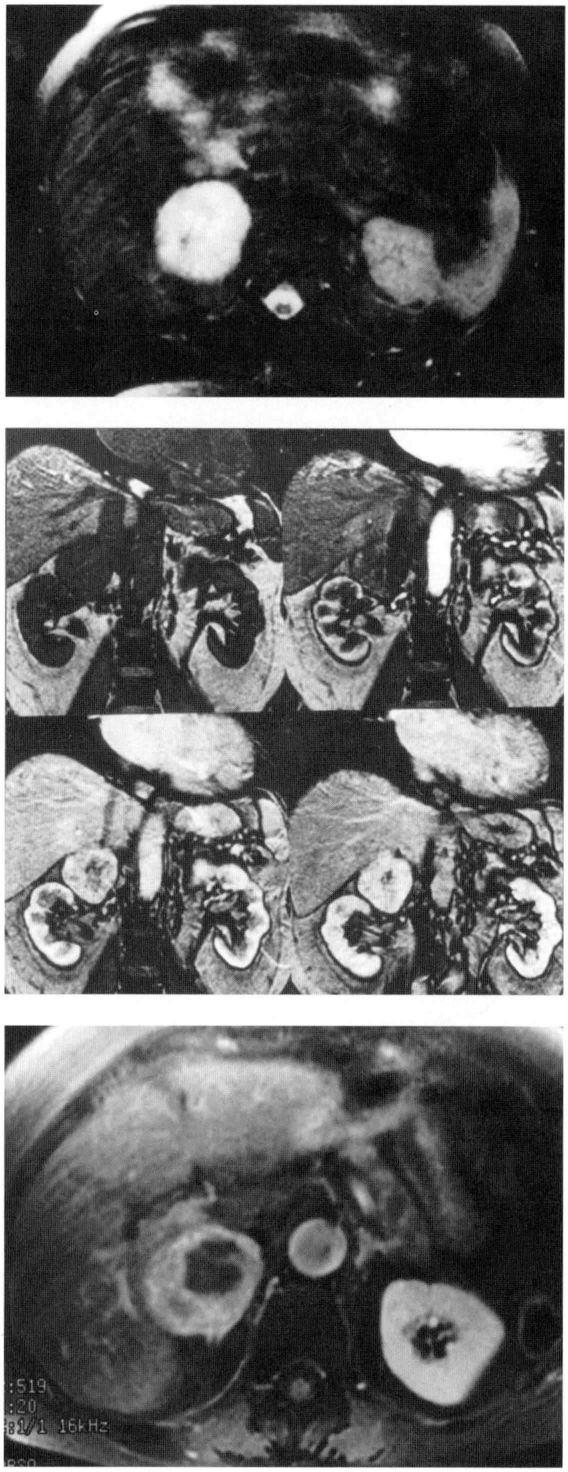

a b c

Fig. 21.14 a–c. Pheochromocytoma of the right adrenal gland. **a** Axial T2-weighted fat-suppressed image in which the adrenal mass presents with homogeneously high signal intensity. **b** Dynamic contrast-enhanced images before (*top left*) and 30 (*top right*), 60 (*bottom left*), and 300 (*bottom right*) s after injection of 0.1 mmol/kg Gd-DTPA, showing strong enhancement of the mass without signs of wash-out. **c** Axial postcontrast T1-weighted fat-suppressed image demonstrating delayed enhancement with central necrotic areas

21.6 Nonhyperfunctioning Adrenal Masses

Differentiation of nonhyperfunctioning adrenal lesions is mainly based on MRI. Some recent articles have, however, reemphasized the role of precontrast or delayed postcontrast CT for differentiating benign and malignant adrenal masses. Overall accuracy of MRI is higher and therefore the method should be described here in more detail (Glazer et al. 1986).

21.6.1 Image Analysis

For characterization of adrenal lesions, various authors have recommended the measurement of signal intensities (SI) in the adrenal lesions themselves as well as in reference tissues such as paraspinal muscle, the liver, or even the spleen. To derive accurate results, it is important that the region of interest for the SI measurement and subsequent calculations be chosen as large as possible while avoiding tissue interfaces, areas of shading, and motion artifacts.

Based on SI measurements of multiecho T2-weighted conventional SE sequences, the T2 relaxation time of a specific tissue can be calculated by the formula:

$$T2 = (TE_2 - TE_1)/(\ln SI_1/SI_2),$$

where SI refers to signal intensity of a given echo (GLAZER et al. 1986).

The lipid contents within a particular adrenal lesion can be quantitated using an SI index based on SI measurements of the lesion in in-phase and opposed-phase GRE images:

$$\text{SI index} = [(\text{SI on IP} - \text{SI on OP})7(\text{SI on IP})] \times 100\%,$$

where IP stands for in-phase and OP for out-of-phase. Some investigators have proposed expressing the SI index relative to other reference tissues such as liver or muscle (MITCHELL et al. 1992; TSUSHIMA et al. 1992).

Finally, the degree of contrast enhancement can be quantitated based on dynamic, contrast-enhanced multiplanar GRE images. Here, too, the use of reference tissues has been suggested (KRESTIN et al. 1989, 1991; SQUILLACI et al. 1993).

21.6.2 Nonhyperfunctioning Adenomas

Adrenal adenomas are often nonhyperfunctioning. Whereas specific clinical symptoms will alert the physician to the possible presence of a hyperfunctioning adenoma, benign nonhyperfunctioning adenomas are usually incidental findings identified in approximately 1% of the adult population.

Most adenomas appear slightly hypointense or isointense to the liver on T1-weighted images and slightly hyper- or isointense on T2-weighted images. Comparing relative lesion-to-fat signal intensities, adenomas show low-to-medium relative signal intensities on MR images regardless of the TR, TE, and flip angle used. It has thus been proposed that lesions with a ratio of less than 1.5 should be classified as benign, while those with a ratio between 1.5 and 2.0 should be considered equivocal (REINIG et al. 1985; KRESTIN et al. 1989) (Fig. 21.15).

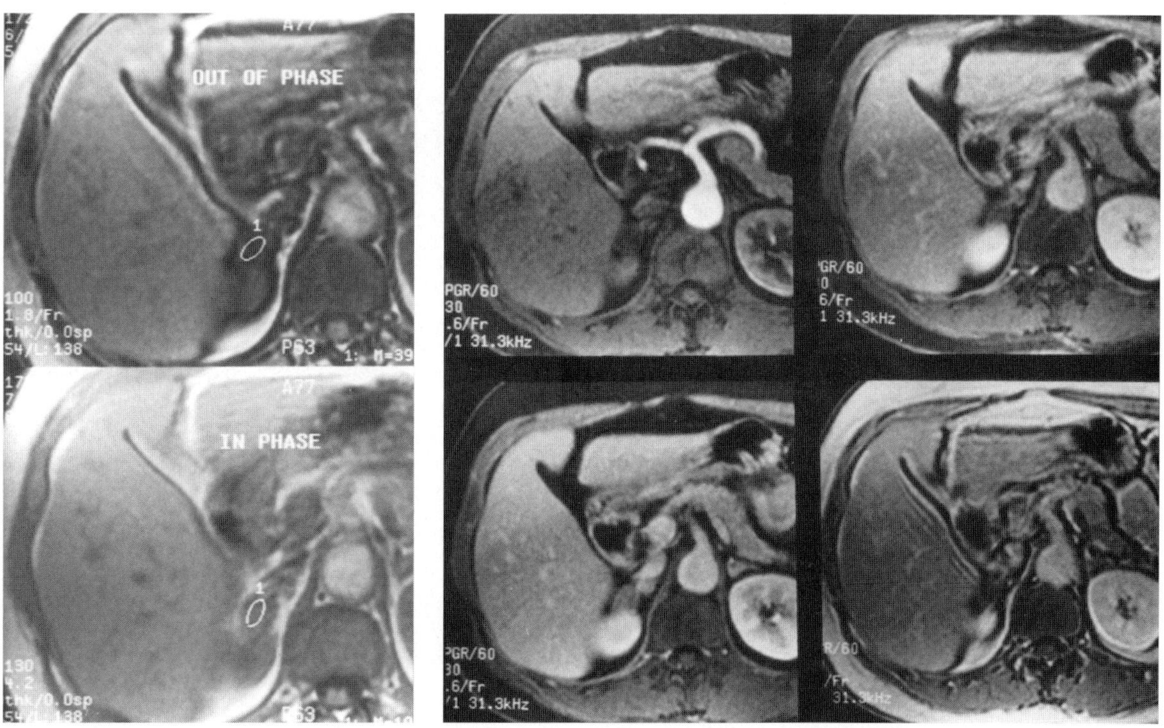

a b

Fig. 21.15 a,b. Nonfunctioning adrenal adenoma. **a** Axial chemical shift images of the adrenal mass with low signal intensity on the opposed-phase (*top*) and high signal intensity on the in-phase (*bottom*) image, demonstrating the presence of lipid within the lesion. **b** Contrast-enhanced examination, with images before (*top left*) and 30 (*top right*), 60 (*bottom left*), and 300 (*bottom right*) s following injection of 0.1 mmol/kg Gd-DTPA, showing early wash-out of the contrast

On chemical shift opposed-phase images, fat-containing adenomas present with low signal intensities compared with the adjacent liver. However, malignant lesions may also demonstrate a loss of signal intensity in certain cases (Mitchell et al. 1992).

On dynamic contrast-enhanced GRE sequences adenomas usually show only mild contrast enhancement and quick wash-out, allowing distinction from malignant lesions or pheochromocytomas. A maximal signal increase after contrast administration of less than 100% and rapid wash-out (<30% at 10 min) have been established as criteria for benign masses on dynamic contrast-enhanced GRE sequences. However, atypical adrenal adenomas have been described as being considerably hyperintense compared with hepatic parenchyma on T2-weighted images and as showing avid, prolonged contrast enhancement on contrast-enhanced T1-weighted images.

21.6.3 Myelolipomas

Myelolipomas are rare, benign neoplasms of the adrenal glands that are composed of variable amounts of fat and muscle tissue. They are usually asymptomatic and thus are found incidentally in most cases. Diagnosis of a myelolipoma is based on the identification of fat within the lesion. This can be easily accomplished with either CT or MRI. Due to its multiplanar imaging capabilites, MRI may, however, be superior to CT in distinguishing large adrenal myelolipomas from a retroperitoneal liposarcoma or a large renal angiomyolipoma. Fat-suppressed MR images may be performed to prove the fatty content, if necessary (Casey et al. 1994; Musante et al. 1991).

21.6.4 Metastases

Certain morphological criteria are suggestive for a malignant adrenal lesion on CT or MRI, including diameter over 5 cm, irregular contours, invasion of neighboring structures, and change in size on follow-up. Additionally, specific MR features may be indicative for malignancy: adrenal metastases appear hypo- or isointense to liver on T1-weighted images and show a strong signal increase on T2-weighted

a

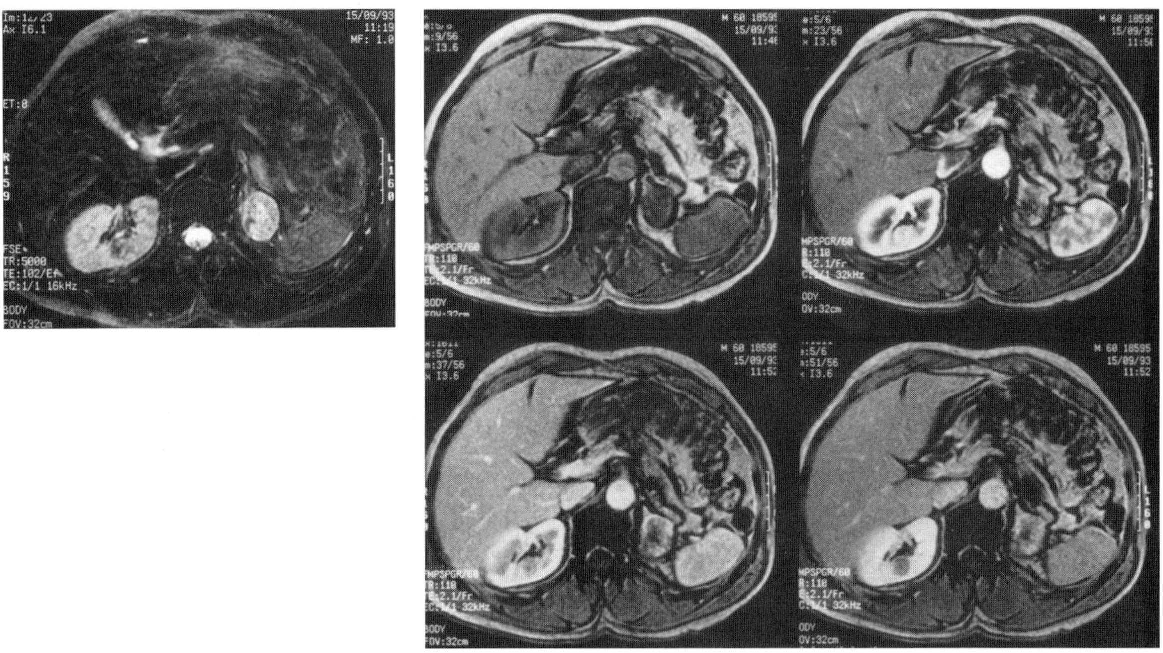

b

Fig. 21.16 a,b. Adrenal metastasis of a renal cell carcinoma of the left kidney. **a** Axial fat-suppressed T2-weighted image demonstrating high signal intensity of a left adrenal mass. **b** Dynamic contrast-enhanced examination, with images before (*top left*) and 30 (*top right*), 60 (*bottom left*), and 300 (*bottom right*) s after injection of 0.1 mmol/kg Gd-DTPA, demonstrating early enhancement and slow wash-out of the lesion. Note an additional renal metastasis in the right kidney with early enhancement and rapid signal decrease images (Fig. 21.16). Comparing relative lesion-to-fat signal intensities, malignant lesions usually present ratios of more than 2.0. Using these criteria, accuracies between 91% and 95% for distinction between adenoma and adrenal metastases were found (REINIG et al. 1994).

On chemical shift opposed-phase images, metastases can be disinguished from fat-containing adenomas by virtue of their higher signal intensites. TSUSHIMA et al. (1993) calculated signal intensity indexes between in-phase and opposed-phase images. In this study, using a cut-off value of 5%, a 100% accuracy was found in the distinction of adenomas from nonadenomatous lesions. Metastases of renal cell carcinoma, hepatocellular carcinoma, and liposarcoma, however, may contain cytoplasmic lipid and thus also present with a loss of signal intensity on opposed-phase images.

Following administration of contrast material, metastases typically show a rapid contrast enhancement with a maximum signal increase >150% and a persistent high signal intensity (>75%) after 10 min (KRESTIN et al. 1991).

21.6.5 Adrenal Carcinoma

While most adrenal carcinomas are nonhyperfunctioning, between 15% and 50% are hyperfunctioning, with the majority of them causing Cushing's syndrome. Adrenal carcinomas are usually larger than 6 cm in diameter and can invade adjacent organs and the inferior vena cava. Calcifications may be present. Relaxation times of carcinomas are not significantly different from those found in metastatic disease and distinction between these two entities thus cannot be made by MRI. However, primary adrenocortical carcinomas are usually unilateral. Due to its multiplanar imaging capabilites. MRI has been reported to be superior to CT in staging of disease, allowing better identification of invasion

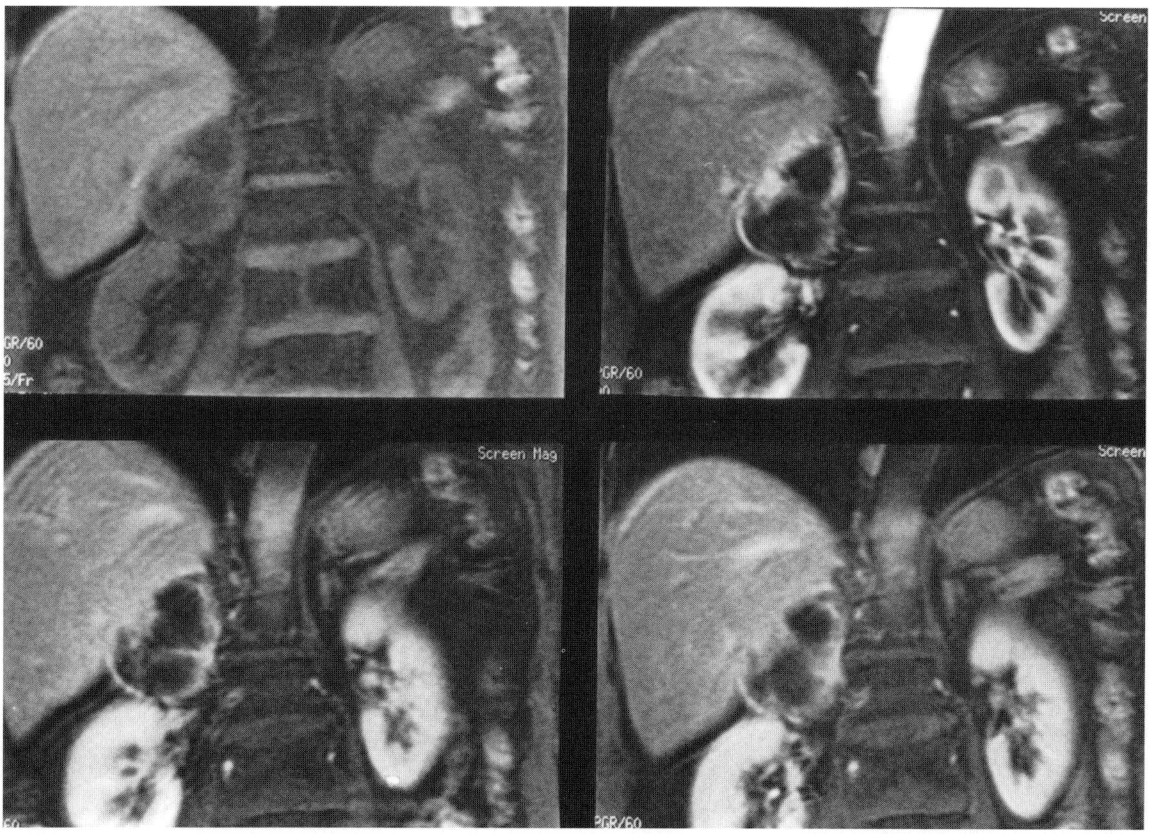

Fig. 21.17. Carcinoma of the right adrenal gland. A dynamic contrast-enhanced examination, with images before (*top left*) and 30 (*top right*), 60 (*bottom left*), and 300 (*bottom right*) s following injection of 0.1 mmol/kg Gd-DTPA, shows a large centrally necrotic inhomogeneous early enhancing malignant mass

into adjacent structures (Fig. 21.17).

21.7 Conclusions

1. Signal intensity alterations of the renal parenchyma after administration of Gd-DTPA are very characteristic and typical for a normal renal excretory function.
2. Dynamic functional studies allow semiquantitative evaluation of the glomerular filtration rate of the kidneys. For the first time, an imaging procedure is therefore available which provides good spatial resolution (and, consequently, good morphological demonstration) and also information about renal function.
3. Dynamic MRI is a highly accurate method for the differentiation of intrarenal and extrarenal masses due to the clear visualization of the corticomedullary junction. Renal cell carcinomas therefore can be better delineated and preoperative staging is improved.
4. In adrenal endocrinopathies MRI plays only a secondary role. It may be used for detection of extra-adrenal pheochromocytomas, but is not helpful in evaluating patients with Cushing's or Conn's syndrome.
5. MRI is the most accurate noninvasive method for differentiation of incidentally detected adrenal masses. Of the many proposed methods, the chemical shift imaging technique provides the best results for differentiation of adrenal adenomas from malignant masses and pheochromocytomas.

References

Casey LR, Cohen AJ, Wilw AG, Dietrich RB (1994) Giant adrenal myelolipomas: CT and MRI findings. Abdom Imaging 19:165–167

Choyke PL, Frank JA, Girton ME, et al. (1989) Dynamic gadolinium-DTPA enhanced MRI of the kidneys: a physiologic correlation. Radiology 170:713–718

Eilenberg S, Lee J, Brown J, Mirowitz S, Rartar V (1990) Renal massses: evaluation with gradient-echo Gd-DTPA-enhanced dynamic MR imaging. Radiology 166:634–649

Glazer GM, Woolsey EJ, Borello J (1986) Adrenal tissue characterization using MR imaging. Radiology 158:73–79

Hricak H, Thoeni RF, Carroll PR, Demas BE, Marotti M, Tanagho EA (1988) Detection and staging of renal neoplasms: a reassessment of MR imaging. Radiology 166:643–649

Kikinis R, von Schulthess GK, Jäger P, et al. (1987) Normal and hydronephrotic kidney: evaluation of renal function with contrast-enhanced MR imaging. Radiology 165:837–842

Krestin GP (1990) Morphologic and functional MRI of the kidneys and adrenal glands. Field and Wood, Philadelphia

Krestin GP (1994) Magnetic resonance imaging of the kidneys: current status. Magn Reson Q 19:2–21

Krestin GP, Steinbrich W, Friedmann G (1989) Adrenal masses: evaluation with fast gradient-echo MR imaging and Gd-DTPA-enhanced dynamic studies. Radiology 171:675–680

Krestin GP, Friedman G, Fischbach R, Neufang KFR, Allolio B (1991) Evaluation of adrenal masses in oncologic patients: dynamic contrast-enhanced MR vs CT. J Comput Assist Tomogr 15:104–110

Krestin GP, Schuhmann-Giamperi G, Haustein J, et al. (1992) Functional dynamic MRI imaging, pharmacokinetics and safety of gadolinium-DTPA in patients with impaired renal function. Eur Radiol 2:16–23

Krestin GP, Fischbach R, Vorreuther R, von Schulthess GK (1993) Alterations in renal morphology and function after ESWL therapy: evaluation with dynamic contrast-enhanced MRI. Eur Radiol 3:227–233

Marotti M, Hricak H, Fritsche P, Crooks LE, Hedgock MW, Tanagho EA (1987) Complex and simple renal cysts: comparative evaluation with MR imaging. Radiology 162:679–683

Mitchell DG, Crovello M, Matteucci T, Petersen RO, Miettinen MM (1992) Benign adrenocortical masses: diagnosis with chemical shift MR imaging. Radiology 185:345–351

Musante F, Derchi LE, Bazzocchi M, Avataneo T, Gandini G, Pozzi Mucelli RS (1991) MR imaging of adrenal myelolipomas. J Comput Assist Tomogr 15:111–114

Reinig JW, Doppman JL, Dwyer AJ, Johnson AR, Knop RH (1985) Distinction between adrenal adenomas and adrenal metastases using MR imaging. J Comput Assist Tomogr 9:898–901

Reinig JW, Stutley JE, Leonhardt CM, Spicer KM, Margolis M, Caldwell CB (1994) Differentiation of adrenal masses with MR imaging: comparison of techniques. Radiology 192:41–46

Rofsky NM, Weinreb JC, Bosniak MA, Libes RB, Birnbaum BA (1991) Renal lesion characterization with gadolinium-enhanced MR imaging. Efficacy and safety in patients with renal insufficiency. Radiology 180:85–89

Roubidoux MA, Dunnick NR, Sostman HD, Leder RA (1992) Renal carcinoma: detection of venous extension with gradient-echo MR imaging. Radiology 182:269–272

Semelka RC, Shoenut JP, Kroeker MA, MacMahon RG, Greenberg HM (1992) Renal lesions: controlled comparison between CT and 1.5 T MR imaging with nonenhanced and gadolinium-enhanced fat-suppressed spin-echo and breath-hold FLASH techniques. Radiology 182:425–430

Semelka RC, Hricak H, Stevens SK, Finegold R, Tomei E, Carroll PR (1993) Combined gadolinium-enhanced and fat-saturation MR imaging of renal masses. Radiology 178:803–809

Squillaci E, Vidiri A, Cresco M, et al. (1993) Characterization of adenomas and metastases in the adrenals: comparison between spin-echo sequences and Gd-DTPA enhanced dynamic studies. Eur Radiol 3:33–37

Tsushima Y, Ishizaka H, Kato T, Matsumota M (1992) Differential diagnosis of adrenal masses using out-of-phase FLASH imaging: a preliminary report. Acta Radiol 33:262–265

Tsushima Y, Ishizaka H, Matsumoto M (1993) Adrenal masses: differentiation with chemical shift, fast low-angle shot MR imaging. Radiology 186:705–709

van Erkel A, van Gils A, Lequin M, Kruitwagen C, Bloem JL, Falke THM (1994) CT and MR distinction of adenomas and nonadenomas of the adrenal gland. J Comput Assist Tomogr 18:432–438

van Gils A, Falke T, van Erkel A, Aerndt JW, Sandler MP, van der Mey AGL, Hoogma RPLM (1991) MR imaging and MIBG scintigraphy of pheochromocytomas and extraadrenal functioning paragangliomas. RadioGraphics 11:37–57

von Schulthess GK (1989) Morphology and function in MRI. Springer, Berlin Heidelberg New York

22 The Musculoskeletal System

P.A. RINCK, A. GRECO, and M.T. MCNAMARA

CONTENTS

22.1 Contrast-Enhanced Musculoskeletal Magnetic Resonance Imaging

22.1.1 Introduction

Magnetic resonance (MR) imaging has made a significant impact upon the diagnosis of musculoskeletal diseases and abnormalities. After the central nervous system, musculoskeletal diseases have become the second most important application of MR imaging (MCNAMARA and GRECO 1995, 1998).

This chapter deals with the indications for intravenous or intra-articular application of gadolinium-based extracellular fluid (ECF) space contrast agents in musculoskeletal imaging. It will only cover these particular indications, without reviewing the indications for plain MR imaging. For applications in the head and spine, see Chap. 18.

Contrast agents are employed in the customary way by intravenous injection in muscle and bone imaging, whereas in imaging of joints both intravenous and intra-articular applications are possible. Most of the intravenous applications are in static contrast-enhanced imaging, although dynamic contrast-enhanced image series have been shown to be useful.

22.1.2 MR Arthrography

Direct MR arthrography requires injection of a contrast agent or saline into the joint. Thus, it is a partly invasive technique. Indirect arthrography exploits the uptake of a contrast agent into the joint cavity after intravenous injection.

22.1.2.1 Direct MR Arthrography

Intra-articular administration of saline or gadolinium-based contrast agents facilitates the distension of a joint. The obvious drawback is the invasiveness of the technique and the associated risks.

Magnetic resonance arthrography comprises the intra-articular injection under x-ray fluoroscopic control of an amount which depends on the capacity of the joint. It is important to exercise the joint prior to scanning to ensure that the contrast medium has had an adequate opportunity to fill all fissures and

P.A. RINCK, MD, PhD, Professor of Diagnastic Imaging, NMR Laboratory, Medical Image Processing Group, Faculty of Medicine and Pharmacy, University of Mons-Hainaut, 24, Avenue du Champ de Mars; B-7000 Mons, Belgium and Centre Hospitalier Princesse Grace, Magnetic Resonance Unit, Avenue Pasteur, BP No. 489, MC-98012 Monte Carlo Cedex, Monaco
A. GRECO, MD, Centre Hospitalier Princesse Grace, Magnetic Resonance Unit, Avenue Pasteur, BP No. 489, MC-98012 Monte Carlo Cedex, Monaco
M.T. MCNAMARA, MD, Centre Hospitalier Princesse Grace, Magnetic Resonance Unit, Avenue Pasteur, BP, No. 489, MC-98012 Monte Carlo Cedex, Monaco

Table 22.1. Current applications of direct MR arthrography

Joint	Assessment or differentiation of:
Shoulder	Rotator cuff undersurface Complete/partial rotator cuff tears Postoperative shoulder Glenohumeral instability Labral lesions
Elbow	Ulnar collateral ligament Osteochondrosis dissecans
Wrist	Ligament injuries
Hip	Tears of the acetabular labrum
Knee	Postoperative residual or recurrent meniscal tear Ganglion of the cruciate ligament Articular cartilage surface in osteochondral injuries and chondromalacia Plica syndrome Osteochondrosis dissecans
Ankle	Injuries to the collateral ligaments in cases of chronic instability Osteochondrosis dissecans

defects. Current indications for direct MR arthrography are listed in Table 22.1.

The examination is performed in two parts: A preinjection T2-weighted sequence is used to identify pathology, such as bursal surface tears, ganglia or cysts, or, possibly, fluid or blood collections. Then the gadolinium-based contrast agent is injected, followed by a T1-weighted fat-saturated sequence (Palmer et al. 1993; Palmer 1996). Details of the injection techniques, pulse sequences and imaging protocols can be found in (Dalinka and Bonvita 1978; Fransson 1993; Hajek et al. 1990; Kopka et al. 1994; Kramer et al. 1997; Recht and Resnick 1994; Tirman et al. 1997a,b).

The contrast agent is diluted between 1/200 and 1/250 of the commercially available concentration, for example 0.1 ml into 20 ml of saline or 0.4 ml into 100 ml of saline. Use of the agent without dilution would cause susceptibility artifacts with resultant low signal on T2-weighted images and, possibly, irritation of the synovia (Recht and Resnick 1994).

Intra-articular application of contrast agents has not yet been approved by the relevant authorities although it is increasingly used. Depending on local laws, written or oral consent of the patient is required. This, the increased costs and the time required for the examination have limited direct arthrography.

The tolerability and the intra-articular kinetics of gadolinium-based contrast agents used for intra-articular injection are not yet completely understood. In Gd-DOTA, no microscopic changes of the joints or bone absorption of the contrast agent were detected. No cytotoxicity for chondrocytes was observed at a concentration of 5 mmol/l, but a decreased cell count was observed at a higher concentration (50 mmol/l). The intra-articular Gd-DOTA concentration decreased with time according to a logarithmic curve with an intra-articular half-life of 103–152 min (Rahmouni et al. 1995).

22.1.2.2
Indirect MR Arthrography

Indirect MR arthrography is achieved by intravenous injection of a paramagnetic MR contrast agent. After the injection, exercising the joint for about 10 min results in considerable signal intensity increase within the joint cavity. Fat-saturated MR sequences then yield arthrographic images (Vahlensieck et al. 1998).

Disadvantages of indirect MR arthrography are lack of distension of the joint, enhancement of juxta-articular structures, and, possibly, insufficient enhancement. However, according to one research group, rotator cuff tears, meniscal tears, and cartilage defects were better delineated with this method than with plain MR imaging and showed a good correlation with arthroscopic results (Vahlensieck et al. 1996).

The answer to the question of optimum contrast agent dose is not yet clear (Rinck and Muller 1998). At 0.2 T, the joint fluid enhancement in unstable shoulders was on average 134% following 0.1 mmol/kg body weight (bw) and 182% after 0.3 mmol/kg bw, whereas corresponding values in the stable shoulder in the same individuals were 69% and 142%, and 65% and 159% in the healthy controls. Enhancement of the joint fluid was higher after the triple dose than after the standard dose in both the unstable shoulders and the controls. Compared with the stable controls, enhancement in the unstable shoulders was higher for the lower dose while there was no significant difference between the groups following the higher dose (Wintzell et al. 1998).

22.2
Upper Extremity

22.2.1
Shoulder

Progress in plain MR imaging of the shoulder did not initially keep pace with the advances in knee imaging. This was largely due to relatively inadequate shoulder coil design.

Investigators have used injection of diluted gadolinium chelate solution in an attempt to improve the diagnostic sensitivity of MR for the detection of tendon injuries and of the glenohumeral ligament-labral complex.

Among tendon injuries, rotator cuff tears are the most common. In the unstable shoulder, evaluation of labral and capsular anatomy is less complicated when the structures are outlined by joint fluid. In the absence of a native joint effusion, MR arthrography is useful for delineating these structures. Several authors have claimed that the MR examination is more sensitive, allowing visualization of cuff defects on T1-weighted images, which have a better signal-to-noise ratio than T2-weighted images. MR arthrography of the shoulder joint enhances the accuracy of MR in the event of an uncertain finding on plain MR images (Kreitner et al. 1994; Palmer 1996; Reinus et al. 1995) (Fig. 22.1).

There are some researchers who claim that high-volume saline-enhanced MR arthrography is accurate in revealing the labrum, the ligaments, and the bony components of the glenohumeral joint. Saline solution is inert and inexpensive, two advantages over gadolinium-based contrast agents (Willemsen et al. 1998). However, other groups state that saline arthrograms in combination with gradient-echo (GRE) and spin-echo (SE) sequences are inferior to gadopentetate arthrograms with GRE sequences (Zanetti and Hodler 1997).

We routinely perform T1-weighted fat-saturated sequences of the shoulder following intravenous infusion of the contrast agent. Strong enhancement of fluid and inflammation produces excellent contrast with adjacent structures (Figs. 22.2–22.4).

Pathology of the glenohumeral joint is another important indication for MR arthrography. Glenohumeral joint instability may result in subluxation, with subsequent lesions of the glenohumeral ligaments and glenoid labrum. In glenohumeral instability MR imaging is superior to computed tomography (CT) in the imaging of all joint structures (Figs. 22.5, 22.6). Optimal surgical approach can be accurately predicted with both imaging methods but special surgical techniques cannot be effectively planned to replace diagnostic arthroscopy in all cases (Bachmann et al. 1998).

In a study evaluating the efficiency of different techniques in detecting tears, the sensitivities were as

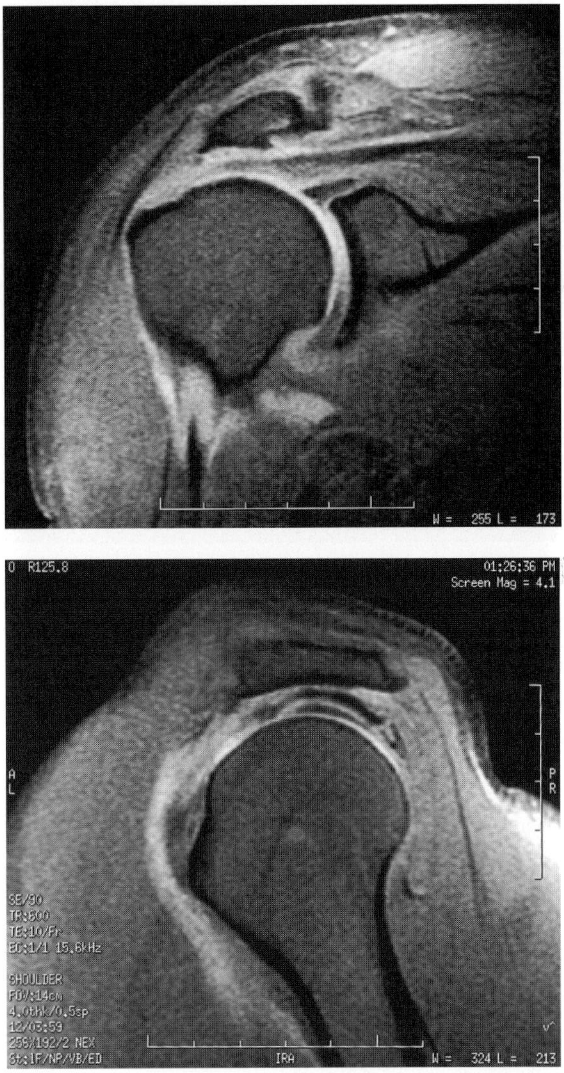

a

b

Fig. 22.1 a,b. Supraspinatus tendon tear. Fat-saturated coronal (**a**) and sagittal (**b**) images following intra-articular administration of a saline-diluted gadolinium-based contrast agent. Supraspinatus tendon tear with enhancement of subacromial and subdeltoid bursae

follows: MR arthrography 96%, plain MR imaging 93%, and CT arthrography 76% (Chandnani et al. 1993).

Use of MR arthrography to evaluate pathologic conditions of the shoulder is becoming widespread. However, normal anatomy or anatomic variations can cause errors in interpretation. The most common variations occur at the origins of the glenohumeral ligaments and the insertion of the joint capsule. Common normal variants of the labrum include a sublabral foramen and the Buford complex. Pitfalls related to the arthrographic technique include (a) visualization of a deep sulcus

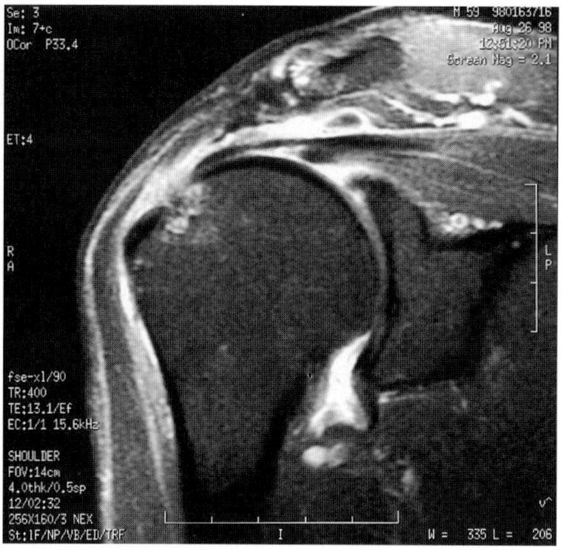

Fig. 22.2. Shoulder trauma. Coronal T1-weighted fat-saturated image following intravenous injection of a gadolinium-based contrast agent. The agent enhances the intra- and periarticular fluid, depicting a supraspinatus tendon tear. There is post-traumatic enhancement of the tuberosity bone marrow

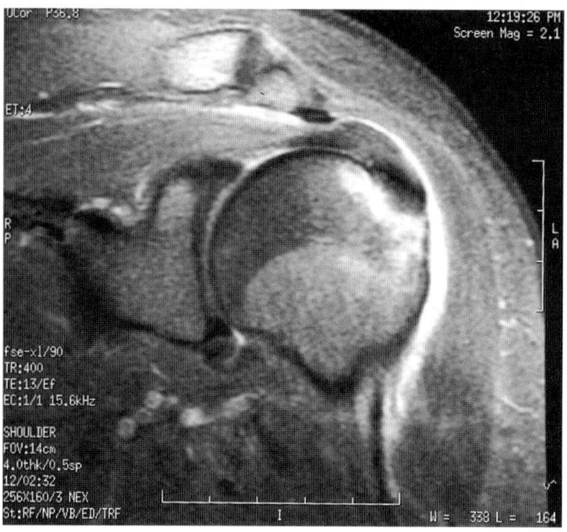

Fig. 22.3. Supraspinatus tendinosis with avulsion. Coronal T1-weighted fat-saturated image following intravenous injection of contrast agent shows thickened hyperintense supraspinatus tendon and strong tuberosity bone marrow enhancement. There is also enhancing subdeltoid fluid effusion

between the insertion of the long head of the biceps tendon and the superior labrum and (b) an apparent type III capsular insertion due to overdistension of the capsule by injected contrast material (Beltran et al. 1997).

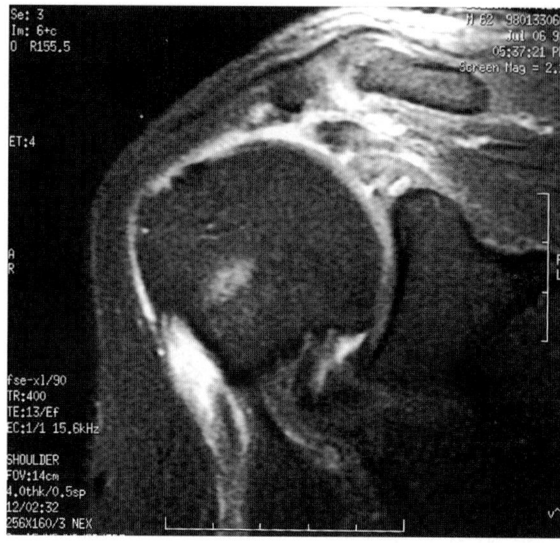

Fig. 22.4. Complete supraspinatus tear with retraction. This coronal fat-saturated T1-weighted image shows retraction of the hypointense supraspinatus tendon

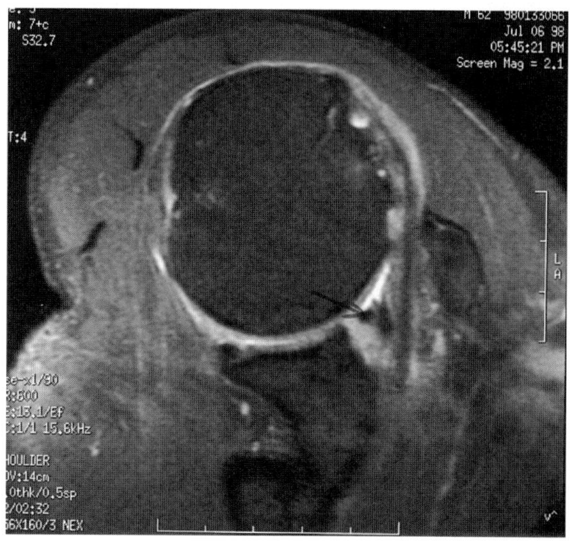

Fig. 22.5. Avulsion of the anterior glenoid labrum. Fat-saturated transverse T1-weighted image following intravenous injection of contrast agent

22.2.2 Elbow, Hand, and Wrist

In the elbow, no reports on studies in patients involving direct arthrography with gadolinium-based contrast agents have been published. Saline administration into the joint in cases of trauma to the ulnar collateral ligament (UCL) has been shown to be very efficient in the detection of partial and complete UCL tears (Schwartz et al. 1995). We often use contrast

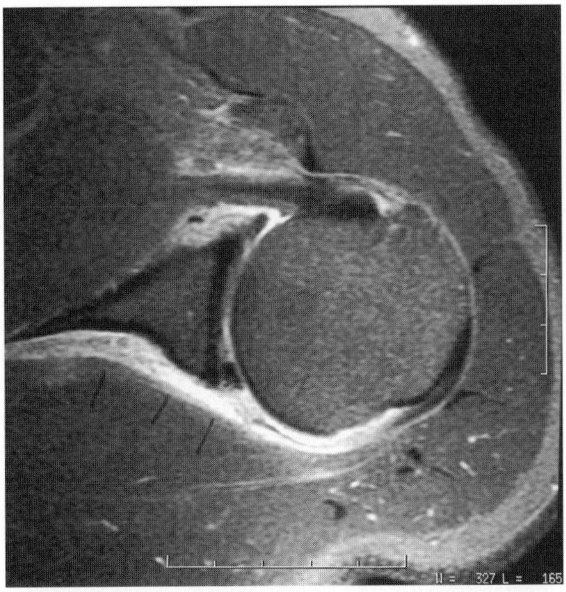
a

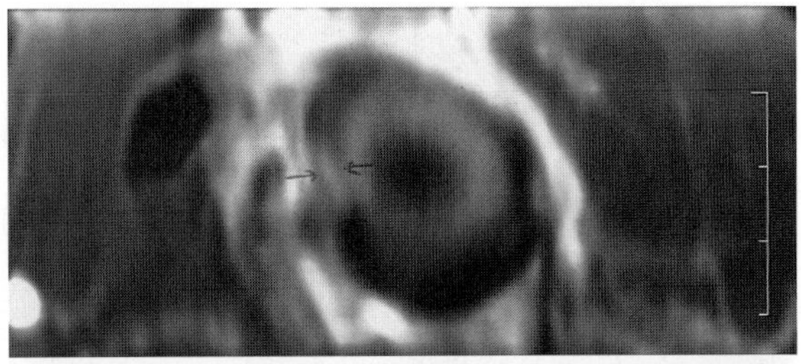
b

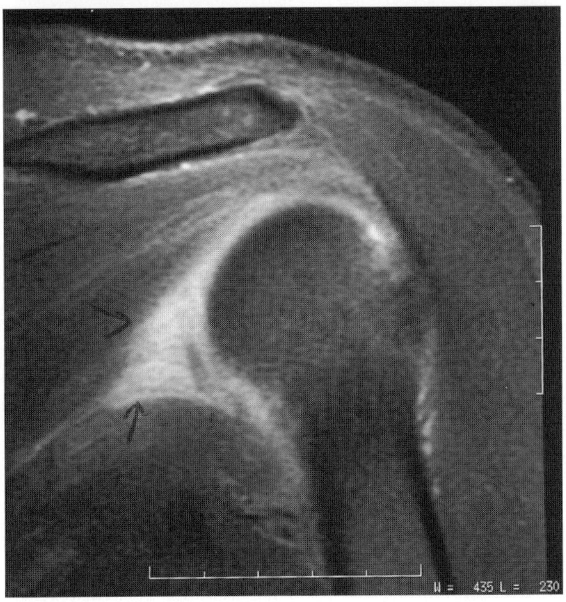
c

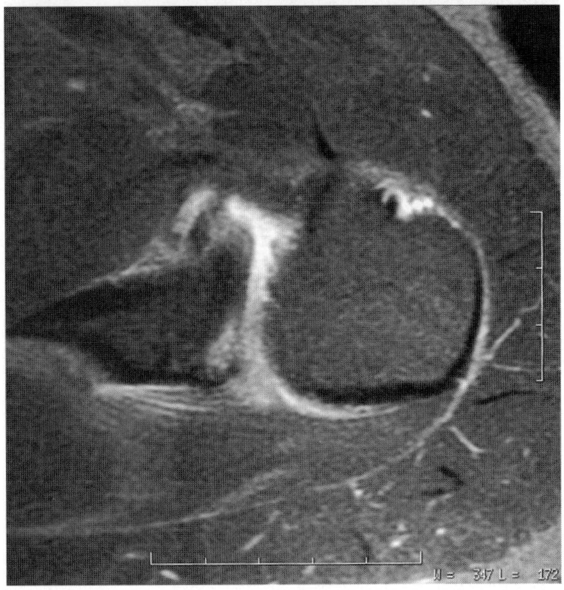
d

Fig. 22.6 a–d. Glenoid labrum tear after intravenous injection of contrast agent. **b** Sagittal reconstruction of three-dimensional GRE images of the glenoid reveal hyperintense labral tear (*arrows*). **a** Transverse fat-saturated T1-weighted image shows a posteroinferior glenoid rim fracture. **c,d** Coronal (**c**) and transverse (**d**) postcontrast fat-saturated T1-weighted images show posterior capsular disruption with leak of enhanced joint fluid

agent for the evaluation of the painful elbow in order to better delineate the source of pain (Fig. 22.7).

Indirect arthrography with gadolinium-based compounds seems to be promising in osteoarthritis, osteonecrosis, and osteochondritis dissecans (LUND et al. 1996; PEISS et al. 1995; VAHLENSIECK et al. 1996).

Magnetic resonance imaging of the hand and wrist is performed primarily for post-traumatic pathology of the carpal bones, usually the scaphoid, the triangular fibrocartilage complex, and the tendons, and for cases of carpal tunnel syndrome.

Early detection of scaphoid fracture is often problematic on plain radiographs. Coronal T1-weighted MR images readily demonstrate acute fractures due to the low signal intensity produced by edema and hemorrhage. STIR images show a conspicuous pattern of high signal intensity. Persistent signal changes on T1-weighted and STIR images are highly suggestive of avascular necrosis. For the evaluation of the vascularity of fracture fragments of the fractured carpal scaphoid in the acute (<4 weeks) and chronic (>3 months) phases, dynamic MR imaging sequences have been proposed. In these examinations it could be shown that in most acute fracture patients, enhancement of the distal pole was greater than that of the proximal. In chronic fracture patients the enhancement pattern was

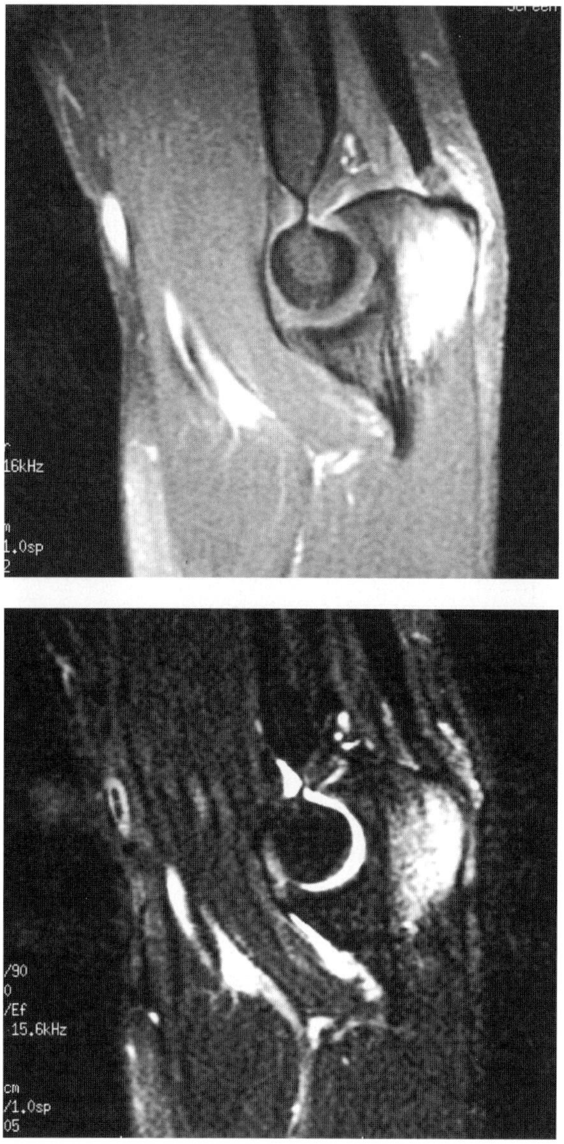

a

b

Fig. 22.7 a,b. Chronic triceps tenosynovitis. **a** Sagittal T1-weighted fat-saturated contrast-enhanced image demonstrates focal enhancement of the distal triceps tendon, peritendinous sheath, and olecranon bone marrow. **b** Sagittal STIR image demonstrates increased signal intensity in the bone marrow. The distal triceps tendon is less well appreciated than on the enhanced T1-weighted image

reversed in most cases, as the proximal pole enhanced to a greater degree than the distal (Munk et al. 1998).

Chronic wrist pain is frequently associated with carpal ligament injury or carpal instability. MR imaging is the only technique that allows direct examination of these structures (Schweitzer et al. 1992).

Well-defined bone lesions with sclerotic borders, especially if they show high signal intensity on T2-weighted images, are readily identified with MR imaging as bone cysts. However, it is noteworthy that bone cysts can enhance with gadolinium depending upon the degree of vascularity of any granulation tissue within the lesion.

22.3 Lower Extremity

22.3.1 Hip and Pelvis

Labral pathology is a major cause of hip pain. None of the conventional and computed imaging methods has solved the diagnostic problem of reliably depicting labral tears, which are believed to be a precursor of osteoarthritis. MR arthroscopy seems to have a far higher diagnostic sensitivity and accuracy in these patients than all formerly applied imaging methods (Czerny et al. 1996; Hodler et al. 1995; Petersilge et al. 1996).

In fractures of the femoral head it has been shown in animal studies (Cova et al. 1991) and in patients that after intravenous administration of a contrast agent it is possible to evaluate whether the perfusion of the femoral head is impaired (Lang et al. 1993).

Bone perfusion of the hip can be studied using dynamic gadolinium-enhanced subtraction MR imaging at the onset of proven Legg-Calvé-Perthes disease with initial negative plain films. Subtraction MR imaging depicts ischemia as a widespread absence of enhancement (Sebag et al. 1997). On static T1-weighted images, gadolinium enhancement occurs in the peripheral regions of the femoral epiphysis in the early stages of the disease. The central part of the epiphysis becomes more enhanced over time and peaks in the period 1–3 years after diagnosis (Hochbergs et al. 1997). In avascular necrosis a diffuse enhancement in the femoral head may be seen, with T2-weighted, STIR, and contrast-enhanced T1-weighted fat saturation imaging (Li and Hiette 1992) (Fig. 22.8).

Other less common lesions of the femoral head include transient osteoporosis of the hip. In these cases there is bone edema which is virtually indistinguishable from that seen in avascular necrosis. It occurs in pregnant women (usually in the third trimester) and also in men, and causes pain that is self-limited, usually resolving after several months (Fig. 22.9).

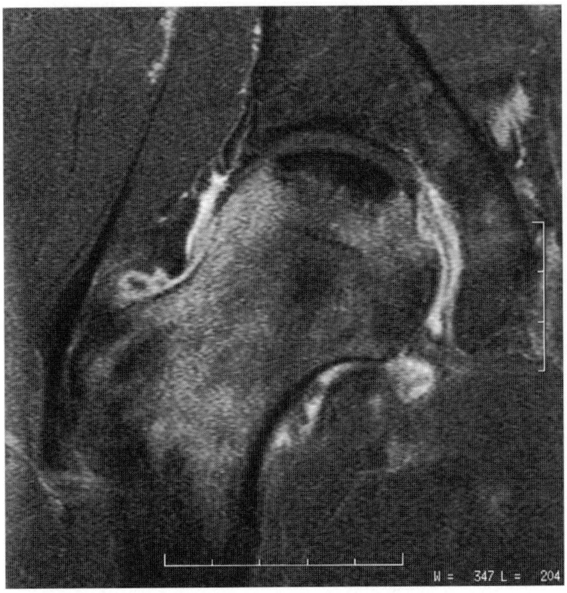

Fig. 22.8. Avascular necrosis. This coronal T1-weighted image with fat saturation following intravenous injection of a contrast agent shows the nonenhancing superior aspect of the femoral head. There is also inflammatory enhancement of the femoral neck bone marrow and of synovial fluid

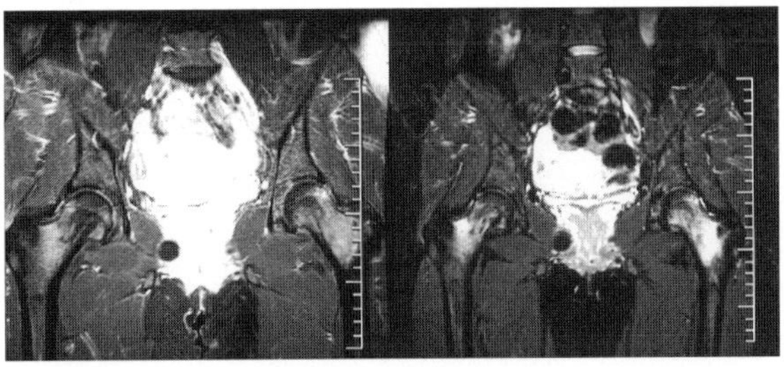

a,b

Fig. 22.9. Transient osteoporosis of the hip. **a** Coronal T1-weighted fat-saturated image following intravenous administration of contrast agent depicts extensive bilateral femoral bone marrow enhancement. **b** On the corresponding STIR image increased signal intensity is seen

22.3.2
Knee

Magnetic resonance imaging of the knee is by far the most frequently performed me examination of the musculoskeletal system, excluding the spine. This technique has rapidly evolved to a point where it is the single most important diagnostic test for internal derangements of the knee. MR of the knee is geared primarily to the evaluation of the menisci (Stoller et al. 1987), the cruciate (Hodler et al. 1992; Remer et al. 1992; Vahey et al. 1991) and collateral (Turner et al. 1985) ligaments, the patellofemoral joint and extensor mechanism (Shellock et al.

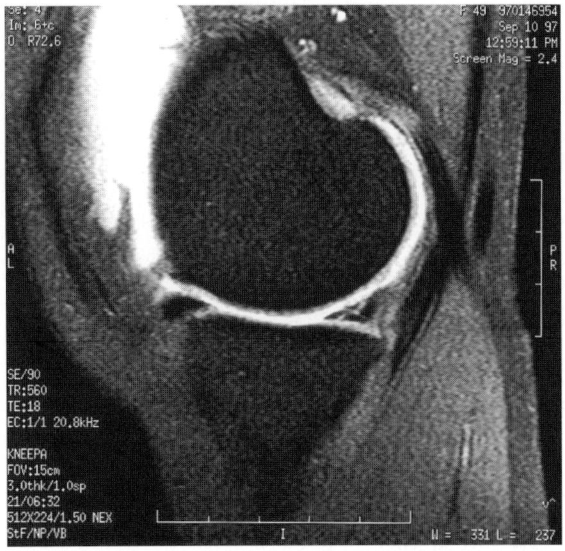

Fig. 22.10. Grade III tear involving the posterior horn of the medial meniscus. Sagittal fat-saturated T1-weighted image following intra-articular injection of contrast agent

1988, 1989), the articular cartilage, and the tendons and osseous structures.

Normal anatomy and normal enhancement behavior after intra-articular injection have been studied in the knee. The extent of contrast enhancement of synovial structures is usually not uniform within the examined joint. In the intercondylar fossa, the thickness of synovial structures is more often pronounced, while in the suprapatellar recess, synovial thickness is constant and minimal. The presence and the varying extent and thickness of synovial structures in asymptomatic knees in middle-aged individuals must be borne in mind in the evaluation of early and mild synovitis of the knee joint with gadolinium-enhanced MR imaging (Boegard et al. 1996).

The injection of fluid that contains contrast agent into the joint seems to ensure a sufficient volume of liquid to highlight meniscal tears (Fig. 22.10); this is especially important in the postoperative diagnostic follow-up, which makes MR arthrography a feasible replacement of arthroscopy in these cases (Applegate et al. 1993; Farley et al. 1991).

Magnetic resonance imaging appears to be an effective and safe, albeit controversial, method for the evaluation of articular cartilage abnormalities, the gold standard being arthroscopy (Kramer et al. 1994; Peterfy et al. 1994a,b; Recht and Resnick 1994). Direct MR arthrography increases the sensitivity for detecting cartilage lesions with the exception of intrachondral abnormalities (Kramer et al.

1994; Chandnani et al. 1991). In one study MR arthrography results were compared with arthrographic findings. Baseline MR imaging had a sensitivity of 25%, a specificity of 77.9% and a diagnostic confidence of 83% in the diagnosis of chondromalacia; these figures increased to 93%, 97.6% and 91.5% after contrast agent injection (Giovagnoni et al. 1995).

Direct MR arthrography has also raised diagnostic accuracy in cases of osteochondrosis dissecans. It seems possible to replace diagnostic arthroscopy in suspected cases of this disease (Kramer et al. 1992).

22.3.3 Foot and Ankle

MR arthrography has high sensitivity in the diagnosis and staging of anterior talofibular and calcaneofibular tears and in the depiction of osteochondral fractures (Chandnani et al. 1994).

One of the early indications for MR imaging of the ankle was evaluation of the Achilles tendon. In chronic Achilles tendon disorder (achillodynia) T1-weighted images following gadolinium contrast medium enhancement has proved to be the best method by which to visualize intratendinous signal abnormality. Histopathologic examination shows an increased noncollagenous extracellular matrix and altered fiber structure in the lesions corresponding to the contrast-enhanced areas. There is a high level of extracellular glycosaminoglycans, which are highly fixed negatively charged macromolecules with an extreme water-retaining capacity and which may contribute to the enhancement by the gadolinium contrast agent (Movin et al. 1998).

22.4 Temporomandibular Joint

Magnetic resonance imaging with intravenous administration of a Gd-based contrast agent is useful in the demonstration of the temporomandibular joint (TMJ) disc. The contrast agent increases intensity in the retrodiscal space, the pterygoid venous plexus, as well as joint effusion. The incidence in marked contrast effect is higher in TMJs with severe internal derangement than in those with normal or mild internal derangement (Takebayashi et al. 1997).

22.5 Other Muscle and Bone Diseases

22.5.1 Trauma

Most muscle injuries occur during a sudden forceful stretching of a contracted muscle. Such injuries result in a spectrum of muscle or musculotendinous lesions with variable amounts of associated edema and hemorrhage. These lesions are readily detected on standard long TR MR images (T2-weighted, STIR) as a high-intensity signal (Greco et al. 1991).

Intravenous administration of gadolinium is recommended in the setting of clinically suspected muscle injuries not visualized on T2 and STIR sequences (el-Noueam et al. 1997).

Early differentiation between intramuscular hematomas and bleeding and surrounding edema and recognition of the divided muscle fibers are possible only after the intravenous injection of an MR contrast agent. It is possible to follow up the healing process after muscle injuries by means of plain MR. Contrast-enhanced MR allows early evaluation of muscle abnormalities and is particularly valuable for recognizing the margins of the injured muscles (Mellerowicz et al. 1997).

22.5.2 Infection and Inflammation

Infection of the musculoskeletal system comprises a number of conditions affecting skin, fascia, muscle, joints, tendon sheaths, and bone. MR imaging with intravenous contrast application has developed into the preferred modality to study complicated extremity infections, since it provides an accurate portrayal of the extent of osseous and nonosseous involvement and identifies areas of necrosis (Towers et al. 1997). It is especially useful in distinguishing abscesses from surrounding cellulitis/myositis. Lack of contrast enhancement rules out infection with a high degree of certainty. However, contrast enhancement cannot be used to reliably distinguish infectious from noninfectious inflammatory conditions (Hopkins et al. 1995).

The administration of gadolinium is useful in distinguishing abscesses from very edematous, inflamed soft tissues, including muscle and fat. This is true for both high- and low-resolution images. In cases where osteomyelitis has developed as a direct extension of a local abscess, the destruction of both cortical and trabecular bone adjacent to the abscess can be easily seen (BELTRAN et al. 1987, MORRISON et al. 1993). Separate osteomyelitic foci due to hematogenous spread can be seen as high signal intensity collections on T2-weighted images, especially with a T2-weighted fat saturation technique. These foci are particularly easy to identify on gadolinium-enhanced T1-weighted fat saturation images if high-resolution techniques are used. Hematogenous foci within bone are seen on high-resolution images as destruction of trabeculae. Enhancing intact bone marrow adjacent to the infectious soft tissue foci does not necessarily indicate osteomyelitis. Enhancement may only reflect the increased vascularity of the marrow as a reaction to the adjacent infection (MORRISON et al. 1993).

Rheumatoid arthritis has become a major indication for contrast-enhanced MR imaging because the extension of inflammatory soft tissue is well demarcated. After administration of contrast agent there is marked enhancement of the pannus. In plain SE or GRE sequences synovitis is indistinguishable from joint effusion. The highly vascular synovitis enhances early after intravenous contrast medium injection; thus rapid imaging is necessary (ADAM et al. 1991; BJORKENGREN et al. 1990; HERVE-SOMMA et al. 1992; JEVTIC et al. 1993, 1997; KURSUNOGLU-BRAHME et al. 1990; KÖNIG et al. 1990; REISER et al. 1989; SUGIMOTO et al. 1996; TAMAI et al. 1994; YAMATO et al. 1993).

The long-term follow-up of rheumatoid synovial proliferation of the small joints in the hand using contrast-enhanced MRI is feasible and may provide additional information regarding disease activity. Important advantages over conventional radiographic methods are its ability to demonstrate (a) qualitative differences of synovial proliferation within bone erosions, and (b) not only early rheumatoid arthritis and deterioration but also the improvement of inflammatory disease (JEVTIC et al. 1997; SUGIMOTO et al. 1996). In examinations of the elbow sometimes gadolinium-enhanced dynamic MR imaging can be used to quantify synovial hyperemia and hence inflammatory activity. In joint inflammation of the wrist contrast-enhanced MR imaging and positron emission tomography allow quantification of volumetric and metabolic changes and comparison of efficacies of anti-inflammatory drugs (PALMER et al. 1995).

A special case of synovitis is pigmented villonodular synovitis, which is most common in the knee joint but may also be seen in the hip (HUGHES et al. 1995). The finding is usually a synovial mass which is heterogeneous with a signal intensity that is iso- or hypointense compared with that of muscle. There is always effusion in the affected joint. The use of intravenous contrast agent increases the heterogeneity of the synovia.

22.5.3 Tumors

Contrast-enhanced MR imaging allows better demarcation of tumors from surrounding tissue. After contrast administration, sclerotic, fibrotic, and avascular necrotic regions of tumors exhibit low signal intensity and are well differentiated from enhancing viable portions of the tumor (ERLEMANN et al. 1990), which is of importance for the selection of a biopsy site (GEIRNAERDT et al. 1998). However, an increase in signal intensity after contrast agent injection is unspecific because reactive tissue, peritumoral edema, and tumorous tissue enhance too. Gadolinium-enhanced T1-weighted fat saturation images will provide information about the vascularity of musculoskeletal tumors (SEEGER et al. 1991).

Contrast-enhanced MR imaging has become the imaging technique of first choice for local staging of bone tumors when limb-saving surgery is envisaged (BLOEM et al. 1997). The same holds true for monitoring possible local recurrence of bone tumors after treatment.

Differentiation between extraosseous tumor and perineoplastic edema remains one of the major pitfalls of MR imaging. Both have high signal on T2-weighted sequences and similar contrast enhancement on conventional postcontrast sequences. On dynamic studies peritumoral edema reveals a more gradual increase in signal intensity than does tumor.

In solitary bone lesions, gadolinium appears to add little to the diagnostic sensitivity or specificity of MR imaging. For selective tumors, such as osteosarcoma, gadolinium offers the potential for determining the efficacy of chemotherapy, by evaluating tumor necrosis prior and subsequent to chemotherapy. In select situations, especially sarcomas close to joints, gadolinium may aid and augment specific pulse sequences in determining whether tumor resection should be intra- or extra-articular (BLOEM et al. 1988; SUNDARAM 1997).

In metastatic disease to bone, after contrast administration, lesion enhancement renders the differentiation of tumor and fatty marrow difficult. The value of gadolinium-enhanced MR imaging may be increased by the supplementary use of fat saturation.

An appearance of a lobulated mass of high signal on T2-weighted images with low signal intensity septa, a ring-and-arc line enhancement pattern, and septal enhancement on MR images after intravenous administration of a gadolinium-based contrast agent improves tissue characterization of cartilaginous tumors and may assist in identifying low-grade chondrosarcoma (De Beuckeleer et al. 1996; Geirnaerdt et al. 1993).

In osteoid osteoma, MR images show bone marrow edema and soft tissue reactive changes that usually enhance after gadolinium administration, producing a misleading aggressive appearance (Assoun et al. 1994). MR angiography promises to be useful for assessing response to chemotherapy in osteogenic sarcoma by detecting treatment-induced changes in tumor neovascularity (Bloem et al. 1988; Lang et al. 1995a,b; Seeger et al. 1991; Swan et al. 1995).

In plasma cell myeloma, on T1-weighted postcontrast images, all the lesions showed a marked enhancement in the arterial phase and no additional lesions were depicted (Rahmouni et al. 1993).

Dynamic imaging techniques can be applied to try to differentiate benign from malignant tumors. Erlemann and collaborators showed that in dynamic imaging, 84% of malignant tumors exhibited slope values higher than 30% per minute and 72% of benign tumors showed slope values lower than 30%. However, overlap exists and only cautious statements on histology can be made (Erlemann et al. 1989).

Another research group has studied slope values of time-intensity curves of postcontrast dynamic sequences and calculated, pixel by pixel, the highest enhancement rates during the first minute after administration of contrast. The highest rate of enhancement was displayed on the first-pass (FP) image. The FP slope value correlated well with tissue vascularization and perfusion rather than with the histopathologic type of lesion. Therefore there will always be highly vascularized or perfused benign lesions with FP slope values in the range of values in malignant tumor (aneurysmal bone cyst, eosinophilic granuloma, giant cell tumor, osteoid osteoma, acute osteomyelitis, subcutaneous abscess, and myositis ossificans). However, the high spatial resolution of the FP images allows easy detection of viable tumor tissue and differentiation from necrosis and inflammation. This is important not only in the planning of the biopsy site but also in the evaluation of response to induction chemotherapy (Verstraete et al. 1994). In primary bone tumors, dynamic contrast enhancement may be helpful in differentiating between viable tumor and edema, benign and malignant tumors, and response to treatment (Bonnerot et al. 1992; Fletcher et al. 1992; Hanna et al. 1992; Lang et al. 1995a).

On dynamic postcontrast T1-weighted images, Erlemann et al. (1990) showed that a reduction in the maximum slope values by at least 60% after chemotherapy was associated with a good response to chemotherapy with an accuracy of 85.7%. Other authors have found a high correlation between tumor slope values after chemotherapy and histologic findings. Fletcher et al. (1992) noted that all histologically responsive tumors had slopes of 40% per minute or less after completion of chemotherapy and only one nonresponsive lesion had a slope of less than 40% per minute. Hanna et al. (1992) found that the slope values correlated with the percentage of tumor necrosis. A critical slope value of 45% per minute correctly predicted histologic response to chemotherapy.

A simple qualitative postprocessing method to evaluate dynamic contrast enhancement is subtraction imaging. These images are created by subtracting precontrast images from enhanced images at the time of maximal tumoral vascular uptake. On the subtraction images, areas with remaining viable tumor cells are highlighted against nonenhancing tissues, as has been shown in osteosarcoma and Ewing's sarcoma (De Baere et al. 1992; Van der Woude et al. 1995).

22.6 Conclusions

Advances in MR software and hardware design have resulted in major improvements in imaging of the musculoskeletal system. MR imaging affords precise depiction of anatomy and sensitive detection of a great variety of diseases and injuries. For most of the joints, tendons, and ligaments of the body, MR imaging has indeed become the imaging modality or diagnostic examination of choice, providing noninvasive or semi-invasive insight where only invasive techniques were previously effective or available. The end result is a significant improvement in diagnosis and a more cost-effective and timely path toward initiation of treatment.

References

Adam G, Dammer M, Bohndorf K, Christoph R, Fenke F, Gunther RW (1991) Rheumatoid arthritis of the knee: value of gadopentetate dimeglumine-enhanced MR imaging. Am J Roentgenol 156:125–129

Applegate GR, Flannigan BD, Tolin BS, Fox JM, Del Pizzo W (1993) MR diagnosis of recurrent tears in the knee: value of intraarticular contrast material. Am J Roentgenol 161:821–825

Assoun J, Richardi G, Railhac JJ, et al. (1994) Osteoid osteoma: MR imaging versus CT. Radiology 191:217–223

Bachmann G, Bauer T, Jurgensen I, Schwab J, Weimar B, Rau WS (1998) The diagnostic accuracy and therapeutic relevance of CT arthrography and MR arthrography of the shoulder. Fortschr Röntgenstr 168:149–156

Beltran J, Noto AM, McGhee RB, Freedy RM, McCalla MS (1987) Infections of the musculoskeletal system: high-field-strength MR imaging. Radiology 164:449–454

Beltran J, Bencardino J, Mellado J, Rosenberg ZS, Irish RD (1997) MR arthrography of the shoulder: variants and pitfalls. Radiographics 17:1403–1412

Bjorkengren AG, Geborek P, Rydholm U, Holtas S, Petterson H (1990) MR imaging of the knee in acute rheumatoid arthritis: synovial uptake of gadolinium-DOTA. Am J Roentgenol 155:329–332

Bloem JL, Taminiau AH, Eulderink F, Hermans J, Pauwels EK (1988) Radiologic staging of primary bone sarcoma: MR imaging, scintigraphy, angiography, and CT correlated with pathologic examination. Radiology 169:805–810

Bloem JL, van der Woude HJ, Geirnaerdt M, Hogendoorn PC, Taminiau AH, Hermans J (1997) Does magnetic resonance imaging make a difference for patients with musculoskeletal sarcoma? Br J Radiol 70:327–337

Boegard T, Johansson A, Rudling O, Petersson I, Forslind K, Jonsson K (1996) Gadolinium-DTPA-enhanced MR imaging in asymptomatic knees. Acta Radiol 37:877–882

Bonnerot V, Charpentier A, Frouin F, Kalifa C, Vanel D, Di Paola R (1992) Factor analysis of dynamic magnetic resonance imaging in predicting the response of osteosarcoma to chemotherapy. Invest Radiol 27:847–855

Chandnani VP, Harper MT, Ficke JR, Gagliardi JA, Rolling L, Christensen KP, Hansen MF (1994) Chronic ankle instability: evaluation with MR arthrography. Radiology 192:189–194

Chandnani VP, Ho C, Chu P, Trudell D, Resnick D (1991) Knee hyaline cartilage evaluated with MR imaging: a cadaveric study involving multiple imaging sequences and intraarticular injection of gadolinium and saline solution. Radiology 178:557–561

Chandnani VP, Yeager TD, DeBerardino T, Christensen K, Gagliardi JA, Heitz DR, Baird DE, Hansen MF (1993) Glenoid labral tears: prospective evaluation with MRI imaging, MR arthrography, and CT arthrography. Am J Roentgenol 161:1229–1235

Cova M, Kang YS, Tsukamoto H, et al. (1991) Bone marrow perfusion evaluated with gadolinium-enhanced dynamic fast MR imaging in a dog model. Radiology 179:535–539

Czerny C, Hofmann S, Neuhold A, Tschauner C, Engel A, Recht MP, Kramer J (1996) Lesions of the acetabular labrum: accuracy of MR imaging and MR arthrography in detection and staging. Radiology 200:225–230

Dalinka MK, Bonvita J (1978) Arthrography. In: Practice of surgery. Haper and Row, Hagerstown, pp 1–67

de Baere T, Vanel D, Shapeero LG, Charpentier A, Terrier P, di Paola M (1992) Osteosarcoma after chemotherapy: evaluation with contrast material-enhanced subtraction MR imaging. Radiology 185:587–592

De Beuckeleer LH, De Schepper AM, Ramon F (1996) Magnetic resonance imaging of cartilaginous tumors: is it useful or necessary? Skeletal Radiol 25:137–141

el-Noueam KI, Schweitzer ME, Bhatia M, Bartolozzi AR (1997) The utility of contrast-enhanced MRI in diagnosis of muscle injuries occult to conventional MRI. J Comput Assist Tomogr 21:965–968

Erlemann R, Reiser MF, Peters PE, et al. (1989) Musculoskeletal neoplasms: static and dynamic Gd-DTPA-enhanced MR imaging. Radiology 171:767–773

Erlemann R, Sciuk J, Bosse A, Ritter J, Kusnierz-Glaz GR, Peters PE, Wuisman P (1990) Response of osteosarcoma and Ewing sarcoma to preoperative chemotherapy: assessment with dynamic and static MR imaging and skeletal scintigraphy. Radiology 175:791–796

Farley TE, Howell SM, Love KF, Wolfe RD, Neumann CH (1991) Meniscal tears: MR and arthrographic findings after arthroscopic repairs. Radiology 180:517–522

Fletcher BD, Hanna SL, Fairclough DL, Gronemeyer SA (1992) Pediatric musculoskeletal tumors: use of dynamic, contrast-enhanced MR imaging to monitor response to chemotherapy. Radiology 184:243–248

Fransson SG (1993) Wrist arthrography. Acta Radiol 34:111–116

Geirnaerdt MJ, Bloem JL, Eulderink F, Hogendoorn PC, Taminiau AH (1993) Cartilaginous tumors: correlation of gadolinium-enhanced MR imaging and histopathologic findings. Radiology 186:813–817

Geirnaerdt MJ, Bloem JL, van der Woude HJ, Taminiau AH, Nooy MA, Hogendoorn PC (1998) Chondroblastic osteosarcoma: characterisation by gadolinium-enhanced MR imaging correlated with histopathology. Skeletal Radiol 27:145–153

Giovagnoni A, Valeri G, Ercolani P, Paci E, Carloni S, Soccetti A (1995) Magnetic resonance arthrography in chondral disease of the knee. Radiol Med (Torino) 90:219–225

Greco A, McNamara MT, Escher RM, Trifilio G, Parienti J (1991) Spin-echo and STIR MR imaging of sports-related muscle injuries at 1.5 T. J Comput Assist Tomogr 15:994–999

Greenspan A (1993) Benign bone-forming lesions: osteoma, osteoid osteoma, and osteoblastoma. Clinical, imaging, pathologic, and differential considerations. Skeletal Radiol 22:485–500

Hajek PC, Sartoris DJ, Neumann CH, Resmick D (1990) Magnetic resonance knee arthrography. Acta Orthop Scand 61(Suppl 240):1–57

Hanna SH, Parham DM, Fairclough DL, Meyer WH, Le AH, Fletcher BD (1992) Assessment of osteosarcoma response to preoperative chemotherapy using dynamic FLASH gadolinium-DTPA-enhanced magnetic resonance mapping. Invest Radiol 27:367–373

Herve-Somma CMP, Sebag GH, Prieur AM, Bonnerot V, Lallemand DP (1992) Juvenile rheumatoid arthritis of the knee: MR evaluation with Gd-DOTA. Radiology 182:92–98

Hochbergs P, Eckervall G, Wingstrand H, Egund N, Jonsson K (1997) Epiphyseal bone-marrow abnormalities and restitution in Legg-Calvé-Perthes disease. Evaluation by MR imaging in 86 cases. Acta Radiol 38:855–862

Hodler J, Haghigh P, Trudell D, Resnick D (1992) The cruciate ligaments of the knee: correlation between MR appearance and gross and histologic findings in cadaveric specimens. Am J Roentgenol 159:357–360

Hodler J, Yu JS, Goodwin D, Haghighi P, Trudell D, Resnick D (1995) Arthrography of the hip: improved imaging of the

acetabular labrum with histologic correlation in cadavers. Am J Roentgenol 165:887–891
Hopkins KL, Li KC, Bergman G (1995) Gadolinium-DTPA-enhanced magnetic resonance imaging of musculoskeletal infectious processes. Skeletal Radiol 24:325–333
Hughes TH, Sartoris DJ, Schweitzer ME, Resnick DL (1995) Pigmented villonodular synovitis: MRI characteristics. Skeletal Radiol 24:7–12
Jevtic V, Watt I, Rozman B, et al. (1993) Precontrast and postcontrast (Gd-DTPA) magnetic resonance imaging of hand joints in patients with rheumatoid arthritis. Clin Radiol 48:176–181
Jevtic V, Watt I, Rozman B, et al. (1997) Contrast enhanced Gd-DTPA magnetic resonance imaging in the evaluation of rheumatoid arthritis during a clinical trial with DMARDs. A prospective two-year follow-up study on hand joints in 31 patients. Clin Exp Rheumatol 15:151–156
König H, Sieper J, Wolf K-J (1990) Rheumatoid arthritis: evaluation of hypervascular and fibrous pannus with dynamic MR imaging Enhanced with Gd-DTPA. Radiology 176:473–477
Kopka L, Funke M, Fischer V, Keating D (1994) MR arthrography of the shoulder with gadopentetate dimeglumine: influence of concentration, iodinated contrast material, and time of signal intensity. Am J Roentgenol 163:621–623
Kramer J, Stiglbauer R, Engel A, Prayer L, Imhof H (1992) MR Contrast arthrography (MRA) in osteochondrosis dissecans. J Comput Assist Tomogr 16:254–260
Kramer J, Recht MP, Imhof H, Stiglbauer R, Engel A (1994) Postcontrast MR arthrography in assessment of cartilage lesions. J Comput Assist Tomogr 18:218–224
Kramer J, Scheurecker A, Mohr E, Engel A, Recht M (1997) Magnetic resonance arthrography: benefits and indications. Advances in MRI Contrast 4:104–119
Kreitner KF, Grebe P, Kersjes W, Runkel M, Kirschner P, Schild HH (1994) Application possibilities of MR arthrography in diseases of the shoulder joint. Fortschr Röntgenstr 160:137–142
Kursunoglu-Brahme S, Riccio T, Weisman MH, Resnick D, Zvaifler N, Sanders ME, Fix C (1990) Rheumatoid knee: role of gadopentetate-enhanced MR imaging. Radiology 176:831–835
Lang P, Mauz M, Schorner W, et al. (1993) Acute fracture of the femoral neck: assessment of femoral head perfusion with gadopentetate dimeglumine-enhanced MR imaging. Am J Roentgenol 160:335–341
Lang P, Grampp S, Vahlensieck M, et al. (1995a) Primary bone tumors: value of MR angiography for preoperative planning and monitoring response to chemotherapy. Am J Roentgenol 165:135–142
Lang P, Honda G, Roberts T, et al. (1995b) Musculoskeletal neoplasm: perineoplastic edema versus tumor on dynamic postcontrast MR images with spatial mapping of instantaneous enhancement rates. Radiology 197:831–839
Li KCP, Hiette P (1992) Contrast-enhanced fat saturation magnetic resonance imaging for studying the pathophysiology of osteonecrosis of the hips. Skeletal Radiol 21:375–379
Lund PJ, Chan KM, Unger EC, Galgiani TN, Pitt MJ (1996) Magnetic resonance imaging in coccidioidal arthritis. Skeletal Radiol 25:661–665
McNamara MT, Greco A (1995) Musculoskeletal applications: joints and sports medicine. In: Rinck PA (ed) The rational use of magnetic resonance imaging. Blackwell, Oxford, pp 217–239
McNamara MT, Greco A (1998) The Role of MR imaging in sports injuries of the muscles. In: Masciocchi C (ed) Radiological imaging of sports injuries. Springer, Berlin Heidelberg, New York, pp 31–47
Mellerowicz H, Lubasch A, Dulce MC, Dulce K, Wagner S, Wolf KJ (1997) Diagnosis and follow-up of muscle injuries by means of plain and contrast-enhanced MRI: experimental and clinical studies. Fortschr Röntgenstr 166:437–445
Morrison WB, Schweitzer ME, Bock GW, Mitchell DG, Hume EL, Pathria MN, Resnick D (1993) Diagnosis of osteomyelitis: utility of fat-suppressed contrast-enhanced MR imaging. Radiology 189:251–257
Movin T, Kristoffersen-Wiberg M, Rolf C, Aspelin P (1998) MR imaging in chronic Achilles tendon disorder. Acta Radiol 39:126–132
Munk PL, Lee MJ, Janzen DL, et al. (1998) Gadolinium-enhanced dynamic MRI of the fractured carpal scaphoid: preliminary results. Australas Radiol 42:10–15
Palmer WE (1996) MR arthrography: is it worthwhile? Top Magn Reson Imaging 8:24–43
Palmer WE, Brown JH, Rosenthal DI (1993) Rotator cuff: evaluation with fat-suppressed MR arthrography. Radiology 188:683–687
Palmer WE, Brown JH, Rosenthal DI (1994) Labral-ligamentous complex of the shoulder: evaluation with MR arthrography. Radiology 190:645–651
Palmer WE, Rosenthal DI, Schoenberg OI, Fischman AJ, Simon LS, Rubin RH, Polisson RP (1995) Quantification of inflammation in the wrist with gadolinium-enhanced MR imaging and PET with 2-[F-18]-fluoro-2-deoxy-D-glucose. Radiology 196:647–655
Peiss J, Adam G, Casser R, Urhahn R, Gunther RW (1995) Gadopentetate-dimeglumine-enhanced MR imaging of osteonecrosis and osteochondritis dissecans of the elbow: initial experience. Skeletal Radiol 24:17–20
Peterfy CG, Majumdar S, Lang P, van Dijke CF, Sack K, Genant HK (1994a) MR imaging of the arthritic knee: improved discrimination of cartilage, synovium, and effusion with pulse saturation transfer and fat-suppressed T1-weighted sequences. Radiology 191:413–417
Peterfy CG, van Dijke CF, Janzen DL, et al. (1994b) Quantification of articular cartilage in the knee with pulsed saturation transfer subtraction and fat-suppressed MR imaging: optimization and validation. Radiology 192:485–491
Petersilge CA, Haque MA, Petersilge WJ, Lewin JS, Lieberman JM, Buly R (1996) Acetabular labral tears: evaluation with MR arthrography. Radiology 200:231–235
Rahmouni A, Divine M, Mathieu D, et al. (1993) Detection of multiple myeloma involving the spine: efficacy of fat-suppression and contrast-enhanced MR imaging. Am J Roentgenol 160:1049–1052
Rahmouni A, Mathieu D, Chambon C, Dao TH, Hernigou P, Vasile N (1995) Intraarticular tolerability and kinetics of gadolinium tetra-azacyclododecane tetraacetic acid. Acad Radiol 2:413–417
Recht MP, Resnick D (1994) MR imaging of articular cartilage: current status and future directions. Am J Roentgenol 163:283–290
Reinus WR, Shady KL, Mirowitz SA, Totty WGMR (1995) Diagnosis of rotator cuff tears of the shoulder: value of using T2-weighted fat-saturated images. Am J Roentgenol 164:1451–1455
Reiser MF, Bongartz GP, Erlemann R, Schneider M, Pauly T, Sittek H, Peters PE (1989) Gadolinium-DTPA in rheumatoid arthritis and related disease: first results with dynamic magnetic resonance imaging. Skeletal Radiol 18:591–597
Remer EM, Fitzgerald SW, Friedman H, Rogers LF, Hendrix

RW, Schafer MF (1992) Anterior cruciate ligament injury: MR imaging diagnosis and patterns of injury. RadioGraphics 12:901–915
Rinck PA, Muller RN (1998) Field strength and dose dependence of enhancement by gadolinium-based MR contrast agents. Eur Radiol (in press)
Schwartz ML, Al-Zahrani S, Morwessel RM, Andrews JR (1995) Ulnar collateral ligament injury in the throwing athlete: evaluation with saline-enhanced MR arthrography. Radiology 197:297–299
Schweitzer ME, Brahme SK, Hodler J, et al. (1992) Chronic wrist pain: spin-echo and short tau inversion recovery MR imaging and conventional and MR arthrography. Radiology 182:205–211
Sebag G, Ducou Le Pointe H, Klein I, Maiza D, Mazda K, Bensahel H, Hassan M (1997) Dynamic gadolinium-enhanced subtraction MR imaging – a simple technique for the early diagnosis of Legg-Calvé-Perthes disease: preliminary results. Pediatr Radiol 27:216–220
Seeger LL, Widoff BE, Bassett LW, et al. (1991) Preoperative evaluation of osteosarcoma: value of gadopentetate dimeglumine-enhanced MR imaging. Am J Roentgenol 157:347–352
Shellock FG, Mink JH, Fox JM (1988) Patellofemoral joint: kinematic MR imaging to assess tracking abnormalities. Radiology 168:551–553
Shellock FG, Mink JH, Deutsch AL, Fox JM (1989) Patellar tracking abnormalities: clinical experience with kinematic MR imaging in 130 patients. Radiology 172:799–804
Stoller DW, Martin C, Crues JV, Kaplan L, Mink JH (1987) Meniscal tears: pathologic correlation with MR imaging. Radiology 163:731–735
Sugimoto H, Takeda A, Masuyama J, Furuse M (1996) Early-stage rheumatoid arthritis: diagnostic accuracy of MR imaging. Radiology 198:185–192
Sundaram M (1997) The use of gadolinium in the MR imaging of bone tumors. Semin Ultrasound CT MR 18:307–311
Swan JS, Grist TM, Sproat IA, Heiner JP, Wiersma SR, Heisey DM (1995) Musculoskeletal neoplasms: preoperative evaluation with MR angiography. Radiology 194:519–524
Takebayashi S, Takama T, Okada S, Masuda G, Matsubara S (1997) MRI of the TMJ disc with intravenous administration of gadopentetate dimeglumine. J Comput Assist Tomogr 21:209–215
Tamai K, Yamato M, Yamaguchi T, Ohno W (1994) Dynamic magnetic resonance imaging for the evaluation of synovitis in patients with rheumatoid arthritis. Arthritis Rheum 37:1151–1157
Tirman PF, Palmer WE, Feller JF (1997a) MR arthrography of the shoulder. Magn Reson Imaging Clin North Am 5:811–839
Tirman PF, Steinbach LS, Belzer JP, Bost FW (1997b) A practical approach to imaging of the shoulder with emphasis on MR imaging. Orthop Clin North Am 28:483–515
Towers JD (1997) The use of intravenous contrast in MRI of extremity infection. Semin Ultrasound CT MR 18:269–275
Turner DA, Prodomos CC, Petasnick JP, Clark JW (1985) Acute injury of the ligaments of the knee: magnetic resonance evaluation. Radiology 154:717–722
Vahey TN, Broome DR, Kayes KJ, Schelbourne KD (1991) Acute and chronic tears of the anterior cruciate ligament: differential features at MR imaging. Radiology 181:251–253
Vahlensieck M, Peterfy CG, Wischer T, et al. (1996) Indirect MR arthrography: optimization and clinical applications. Radiology 200:249–254
Vahlensieck M, Sommer T, Textor J, Pauleit D, Lang P, Genant HK, Schild HH (1998) Indirect MR arthrography: techniques and applications. Eur Radiol 8:232–235
van der Woude HJ, Bloem JL, Verstraete KL, Taminiau AH, Nooy MA, Hogendoorn PC (1995) Osteosarcoma and Ewing's sarcoma after neoadjuvant chemotherapy: value of dynamic MR imaging in detecting viable tumor before surgery. Am J Roentgenol 165:593–598
Verstraete KL, Dierick A, De Deene Y, Uyttendaele D, Vandamme F, Roels H, Kunnen M (1994) First-pass images of musculoskeletal lesions: a new and useful diagnostic application of dynamic contrast-enhanced MRI. Magn Reson Imaging 12:687–702
Willemsen UF, Wiedemann E, Brunner U, Scheck R, Pfluger T, Kueffer G, Hahn K (1998) Prospective evaluation of MR arthrography performed with high-volume intraarticular saline enhancement in patients with recurrent anterior dislocations of the shoulder. Am J Roentgenol 170:79–84
Wintzell G, Haglund-Akerlind Y, Larsson H, Zyto K, Larsson S (1998) Joint fluid enhancement at MRI of the glenohumeral joint with intravenous injection of gadodiamide in standard and triple dose: a prospective comparative study of stable and unstable shoulders. Skeletal Radiol 27:87–91
Yamato M, Tamai K, Yamaguchi T, Ohno W (1993) MRI of the knee in rheumatoid arthritis: Gd-DTPA perfusion dynamics. J Comput Assist Tomogr 17:781–785
Zanetti M, Hodler J (1997) Contrast media in MR arthrography of the glenohumeral joint: intra-articular gadopentetate vs saline: preliminary results. Eur Radiol 7:498–502

23 Contrast-Enhanced Magnetic Resonance Angiography

G. Marchal and H. Bosmans

CONTENTS

23.1 Introduction

Magnetic resonance imaging (MRI) of blood vessels has always been a special topic. In conventional MRI, the pulsatility of the blood usually causes artifacts. Not only can the signal intensity (SI) in the vessel be very variable, it can also spread along the phase-encoded direction and overlay important image details. More importantly, the signal intensities can appear as a ghost and mimic a lesion. The understanding of these phenomena and a few techniques to counter these artifacts led in the late 1980s to the development of the so-called MR angiography (MRA) sequences. With these sequences, the signal intensities in the blood vessels are hyperintense and most artifacts are overcome. Two groups of sequences were developed in parallel and are still extensively used today: time-of-flight and phase contrast imaging. The hyperintense signal intensities in the first group are derived from inflow effects, whereas for phase contrast imaging, flow-induced phase effects play a major role. In both methods, the basic sequence is a gradient recalled echo technique with short repetition time (TR)/echo time (TE), enabling the acquisition of 2D or 3D images in a reasonable time period. The artifacts along the phase-encoded direction are overcome by using dedicated gradient schemes ("gradient motion refocusing gradients" or "first-order flow-compensating gradients"). The use of these gradients does not enforce the signal intensity but rather avoids the signal voids or the spread of the signal along the phase-encoded direction.

G. Marchal, MD, PhD, Professor, Department of Radiology, University Hospitals Gasthuisberg, Catholic University of Leuven, Herestraat 49, B-3000 Leuven, Belgium
H. Bosmans, PhD, Professor, Department of Radiology, University Hospitals Gasthuisberg, Catholic University of Leuven, Herestraat 49, B-3000 Leuven, Belgium

23.1.1 Inflow Enhancement

Hyperintense signal intensities in the blood vessel are not expected in T1-weighted acquisitions, since the T1 of the blood is long. The paradoxical enhancement due to inflow phenomena in the time-of-flight techniques can be understood as follows: the spins in the blood vessels are different from the surrounding tissues because they continuously enter (inflow) and leave the imaging volume. Therefore, they are subjected only to a small succession of radiofrequency (RF) excitation pulses, after which they are replaced by fresh blood. The surrounding tissues, on the other hand, are stationary and therefore experience the complete series of RF pulses. The crucial fact is that in gradient-echo acquisitions, the signal intensity changes during the series of RF pulses (Fig. 23.1). After a first RF pulse, the signal intensity is high. After the second pulse, the signal intensity is already lower, and this effect continues until a (low) steady state signal intensity is reached. In a 2D acquisition with, for example, a matrix of 192 × 256, the tissues in the imaging plane are subjected to 192 RF pulses. Stationary tissues experience all of them. The averaged signal provided by these tissues will be low. On

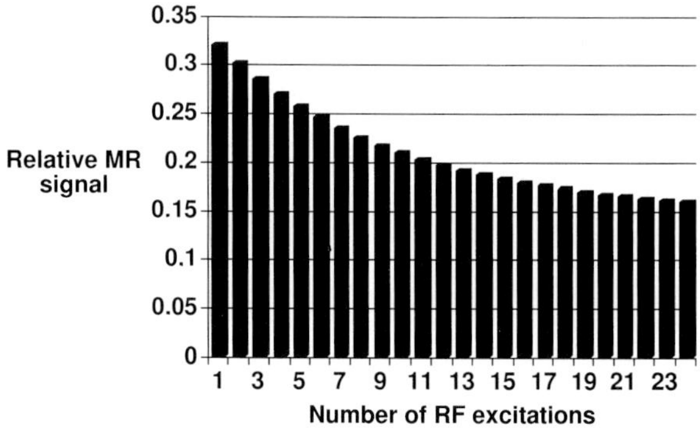

Fig. 23.1. MR signal intensity as a function of the number of successive excitation pulses

the other hand, flowing spins which enter the slice experience only a few RF pulses and hence cause a large signal intensity. The blood then leaves the imaging plane and is replaced by fresh blood that will again experience only a few pulses. Under these conditions, the signal intensity in the blood vessel will be rather high since a steady state value is never reached.

Figure 23.2a illustrates the specific signal intensities due to the inflow effect. Near the entrance plane, the spins in the blood vessel provide the highest signal. Deeper in the imaged volume, this signal gradually decreases until eventually it reaches the steady state. At this point, the contrast with the surrounding tissue will be lost and the spins are said to be saturated. This saturation effect can also be understood with a model (Fig. 23.2b): the stationary tissue is seen as a warm water bath, in which the vessel (a tube filled with flowing cold water) is submersed. The temperature difference between the vessel and the stationary tissue is a measure for the image contrast. In practice, the temperature difference between the tube and the warm water bath will progressively decrease, until the temperature of the water in the tube reaches the value of the warm water bath and the temperature difference between the two substances is lost.

The hyperintense signal intensities in the blood vessels depend not only on the inflow effect, but also on the type of flow. Only with laminar flow do the special flow rephasing gradients perform properly. In practice, the success of the technique depends on the velocity of the blood in the vessel, the length of the vessel in the imaging slab, the flow pattern, and the sequence parameter setting. Whenever the blood remains in the slice or slab for a long time, the signal gets saturated. It is particularly difficult to visualize veins and slow-flowing arterial blood in patients with low cardiac output, in obstructive diseases, or in high-resistance vessels. Other determining factors are artifacts due to respiratory motion or intrinsic organ motion.

In practice, 2D and 3D time-of-flight techniques can be used routinely for MRA of the carotids – although the real specificity may be lower than has been reported (Kallmes et al. 1996) – and also for MRA of the vertebral arteries and intracranial vessels (Stock et al. 1996; Furst et al. 1996). A successful time-of-flight acquisition requires that care be taken to optimize slice or slab orientations and slab thicknesses, and additional techniques, such as magnetization transfer pulses, in order to reduce further the contribution of the stationary tissues. High-resolution 3D acquisitions can be obtained, from which projections in any direction and of user-defined subvolumes can be calculated (Fig. 23.2c,d).

Using time-of-flight techniques, the high-resistance peripheral vessels can only be visualized with 2D slices perpendicular to the vessels. Some reports are optimistic about the results of this approach (Cortell et al. 1996), while others are less enthusiastic: in obstructive iliac artery lesions, its sensitivity and specificity is often too low to replace conventional diagnostic arteriography (Snidow et al. 1996a). More specialized techniques are based on ECG triggering, or gating of the acquisition process to the systolic phase during which flow is maximal (Yucel et al. 1994). Another non-invasive MRI approach is phase contrast imaging (Schmiedl et al. 1996), as discussed in a separate section.

Fig. 23.2. a The result of inflow enhancement is shown in the representation of a vessel. Where the blood enters the slab, the signal intensity is hyperintense (the spins underwent only one excitation pulse). More distal in the vessel, the spins are subjected to successive excitations, and their signal intensity decreases gradually. **b** The inflow enhancement can be compared to the model with a warm water bath. The vessel contrast-to-noise ratio in the MRA images behaves like the temperature difference across a cold water "vessel" that crosses a warm water bath. Initially, the temperature difference is high. This difference decreases along the tube. It is lost more rapidly when the water moves slowly through the vessel. Under certain conditions, the temperature difference can be zero. In MRA terminology, this condition is called "saturation," and, in the images, the vessel at that point is no longer visible **c, d** The data of a high-resolution 3D nonenhanced MRA acquisition of the intracranial vessels can be projected along any direction: **c** axial direction and **d** coronal view of a smaller subvolume

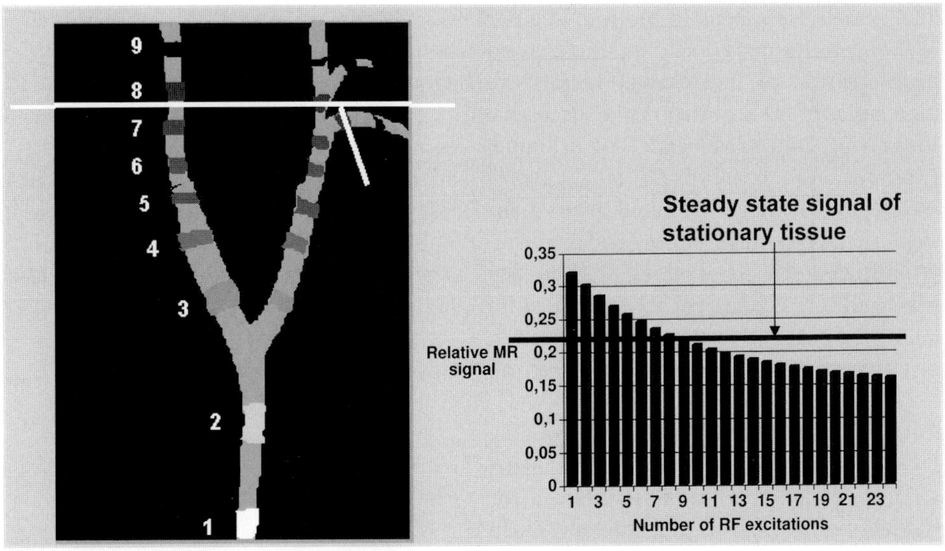
9
8
7
6
5
4
3
2
1
Steady state signal of stationary tissue
Relative MR signal
0,35
0,3
0,25
0,2
0,15
0,1
0,05
0
1 3 5 7 9 11 13 15 17 19 21 23
Number of RF excitations

a

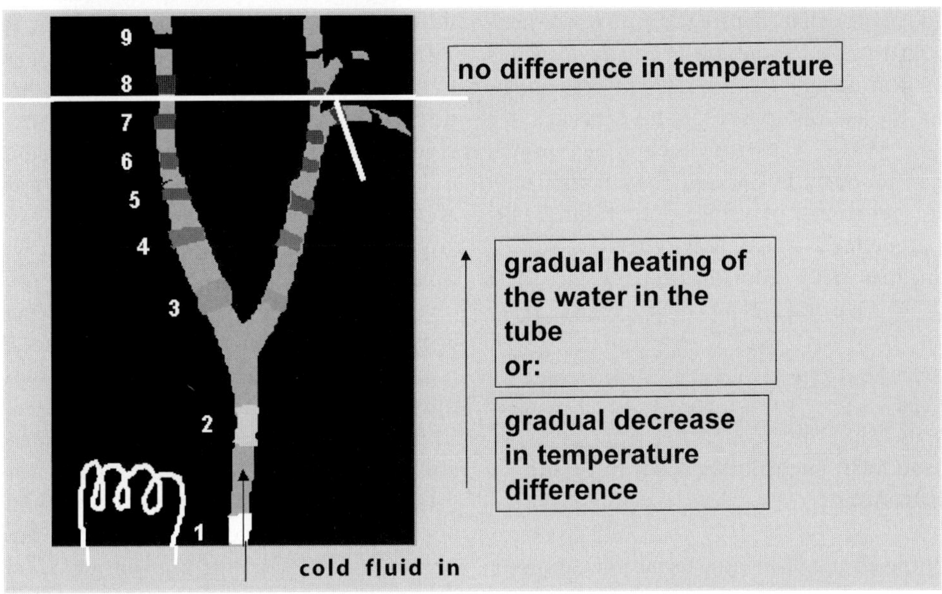
9
8
7
6
5
4
3
2
1
no difference in temperature
gradual heating of the water in the tube or:
gradual decrease in temperature difference
cold fluid in

b

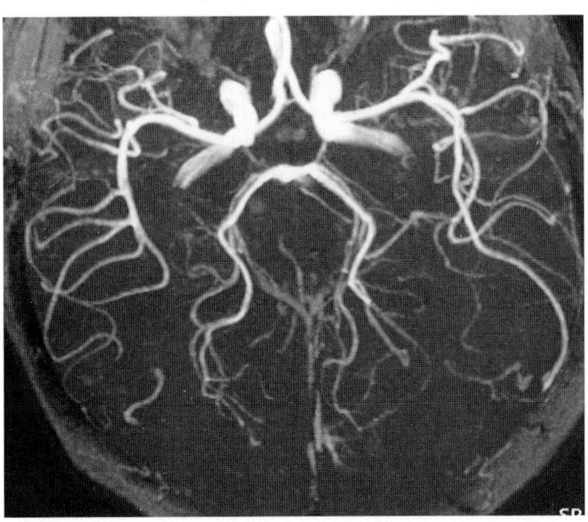

c

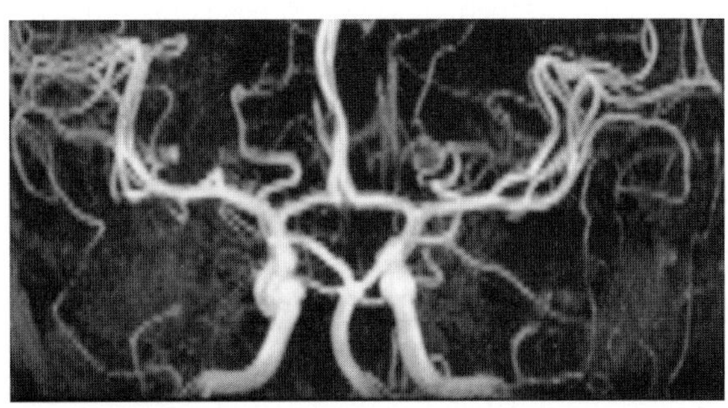

d

Abdominal vessels are subject to motion. Regular 3D time-of-flight techniques such as those used for imaging of carotid or intracranial vessels are not optimal. A series of 2D acquisitions in successive breath-holds can be used to visualize, for example, the portal venous system (Nghiem et al. 1996). Improved strategies to image the renal arteries include the use of background suppression pulses, labeling of inflowing blood, systolic gating, the acquisition of multiple echoes per excitation pulse (echo planar type acquisition), and subtraction techniques (Wielopolski et al. 1995;Li et al. 1994).

Coronary and pulmonary vessels are probably the most challenging vessels to study with MRA techniques. High spatial resolution is required for tortuous vessels with highly pulsatile flow. In addition, substantial motion is present due to respiration and myocardial contraction. Two-dimensional, ECG-triggered gradient-echo acquisitions have been performed in breath-hold, with an acquisition during the systolic phase of the cardiac cycle (Duerinckx 1997). Navigator techniques, which measure continuously but accept data points only when the position of the diaphragm falls within a predefined range, have been a breakthrough in this field (McConnell et al. 1997; Li et al. 1996; Oshinski et al. 1996; Wang et al. 1996).

23.1.2 Inflow-Based MRA Techniques After Injection of a Contrast Agent

After the intravenous or intra-arterial injection of a T1 relaxation agent, the T1 of the blood and perfused tissues is shortened. In T1-weighted acquisitions, the associated signal intensity of these tissues therefore increases. As most gradient-echo acquisitions, including the currently used techniques for MRA, provide images with a certain degree of T1-weighting, the signal intensity of the vessels during and after the injection of a contrast agent will be increased compared with a plain acquisition. The signal intensity for a typical gradient-echo acquisition as a function of the number of RF pulses for tissues with different T1 is schematically drawn in Fig. 23.3a. It can be seen that for tissues with a very short T1, the global signal intensities are markedly higher than those of tissues with a longer T1. In particular, the steady state signal intensity after a contrast injection in perfused tissues is higher than that in other tissues. This effect offers an alternative mechanism to obtain a positive blood vessel contrast. Figure 23.3b shows a model that can be used to better understand the effect of contrast agent injection.

The injection of contrast agents can be used to complement the time-of-flight effect. The major advantage of this approach is that MRA becomes less dependent on flow velocity, and more optimal slab thicknesses and orientations can be chosen since saturation of the blood is largely eliminated. Figure 23.3c shows a contrast-enhanced MRA acquisition that visualizes intracranial veins in a sagittal subvolume of the brain.

23.1.3 Phase Contrast Imaging

Dedicated gradient schemes can be used to overcome flow artifacts, such as in time-of-flight techniques. These basic tools, however, can be also used to intentionally create flow-related effects to which the stationary tissues are insensitive. In practice, the image is scanned at least twice (but usually 4 times) making a reference scan without flow-induced phase effects, and one to three acquisitions with phase effects that are proportional to the flow along a particular direction in space. After the measurement, the reference image is subtracted from the phase-"encoded" images and reveals only the flowing spins. The signal intensity in the blood vessels is a function of the intrinsic signal intensity and the velocity of the spins. In practice, different acquisition schemes are available, creating different phase effects for different mean velocities of the spins. An optimal effect is observed for sequences that achieve a flow-induced phase angle of 180° for a given mean velocity in a vessel. The appropriate velocity encoding gradient (the VENC) has to be chosen prior to the acquisition.

The vessel contrast to noise ratios in phase contrast acquisitions are greater than those in time-of-flight techniques, as there is no surrounding tissue left in the images. For the same reason, saturation is less of a problem. A major disadvantage is the longer acquisition time, since the basic acquisition has to be repeated 2–4 times. However, phase contrast imaging can be an alternative technique to time-of-flight acquisitions in imaging of, for example, carotid arteries. It is complementary to, or offers substantial advantages over, time-of-flight techniques in the evaluation of venous anomalies in the brain (Pernicone et al. 1990), renal arteries (Loubeyre et al. 1996a), peripheral arteries (Schmiedl et al. 1996), portal venous system (Nghiem et al. 1996; Hara et al. 1996), and vascular malformations of

a
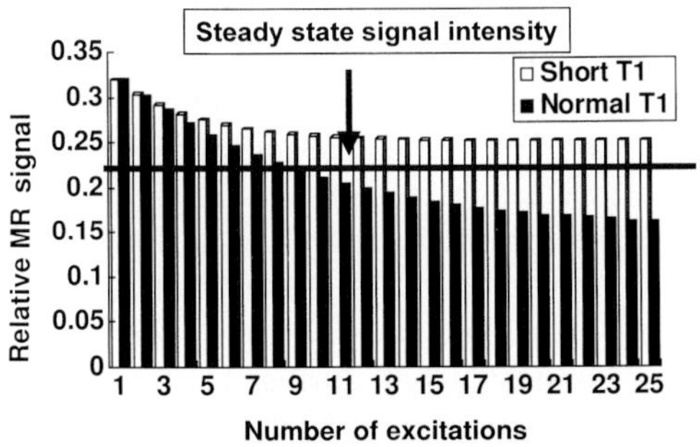

b
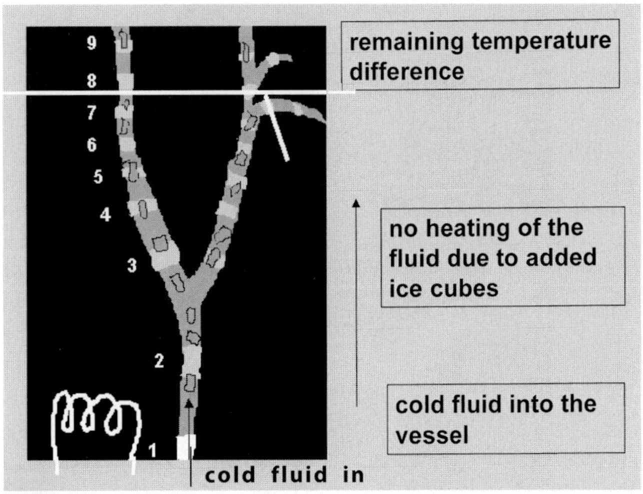

c
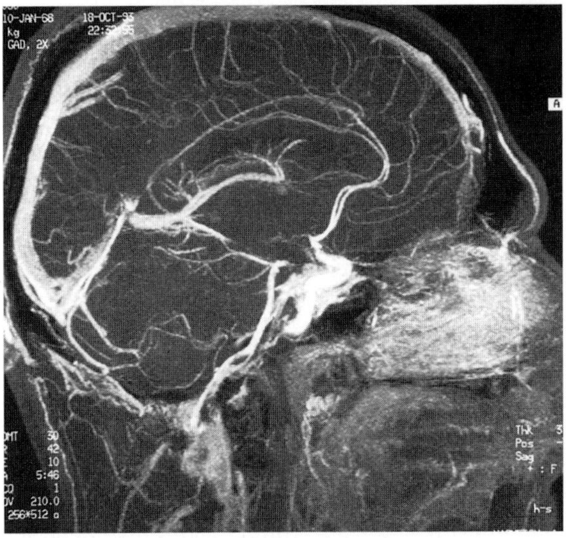

Fig. 23.3. **a** This graph compares the signal intensities in vessels before (normal T1) and after the injection of a contrast agent (short T1). The signal intensity after the injection of a contrast agent remains higher than a nonenhanced acquisition. In particular, the signal always remains higher than the steady state signal intensity in adjacent tissues. **b** This model for contrast enhancement is identical to that in Fig. 23.2b, but ice cubes are injected into the tube such that the temperature difference remains significant. Saturation will no longer occur. **c** A 3D mid-sagittal time-of-flight acquisition in a normal volunteer after a dose of 0.2 mmol/kg Gd-DTPA (acquisition time of 5min) shows that both arteries and veins are visualized

the spinal cord (Mascalchi et al. 1995; Gelbert et al. 1992). As with time-of-flight techniques, gating of the acquisition to specific phases of the cardiac cycle has been proposed to improve image quality (Silverman et al. 1996; de Haan et al. 1996; Wasser et al. 1997). In a further evolution, the VENC has been adapted to the cardiac phase (Swan et al. 1994).

23.1.4 Phase Contrast Techniques After Injection of a Contrast Agent

The injection of contrast agents has no effect on the flow-induced phase effects. An optimal choice of VENC remains mandatory for a successful acquisition. The influence of contrast injections will be restricted to enhancement of the intrinsic signal strength of the spins. Therefore, it is possible to better visualize smaller vessels or to increase the resolution. This effect has been shown for phase contrast acquisitions of the renal arteries (Bass et al. 1997) and for studies of the portal venous system (Nghiem et al. 1995).

23.2 The Need for Fast Acquisition Schemes in Contrast-Enhanced MRA

The acquisition time of regular 3D time-of-flight images can be calculated from the same formulas as are used for conventional MRI:

$$\text{Acquisition time} = \text{TR} \times N_{ph} \times N_{part} \times N_{av},$$

where TR is the repetition time; N_{ph}, the number of in-plane phase-encoded scans; N_{part}, the number of partitions and N_{av}, the number of signal averages.

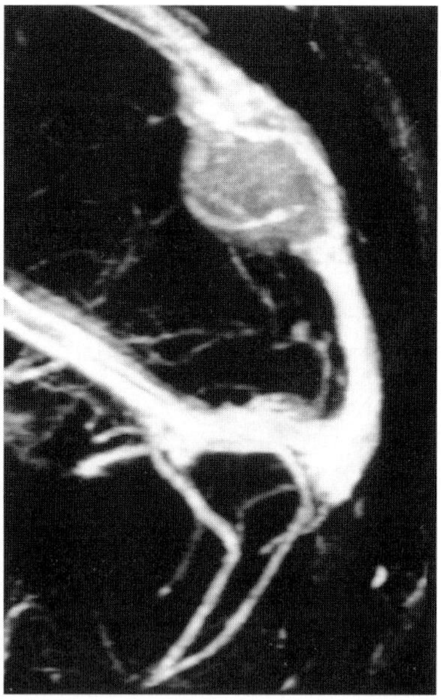

Fig. 23.4. A contrast-enhanced time-of-flight study shows how the meningioma grows into the superior sagittal sinus

Using a TR of 40 ms, an in-plane matrix of 192 × 256, 64 partitions (which makes it possible to reconstruct a volume of 64 mm into 64 slices of 1 mm), and one signal averaging, a total acquisition time of 8 min is needed. This would be a typical measurement time for an MRA examination of the intracranial vessels or the carotid arteries. Phase contrast imaging with the same pixel sizes takes 2–4 times longer and is therefore usually performed at a lower resolution.

Compared with the duration of the passage of a bolus of contrast agent, this acquisition time of 8 min is long. During the measurement, the contrast agent will first opacify the arteries, later the veins, and then be diluted in the blood pool and enhance the soft tissue. With an 8-min acquisition, an average picture will be obtained, showing the arteries, veins, and perfused tissues.

Intracranial vessels have been studied with this technique: as the T1 of blood is significantly shortened during an 8-min acquisition while the contrast uptake of the brain parenchyma is negligible, blood vessel contrast can be markedly increased. Contrast-enhanced time-of-flight MRA is an appropriate tool to visualize the intracranial veins (Fig. 23.4) and smaller arteries (Marchal et al. 1992; Runge et al. 1993; McLachlan et al. 1994). In other regions of the body, the effects are less beneficial. In the neck, for example, the contrast uptake of soft tissue and the fact that arteries and veins are overlapping in projected images restrict its use for the visualization of the carotid arteries. Although saturation problems are overcome, new postprocessing tools would be required to segment the vessels out of the acquisition volume (Cloft et al. 1996). In the abdomen, the uptake of the soft tissues and the venous enhancement also reduce the potential use of this approach for improved imaging of the renal arteries. Venous overlap is a major problem in the study of peripheral arteries.

In 1993, a new method was proposed (Prince et al. 1993) to improve time-of-flight MRA of abdominal vessels. The authors used a continuous, slow injection of contrast agent during a 3- to 5-min time-of-flight measurement. In this way, the T1 in the arteries was kept short during the entire measurement and the venous enhancement was relatively low because of a slow progressive tissue uptake after the first pass. This method seemed very promising to image large abdominal vessels and it improved the visualization of the renal arteries. A major disadvantage of the technique was the need for high doses.

In a further evolution, other injection schemes were studied. It is a basic characteristic of MRI that the contribution of successive signals acquired during a particular measurement depends on the amount of phase encoding in the signal. In practice, the measurements that have to be written in the center of the k-space (where minimal phase encoding occurs) are most determining for the signal intensity. The signals near the periphery of the k-space (with most position encoding) make a major contribution to the image resolution (Fig. 23.5). This effect is well known from, for example, fast spin-echo measurements, where the peripheral lines in the k-space are acquired near the beginning or the end of the echo train. The effective T1- or T2-weighting in a fast spin-echo image is determined by the time in between the excitation and the acquisition of the center of the k-space. With a contrast injection timed to have the bolus passage in the vessels during the acquisition of the data of the center of the k-space, an optimal exploitation of the T1 contrast agent can be expected. A careful timing of the bolus can therefore be used to reduce the total dose needed or to further increase the signal intensity of the blood (Earls et al. 1996).

Most acquisition schemes fill the k-space from bottom to top. In this way, the center of the k-space is scanned half way through the measurement. At that moment, the bolus has to pass. In practice, correct timing requires some prior knowledge of the

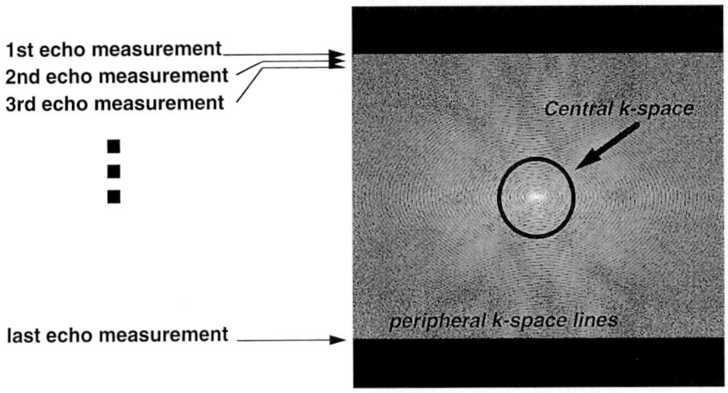

Fig. 23.5. In k-space, the data in the center determine the gray values in the image, while the data near the periphery contribute to the image resolution

circulation time in the patient. With the information obtained from a test bolus injection, it is possible to have the bolus arrive a few seconds before scanning the center of the k-space.

In a further evolution of this work, a preparation scan has been developed that tracks the arrival of the bolus and initiates the MRA acquisition subsequently (Foo et al. 1997; Prince et al. 1997).

Other k-space filling schemes, acquiring the center lines near the beginning of the measurement, have been studied. The passage of the bolus then has to occur at the very beginning of the measurement and the remaining part of the k-space is imaged with vessels containing at least a minimal amount of contrast agent. Although this is a better approach in theory, the image quality can be compromised by artifacts due to the fact that the center of the k-space is scanned when the steady state values have not yet been reached. In practice, this type of acquisition is preceded by a series of prepulses. Differences between these adapted schemes and the regularly available ones are sometimes very limited. Another aspect of this type of optimization is that large changes in the concentration of the contrast agent when scanning the center lines of the k-space can result in image artifacts (Ito et al. 1997; Maki et al. 1996). Therefore, optimization has still to be verified in larger groups of patients.

Recently, with the advent of a more powerful generation of MR scanners, a new contrast-enhanced approach has been achieving rapid acceptance in clinical practice. New gradient-echo acquisitions have been proposed with an ultrashort TE, namely in the order of 1–2 ms. With these sequences, at least the majority of possible flow-induced dephasing effects do not appear, and therefore flow rephasing gradients are not necessary. Associated with the short TE is a short TR, and this directly influences the total measurement time. This scheme provides

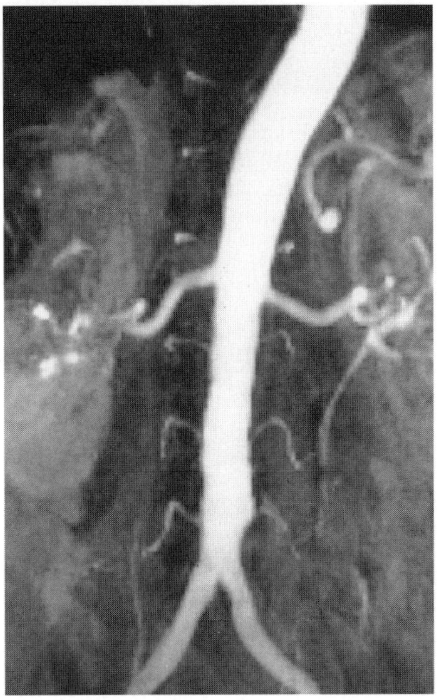

Fig. 23.6. A contrast-enhanced 27-s acquisition (TR/TE/FL 4.4 ms/1.4 ms/30°, 64 partitions after zero filling of the raw data) of the abdominal vessels shows motion-free images with an impressive image detail

T1-weighted acquisitions with very poor contrast due to the very unfavorable combination of TR, TE, and flip angle. However, tissues with an ultrashort T1 show up bright. Hyperintense signal intensities in the blood vessels are obtained only via the injection of a positive contrast agent (Talagala et al. 1995). Using, as an example, TR/TE 4 ms/2 ms, matrix 192 × 256, and 32 partitions, this acquisition results in a total measurement of only 24 s. In practice, this acquisition can be run with a similar parameter setting during a breath-hold, and it is therefore a candidate for abdominal (Fig. 23.6) and even thoracic MRA (Fig. 23.7). The first clinical comparisons

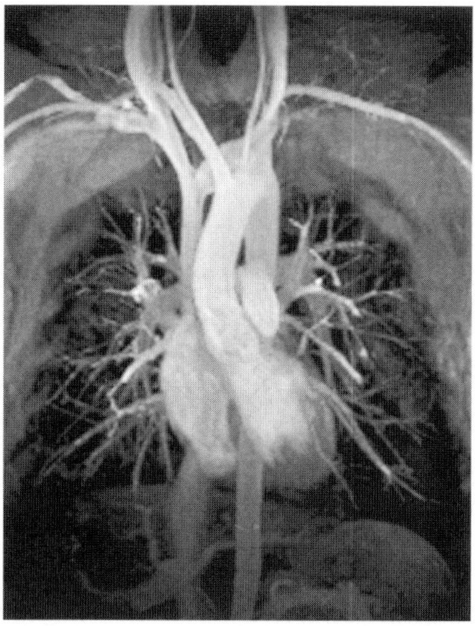

Fig. 23.7. Patient with an acute thoracic pain syndrome. A complete evaluation of all thoracic vessels obtained with an ultrafast contrast-enhanced MRA acquisition (TR/TE/FL 3.8 ms/1.3 ms/25°, acquisition time 14 s) shows no abnormal findings

between the fast contrast-enhanced time-of-flight acquisitions and the previous approaches for MRA of the renal, celiac, and superior mesenteric arteries (Prince et al. 1995; Holland et al. 1996) show a clear superiority of the new methods.

Any additional technique to further shorten the acquisition time makes the sequence more feasible in clinical routine (see below). Subtraction of precontrast from postcontrast images can always be considered to increase the vessel contrast-to-noise ratios, and the technique is particularly appealing with the ultrafast acquisition schemes where a constant level of breath-holding can be easily achieved or in anatomical regions that are not subjected to substantial motion.

There has so far not been renewed interest in contrast-enhanced, phase contrast images. The acquisition time of phase contrast imaging cannot be significantly shortened. A major problem is that dedicated phase-encoding gradients with a certain strength, duration, and time spacing have to be applied in between excitation pulse and signal read-out to induce the phase effects. These pulses determine the underlimits to the TE. The necessary echo time is so long that flow refocusing gradients remain mandatory, which further prolongs the TE. As a result, the TR is much longer than that which can be achieved with ultrafast gradient-echo techniques.

23.3 The Implementation of Fast Acquisitions

The most commonly used reconstruction method in MRI is based on the Fourier theorem. Using this technique, MR images are obtained after fast Fourier transform of the k-space data. This unique procedure is made possible by the use of a minimal number of magnetic field gradients. They are applied during the excitation pulse (to excite a specific slice or slab), during the signal read-out (to encode the columns in an image), and in between the excitation pulse and the signal read-out (to encode the rows in the image and, in the case of 3D MRI, also the planes). Every individual data point in the k-space has to be obtained after a unique combination of the magnetic field gradient durations. One echo read-out provides one row in the k-space.

An acquisition scheme of ultrafast contrast-enhanced MRA is not different from the schemes of conventional spin-echo measurements. The same number of gradients have to be applied and the same number of echoes have to be generated. However, instead of using slow magnetic field gradients with restricted amplitude, ultrafast acquisition schemes are fully demanding of the gradient system. Frequency and phase encoding are performed with strong and short gradients. The minimal TE that can be obtained depends on: (a) the time to encode the slices and refocus this magnetic field gradient, (b) the time to perform phase and through-plane encoding, and (c) the time to first dephase the spins with a gradient along the frequency-encoded direction and subsequently create the rephased echo (Fig. 23.8).

Techniques to further shorten the acquisition time follow the same basic rule: all k-space points have experienced a different amount of magnetic field gradients. Keyhole imaging further relies on the fact that the peripheral lines in the k-space are not very sensitive to variations caused by T1 and T2 differences. Excellent image quality can be obtained with the center of the k-space scanned during the passage of the bolus and the peripheral lines used from measurements at other time points. In practice, this means that the temporal resolution can be increased significantly, such that 3D slabs can be reconstructed every 2 s (Korosec et al. 1996). A limitation that will be overcome with future computer systems is the extremely long image reconstruction times for the 3D versions of this technique, due to the necessary data reordering. The use of powerful gradient systems is mandatory

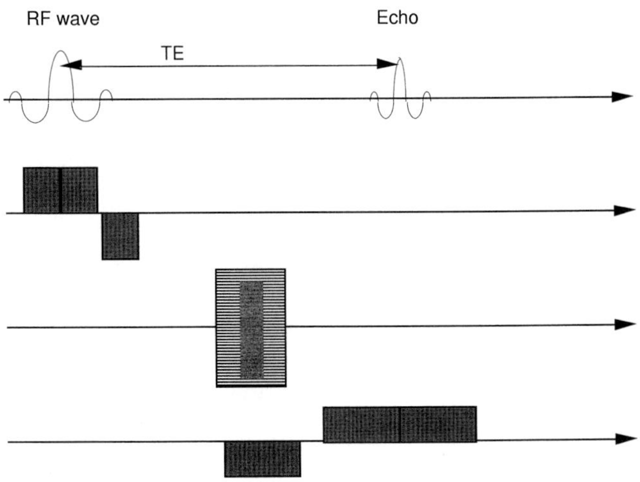

Fig. 23.8. Depiction of magnetic field gradients have to be applied during a measurement, irrespective of the type of acquisition

as all the different encodings still have to be performed within a time period that is as short as possible.

The scheme of techniques with longer echo trains for contrast-enhanced MRA is very similar to echo planar imaging (EPI) or fast spin-echo techniques. As long as each echo is differently encoded and the entire k-space is filled, images can be calculated. Since gradient-echo acquisitions are used, such images also require a fast gradient slew rate. Hence, it is well known from echo planar type acquisitions that slower echo trains are hampered by disturbing susceptibility-induced artifacts. In an animal experiment (Fig. 23.9), it was shown that the segmented 3D images have an improved T1 contrast, but suffer from increased dephasing effects. They are also markedly more sensitive to susceptibility effects. This limits their use in clinical practice. The same artifacts may be observed in MR angiograms acquired with related techniques and were confirmed in a study using EPI-based phase contrast images of the carotid arteries (Wildermuth et al. 1995). The potential of EPI-based techniques remains to be studied.

Postprocessing can further reduce the imaging time per pixel. Most algorithms fill in incompletely acquired k-spaces prior to image reconstruction. A well-known postprocessing technique is zero filling, which reduces the signal loss due to partial volume effects and increases the continuity of the vessels (Du et al. 1994). In practice, twice the number of partitions can be reconstructed from the same acquisition. This may improve the through-plane resolution, which is appreciated when the vessels are studied from different projective views (Fig. 23.10).

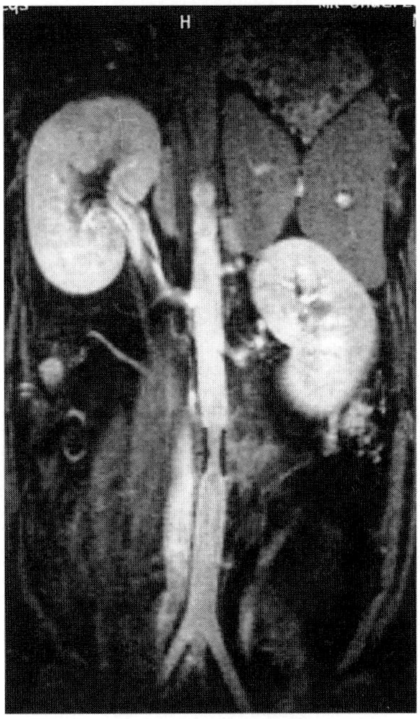

Fig. 23.9. Image acquired with a segmented gradient-echo sequence (echo train length 12, a fat suppression preparation pulse, 24 partitions, TR 41 ms, acquisition time only 17 s) showing an impressive T1-weighted contrast. The image was obtained 10 min after the injection of a contrast agent. The clinical value of this technique, however, remains uncertain due to the possible problems with susceptibility effects and an increased sensitivity for dephasing effects as seen on the stenosis of the left renal artery (*arrow*) in this dog

23.4 Optimization of Contrast-Enhanced MRA

In both time-of-flight and phase contrast acquisitions, image quality strongly depends on the flow in

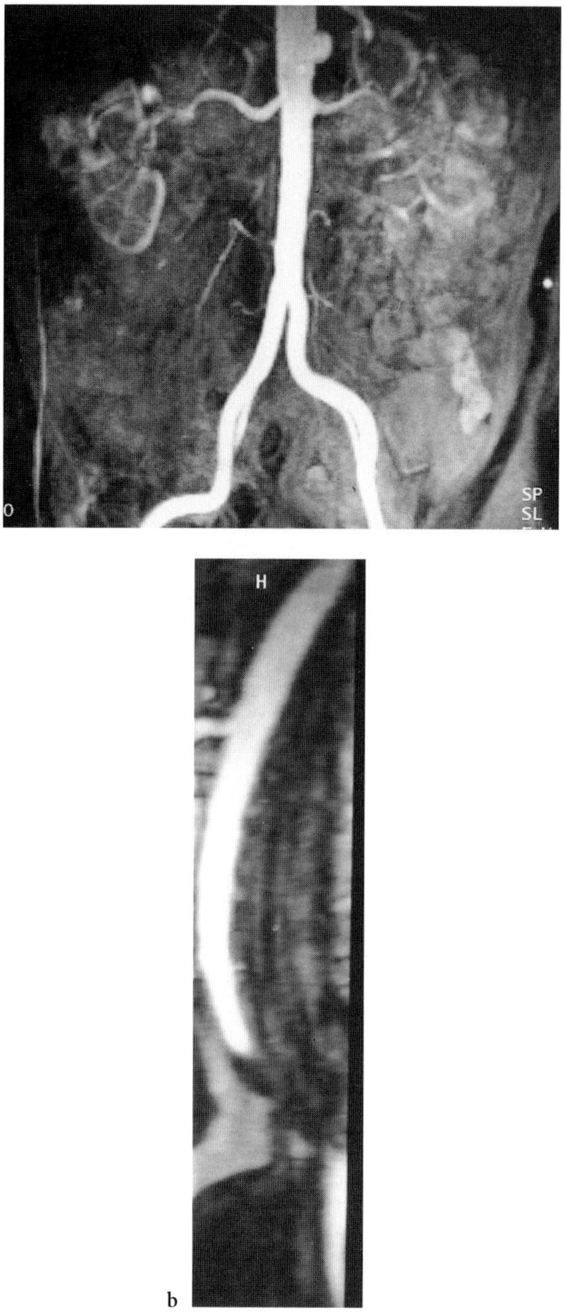

a

b

Fig. 23.10. The coronal projection (**a**) and sagittal reconstruction (**b**) are obtained from a data set acquired with a slice thickness of 5 mm (total acquisition time 7 s only), but after zero filling calculated with an effective slice thicknesses of 2.5 mm. The image resolution for the sagittal image is acceptable

the vessels and on the sequence parameters (Urchuk and Plewes 1992; Du et al. 1996). As stated above, a first requirement for time-of-flight MRA is a sufficient refreshment of the spins in the slice or slab, ensuring the inflow-related signal enhancement. The following sequence parameters can be set to maximally preserve this effect (Atkinson et al. 1994; Tkach et al. 1993):

- The slab orientation has to be perpendicular to the vessel.
- The use of multiple overlapping thin slabs, rather than one large 3D volume.
- A repetition time that is not too short, to reduce the number of pulses that the spins experience per transition through the volume.
- An echo time that is sufficiently short to decrease flow-induced dephasing and possibly fit to the opposed phase condition between water and fat (e.g., 7 ms on a 1.5-T system); flow rephasing gradients have to be applied.
- A flip angle that is not too large, to preserve the inflow-related signal enhancement after a large number of pulses, but that is nevertheless large enough to suppress the background tissue.
- Magnetization transfer pulses or fat suppression techniques to suppress the background tissue.
- Pixel sizes that are chosen as a function of the required image detail.
- In specific regions of the body, triggering of the acquisitions to the ECG cycle in order to catch the blood in the optimal cardiac phase (e.g., to the systolic phase when inflow is required or to the diastolic phase to reduce flow-induced artifacts).

In phase contrast imaging, the inflow effect is only of secondary importance. Determining parameters for this type of imaging are:

- The VENC (which is an estimate of the average velocity in the vessels, in order to adequately dephase the flowing spins)
- The image resolution, which has a strong influence on the total acquisition time
- As with time-of-flight techniques, triggering of the acquisition to the ECG, or, alternatively, use of a different VENC over the cardiac cycle

Many of the above optimizations are not necessary with ultrafast contrast-enhanced MRA. Slab orientations can be set arbitrarily, have an arbitrary thickness, and therefore in practice include a maximal vessel segment. Repetition time and echo time have to be as short as possible. From Ernst angle calculations, optimal flip angles can be smaller than with plain time-of-flight techniques and much smaller than those for contrast-enhanced 5-min acquisitions in the brain (Bosmans et al. 1995a). Prepulses are not applied, as they would currently at least double the acquisition time.

The optimal protocol, however, has not yet been proposed, as new factors have an influence on image

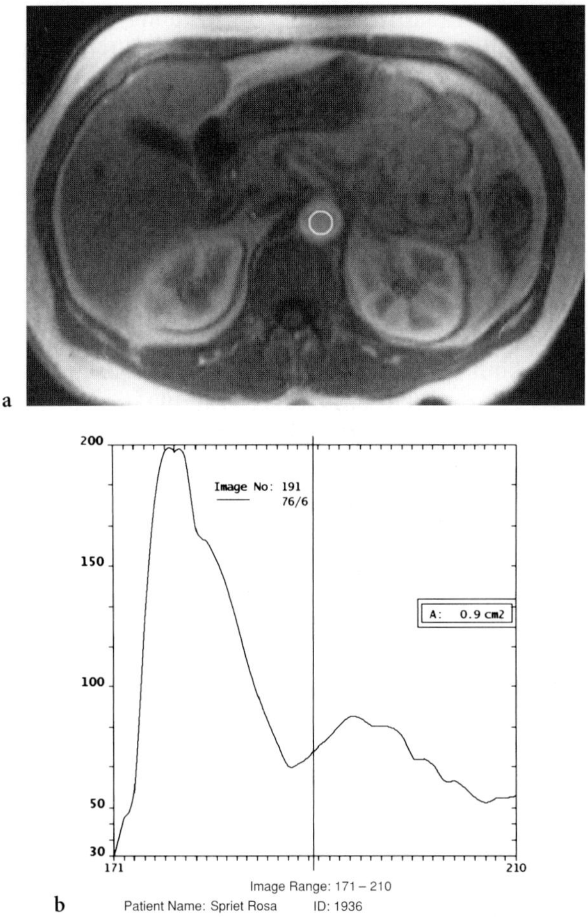

Fig. 23.11. **a** Typical 1-s turboFLASH acquisition used during the test bolus. The plot in **b** shows the signal intensities in the aorta as a function of time, allowing the calculation of the bolus arrival time

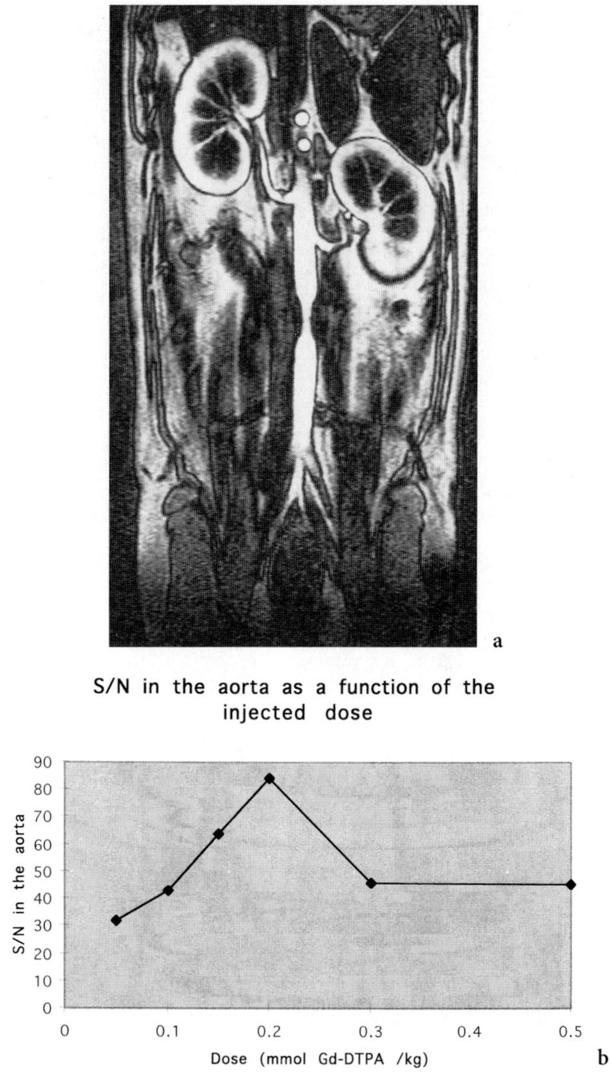

Fig. 23.12. **a** Fast MR angiogram of the abdominal vessels in a dog, using a dose of 0.1 mmol/kg Gd-DOTA (TR/TE/FL 5 ms/2 ms/30°, high resolution, 8 partitions, bandwidth 390 Hz/pixel, acquisition time 10 s). **b** A comparative study shows an optimal contrast-to-noise ratio in the aorta at a dose of 0.2 mmol/kg

quality. Whereas the acquisition has to be short, it is not clear how short it should be. As with other MRI techniques, a trade-off exists between measurement time and image resolution. The following factors would have to be considered:

- Is there a need for an acquisition during breath-hold? How detrimental is an incomplete breath-hold?
- Which image resolution is required for a particular vessel?
- Is it necessary to visualize arteries without the slightest venous overlap?
- Is interpolation or zero filling in the k-space acceptable to improve image resolution?
- Can a high-resolution acquisition be performed at the cost of a slightly longer echo time and repetition time?

Another aspect under investigation is the scheme of contrast injection. The arrival of the test bolus in the artery under study can be timed with a so-called test bolus acquisition (Earls et al. 1996). This is usually a fast T1-weighted MRI technique, performed during the injection of a small amount of contrast agent (e.g., 2 ml), and provides a cross sectional image of the vessel every second (Fig. 23.11). The following aspects are currently being studied by several groups:

- Which total dose is optimal? What is the success rate when using only small doses? In Fig. 23.12, different doses are compared in an animal study using a 10-s 3D MRA technique (TR/TE 5.9 ms/

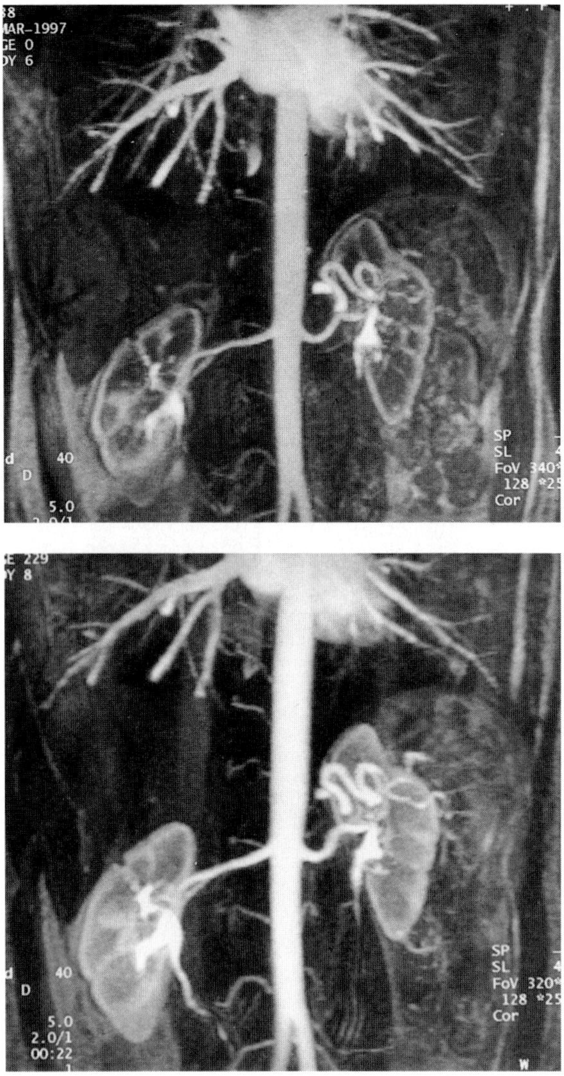

a

b

Fig. 23.13 a,b. Angiograms in a normal volunteer obtained using the same amount of injected contrast agent but with a different bolus duration. In **a** the duration was 8.8 s and in **b**, 4.4 s. A test bolus acquisition was performed prior to the measurement to ensure a bolus well centered around the scanning of the center of k-space. Using a faster injection rate, the vessel contrast-to-noise ratio in the aorta increased from 43 to 50

2.4 ms, 8 partitions). The optimal dose was found to be 0.2 mmol/kg.

- At which rate should the dose be injected? A first investigation is reported in STROUSE et al. (1996). The state that the dose injection rate can be a determining parameter. Figure 23.13 shows the difference between an injection during an 8.8-s and a 4.4-s bolus in the same volunteer after a test bolus acquisition. This preliminary study shows a clear preference for a high injection rate.
- When should the bolus arrive?

Considerable work needs to be done on these topics, as the optimal solutions can even differ from technique to technique. It may very well be that the optimal dose for a 7-s acquisition is different from that of a 20-s session or that acquisitions with higher resolution require increased doses.

Finally, the images have to be inspected for image artifacts. High slew rates are used which increase the risk of zipper artifacts and spikes. More typical artifacts are related to the sudden passage of a bolus when scanning the central k-space lines and show up as a kind of ghost artifact in the phase-encoding direction (MAKI et al. 1996; ITO et al. 1997). After the injection of a contrast agent, these artifacts become more visible due to the large signal-to-noise ratios in the vessels.

23.5 Current Clinical Applications of Contrast-Enhanced MRA

The first studies to use contrast-enhanced time-of-flight MRA mainly focused on intracranial applications. This is not surprising since other regions under study with time-of-flight or phase contrast techniques benefitted less from contrast enhancement. For example, the vessel contrast-to-noise ratios of carotid arteries decreased because of the contrast agent uptake in soft tissues and the venous overlap. The same problems also applied for abdominal and peripheral vessels. Contrast-enhanced time-of-flight acquisitions of the intracranial vessels improve the detection and the visualization of venous anomalies, and the evaluation of sinus thrombosis and the venous drainage in arteriovenous malformations (MARCHAL et al. 1990; RUNGE et al. 1993). The visualization of arteries is not significantly improved (JUNG et al. 1995). In patients with intracranial aneurysms, the presence of stagnant flow or the reduced flow distal to an aneurysm can be better appreciated (BOSMANS et al. 1995b). Whenever the arterial intracranial system has to be evaluated, however, a contrast-enhanced acquisition should never be applied as the technique of choice since the veins and the plexus choroideus also enhance after a contrast injection and superimpose, for instance, on the arteries of the circle of Willis.

Another indication for contrast-enhanced time-of-flight MRA is the visualization of brain tumors with their feeding and draining vessels. An evaluation of contrast-enhanced time-of-flight acquisitions showed that most large vessels could be very well visualized but smaller arteries were not appropriately seen (WILMS et al. 1993).

The new ultrafast acquisitions are just very fast and poorly T1-weighted acquisitions. Before they recently became available, many authors combined contrast injections with more conventional T1-weighted acquisitions. SIVANANTHAN et al. (1993) used a T1-weighted 2D turboFLASH method to assess the arterial anatomy in patients with advanced atherosclerotic aortoiliac disease. This MRA technique accurately detected all aortic occlusions, their sites and extent. All iliac occlusions were also correctly identified. The stenoses were seen, but often overgraded, probably due to an echo time that was too long, in the absence of refocusing gradients. The 3D version of this technique has also been used for imaging of the portal venous system (YAMASHITA et al. 1996). Pulmonary vessels were studied with a routine contrast-enhanced T1-weighted (non-inflow-related) technique by LOUBEYRE et al. (1994). They exploited a multiplanar T1-weighted dynamic acquisition to image pulmonary emboli and concluded that the technique was appropriate for thrombi in the proximal portions of the pulmonary arteries but not for detecting more peripheral ones. A similar technique was used by LAISSY et al. (1995), showing that the association of segmented gradient-echo images and contrast-enhanced turboFLASH images can provide information on normal and diseased pulmonary arteries within the mediastinum until the subsegmental branches. PRINCE et al. (1996) applied a 3- to 5-min contrast-enhanced time-of-flight MRA technique without breath-holding. Aortic dissection, coarctation, and aneurysms could be correctly assessed.

The real breakthrough of contrast-enhanced MRA came with the introduction of the ultrafast acquisition schemes that were easier to use and required less cooperation from the patient. They were first applied for abdominal MRA, including renal and mesenteric arteries.

For carotid and intracranial arteries, correct timing of the acquisition is a prerequisite. In practice, this protocol is also quite robust (LEVY and PRINCE 1996). A typical result is shown in Fig. 23.14.

Aortoiliac inflow was evaluated by SNIDOW et al. (1996b). Sensitivity and specificity for obstructive lesions were, respectively, 100% and 100% for the aorta, 100% and 98% for the common iliac arteries, 100% and 89% for the external iliac arteries, 100% and 89% for the main renal arteries, and 100% and 62% for the accessory renal arteries. The low resolution limited the evaluation of the small renal arteries. HOLLAND et al. (1996) claimed that when using both a 2D time-of-flight and a contrast-enhanced ultrafast MRA acquisition, stenotic segments or occlusions of renal, celiac, superior mesenteric, and inferior mesenteric arteries can be accurately defined and graded. Similar results were obtained using an ultrafast segmented contrast-enhanced MRA acquisition scheme (DOUEK et al. 1995).

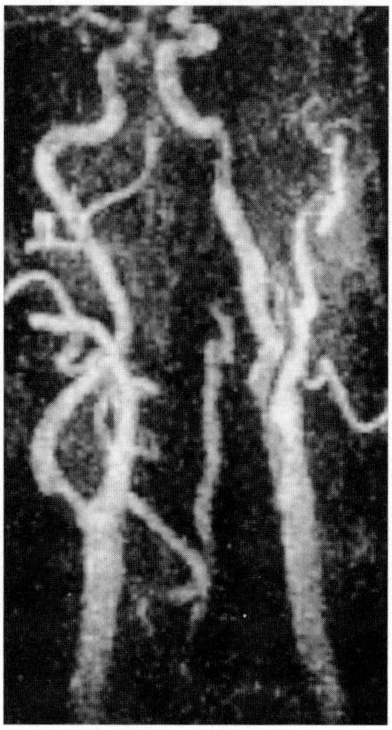

Fig. 23.14. This example shows an ultrafast contrast-enhanced acquisition of the carotid arteries (TR/TE/Fl 4.2 ms/1.7 ms/30° total acquisition time 25 s). The image shows a moderate- to high-grade stenosis of the ostium of the right internal carotid artery

The larger thoracic vessels have also been studied with ultrafast contrast-enhanced MRA. Image quality is also excellent, notwithstanding the difficult flow conditions and sources of motion artifacts in this region. PRINCE et al. (1996) and KRINSKY et al. (1997) showed that ultrafast MRA is an accurate imaging modality in the diagnosis of thoracic aortic disease. The latter study showed a sensitivity of 92% and specificity of 100% for acute and chronic aortic dissection and was as useful as conventional MRI for diagnosis of aneurysms and arch vessel disease.

VRACHLIOTIS et al. (1997) applied a related technique to evaluate the patency of coronary artery bypass grafts and found good agreement with coronary angiography.

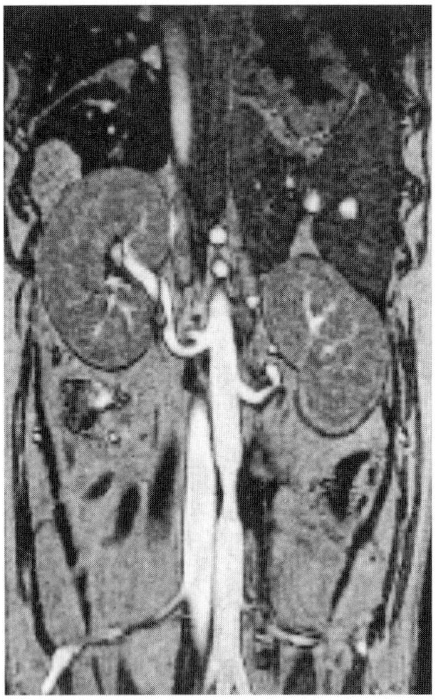

Fig. 23.15. This image was obtained 5 min after the injection of AMI-227, in the same animal model as in Figs. 23.9, 23.12, and 23.17 (dose of 40 μmol/kg). Acquisitions up to 20 min after the injection show no major differences. Even 30 min after the injection there was still an impressive contrast enhancement in the vessels. Arteries and veins enhance equally well

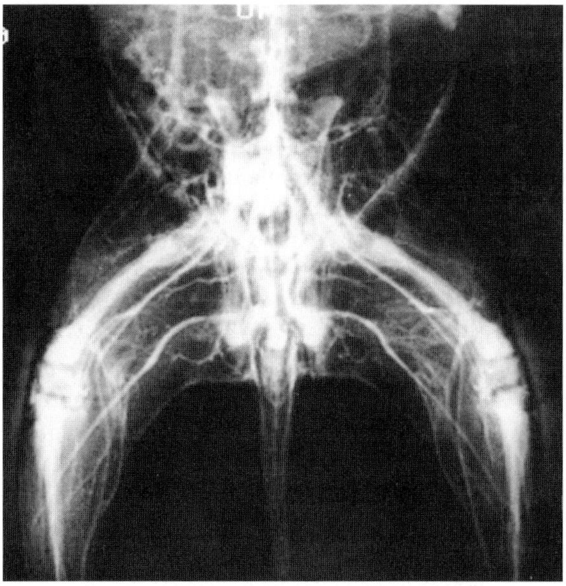

Fig. 23.16. This projective MR angiogram of a rabbit was obtained after a high dose of Gd-DTPA-polylysine using a technique that suppressed the fat and all other tissues with longer T1

23.6 The Use of Blood Pool Agents for Contrast-Enhanced MRA

Blood pool agents for MRI can be categorized into two classes: ultrasmall ferrite particles, on the one hand, and large polymers, on the other. Both are characterized by different pharmacological or toxicological properties. In this section we restrict the discussion to the use of these agents for MRA purposes.

Blood pool agents remain in the blood for a significantly longer time than do regular contrast agents and the uptake in the tissues is limited. These characteristics can be used to solve certain shortcomings of currently used contrast agents. First, compared with currently available nonspecific agents, blood pool agents permit images to be acquired during a longer period after injection of the agent. This feature can be advantageous to repeat certain measurements or to acquire images in different regions of the body without the need to inject a new bolus of contrast agent. The time window that is available depends on the specific agent. In Fig. 23.15, an example is shown of an ultrafast contrast-enhanced MRA acquisition 5 min after the injection of 40 μmol of AMI-227 (Guerbet, France). A (small!) drop in image quality was observed between the first and the second acquisition after the injection of the contrast agent. The image quality then remained nearly identical for about half an hour. In dedicated applications, the use of these agents would enable MR angiograms to be obtained at any time during, for example, an interventional angiographic procedure.

The reduced uptake in the soft tissues increases the vessel to background contrast-to-noise ratio. This feature could be beneficial for the visualization of abdominal or carotid arteries. It must be stressed, however, that the relatively high concentration of contrast agents in the veins counteracts this potential benefit. On the other hand, it is a good method to visualize the veins.

Other applications for blood pool agents would be dose reductions, achieved due to stronger relaxation characteristics (Bogdanov et al. 1993; Vogl et al. 1996; Mayo-Smith et al. 1996; Loubeyre et al. 1996b) or further shortened T1 values. In our earlier work (Marchal et al. 1991), Gd-DTPA-polylysine was used with MRA techniques that relied on the extremely short T1 of the blood. In Fig. 23.16 we show an example of an acquisition in a rabbit using two preparation pulses, one to suppress the soft tissues and one to suppress the fat, followed by a flow-compensated spin-echo read-out. With the regular

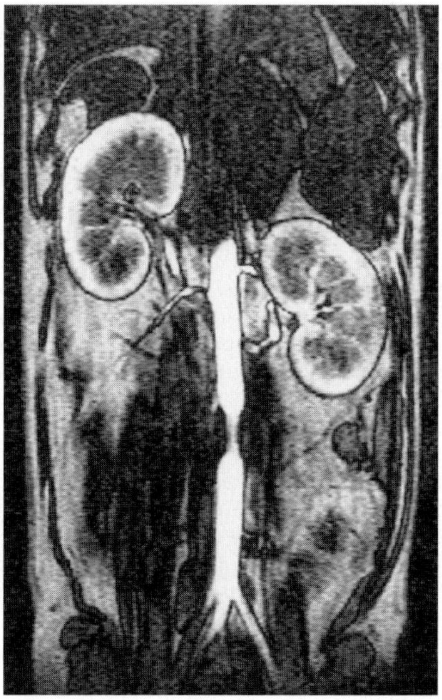

Fig. 23.17. MR angiogram in a dog model obtained with an ultrafast MRA technique during intra-arterial delivery of 0.01 mmol/kg Gd-DOTA

Gd-chelates we could never obtain similar MR angiograms.

23.7 Future Perspectives

MRA and, more precisely, contrast-enhanced MRA is rapidly gaining acceptance in clinical routine. The technique is quite robust and ultrafast. Currently, most centers are evaluating these techniques for diagnostic or screening purposes. In the meantime, in new dedicated open MR systems the first steps are being taken in the direction of interventional MR procedures and the necessary instruments are being developed. Using MR-compatible catheters and ever shorter acquisition schemes to guide the placement of the catheters and to acquire MR angiograms, interventional MR angiography procedures may become a reality in the future. In Fig. 23.17, an MR angiogram of a dog is shown. It was obtained with a fairly conventional 10-s acquisition sequence and an intra-arterially injected dose of Gd-DTPA as low as 0.01 mmol/kg.

Acknowledgements. We would like to express our gratitude to a number of persons for their assistance in the areas specified: experimental work in animals: Prof. Dr. Y. Ni, Dr. Y. Miao, and Dr. F. Raat; neuro-MRA applications: Prof. Dr. P. Demaerel and Prof. Dr. G. Wilms; abdominal MRA applications: Prof. Dr. L. Van Hoe and Dr. T. Dejaegere; thoracic MRA applications: Prof. Dr. J. Bogaert and Dr. S. Dymarkowski.

References

Atkinson D, Brant-Zawadzki M, Gillan G, Purdy D, Laub G (1994) Improved MR angiography: magnetization transfer suppression with variable flip angle excitation and increased resolution. Radiology 190:890–894

Bass JC, Prince MR, Londy FJ, Chenevert TL (1997) Effect of gadolinium on phase-contrast MR angiography of the renal arteries. AJR 168:261–266

Bogdanov AA Jr, Weissleder R, Frank HW, Bogdanova AV, Nossif N, Schaffer BK (1993) A new macromolecule as a contrast agent for MR angiography: preparation, properties and animal studies. Radiology 187:701–706

Bosmans H, Marchal G, Lukito G, Ni Y, Wilms G, Laub G, Baert AL (1995a) Time-of-flight MR angiography of the brain: comparison of acquisition techniques in healthy volunteers. AJR 164:161–167

Bosmans H, Wilms G, Marchal G, Demaerel P, Baert AL (1995b) Characterisation of intracranial aneurysms with MR angiography. Neuroradiology 37:262–266

Cloft HJ, Murphy KJ, Prince MR, Brunberg JA (1996) 3D gadolinium-enhanced MR angiography of the carotid arteries. Magn Reson Imaging 14:593–600

Cortell ED, Kaufman JA, Geller SC, Cambria RP, Rivitz SM, Waltman AC (1996) MR angiography of tibial runoff vessels: imaging with the head coil compared with conventional arteriography. AJR 167:147–151

de Haan MW, Kouwenhoven M, Thelissen RP, Koster D, Kessels AG, de Leeuw PW, van Engelshoven JM (1996) Renovascular disease in patients with hypertension: detection with systolic and diastolic gating in three-dimensional phase-contrast MR angiography. Radiology 198:449–456

Douek PC, Revel D, Chazel S, Falise B, Villard J, Amiel M (1995) Fast MR angiography of the aortoiliac arteries and arteries of the lower extremities: value of bolus-enhanced whole-volume subtraction technique. AJR 165:431–437

Du YP, Parker DL, Davis WL, Cao G (1994) Reduction of partial volume artifacts with zero-filled interpolation in three-dimensional MR angiography. J Magn Reson Imaging 4:733–741

Du YP, Parker DL, Davis WL, Cao G, Buswell HR, Goodrich KC (1996) Experimental and theoretical studies of vessel contrast-to-noise ratio in intracranial time-of-flight MR angiography. J Magn Reson Imaging 6:99–108

Duerinckx AJ (1997) MRI of coronary arteries. Int J Card Imaging 13:191–197

Earls JP, Rofsky NM, DeCorato DR, Krinsky GA, Weinreb JC (1996) Breath-hold single-dose gadolinium-enhanced three-dimensional MR aortography: usefulness of a timing examination and MR power injector. Radiology 201:705–710

Foo TK, Saranathan M, Prince MR, Chenevert TL (1997) Automated detection of bolus arrival and initiation of data acquisition in fast, three-dimensional, gadolinium-enhanced MR angiography. Radiology 203:275–280

Furst G, Hofer M, Steinmetz H, et al. (1996) Intracranial stenoocclusive disease: MR angiography with magnetization transfer and variable flip angle. Am J Neuroradiol 17:1749–1757

Gelbert F, Guichard JP, Mourier KL, et al. (1992) Phase-contrast MR angiography of vascular malformations of the spinal cord at 0.5T. J Magn Reson Imaging 2:631–636

Hara AK, Burkart DJ, Johnson CD, Ehman RL, Ilstrup DM (1996) Abdominal phase-contrast MR angiography: breath-hold versus non-breath-hold techniques. J Magn Reson Imaging 6:94–98

Holland GA, Dougherty L, Carpenter JP, et al. (1996) Breath-hold ultrafast three-dimensional gadolinium-enhanced MR angiography of the aorta and the renal and other visceral abdominal arteries. AJR 166:971–981

Ito K, Kato J, Okada S, Kumazaki T (1997) K-space filter effect in three-dimensional contrast MR angiography. Acta Radiol 38:173–175

Jung HW, Chang KH, Choi DS, Han MH, Han MC (1995) Contrast-enhanced MR angiography for the diagnosis of intracranial vascular disease: optimal dose of gadopentetate dimeglumine. AJR 165:1251–1255

Kallmes DF, Omary RA, Dix JE, Evans AJ, Hillman BJ (1996) Specificity of MR angiography as a confirmatory test of carotid artery stenosis. Am J Neuroradiol 17:1501–1506

Korosec FR, Frayne R, Grist TM, Mistretta CA (1996) Time-resolved contrast-enhanced 3D MR angiography. Magn Reson Med 36:345–351

Krinsky GA, Rofsky NM, DeCorato DR, et al. (1997) Thoracic aorta: comparison of gadolinium-enhanced three-dimensional MR angiography with conventional MR imaging. Radiology 202:183–193

Laissy JP, Bancal C, Sekkal S, et al. (1995) Pulmonary MR angiography at 1.0 T: early results with k-space segmented and post-contrast TurboFLASH two-dimensional time-of-flight sequences. Eur J Radiol 20:9–15

Levy RA, Prince MR (1996) Arterial-phase three-dimensional contrast-enhanced MR angiography of the carotid arteries. AJR 167:211–215

Li D, Haacke EM, Mugler JP-3rd, Berr S, Brookeman JR, Hutton MC (1994) Three-dimensional time-of-flight MR angiography using selective inversion recovery RAGE with fat saturation and ECG-triggering: application to renal arteries. Magn Reson Med 31:414–422

Li D, Kaushikkar S, Haacke EM, et al. (1996) Coronary arteries: three-dimensional MR imaging with retrospective respiratory gating. Radiology 201:857–863

Loubeyre P, Revel D, Douek P, Delignette A, Baldy C, Genin G, Amiel M (1994) Dynamic contrast enhanced MR angiography of pulmonary embolism: comparison with pulmonary angiography. AJR 162:1035–1039

Loubeyre P, Trolliet P, Cahen R, Grozel F, Labeeuw M, Minh VA (1996a) MR angiography of renal artery stenosis: value of the combination of three-dimensional time-of-flight and three-dimensional phase-contrast MR angiography sequences. AJR 167:489–494

Loubeyre P, Canet E, Zhao S, Benderbous S, Amiel M, Revel D (1996b) Carboxymethyl-dextran-gadolinium-DTPA as a blood-pool contrast agent for magnetic resonance angiography. Experimental study in rabbits. Invest Radiol 31:288–293

Maki JH, Prince MR, Londy FJ, Chenevert TL (1996) The effects of time varying intravascular signal intensity and k-space acquisition order on three-dimensional MR angiography image quality. J Magn Reson Imaging 6:642–651

Marchal G, Bosmans H, Van Fraeyenhoven L, Wilms G, Van Hecke P, Plets C, Baert AL (1990) Intracranial vascular lesions: optimization and clinical evaluation of three-dimensional time-of-flight MR angiography. Radiology 175:443–448

Marchal G, Bosmans H, Van Hecke P, Jiang Y, Aerts P, Bauer H (1991) Experimental Gd-DTPA polylysine enhanced MR angiography: sequence optimization. J Comput Assist Tomogr 15:711–715

Marchal G, Michiels J, Bosmans H, Van Hecke P (1992) Contrast-enhanced MRA of the brain. J Comput Assist Tomogr 16:25–29

Mascalchi M, Bianchi MC, Quilici N, Mangiafico S, Ferrito G, Padolecchia R, Bartolozzi C (1995) MR angiography of spinal vascular malformations. AJNR 16:289–297

Mayo-Smith WW, Saini S, Slater G, Kaufman JA, Sharma P, Hahn PF (1996) MR contrast material for vascular enhancement: value of superparamagnetic iron oxide. AJR 166:73–77

McConnell MV, Khasgiwala VC, Savord BJ, Chen MH, Chuang ML, Manning WJ, Edelman RR (1997) Prospective adaptive navigator correction for breath-hold MR coronary angiography. Magn Reson Med 37:148–152

McLachlan SJ, Francisco JC, Pernicone JR, Hasso AN (1994) Efficacy evaluation of gadoteridol for MR angiography of intracranial vascular lesions. J Magn Reson Imaging 4:405–411

Nghiem HV, Winter TC 3rd, Mountford MC, et al. (1995) Evaluation of the portal venous system before liver transplantation: value of phase-contrast MR angiography. AJR 164:871–878

Nghiem HV, Winter TC, Schmiedl UP, Freeny PC (1996) MR angiography of the portal venous system. Semin Ultrasound CT MR 17:360–373

Oshinski JN, Hofland L, Mukundan S Jr, Dixon WT, Parks WJ, Pettigrew RI (1996) Two-dimensional coronary MR angiography without breath holding. Radiology 201:737–743

Pernicone JR, Siebert JE, Potchen EJ (1990) Three dimensional phase-contrast MR angiography in the head and neck: preliminary report. AJR 155:167–176

Prince MR, Yucel EK, Kaufman JA, Harrison DC, Geller SC (1993) Dynamic gadolinium-enhanced three-dimensional abdominal MR arteriography. J Magn Reson Imaging 3:877–881

Prince MR, Narasimham DL, Stanley JC, Chenevert TL, Williams DM, Marx MV, Cho KJ (1995) Breath-hold gadolinium-enhanced MR angiography of the abdominal aorta and its major branches. Radiology 197:785–792

Prince MR, Narasimham DL, Jacoby WT, Williams DM, Cho KJ, Marx MV, Deeb GM (1996) Three-dimensional gadolinium-enhanced MR angiography of the thoracic aorta. AJR 166:1387–1397

Prince MR, Chenevert TL, Foo TK, Londy FJ, Ward JS, Maki JH (1997) Contrast-enhanced abdominal MR angiography: optimization of imaging delay time by automating the detection of contrast material arrival in the aorta. Radiology 203:109–114

Runge VM, Kirsch JE, Lee C (1993) Contrast enhanced MR angiography. J Magn Reson Imaging 3:233–239

Schmiedl UP, Yuan C, Nghiem HV, Winter TC, Freeny PC (1996) MR angiography of the peripheral vasculature. Semin Ultrasound CT MR 17:404–411

Silverman JM, Friedman ML, Van Allan RJ (1996) Detection of main renal artery stenosis using phase contrast cine MR angiography. AJR 166:1131–1137

Sivananthan UM, Ridgway JP, Bann K, Verma SP, Cullingworth J, Ward J, Rees MR (1993) Fast magnetic resonance angiography using turbo-FLASH sequences in advanced aortoiliac disease. Br J Radiol 66:1103–1110

Snidow JJ, Harris VJ, Johnson MS, Cikrit DF, Lalka SG, Sawchuk AP, Trerotola SO (1996a) Iliac artery evaluation

with two-dimensional time-of-flight MR angiography: update. J Vasc Interv Radiol 7:213–220
Snidow JJ, Johnson MS, Harris VJ, et al. (1996b) Three-dimensional gadolinium-enhanced MR angiography for aortoiliac inflow assessment plus renal artery screening in a single breath hold. Radiology 198:725–732
Stock KW, Wetzel S, Kirsch E, Bongartz G, Steinbrich W, Radue EW (1996) Anatomic evaluation of the circle of Willis: MR angiography versus intraarterial digital subtraction angiography. AJNR 17:1495–1499
Strouse PJ, Prince MR, Chenevert TL (1996) Effect of the rate of gadopentetate dimeglumine administration on abdominal vascular and soft-tissue MR imaging enhancement patterns. Radiology 201:809–816
Swan JS, Grist TM, Weber DM, Sproat IA, Wojtowycz MM (1994) MR angiography of the pelvis with variable velocity encoding and a phased-array coil. Radiology 190:363–369
Talagala SL, Jungreis CA, Kanal E, Meyers SP, Foo TK, Rubin RA, Applegate GR (1995) Fast three-dimensional time-of-flight MR angiography of the intra-cranial vasculature. J Magn Reson Imaging 5:317–323
Tkach JA, Ruggieri PM, Ross JS, Modic MT, Dillinger JJ, Masaryk TJ (1993) Pulse sequence strategies for vascular contrast in time-of-flight carotid MR angiography. J Magn Reson Imaging 3:811–820
Urchuk SN, Plewes DB (1992) Mechanisms of flow-induced signal loss in MR angiography. J Magn Reson Imaging 2:453–462
Vogl TJ, Hoffmann Y, Juergens M, Weinmann HJ, Muhler A, Yucel S, Felix R (1996) Experimental evaluation of contrast medium enhanced high resolution MR angiography in the animal model. Gd-DTPA compared with Gd-DTPA-Polylysine. Radiologe 36:254–262
Vrachliotis TG, Bis KG, Aliabadi D, Shetty AN, Safian R, Simonetti O (1997) Contrast-enhanced breath-hold MR angiography for evaluating patency of coronary artery bypass grafts. AJR 168:1073–1080
Wang Y, Rossman PJ, Grimm RC, Wilman AH, Riederer SJ, Ehman RL (1996) 3D MR angiography of pulmonary arteries using real-time navigator gating and magnetization preparation. Magn Reson Med 36:579–587
Wasser MN, Westenberg J, van der Hulst VP, van Baalen J, van Bockel JH, van Erkel AR, Pattynama PM (1997) Hemodynamic significance of renal artery stenosis: digital subtraction angiography versus systolically gated three-dimensional phase-contrast MR angiography. Radiology 202:333–338
Wielopolski PA, Adamis M, Prasad P, Gaa J, Edelman R (1995) Breath-hold 3D STAR MR angiography of the renal arteries using segmented echo planar imaging. Magn Reson Med 33:432–438
Wildermuth S, Debatin JF, Huisman TA, Leung DA, McKinnon GC (1995) 3D phase contrast EPI MR angiography of the carotid arteries. J Comput Assist Tomogr 19:871–878
Wilms G, Bosmans H, Marchal G, Demaerel P, Goffin J, Plets C, Baert AL (1993) Magnetic resonance angiography of supratentorial tumours: comparison with selective digital subtraction angiography. Neuroradiology 37:42–47
Yamashita Y, Mitsuzaki K, Miyazaki T, et al. (1996) Gadolinium-enhanced breath-hold three-dimensional MR angiography of the portal vein: value of magnetization-prepared rapid acquisition gradient-echo sequence. Radiology 201:283–288
Yucel EK, Silver MS, Carter AP (1994) MR angiography of normal pelvic arteries: comparison of signal intensity and contrast-to-noise ratio for three different inflow techniques. AJR 163:197–201

24 Dynamic Contrast-Enhanced Magnetic Resonance Imaging and Image Processing

G. TORHEIM and P.A. RINCK

CONTENTS

24.1 Introduction

Magnetic resonance (MR) images of the same slice through the human body taken at set time intervals before and after the administration of a contrast agent are commonly described as "dynamic" images. These dynamic images follow the passage of the contrast agent through the human body and allow the discrimination of different uptake patterns in different tissues or lesions.

However, the individual images of a dynamic time series will, in some cases, not yield all information contained in them. Thus, the combination of dynamic MR imaging and of mathematical image manipulation has attracted many researchers to try and highlight anatomical and pathological structures and processes which, per se, are invisible on single plain or single enhanced images. This chapter gives an overview of some of the techniques which combine the mathematical power of computers with the biophysical power of contrast agents. It also shows that dynamic MR imaging is a modality with an enormous potential, but also replete with pitfalls.

This description cannot be exhaustive given the wide spectrum of the field. For the basics of image processing we refer to standard textbooks of general image processing methods (e.g., GONZALES and WINTZ 1987; RUSS 1995), and for the basics of MR contrast agents to RINCK (1995), RINCK and MULLER (1998), and WATSON et al. (1992).

For some clinical applications of dynamic imaging we refer to the contributions by PAVONE (liver and pancreas), LOMBARDI (heart), KRESTIN (kidneys and adrenals) RINCK (musculoskeletal system), and MARCHAL (angiography) in this volume.

In addition, we refer to the following publications, listed according to subject area: overviews of all dynamic applications (BARENTSZ et al. 1995; RINCK 1995; RINCK and MYHR 1998; VILLA et al. 1995); bladder (KIM et al. 1994); brain (GOWLAND et al. 1992; KORNMESSER et al. 1986; ROSEN et al. 1990, 1991; VILLRINGER et al. 1988); breast (BOETES et al. 1994; FLICKINGER et al. 1993; GRIBBESTAD et al. 1994; HAYTON et al. 1996; HEYWANG-KÖBRUNNER and BECK 1995; KAISER 1990; KNOPP et al. 1996; MÜLLER-SCHIMPFLE et al. 1997; STACK et al. 1990; TOFTS et al. 1995); heart (EICHENBERGER et al. 1994; HIGGINS and SAKUMA 1996; LOMBARDI et al. 1997; WILKE et al. 1994); kidneys (KRESTIN 1994; VON SCHULTHESS et al. 1991); liver (MARTÍ-BONMATÍ et al. 1994); musculoskeletal applications (ERLEMANN et al. 1989; VERSTRAETE et al. 1994, 1996).

In this chapter we will focus our attention on the particular combination of computer algorithms and contrast studies and discuss image processing methods of dynamic contrast-enhanced MR images step by step. Although we concentrate on the postprocessing phase, we emphasize that postprocessing methods and parameters should always be selected on the basis of the image acquisition protocol.

G. TORHEIM, MS, MR-Center, Medical Section, University of Trondheim, Trondheim, Norway and NMR Laboratory, Medical Imaging Processing Group, Faculty of Medicine and Pharmacy, University of Mons-Hainaut; 24, Avenue du Champ de Mars, B-7000 Mons, Belgium
P.A. RINCK, MD, PhD, Professor of Diagnostic Imaging, NMR Laboratory, Medical Image Processing Group, Faculty of Medicine and Pharmacy, University of Mons-Hainaut; 24, Avenue du Champ de Mars, B-7000 Mons, Belgium and Centre Hospitalier Princesse Grace, Magnetic Resonance Unit, Avenue Pasteur, BP No. 489, MC-98012 Monte Carlo Cedex, Monaco

Some Fundamentals. In the early days of MR contrast agents, one would typically acquire one precontrast and one postcontrast image with a spin-echo pulse sequence and visually compare the two images. Postprocessing by computers was usually limited to creating a subtraction image, subtracting on a pixel-by-pixel basis (Fig. 24.1).

By acquiring a series of images while the contrast agent passes through the body, one can create curves describing their signal intensity as a function of time. This simple observation is the basis for the added information value of dynamic contrast-enhanced MR studies.

In general, the entire dynamic acquisition and image processing procedure consists of the following steps:

1. Acquisition of a time series of images before and after the contrast agent is administered
2. Noise filtering of the acquired images (optional)
3. Motion correction (optional)
4. Definition of time-intensity curves
5. Processing of time-intensity curves
6. Presentation of the data

The noise filtering and motion correction steps are optional but in many instances necessary and fairly complicated.

a,b

c

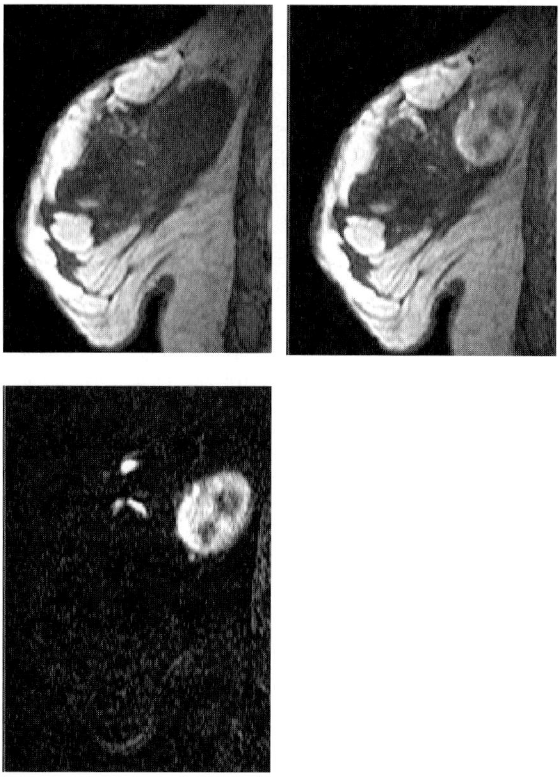

Fig. 24.1a–c. Image subtraction applied to contrast-enhanced breast images. A gadolinium-based ECF was injected. **a** Precontrast image; **b** Postcontrast image, approximately 50 s after injection; **c** subtraction image. Negative intensity values were set to zero. Processed and visualized by the software program Dynalize 1.0. (Images courtesy of Dr. Kjell-Arne Kvistad, MR-Center, Medical Section, Trondheim, Norway)

24.2 Acquisition of Dynamic Contrast-Enhanced MR Images

The chosen pulse sequence and pulse sequence parameters (including field of view, slice thickness, etc.), the type of contrast agent (e.g., extracellular fluid space or blood pool agent; relaxation and/or susceptibility agent), the manner of administration of the contrast agent (injection site; bolus or infusion), and the concentration of contrast agent are all important factors which influence the contrast in the images and/or temporal intensity change. Therefore, they also influence the selection of postprocessing techniques and parameters.

The strength of the magnetic field and the concentration of the contrast agent are important factors modulating the contrast change after the administration of a contrast agent (Rinck et al. 1988; Rinck and Muller 1998). For instance, a high concentration of a gadolinium-based extracellular fluid (ECF) space agent can lead to strong T2* effects in gradient-echo sequences, causing a damping of the higher parts of the time-intensity curve. High concentration can also put the system in a slow to intermediate water exchange range (Donahue et al. 1997).

24.3 Noise Filtering

Standard noise reduction filters like median, Butterworth, etc. can be applied to each image. For details on this topic we refer to the standard image processing textbooks mentioned above since most of the general theory is also applicable to MR images.

Although conventional MR images often have a very good contrast-to-noise ratio, dynamic contrast-enhanced image series may have a lower contrast-to-noise ratio, in spite of the enhancement by the contrast agent. This is due to shorter acquisition times or acquisition procedures per image (Jones et al. 1993) in order to display the dynamics of the contrast agent uptake.

Thus, these images may benefit from application of noise reduction methods. Both standard filters and Bayesian approaches have been successfully applied (GODTLIEBSEN 1991; GODTLIEBSEN and SEBASTIANI 1994; SEBASTIANI et al. 1996).

24.4 Motion Correction

In order to perform a sound pixel-by-pixel analysis, all images in the series must be spatially aligned.

The importance of this problem depends on the application. While organs like the brain can be kept virtually motionless by fixing the head, other organs, in particular the heart, but also the lungs, the liver, and the breasts, will often move between images, mainly due to respiration, cardiac contraction, or involuntary patient movement.

Physical fixation of the body, ECG gating, and breath-holding techniques can reduce the motion within and between images. Outside markers for the realignment of images are of use only in limited applications. To minimize inherent motion during image acquisition, one can perform motion correction by means of navigator echoes. Still, automatic correction for motion between images remains one of the main problems for dynamic MR imaging of many organs and there is a need for postprocessing techniques to realign images.

Most of the currently available methods have not been developed to align temporal image series, but rather intermodality data, e.g., single-photon emission computed tomography/positron emission tomography (SPECT/PET) and MR/computed tomography (CT) images (WOODS et al. 1993), or intramodality data, such as MR images with different T1- and T2-weighting (WELLS et al. 1996).

Typically, these algorithms are designed to align one image to another. However, by applying the same algorithm iteratively, these methods can be used on temporal image series. A technique now considered classical is reported in WOODS et al. (1993).

Pixel-Based Methods. In this approach one assumes that there is a correlation between the intensities of corresponding regions in the two images to be aligned. Based on this assumption, one seeks to minimize, for example, the standard deviation of pixel intensities of corresponding regions in the two images. This method is attractive since it does not require external markers and does not rely on recognizing structures in the images. However, one should remove as many irrelevant features as possible, such as anatomical structures of no interest and the background. The cutting may require user interaction.

Several authors have reported similar methods, which can be viewed as a generalization of the Woods technique. These methods are based on the concepts of entropy and mutual information (COLLIGNON et al. 1995; MEYER et al. 1996; STUDHOLME et al. 1995; WELLS et al. 1996). Some authors claim that their methods are more robust than the one reported by Woods (WELLS et al. 1996), and that they also facilitate almost completely automatic processing (MEYER et al. 1996). However, these methods have not been specifically designed for dynamic contrast-enhanced image series.

As pointed out by HAYTON et al. (1996), although all slices in the dynamic scan are limited to one modality, contrast behavior is changing due to the contrast agent, potentially creating multimodal distribution of values in the data set. This means that, since different tissue types have different uptake patterns and velocities of a contrast agent, tissues A and B with no contrast at time zero may reveal positive or negative contrast after contrast enhancement and thereby confuse the algorithm. However, since these pixel-based methods will work on large groups of pixels and since one can apply the method iteratively to neighboring slices with small contrast differences, successful alignment should still be possible, as demonstrated by ZUO et al. (1996).

Another solution is to fit the time-intensity curves (or curves derived from the time-intensity curves) to a mathematical model and to align the images by minimizing the sum of the errors of the fits (HAYTON et al. 1996).

The disadvantage of this method is that it assumes the data can be fitted to the model. Thus, pixels with low uptake of contrast agent will be difficult or impossible to fit and may confuse the algorithm.

24.5 Definition of Time-Intensity Curves

The time-intensity curves can be defined using average intensities from manually, semiautomatically, or automatically defined ROIs (TORHEIM et al. 1997), or on a pixel-by-pixel basis. To be clinically useful, the system should be as user-independent and with as high a spatial (anatomical) resolution as possible. This gives priority to the use of an automatic pixel-by-pixel approach, producing one time-intensity

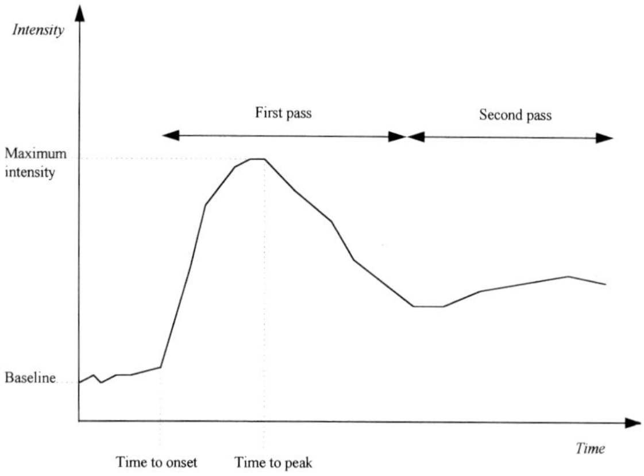

Fig. 24.2. Example of a time-intensity curve. Note that with ECF space contrast agents one seldom sees the second pass. The figure illustrates a curve obtained from a T1-weighted pulse sequence; this can be seen from the fact that the intensity *increases* upon arrival of the contrast agent. For a T2- or T2*-weighted pulse sequence, the arrival of contrast agent can produce a *decrease* in signal intensity, as shown in Fig. 24.3

curve for every pixel in the image. In order to reduce noise in the curves, they can be processed by "moving average" or similar filters. Noise reduction can also be combined with interpolation, as described in SEBASTIANI et al. (1996). Figure 24.2 shows a time-intensity curve with some definitions; clinical examples are provided in Figs. 24.3 and 24.4.

24.6 Processing of Time-Intensity Curves

Two main approaches to the processing of time-intensity curves have been proposed and described in the literature. Processing is possible (a) according to the principles of tracer kinetics and (b) by calculating parameters derived directly from the curves. The goal of the application of tracer kinetics is to reach quantitative measurements, whereas "simple" models of parameters derived directly from the time-intensity curves allow only qualitative measurements. Such qualitative statements might suffice for most clinical evaluations.

It is difficult to say which role tracer kinetics methods will play in dynamic MR imaging in the future. We believe that, at present, the methods described below add little or no clinical information. One potential use of quantifying parameters is in monitoring therapy. However, for standard diagnostic purposes these complicated methods are of a more academic value. This may change in the future. Blood pool agents, for instance, could allow more accurate estimates than those available today.

Because of all the assumptions, uncertainties in the estimated parameters will be big. In addition, one may run into technical/practical problems when estimating T1 and T2 (see Sect. 24.6.1) on equipment available today, related to change in gain settings and scaling of the signals. These problems must be solved before applying these theories.

24.6.1 Tracer Kinetics: Mathematical Models

The following two groups of mathematical models applied on dynamic MR images are both "tracer kinetics models."

The first group of models is sometimes described as "perfusion imaging methods" or "flow imaging methods." These models have been applied successfully using other modalities like PET and CT. They aim at estimating quantities like regional blood flow (perfusion) and mean transit time.

The second group comprises "pharmacokinetic models" (DEN BOER et al. 1997). These models apply principles used in pharmacology to describe the distribution of drugs. They aim at estimating parameters like permeability and extravascular extracellular volume.

Most models make the following assumptions (LASSEN and PERL 1979; TOFTS 1997):

1. Compartments exist that contain the well-mixed tracer in a uniform concentration throughout the compartment.
2. The parameters describing the compartments are constant during the time the system is observed (time invariance).
3. Relaxivity remains constant, i.e., the increase in T1 and/or T2 relaxation rates is proportional to the concentration of the contrast agent (see Eqs. 24.1a and b).
4. T1 or T2 changes can be calculated or estimated on the basis of signal intensity values, making it possible to obtain concentration values.
5. Assumptions regarding the proton exchange rate between compartments have to be made. In most cases, one assumes fast exchange between tissue compartments, and between red blood cells and plasma.
6. The input function which supplies the compartment of interest with contrast agent can be described. This description may be a measured

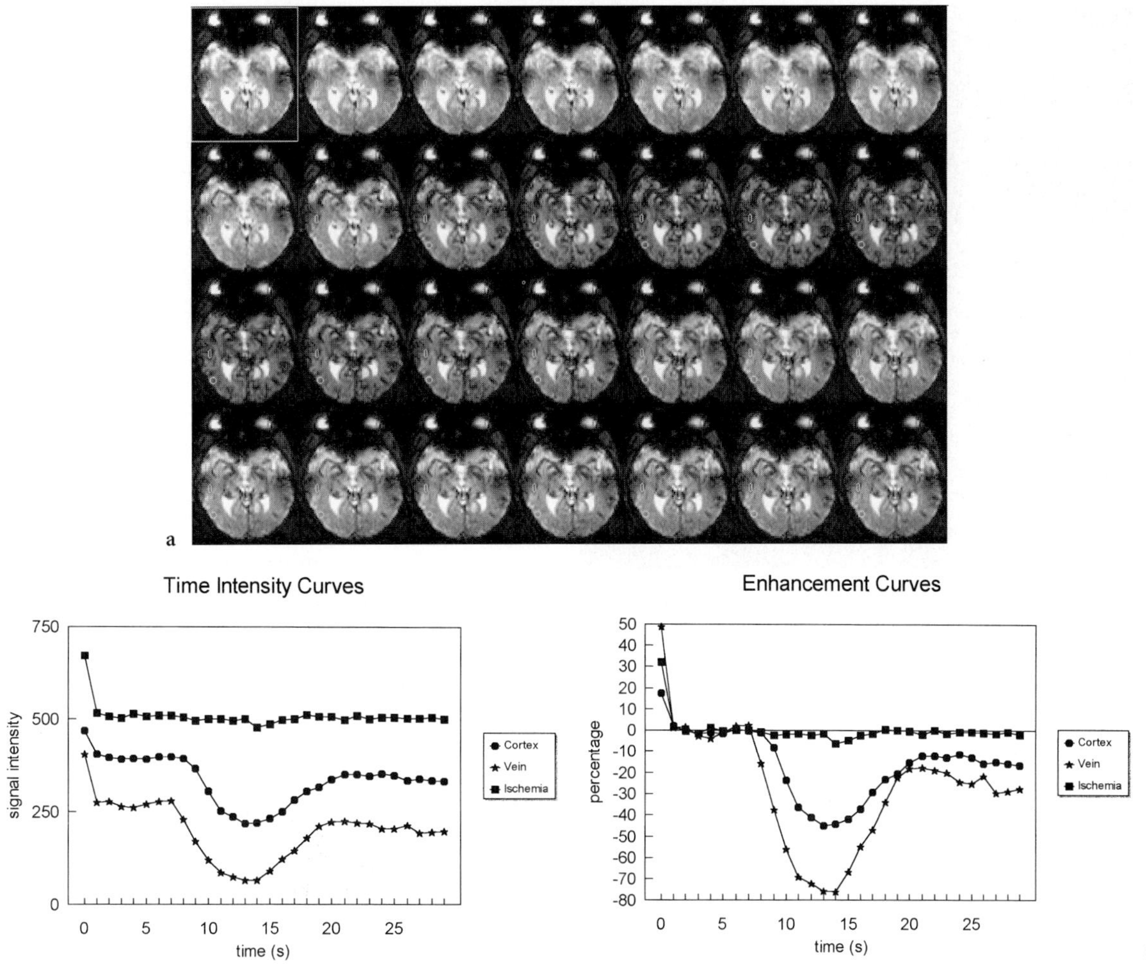

Fig. 24.3 a–c. Patient with right-field hemianopsia. MR imaging was performed 30 h after onset of symptoms. Dynamic sequence during which a gadolinium-based ECF agent (Omniscan) was injected. Several foci of high signal intensity in the occipital cortex were highlighted. **a** From defined ROIs in each image time-intensity curves were generated; **b** time-intensity curves from the ROIs in **a**; **c** corresponding enhancement curves. Images and curves were processed and visualized by the software program Dynalize 1.0. (Images courtesy of Dr. Olav Haraldseth, MR-Center, Medical Section, Trondheim, Norway)

time-concentration curve representing the input, an assumed normal curve, or a mathematical model (Tofts 1997).

Both groups of models require the calculation (or estimation) of time-concentration curves on the basis of time-intensity curves. Assumption 3 is expressed mathematically in Eq. 24.1.

$$R_{1CA} = R_{1NO} + r_1 \times C \quad (24.1a)$$

$$R_{2CA} = R_{2NO} + r_2 \times C \quad (24.1b)$$

where R_{1CA} is the T1 relaxation rate ($T1^{-1}$) of the compartment in the presence of the contrast agent (s^{-1}), R_{1NO} is the T1 relaxation rate ($T1^{-1}$) of the compartment without contrast agent (s^{-1}), r_1 is the T1 relaxivity of the contrast agent ($s^{-1} \times mmol^{-1} \times L$); C is the mean concentration of the contrast agent (mmol/L) in the target tissue, and R_{2CA}, R_{2NO}, and r_2 are the corresponding T2-related parameters [cf. Emrf (1997) for recent recommendations for contrast agent terms].

Furthermore, in order to estimate concentration, one needs a way of calculating changes in T1 and/or T2. The method of choice depends on the pulse sequence applied.

Some tracer kinetics models – typically those which estimate parameters related to permeability, i.e., pharmacokinetics-based models – rely on determining T1. For a gradient-echo sequence one can estimate T1 by running two scans with different flip

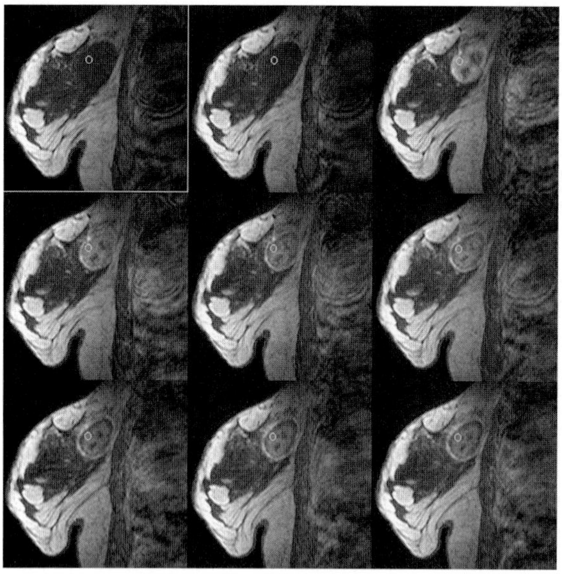

a

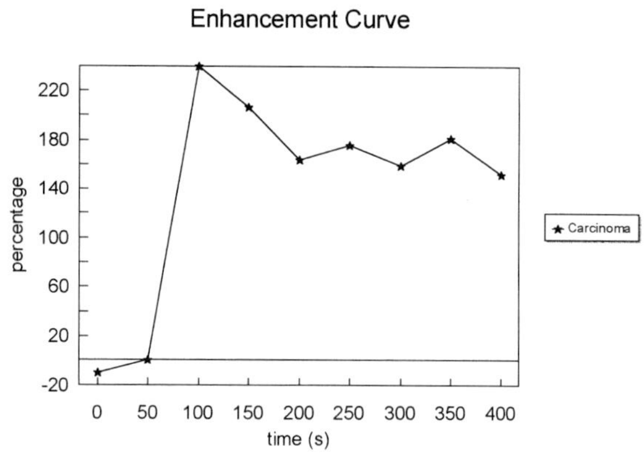

b

Fig. 24.4 a,b. Patient with an invasive breast carcinoma. Dynamic sequence during which a gadolinium-based ECF agent (Omniscan) was injected. **a** Images and ROI definitions; note the strong rim enhancement; **b** enhancement curve obtained from the images in **a**. Images and curves were processed and visualized by the software program Dynalize 1.0. (Images courtesy of Dr. Kjell-Arne Kvistad, MR-Center, Medical Section, Trondheim, Norway)

angles α and β, and keep all other sequence parameters the same.

The following equation is an estimate of (precontrast) T1 (den Boer et al. 1997):

$$T1 = TR/\ln[(SI_\alpha \sin\beta \cos\alpha - SI_\beta \sin\alpha \cos\beta)/ (SI_\alpha \sin\beta - SI_\beta \sin\alpha)], \quad (24.2)$$

where SI is signal intensity and α and β the respective pulse angles.

With further mathematical manipulation, one can use the precontrast T1 value and subsequent intensity measurements to estimate T1 in contrast agent-enhanced tissues. By applying Eq. 24.1a one can then estimate the concentration.

For changes in T2 relaxation rate, some authors have used the following equation to determine $\Delta R2$ as a function of time t:

$$\Delta R2(t) = -\ln[(SI(t)/SI(0))/TE], \quad (24.3)$$

where $\Delta R2(t)$ is change in T2 relaxation at time t, TE is echo time, SI(t) is signal intensity at time t, and SI(0) is the reference signal intensity.

This equation has been applied with echo planar imaging (EPI) sequences (Østergaard et al. 1996) and gradient-echo sequences (Rempp et al. 1994). In the latter one is estimating changes in T2*, not T2.

Typically, perfusion imaging methods will apply Eq. 24.3 since they work with fast T2- or T2*-weighted images in order to monitor faster phenomena.

24.6.1.1
Perfusion/Flow Imaging Methods

Perfusion/flow imaging methods are based on the central volume theorem which states that:

$$MTT = V/F, \quad (24.4)$$

where MTT is the mean transit time, V is the volume of the region of interest, and F is the flow through this region.

Normally, in a brain with an intact blood-brain barrier (BBB), one assumes that the tracer stays intravascularly. If this assumption holds, one can model the system using standard tracer kinetics models (Lassen and Perl 1979). As observed by Weisskoff et al. (1993), the signal in MR imaging is related to the contrast agent (CA) that *remains* in the tissue, while standard tracer kinetics methods usually measure the concentration of tracer *leaving* the tissue. Assuming that we are observing the tracer *leaving*, it can be shown that the MTT of the tissue equals the normalized first moment of the time-concentration curve. However, this is not correct for MR imaging, since, as noted, we are observing the contrast agent remaining in the tissue.

Instead, one can calculate the flow by deconvolving the time-concentration curve with the arterial input function (AIF) and then applying standard tracer kinetics formulas as described in LASSEN and PERL (1979). However, obtaining the deconvolved time-concentration curve presents a problem. Several mathematical approaches exist, but all of them are quite sensitive to noise. ØSTERGAARD et al. (1996) give an overview of different deconvolution approaches and their shortcomings.

Another major problem is to obtain a good input function. This is very difficult since one does not know exactly from where the blood is coming to a particular voxel. The input function should be measured as close to the area of interest as possible and can be obtained either by serial blood samples as in PET studies, or from the dynamic image data (ØSTERGAARD et al. 1996; REMPP et al. 1994) by monitoring an artery. In addition to the above-mentioned problems, one also has to face the issue of estimating the time-concentration curves from the time-intensity curves (see previous section).

Some authors claim that the only reliable parameter that indicator dilution theory can provide from methods like dynamic MR imaging, is relative blood volume. By assuming a constant area under the AIF, the relative blood volume can be estimated by calculating the area under the time-concentration curve.

24.6.1.2 Pharmacokinetics

The methods based on pharmacokinetics try to model diffusion of a substance across membranes. The body is seen as a set of compartments separated by membranes. It is assumed that the flow of contrast agent between the compartments is due to concentration gradients across the membranes (diffusion). This is described using mathematical equations. By estimating time-concentration curves these equations can be solved numerically. Often a combination of three parameters is estimated: influx volume transfer constant between plasma and extravascular extracellular space (EES), the volume of EES per unit volume of tissue, and the efflux ratio. These models have been tested in brains with BBB disruptions (LARSSON et al. 1990), retina (BERKOWITZ et al. 1994), and breast (MUSSURAKIS et al. 1997).

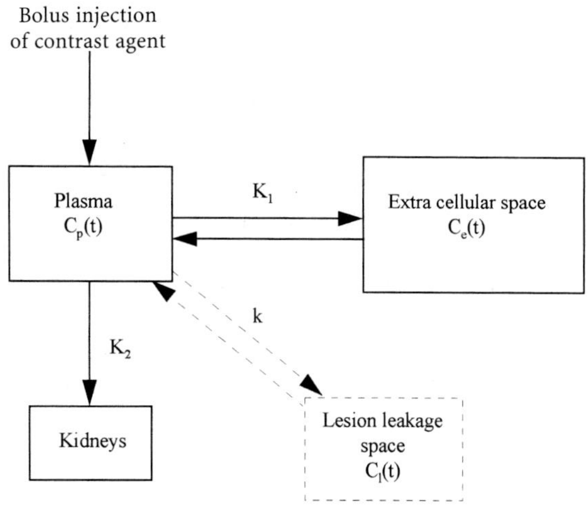

Fig. 24.5. Compartmental model of ECF space contrast agent distribution. Modified after TOFTS (1991). The transfer rate k between the lesion leakage space and the plasma is considered to be isodirectional

We use the model of TOFTS and KERMODE (1991) as an example, and refer to BRIX et al. (1991) and LARSSON et al. (1990) for description of other, similar models. TOFTS (1997) gives a good review of these three models.

The original model of Tofts and Kermode consisted of three compartments (Fig. 24.5):

1. A plasma volume
2. A large extracellular space which is distributed throughout most of the body (e.g., muscle, soft tissue), but does not exist in the brain due to the BBB
3. The kidneys, which eliminate the contrast agent from the plasma, and hence from the extracellular space

In addition to these three compartments, a lesion is added which is connected to the plasma through a permeable membrane. This compartment is small enough not to influence the overall plasma concentration. The time-concentration curve for the plasma can be described with the following biexponential function:

$$C_p(t) = D\left(a_1 e^{-m_1 t} + a_2 e^{-m_2 t}\right), \tag{24.5}$$

where C_p is the plasma concentration, D is the dose of the gadolinium-based contrast agent, a_1 and a_2 are amplitudes of the components, and m_1 and m_2 are their rate constants.

The lesion (e.g., the area of defective BBB or a vascular breast tumor) is modeled containing a leakage space which is defined as part of the tissue to which the plasma tracer has access. The amount of tracer in the leakage space is $v_1 V_t C_1$, where v_1 is the fraction of lesion tissue which the leakage space occupies, V_t is the lesion tissue volume, and C_1 is the tracer concentration in the leakage space. The flow of tracer from plasma into the leakage space is then described with the following equation:

$$v_1 V_t (dC_1/dt) = PS(C_p - C_1), \qquad (24.6)$$

where P is the permeability coefficient, S is the surface area of the membrane, and C_p is the plasma concentration. By defining the transfer coefficient $k = PS/V_t$ and performing mathematical manipulation and combination with Eq. 24.5, one obtains the following equation for the tissue concentration:

$$C_t(t) = D[b_1 \exp(-m_1 t) + b_2 \exp(-m_2 t) + b_3 \exp(-m_3 t)], \qquad (24.7)$$

where $m_3 = k/v_1$, $b_1 = ka_1/(m_3 - m_1)$, $b_2 = ka_2/(m_3 - m_2)$, $b_3 = -(b_1 + b_2)$.

a_1, a_2, m_1, and m_2 have been determined empirically from a "normal" plasma curve. Thus, when $C_t(t)$ is available, one can perform a least squares fit of Eq. 24.7 to obtain k and v_1.

This earlier Tofts model has been criticized, since it assumes that all patients have the same plasma concentration curve, although this may not be the case. Other assumptions are that the transfer coefficient between the lesion space and the plasma space is the same in both directions, and that the flow F is sufficient to replace tracer leaked through the membranes ($F \gg PS$). However, this simple model illustrates many important aspects of pharmacokinetics modeling.

24.6.2
Parameters Derived Directly from the Curves ("Simple" Models)

Intensive research has been devoted to deriving parameters directly from the time-intensity curves. In this approach one does not consider a tracer kinetics model and avoids many of the problems described above simply by not making too many assumptions.

Although this implies that the analysis can be, at best, semiquantitative, from a pragmatic clinical point of view the results can be surprisingly good.

In a recently published paper (Müller-Schimpfle et al. 1997) the authors compared tracer kinetics with simple parameter models and concluded that the parameters derived from the tracer kinetics model gave no advantage compared with the standard evaluation method for clinical applications. However, it is still too early to draw any final conclusions. If the problems encountered in the current settings are solved, dynamic MR imaging and tracer kinetics theories may one day be able to reliably give high-resolution measurements on therapeutically important parameters like perfusion.

Most authors transform the time-intensity curves into enhancement curves by applying the following (or similar) formula:

$$E(t) = (\mathrm{SI}(t) - b)/b \times 100, \qquad (24.8)$$

where $E(t)$ is enhancement at time t, $\mathrm{SI}(t)$ is signal intensity at time t, and b is the baseline value for the time-intensity curve. Refer to Figs. 24.3 and 24.4 for examples. From these curves, parameters like maximum slope, maximum intensity, wash-in slope, and wash-out slope are calculated. Other parameters like time-to-peak and time-to-onset can be derived either from the enhancement curves or directly from the time-intensity curves. These more simple parameters also have the advantage that calculations of parametric maps are, in general, fairly straightforward and very fast (Rinck and Torheim 1997). The interpretation of the different parameters and their significance depends highly on the target organ and disease studied. However, the rich experience gathered during the past 10 years has proven the viability of the approach.

Another empirical approach is to calculate the cross-correlation (CC) or cross-correlation coefficient (CCC) (Rogowska and Wolf 1992), which has been reported to be the most clinically significant parameter of all (Lombardi et al. 1997). However, this method requires the definition of a reference curve.

24.7
Presentation of Parametric Data

Parametric maps are the preferred way of presenting dynamic data. A parametric map combines parametric with spatial information. This is easily done by creating time-intensity curves on a pixel-by-pixel basis and deriving parameters from each curve. Then, a new image is created, in which each pixel intensity value is related to the calculated parameter value from the corresponding time-intensity curve. The simplest way of creating such an image is to use a gray scale, mapping the range of parameter values to different intensity values. Gray-scale images are

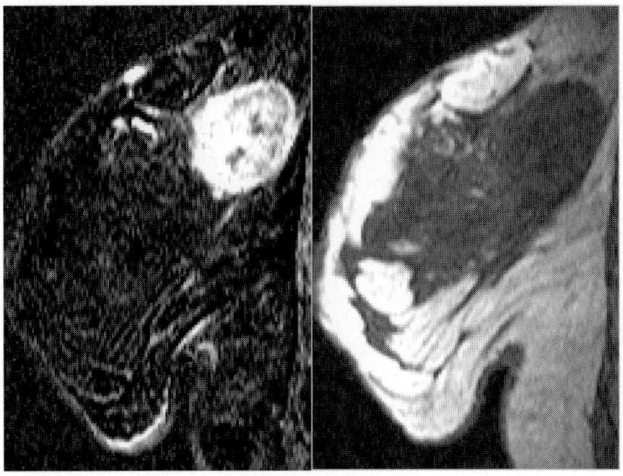

Fig. 24.6. Parametric map (*left*) created by the software program Dynalize 1.0. Each pixel in this map represents a parametric value, in this case the area under the corresponding enhancement curve. The image to the *right* is one of the original images used to create the parametric map

normally easy to interpret, and radiologists are used to them. Figure 24.6 shows a parametric gray-scale image.

The gray-scale representation, however, has some limitations, the most important being that the human eye can separate no more than about 30 gray levels (Russ 1995). Alternatively, the maps can be presented in colors, making it easier to separate more parameter values. Unfortunately, color scales have not been standardized yet. Thus, they can be more difficult to interpret since the mapping from parameter values to colors may not be intuitive. Color coding also opens up other new possibilities, e.g., it allows the combination of several different parameter values in one image by creating two-dimensional color maps. This can be done, for instance, by coding one parameter as change in intensity while the other is coded using different colors (hues) (Degani et al. 1997; Hawighorst et al. 1996).

A third alternative is to combine both of the aforementioned methods by creating a gray-scale map and an overlay using one or many colored regions with parameter values of particular interest, for instance above or below a certain threshold. However, the parametric image requires that the data be analyzed in a pixel-by-pixel fashion. Due to factors like motion this is not always feasible, and processing must be based on time-intensity curves created from ROIs. In this case, one will obtain a limited number of parametric values which can be presented as numerical values or can be used to color the ROIs on one of the original images according to their parametric values (Torheim et al. 1997).

References

Barentsz JO, Boetes C, Verstraete KL, Jager GJ, Mus RDM, Ruijs SHJ (1995) Dynamic gadolinium-enhanced MR imaging of the body. Clin Magn Reson Imaging 5:88–93

Berkowitz BA, Wilson CA, Tofts PS, Peshock RM (1994) Effect of vitreous fluidity on the measurement of blood-retinal barrier permeability using contrast-enhanced MRI. Magn Reson Med 31:61–66

Boetes C, Barentsz JO, Mus RD, et al. (1994) MR Characterization of suspicious breast lesions with a gadolinium enhanced TurboFLASH subtraction technique. Radiology 193:777–781

Brix G, Semmler W, Port R, Schad LR, Layer G, Lorenz WJ (1991) Pharmacokinetic parameters in CNS Gd-DTPA enhanced MR imaging. J Comput Assist Tomogr 15:621–628

Collignon A, Maes F, Delaere D, Vandermeulen D, Suetens P, Marchal G (1995) Automated multimodality image registration using information theory. Computational imaging and vision. Proceedings, 13th International Conference. IPMI. Kluwer Academic, Dordrecht; 3:263–274

Degani H, Gusis V, Weinstein D, Fields S, Strano S (1997) Mapping pathophysiological features of breast tumors by MRI at high spatial resolution. Nature Med 3:780–782

den Boer JA, Hoenderop RKKM, Smink J, et al. (1997) Pharmacokinetic analysis of Gd-DTPA enhancement in dynamic three-dimensional MRI of breast lesions. J Magn Reson Imaging 7:702–715

Donahue KM, Weisskoff RM, Burstein D (1997) Water Diffusion and Exchange as They Influence Contrast Enhancement. J Magn Reson Imaging 7:102–110

Eichenberger AC, Schuiki E, Köchli VD, Amann FW, McKinnon G, von Schulthess GK (1994) Ischemic heart disease: assessment with gadolinium-enhanced ultrafast MR imaging and dipyridamole stress. J Magn Reson Imaging 4:425–431

EMRF (European Magnetic Resonance Forum Foundation) (1997) Recommendations for the nomenclature of MR imaging contrast agent terms. Acta Radiol 38(Suppl 412):5

Erlemann R, Reiser MF, Peters PE, et al. (1989) Musculoskeletal neoplasms: static and dynamic Gd-DTPA-enhanced MR imaging. Radiology 171:767–773

Flickinger FW, Allison JD, Sherry RM, Wright JC (1993) Differentiation of benign from malignant breast masses by time-intensity evaluation of contrast enhanced MRI. Magn Reson Imaging 11:617–620

Godtliebsen F (1991) Noise reduction using Markow random fields. J Magn Reson 92:102–114

Godtliebsen F, Sebastiani G (1994) Statistical methods for noisy images with discontinuities. J Appl Stat 21:459–477

Gonzalez RC, Wintz P (1987) Digital image processing, 2nd edn. Addison-Wesley, Reading, USA

Gowland P, Mansfield P, Bullock P, Stehling M, Worthington B, Firth J (1992) Dynamic studies of gadolinium uptake in brain tumors using inversion-recovery echo-planar imaging. Magn Reson Med 26:241–258

Gribbestad IS, Nilsen G, Fjøsne HE, Kvinnsland S, Haugen OA, Rinck PA (1994) Comparative signal intensity measurements in dynamic gadolinium-enhanced MR mammography. J Magn Reson Imaging 4:447–480

Hawighorst H, Knapstein PG, Weikel W, et al. (1996) Cervical carcinoma: comparison of standard and pharmacokinetic MR imaging. Radiology 201:531–539

Hayton P, Brady M, Tarassenko L, Moore N (1996) Analysis of dynamic MR breast images using a model of contrast enhancement. Med Image Anal 1:207–224

Heywang-Köbrunner SH, Beck R (1995) Contrast-enhanced MRI of the breast. 2nd edn. Springer, Berlin, Heidelberg, New York

Higgins CB, Sakuma H (1996) Heart disease: functional evaluation with MR imaging. Radiology 199:307–315

Jones RA, Haraldseth O, Muller TB, et al. (1993) K-space substitution: a novel dynamic imaging technique. Magn Reson Med 29:830–834

Kaiser WA (1990) Dynamic magnetic resonance breast imaging using a double breast coil: an important step towards routine examinations of the breast. Front Eur Radiol 7:39–68

Kim B, Semelka RC, Ascher SM, Chalpin DB, Caroll PR, Hricak H (1994) Bladder tumor staging: comparison of contrast-enhanced CT, T1- and T2-weighted MR imaging, dynamic gadolinium-enhanced imaging, and late gadolinium-enhanced imaging. Radiology 193:239–245

Knopp MV, Junkermann HJ, Hoffmann U, et al. (1996) Fast dynamic MR imaging for characterization of breast lesions. Experiences in functional MR-mammography. Proceedings, Annual Meeting (New York). International Society of Magnetic Resonance, p 353

Kornmesser W, Laniado M, Deimling M, Felix R (1986) Dynamic MRI of intracranial and intraspinal tumors with fast imaging sequences and intravenous Gd-DTPA. Book of Abstracts. Society of Magnetic Resonance in Medicine. 5th Annual Meeting, Montreal, 317–318

Krestin GP (1994) Magnetic resonance imaging of the kidneys: current status. Magn Reson Q 19:2–21

Larsson HBW, Stubgaard M, Frederiksen JL, Jensen M, Henriksen O, Paulson OB (1990) Quantitation of blood-brain barrier defect by magnetic resonance imaging and gadolinium-DTPA in patients with multiple sclerosis and brain tumors. Magn Reson Med 16:117–131

Lassen NA, Perl W (1997) Tracer kinetic methods in medical physiology. Raven Press, New York

Lombardi M, Jones RA, Westby JW, et al. (1997) Magnetic resonance imaging for the evaluation of the regional myocardial perfusion in an experimental animal model. J Magn Reson Imaging 7:987–995

Martí-Bonmatí L, Masiá L, Torrijo C, Casillas C, Ferrer MD (1994) Dynamic MR imaging of liver tumors: analysis with temporal reconstruction images. Radiology 193:677–682

Meyer CR, Boes JL, Boklye K, et al. (1996) Demonstration of accuracy and clinical versatility of mutual information for automatic multimodality image fusion using affine and thin-plate spline warped geometric deformations. Med Image Anal 1:195–206

Müller-Schimpfle M, Ohmenhauser K, Sand J, Stoll P, Claussen C (1997) Dynamic 3D-MR mammography: is there a benefit of sophisticated evaluation of enchancement curves for clinical routine? J Magn Reson Imaging 7:236–240

Mussurakis S, Buckley DL, Drew PJ, Fox JN, Carleton PJ, Turnball LW, Horsman A (1997) Dynamic MR imaging of the breast combined with analysis of contrast agent kinetics in the differentiation of primary breast tumours. Clin Radiol 52:516–526

Østergaard L, Sorensen AG, Kwong K, Weisskoff RM, Gyldensted C, Rosen BR (1996) High resolution measurement of cerebral blood flow using intravascular tracer bolus passages. Part II. Experimental comparison and preliminary results. Magn Reson Med 36:726–736

Rempp KA, Brix G, Wenz F, Becker CR, Glückel F, Lorenz WJ (1994) Quantification of regional cerebral blood flow and volume with dynamic susceptibility contrast-enhanced MR imaging. Radiology 193:637–641

Rinck PA (ed) (1993) Magnetic resonance in medicine. The basic textbook of the European Magnetic Resonance Forum, 3rd edn. Blackwell Scientific, Oxford

Rinck PA (1995) Some future perspectives of contrast agent development. Clin Magn Reson Imaging 5:129–139

Rinck PA, Muller RN (1998) Field strength and dose dependence of enhancement by gadolinium-based MR contrast agents. Eur Radiol (in press)

Rinck PA, Myhr G (1998) The gadolinium chelates: clinical applications. In: Dawson P, Cosgrove D, Allison D (eds) Textbook of contrast media. Isis Medical Media, Oxford

Rinck PA, Torheim G (1997) Image postprocessing and contrast agents in clinical MR imaging – an introductory overview. Acta Radiol 38(Suppl 412):7–19

Rinck PA, Fischer HW, Vander Elst L, Van Haverbeke Y, Muller RN (1988) Field-cycling relaxometry: medical application. Radiology 168:843–849

Rogowska J, Wolf GL (1992) Temporal correlation images derived from sequential MR scans. J Comput Assist Tomogr 16:784–788

Rosen BR, Belliveau JW, Vevea JM, Brady TJ (1990) Perfusion imaging with NMR contrast agents. Magn Reson Med 14:249–265

Rosen BR, Belliveau JW, Buchbinder BR, et al. (1991) Contrast agents and cerebral hemodynamics. Magn Reson Med 19:285–292

Russ JC (1995) The image processing handbook. 2nd edn. CRC Press, Boca Raton, FL., USA

Sebastiani G, Godtliebsen F, Jones RA, Haraldseth O, Muller TB, Rinck PA (1996) Analysis of dynamic magnetic resonance images. IEEE Trans Med Imag 15:268–277

Stack JP, Redmond OM, Codd MB, Dervan PA, Ennis JT (1990) Breast disease: tissue characterization with Gd-DTPA enhancement profiles. Radiology 174:491–494

Studholme C, Hill D Hawkes D (1995) Multiresolution voxel similarity measures for MR-PET registration. Computational imaging and vision. Proceedings, 13th International Conference. IPMI. Kluwer Academic, Dordrecht; 3:287–298

Tofts PS (1997) Modeling tracer kinetics in dynamic Gd-DTPA MR imaging. J Magn Reson Imaging 7:91–101

Tofts PS, Kermode AG (1991) Measurement of the blood-brain barrier permeability and leakage space using dynamic MR imaging. 1. Fundamental concepts. Magn Res Med 17:357–367

Tofts PS, Berkowitz B, Schnall MD (1995) Quantitative analysis of dynamic Gd-DTPA enhancement in breast tumors using a permeability model. Magn Res Med 33:564–568

Torheim G, Lombardi M, Rinck PA (1997) An Independent software system for the analysis of dynamic MR images. Acta Radiol 38:165–172

Verstraete KL, De Deene Y, Roels H, Dierick A, Uyttendaele D, Kunnen M (1994) Benign and malignant musculoskeletal lesions: dynamic contrast-enhanced MR imaging – parametric "first-pass" images depict tissue vascularization and perfusion. Radiology 192:835–843

Verstraete KL, Van der Woude H-J, Hogendoom PCW, De Deene Y, Kunnen M, Bloem JL (1996) Dynamic contrast-enhanced MR imaging of musculoskeletal tumors: basic principles and clinical applications. J Magn Reson Imaging 6:311–321

Villa A, Van Steenwinkel C, Meloni G, Campani R (1995) Dynamic contrast enhancement in magnetic resonance imaging of the Body. In: Rinck PA (ed). The rational use of magnetic resonance imaging. Blackwell, Oxford, pp 257–278

Villringer A, Rosen BR, Belliveau JW, et al. (1988) Dynamic imaging with lanthanide chelates in normal brain: contrast due to magnetic susceptibility effects. Magn Res Med 6:164–174

von Schulthess GK, Kuoni W, Gerig G, Wüthrich R, Duewell S, Krestin G (1991) Semiautomated ROI analysis in dynamic MR studies. Part II. Application to renal function examination. J Comput Assist Tomogr 15:733–741

Watson AD, Rocklage SM, Carvlin MJ (1992) Contrast agents. In: Stark DD, Bradley WG (eds) Magnetic resonance imaging, 2nd edn. Mosby Year Book, St Louis, pp 372–437

Weisskoff RM, Chesler D, Boxerman JL, Rosen BR (1993) Pitfalls of MR measurements of tissue blood flow with intravascular tracers: which mean transit time? Magn Reson Med 29:553–559

Wells WM, Viola P, Atsumi H, Hakajima S, Kikinis R (1996) Multimodal volume registration by maximization of mutual information. Med Image Anal 1:35–51

Wilke N, Jerosch-Herold M, Stillman AE, et al. (1994) Concepts of myocardial perfusion imaging in magnetic resonance imaging. Magn Reson Q 10:249–286

Woods RP, Mazziotta JC, Cherry SR (1993) MRI-PET registration with automated algorithm. J Comput Assist Tomogr 17:536–546

Zuo CS, Jiang A, Buff BL, Mahon TG, Wong TZ (1996) Automatic motion correction for breast MR imaging. Radiology 198:903–906

III
Ultrasound Contrast Media

25 Ultrasound Contrast Media: Past, Present, and Future

R.F. MATTREY

CONTENTS

25.1 Introduction

Contrast agents have played an important role in diagnostic radiology. Aside from angiography and nuclear medicine techniques that are, by definition, contrast examinations, contrast agents have added significantly to the diagnostic capabilities of all imaging modalities. Sonography is the last technique that has not gleaned the benefits of contrast media administration.

This chapter reviews the history and major milestones, concepts, current status, and future direction of this field, the explosion of which can be seen from the number of yearly publications (Fig. 25.1).

25.2 History

Serious attempts to develop intravenous (IV) contrast agents for ultrasound began in the late 1970s and early 1980s. A successful IV agent for solid organ imaging, reported by MATTREY et al. in 1982, consisted of a fluorocarbon liquid emulsion. The fluorocarbon used was perfluoro-octyl bromide, which was emulsified and made into an IV product by Alliance Pharmaceutical Corp. (San Diego, Calif.). This agent had a biological half-life of several days (MATTREY et al. 1982). It enhanced the venous system for several hours (COLEY et al. 1994) and the liver, spleen, and tumors for 3–4 days, dependent on dose. The agent was developed to a phase II trial that produced similar imaging results in cancer patients (BEHAN et al. 1993). The development of this product has continued, but it has been optimized for oxygen transport rather than for contrast applications.

Microbubble agents were first described by GRAMIAK and SHAH in 1968. They were discovered during the injection of indocyanine green as M-mode echocardiography was being performed. This effect was shown to be due to microbubble formation at the catheter tip by KREMKAU et al. in 1970. These free air bubbles were large and short-lived, as the plasma surface tension forced the air back into solution. Bubbles were optimized for consistent right heart opacification and reported by SMITH et al. 1984. heralding a flurry of reports, mostly in the cardiology literature. They used a galactose-based contrast agent called SHU-454 (Echovist, Schering AG, Berlin, Germany) that released bubbles trapped in the crevasses of the crystal.

Successful transpulmonary delivery of microbubbles was achieved in the mid 1980s, using an agent similar to SHU-454 with the addition of palmitic acid as a surfactant, and was reported by SMITH et al. in 1989. This agent, SHU-508A (Levovist, Schering AG, Berlin, Germany), is currently approved for clinical use in Europe and Canada. Feinstein and co-workers, following microbubble investigations in many liquids, developed a sonicated albumin solution in the mid 1980s and in 1990 reported their clinical experience in opacifying the left ventricle with IV injections (FEINSTEIN et al. 1990). This agent, developed by Molecular Biosystems Inc. (San Diego, Calif.) and given the name Albunex, is now approved for clinical use worldwide. Albunex, made of a more rigid shell, is short-lived in plasma, lasting one circulation time (HILPERT et al. 1989). Levovist

R.F. MATTREY, MD, Department of Radiology, University of California, San Diego Medical Center, 200 W. Arbor Drive, San Diego, CA 92109-8756, USA

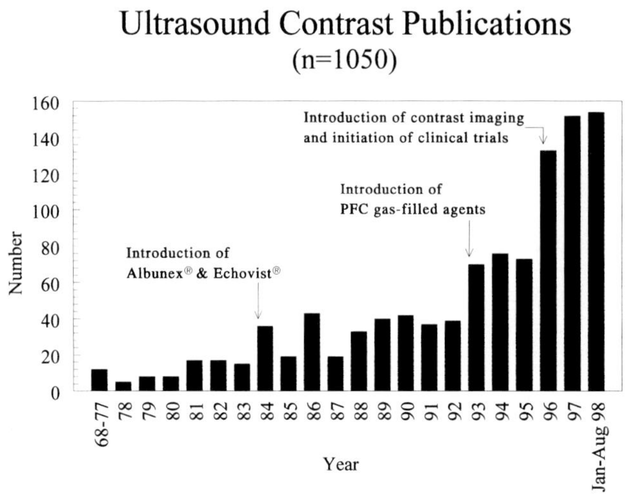

Fig. 25.1. Bar graph displaying the number of indexed publications in the field of ultrasound contrast

has a longer plasma half-life and lasts for a few minutes. Neither agent is visible on standard gray-scale imaging outside the left ventricle because of the low concentration achieved in the systemic circulation.

Perfluoro-octyl bromide emulsion, which successfully enhanced liver, spleen, and tumors for days, remains liquid at body temperature (MATTREY et al. 1982, 1983). In contrast, the fluorocarbon dodecafluoropentane has a low boiling point such that, when an emulsion of this fluorocarbon is injected IV, the liquid turns to vapor in vivo, increasing particle size from submicron to several microns (μm) in diameter and, more importantly, increasing its elasticity. The increase in diameter and elasticity increase its reflectivity from 7 times to 10^{10} times that of red blood cells. This fluorocarbon, developed by Sonus Pharmaceuticals in the early 1990s, was given the name Echogen. Although this agent is visible on gray-scale, it is only detectable on Doppler sonography at the approved human dose.

Also in the early 1990s, the understanding of bubble dynamics led to the development of the new-generation agents. These agents are microbubbles prior to injection that contain both fluorocarbon vapor and nitrogen or air. The presence of fluorocarbon vapor acts as an osmotic stabilizer (SCHUTT et al. 1996). Because the fluorocarbon cannot exit the bubble rapidly, it acts to limit the collapse of the bubble, allowing it to survive the surface tension and ambient and mechanical pressures. As the microbubble enters a high-pressure region, the increased pressure within the bubble forces the air into the plasma; as the microbubble enters a low-pressure region, air reenters because of the difference in the partial pressure of air between the plasma and the bubble interior. The presence of fluorocarbon within the bubble rendered practical the development of small bubbles with sufficient plasma half-life.

The first of these agents was reported in 1994 by MATTREY et al., who found that blood and tissue echogenicity was increased on standard gray-scale imaging for several minutes. They suggested that, at comparable efficacy, the diagnostic dose of the microbubble agent was 25 times less than that of the liquid fluorocarbon agent (MATTREY et al. 1994 a,b). There are now several products in clinical development, with at least one agent from each of the major contrast pharmaceutical companies. The first of these agents to be approved for clinical use for endocardial border delineation in the United States and Europe is FS069 (Optison, Molecular Biosystems, San Diego, Calif.), which is being co-developed and marketed by Mallinckrodt Inc. (St. Louis, MO).

It is doubtful that new agents with significant improvement on the existing new-generation products will be forthcoming. The major areas of expansion will be in specific agents that target tissues, either for diagnostic or, more importantly, therapeutic use. The other area of significant expansion in this field is instrumentation technology, where specific pulsing and/or post-processing techniques will be developed to take advantage of the presence of microbubbles in the circulation.

25.3 The Concept of Ultrasound Contrast

The goal of an ultrasound contrast agent is to increase reflectivity from regions where it is present or where it accumulates. Reflectivity is caused by an impedance mismatch as the sound wave propagates across tissue interfaces. As impedance is dependent upon the mass density of the tissue and the speed of sound through that tissue, alterations in density and/or speed of sound are necessary to increase backscatter. Successful agents have been particles of liquid, solid, or gas. The particle characteristics that affect its backscattering properties are size, density, and compressibility. It is estimated that solid particles (Ophir and Parker 1989) and liquid fluorocarbon particles (Mattrey and Steinbach 1991) are several times more reflective than a red blood cell, but that the elasticity of a gas body makes the bubble 10^{10} times more reflective than a red blood cell (Ophir and Parker 1989).

Although backscatter is highly dependent upon bubble size, microbubbles of successful intravenous agents have a limited size range. If the bubble is too small, it will be short-lived. Because of the high internal pressure of a small bubble, it will collapse under cardiac and systemic pressures and plasma surface tension or lose its contents to a larger bubble or the alveolar space because of the high partial pressure gradient of the gas they carry. If it is large, the pulmonary capillaries will trap it. Therefore, microbubble size in vivo is limited to those bubbles from 1 to 5 μm in diameter and is difficult to control following the first pass, except if the shell is made rigid. Although the density of the particle can be manipulated if it is made liquid, solid, or gaseous, elasticity is the dominant factor, outweighing the effect of low density of a gas bubble.

In addition to increasing backscatter signals, ultrasound contrast agents also influence attenuation. Although tissue attenuation before and after the administration of a contrast agent could provide diagnostic information (Ophir and Parker 1989), attenuation is a hindrance that prevents the assessment of deeper tissues.

25.4 Current Status

25.4.1 Agents

25.4.1.1 Agents of Historical Interest

Early in the development of contrast media, several liquids were used that carried free bubbles downstream of the injection site or the right heart. Those liquids that were more viscous were preferred, such as renografin, sorbitol, 5% dextrose, or albumin solutions. In the early to mid 1980s, sonication was introduced to produce more consistent and uniform microbubbles (Feinstein et al. 1984; Keller et al. 1986). These agents were used for intra-arterial injection to assess the perfusion bed, or for intravenous injection to image the right cardiac chambers or intracardiac shunts.

Liquid agents were attempted, and some agents were identified that could affect backscatter (Ophir et al. 1979). They showed in vivo and in vitro the effect of such agents on kidney enhancement. Tyler found that increased backscatter was dependent upon differences in speed of sound, which was affected by molarity (Tyler et al. 1981). However, because of the low effectiveness of liquid agents (Ophir and Parker 1989), this approach was abandoned.

Liquid fluorocarbon emulsions were first described in 1982 as effective agents for solid organ imaging (Mattrey et al. 1982, 1983). The fluorocarbon perfluoro-octyl bromide (PFOB) was emulsified into 0.25-μm particles and administered intravenously at 2–5 g of PFC/kg or 2–5 ml of a 100% (weight/volume) emulsion/kg. The particles accumulated in the reticuloendothelial system, including circulating macrophages, to render these cells reflective. PFOB emulsions enhanced the liver, spleen, and tumors for several days. The fluorocarbon was shown to be the active ingredient that allowed for the increased backscatter owing to its very low acoustic velocity of approximately 600 m/s (Andre et al. 1990). Because Fluosol, an emulsion of two different fluorocarbons, was in clinical trials as an artificial oxygen carrier, it was tested in man as an ultrasound contrast agent (Mattrey et al. 1987a). It improved the visualization of tumors and allowed the detection of lesions not seen prior to injection. Tumor visualization with this agent was due to the leak of particles across tumor capillaries that were subsequently phagocytosed by macrophages (Mattrey 1989). Macrophage imaging was possible in any abnormally leaky capillary bed, including the heart, where infarction became visible (Mattrey and Andre 1984).

Fluosol and the early formulations of PFOB were invisible in the vascular space. It was discovered during the development process of PFOB that certain formulations were visible in the venous system but not in the arterial space. The sonographic properties of these formulations were compared, and it was discovered that not only the venous system was enhanced but also perfused tissues, such as the kidney

(Satterfield et al. 1993). Filling the veins with echoes allowed Coley and co-workers to show improved detection and definition of venous clots (Coley et al. 1994) and the enhancement of perfused tissues allowed the detection of renal infarction (Coley et al. 1990a). Because of the weak backscatter effect of liquid fluorocarbon particles, the large dose, approximately 120 ml, that was required increased the potential for side-effects and made them impractical for routine use. More importantly, the large particle load activated macrophages to produce a flu-like syndrome in a small percentage of patients (Behan et al. 1993). The development of the liquid fluorocarbons as ultrasound contrast was redirected to their use as oxygen carriers.

The only solid particle tested was iodipimide ethyl ester, which had been developed as a liver- and spleen-specific computed tomography (CT) agent (Violante et al. 1980). Its use as an ultrasound contrast agent was shown in rabbits with Vx2 tumors (Parker et al. 1987). It was also found that surface irregularities and fractures trapped gas, thus increasing backscatter severalfold (Violante et al. 1991; Phillips et al. 1998).

25.4.1.2 Agents Approved or in Clinical Development

Once sonication was used to decrease bubble size and to narrow bubble-size distribution, and sonication of albumin was attempted, the heat generated from the ultrasound energy denatured the albumin and stiffened the shell. The transformation of albumin stabilized the bubbles, and the smaller bubble size generated with sonication allowed their transpulmonary passage to the left ventricle. The stability was sufficient to fill the left ventricle with echoes (Feinstein et al. 1990) and to produce first-pass effects in the systemic circulation (Hilpert et al. 1989). The sonicated albumin product was developed by Molecular Biosystems, Inc. (San Diego, Calif.) for cardiac imaging and given the trade name Albunex. Although Albunex filled the left ventricle, it had no radiologic application, as the product lasted only for the first pass.

Albunex has been updated by its successor FS069, a similar formulation to Albunex, except that fluorocarbon gas was added. FS069 has been given the trade name Optison and approved for endocardial border delineation in the United States and Europe. Albunex has essentially been replaced by FS069 for this indication because of the greater longevity of the latter product and the more consistent filling of the left ventricle. Optison is now under development for myocardial perfusion imaging and radiologic applications. Early data suggest that it may play a role in liver imaging (Moriyasu et al. 1998). Albunex use has now been diverted to intracavitary applications.

SHU 454 (Echovist, Schering AG, Berlin Germany) was developed slightly earlier than Albunex to produce a more consistent and reproducible filling of the right ventricle. It was shortly followed by SHU 508A (Levovist, Schering AG, Berlin Germany), which had a similar formulation to SHU 454 except for the addition of palmitic acid, which stabilized the air bubble and allowed transpulmonary passage for left ventricular opacification. Levovist lasts for minutes in the systemic circulation, allowing Doppler enhancement. Although its radiologic applications had been limited to Doppler enhancemet, the late-generation instruments with wideband harmonics and intermittent imaging have allowed liver imaging during the late phase (Blomley et al. 1998). A new agent, SHU 563A, was developed as an air-filled hard-shelled product that is approximately 1 μm in diameter. This agent has a vascular phase, but is then removed by the reticuloendothelial system to accumulate in the liver and spleen. Its unique shell allows for increased backscatter at low power and large backscatter, with harmonic signal generation at high power when the bubble is disrupted (Burns et al. 1995). This agent is best used in harmonic Doppler or wideband modes, where it has produced precise definition of small liver lesions (Hauff et al. 1997). Because of the ability to recognize the presence of even a single bubble, it was proposed that SHU 563A could be used to quantitate bubble concentration and therefore fractional blood volume.

Although liquid fluorocarbon agents such as PFOB emulsion and Fluosol were effective tissue-enhancing agents, their backscattering properties were weak, requiring relatively large dosages. It was proposed that, if the fluorocarbon had a boiling point below 37°C, the liquid would convert to gas at body temperature, dramatically increasing bubble size, elasticity, and, therefore, reflectivity. These results were demonstrated when dodecafluoropentane emulsion was administered intravenously (Correas and Quay 1996). This product, developed by Sonus Pharmaceuticals in the mid to late 1990s, was given the name Echogen and has been approved for use in Europe. It has been submitted for approval in the United States for endocardial border delineation. Its radiologic applications are still under development. Although this agent is visible on gray-scale (Sehgal et al. 1995), it has been tested in man at low dosages that have only been detectable on Doppler sonography (Robbin and Eisenfeld 1998).

A series of products are now under development that are fluorocarbon gas and air filled: AF0150 (Imagent, Alliance Pharmaceuticals Corp., San Diego, Calif.), BR1 (Bracco Diagnostics), DMP115 (Dupont), and NC100100 (Nycomed-Amersham). The predecessor of DMP115, Aerosome, was abandoned because of its lesser efficacy, as it was an air-filled liposome. Optison, approved for endocardial border delineation, is under development for radiologic applications. These are the products that this author is aware of. It should be noted that this field is changing rapidly, and that changes are quite likely by the time this book is in print. Although some of these agents may reach the end user, several patent issues need to be resolved. It is not clear which agents will ultimately reach fruition. What is clear, however, is that a highly effective class of agents is in its final phases of development, and that these agents should impact clinical practice.

25.4.2 Indications

The need for contrast agents to visualize the endocardiac border, and to enhance the myocardium to detect perfusion abnormalities, has driven the field and led the development. Although transpulmonary agents became available in the mid 1980s for research and in the early 1990s for clinical use, the major effort began when the late-generation agents were shown to enhance the myocardium and depict perfusion defects. In fact, the majority of publications shown in Fig. 25.1 relate to cardiac applications. The major research effort at the present time is to assess coronary atherosclerotic disease by demonstrating diminished coronary reserve during stress echocardiography. This topic and its history are covered in Chap. 33.

Radiologic applications began to appear in the early 1980s, when fluorocarbon emulsions were described. Most of the original effort was aimed at liver and tumor imaging (Mattrey et al. 1982, 1983, 1987a,b; Parker et al. 1987; Behan et al. 1993). The radiologic applications will be described here by mode of administration: intravenous, oral, intracavitary, and interstitial.

25.4.2.1 Intravenous

Intravenous administration of contrast media allows the imaging of the vascular space and solid organs. As microbubbles are too large to escape the capillaries, the agent remains intravascular to enhance the blood pool. Agents not visible on gray-scale enhance Doppler signals, thus increasing the visualization of smaller and deeper vessels that could not be imaged before. These agents, Levovist and Echogen, could then be used to assess Doppler flow. Some investigators have emphasized quantitation and have shown distinct time/intensity curve characteristics in benign and malignant disease. This topic is discussed in more detail in Chap. 29 and 31.

The latest-generation agents are visible on gray-scale, providing new capabilities and potential. In fact, these agents permit high-resolution imaging of the intravascular space, which is not possible with the Doppler agents. These applications are covered in more detail in Chap. 30. It should be noted that gray-scale filling of vessels is potentially more powerful than filling the vessel with Doppler signal. This is because Doppler information is being used to fill vessels to provide anatomical detail. Although this method is reasonable in a significant number of situations, flow and stucture no longer overlap in conditions when flow is disturbed by plaque, aneurysm, clot, or vascular tortuosity. In these situations, turbulence and flow heterogeneity no longer follow structure, resulting in either over- or underestimation of atherosclerotic disease. Gray-scale filling of vessels should be able to depict intraluminal clot and define whether the vessel is completely or partially filled and whether the clot is recanalized (Coley et al. 1994). The interior and the exterior arterial wall will be clearly depicted, allowing the accurate assessment of plaque and atherosclerotic disease. In fact, this technique may become the standard method for the assessment of carotid disease, rather than estimation of stenosis by the presence of abnormal velocity. This topic is covered in more detail in Chapter 30.

The applications for solid organ and tumor imaging will likely become an important role for contrast media. The detection of liver and spleen space-occupying lesions was demonstrated in 1982 by Mattrey et al. because of liver-specific accumulation of echogenic particles. As some microbubble systems, such as Levovist, NC100100, SHU563A, and others, accumulate in the liver and spleen this application appears to be possible with the newer, more effective agents. However, except for NC100100 and SHU 563A, the mechanism of liver entrapment is not yet clear. It appears to be likely related to the slowing of bubbles in the sinusoids of the liver, where flow is too slow to counteract the gravitational effect that causes layering of the bubbles along the non-dependent portion of the sinusoids. Because bubbles are destroyed by ultrasound, liver enhancement lasts for 1 or 2 frames as the transducer is swept across the bubble-filled liver. It is, therefore, important to freeze the images and review them in memory one frame at a time. Liver imaging will be possible with most agents; however, Levovist and SHU563A appear to have greater liver accumulation. Because space-occupying lesions lack sinusoids and reticuloendothelial cells, they appear hypoechoic relative to the enhanced background of the liver. The disadvantage of this technique is the creation of destruction waves that could mimic lesions, and vessels could also mimic small lesions. However, the latter can be recognized as cylindrical structures when consecutive frames are reviewed in the cine mode.

The major indication for solid organ imaging is the enhancement of perfused tissues, which allows the detection of perfusion defects or alterations in perfusion. More than likely, the presence of particles in tissue vessels shortly after infusion enhances tissue echogenicity to a degree comparable to the blood content of the tissue. Although this was true with PFOB emulsion, because the liquid particles were not affected by the sound beam (Munzing et al. 1990), the new agents are destroyed by ultrasound. Destruction adds an unknown element that is bubble- and flow-dependent. If bubbles are fragile, or if the transit time through the tissue is slow, they will be destroyed, affecting tissue enhancement. Because of bubble destruction image contrast will be dependent on blood flow, transmit power (which is focal zone- and frequency-dependent), blood volume, and the sensitivity of the agent to ultrasound. Further, if intermittent imaging is used, image contrast is also dependent on the interframe delay, as the time between frames influences the number of bubbles that could be delivered to the region. For more detail on this topic, please refer to Chap. 32.

One potentially important application that was described with PFOB emulsion was lost with microbubble systems: PFOB permitted the determination of whether kidneys had normal or abnormal concentrating ability. Because PFOB is radiopaque and served as a blood pool agent for CT for several hours (Mattrey 1989), we observed that the renal medulla appeared brighter than cortex. This result was obtained despite the fact that animals were normotensive, PFOB is neither eliminated nor entrapped by the kindney, and the renal cortex contains more blood per gram of tissue than the medulla. Using a dog model, Coley et al. (1990b) showed that the medulla was brighter than cortex because of the osmotic gradient across the papillae. When animals were given Lasix, the medulla lost its signal, becoming less dense than cortex. We believe that the osmotic gradient in the papilla decreases the water content in the interstitium and the vascular space, increasing PFOB concentration and resulting in a higher CT attenuation. Because PFOB particles are visible sonographically, we speculated that sonography may be able to distinguish the normal from the abnormal osmotic gradient. Conditions that affect the osmotic gradient include acute tubular necrosis (ATN), renal artery stenosis, ureteral obstruction, and drugs. A unilateral ATN rabbit model was used to test this hypothesis. Although the ATN kidney was indistinguishable from the normal kidney prior to contrast administration, the administration of PFOB emulsion allowed the recognition of the affected kidney in all rabbits (Munzing et al. 1990). This was possible because the medulla of the ATN kidney failed to enhance following contrast administration.

When microbubbles are given IV, the cortex enhances dramatically and the medulla does not. This result was thought to be due to the fact that the cortex is more vascular than the medulla and cortical enhancement shadows the medulla. However, because bubble destruction is more effective when transit time is long, lack of medullary enhancement is likely due to microbubble destruction since bubbles must travel down and then back up the capillaries paralleling Henle's loop. As intermittent imaging is one technique to image bubbles in capillaries, it may allow the recognition of the medullary enhancement and likely concentrating ability of the kidney. This hypothesis, however, has not yet been tested.

25.4.2.2
Oral

Often ultrasound images of the pancreas, stomach wall, duodenum, and retroperitoneal structures are degraded by bowel gas, and as a result the diagnostic confidence is diminished. Safe, inexpensive oral agents have been proposed (SISLER and TILCOCK 1995; MURADALI et al. 1998; LUND et al. 1992) that are capable of reducing gas artifact, thus improving visualization of bowel wall and surrounding structures. These agents have been shown in animals and in man to be superior to water. Two of these agents have completed the clinical development process, but have not yet been approved for marketing. One agent was developed by ImaRx and licensed to Bracco Diagnostics, and the other was developed by Molecular Biosystems.

25.4.2.3
Intracavitary

MEYER-SCHWICKERATH and FRITSCH in 1986 explored urologic applications of contrast when they imaged the renal pelvis following instillation of with SHU454 in the urinary bladder. This concept was extended to Albunex, and similar results were shown in vitro and in vivo when a 1:100 dilution was used (ATALA et al. 1993). A clinical study performed in the pediatric age group demonstrated the safety and effectiveness of the procedure, with vesicoureteric reflux being diagnosed in 100% of cases (BOSIO 1998). The ultrasound study detected 14 refluxing units out of 100 units that were not detected during a voiding cystourethrogram. Although the 14% false-positive rate relative to the cystogram sounds negative, the question is: which of these studies is the true gold standard?

An application that has become more established is the assessment of tubal patency under ultrasound guidance. This technique was first introduced by DEICHERT et al. in 1989. It consists in filling the uterine cavity with saline to assess the endometrial surface, followed by the injection of either Echovist or Albunex while observing the tubes. The goal is to observe spill at the fimbriae on both sides. The benefit of this technique is the lack of ionizing radiation in patients attempting to conceive. X-ray hysterosalpingography has been shown on meta-analysis investigation to be 65% sensitive and 85% specific, indicating that tubal occlusion is more accurately detected than patency (SWART et al. 1995). The ultrasound contrast technique has been referred to as either HyCoSy (hysterocontrast sonography) or sonoHSG. Several studies have demonstrated not only the feasibility of such a technique, but also its accuracy. A meta-analysis combining the existing clinical data showed that HyCoSy, as compared to laparoscopy, had identical results in 688 of 828 (83.1%) individual tubes, with "false" occlusion in 10.3% and "false" patency in 6.7% (HOLZ et al. 1997). That same study reported that HSG, compared to laparoscopy, had identical results in 116 of 152 tubes (76.3%), with "false" occlusion in 12.5% and "false" patency in 11.2%. Therefore, it appears that this technique is comparable to HSG. Comparable results were shown with Albunex (HOLTE et al. 1995).

25.4.2.4
Interstitial

A potential application that has not been explored is the subcutaneous injection of ultrasound contrast for lymph node imaging. The feasibility of this application was demonstrated when PFDB emulsion was injected subcutaneously. It was known that the emulsion particles accumulate within macrophages in local lymph nodes (HANNA et al. 1994; WOLF et al. 1994). (IKOMI et al. 1994). Because PFDB emulsion is echogenic, it served as an ultrasound lymphographic agent, allowing the recognition of normal from hyperplastic nodes and the latter from nodes with V×2 metastases (WRIGLEY et al. 1993). The normal portions of the node enhanced intensely, whereas V×2 deposits remained unenhanced, appearing as filling defects. With the increased popularity of sentinel node surgery to limit or minimize lymph node dissection in melanoma (KELLEY et al. 1998) and breast cancer patients (GIULIANO et al. 1997), preoperative localization could revolutionize the field. Ultrasound lymphography could serve that role, particularly if the microbubble has an affinity to lymph node tissues to limit the enhancement to the sentinel node. Microbubble systems have not been tested for this application because of the fragility of the microbubbles and their relatively large size, which may inhibit their entry into the lymph vessel. The use of fluorocarbon emulsion or microbubble systems, should they be able to gain access to the lymphatics, should improve the preoperative localization of the sentinel node.

25.4.3
Instrumentation

25.4.3.1
Standard Imaging

Current systems are optimized to image tissues with low impedance differences across an interface.

Except for fat, which offers a 15% difference in impedance mismatch, most tissues differ by a few percent. When microbubbles are introduced into the system, they create interfaces that are orders of magnitude more reflective than tissues. Further, at resonance, microbubbles become emitters themselves, flooding the transducer with signal. Therefore, current systems that are optimized for low reflectivity become saturated with signal. Although many systems now offer a wider dynamic range than past systems, none of the current systems are properly optimized for contrast imaging in standard gray-scale.

In addition to signal saturation, microbubbles have a negative influence on the ultrasound beam and image quality that will be more difficult to resolve. The passage of the sound beam through a field where microbubbles exist creates phase aberrations, as small areas of the beam front slow when traveling through bubbles, whereas other parts of the beam front traveling between bubbles are unaffected. This process creates an irregular beam front that, within a voxel, can result in destructive and constructive interference. In an experiment using Albunex, Mobley et al. (1998) showed that the dispersion of phase velocities grew with increasing bubble concentration.

The impact of contrast media on Doppler imaging has had a positive as well as a negative influence. Contrast media have boosted signal and allowed the visualization of smaller and deeper vessels, as well as vessels with slow flow velocity. However, because of the low spatial resolution of color Doppler and the dramatic increase in signal from the contrast agent, blooming artifacts result, degrading structural detail. In addition, because motion remains a requirement for the generation of color signal, visualization of small microvascular channels is lost as blood velocity becomes equal to or less than that of tissue motion. Increase in color signal with Doppler imaging in the presence of microbubbles is also observed, even in the absence of flow (Burns et al. 1995). This is because Doppler is a multipulse technique that compares the signal between two consecutive pulses. Because bubbles are destroyed by sound, the first pulse destroys the bubble and the second pulse detects its disappearance, resulting in loss of correlation between the two pulses; a color pixel is assigned to the voxel where the bubble resided. In the pulse-wave mode, the increased backscatter affects the gray-scale lookup table, filling the entire velocity spectrum with signal and increasing peak velocity signal. If the gain setting is kept high, then the wave form displays a higher peak velocity. The gray-scale lookup table, adjusted for backscatter from blood, is inappropriate for contrast media. The lookup table could be adjusted by instrument manufacturers to obviate potential errors.

It should be clear from the above discussion that improvements in instrumentation to achieve standard imaging that is appropriate for microbubble systems should improve image quality and contrast performance. However, the recent development of contrast-specific imaging techniques will likely push optimization of standard B-mode and Doppler imaging to a lower priority level.

25.4.3.2 Contrast-Specific Imaging

A full chapter (see Chap. 27) is dedicated to this important topic, as it is critical for the success of contrast media application. Second-harmonic, wideband harmonic (also called pulse inversion), transient response imaging, and so on have leveled the playing field for many contrast agents. Levovist, which was invisible on gray-scale imaging, is visible with these specific techniques. These new imaging techniques are mostly software upgrades on digital systems. Their impact on radiologic applications will be analogous to color and power Doppler and will make them indispensable upgrades. The greatest need for these techniques will be in liver and spleen imaging, where there is a delicate balance between dose, efficacy, and attenuation.

25.5 Future Direction

It is clear from the excitement that has been generated, both in the literature and at scientific meetings, that ultrasound contrast media will be as critical in clinical practice as contrast media have been for CT and magnetic resonance (MR) imaging. The field is burgeoning, with many more innovations yet to come. Given the high cost and the very slow cycle of drug development, as compared with the rapid instrument development cycle, many more innovations will occur in instrumentation.

The highly efficacious current-generation agents, and the revival of the older-generation agents with new contrast-specific imaging techniques, will inhibit the development of products with similar performance. However, should the ultrasound contrast market be as large as anticipated, where even a small market share translates into large returns, new or slightly improved agents will continue to be introduced. It is also possible that, with increased understanding of microbubble behavior in an ultrasound field and the availability of specific imaging or quantitation techniques, specific microbubble systems will be developed. For instance, if bubble destruction is important, more fragile bubbles might have an advantage. Such bubbles, if made resistant to plasma and ambient pressure variations but sensitive to the ultrasound pressures, could deliver sufficient concentrations to the tissue of interest to provide the needed imaging performance.

The future needs for ultrasound contrast are targeting to specific sites for improved diagnostic yield, therapeutic intervention, or drug delivery. Because of the importance of this potential, a full chapter is dedicated to this topic (see Chap. 34).

The development of instrumentation technology will continue to improve and expand at a rapid pace because of the short development cycle, the fierce competition among instrument manufacturers, and the unique synergism between microbubbles and the ultrasound beam. No other imaging modality can make that claim. Although x-ray agents perform better if the x-ray energy matches their K-edge, and a particular MR pulsing sequence takes advantage of the T1 or T2 shortening or susceptibility effects of an MR agent, microbubble behavior during ultrasound radiation is not shared with tissues and is more easily exploited in ultrasound systems.

25.6 Summary

The current status of ultrasound contrast agents and the flurry of unique ultrasound imaging techniques have sparked excitement in this field. This advance should be credited to the pioneers who kept the excitement alive and continued to attract support from pharmaceutical and instrument companies and funding agencies. It is through the understanding of pharmacokinetics, contrast agent and ultrasound interaction, and potential impact on clinical practice that the field developed to its current status and assumed an equal position with the x-ray and MR agents. Ultrasound contrast research was a curiosity from the practitioner's perspective. It was driven by a few and was included in meetings for completion of the program. This field has now burgeoned into a powerful potential contributor to the care of patients. New investigators, in both industry and academia, continue to flock to this new well of opportunity. This field has long needed the critical mass to push it forward. I can safely say we are there.

References

Andre M, Nelson T, Mattrey RF (1990) Physical and acoustical properties of perfluorooctylbromide, an ultrasound contrast agent. Invest Radiol 25:983–987

Atala A, Wible JH, Share JC, Carr MC, Retik AB, Mandell J (1993) Sonography with sonicated albumin in the detection of vesicoureteral reflux. J Urol 150(2 Pt 2):756–758

Behan M, O'Connell D, Mattrey RF, Carney DN (1993) Perfluorooctylbromide as a contrast agent for sonography and computed tomography. AJR 160:399–405

Blomley M, Albrecht T, Cosgrove DO, et al. (1998) Improved imaging of liver metastases using stimulated acoustic emission in the late enhancement phase of the ultrasound contrast agent Levovist. Radiology (in press)

Bosio M (1998) Cystosonography with echocontrast: a new imaging modality to detect vesicoureteric reflux in children. Pediatr Radiol 28:250–255

Burns PN, Fritzsch T, Weitschies W, Uhlendorf V, Hope-Simpson D, Powers JE (1995) Pseudo-Doppler shifts from stationary tissues due to the stimulated emission of ultrasound from a new microsphere contrast agent. Radiology 197(P):402

Clark LC, Gollan F (1966) Survival of mammals breathing organic liquids equilibrated with oxygen at atmospheric pressure. Science 152:1755–1756

Coley BD, Mattrey RF, Roberts A, Keane SF (1990a) The potential role of PFOB enhanced sonography of the kidney. Part II. Detection of partial infarction. Kidney Int 39:740–745

Coley BD, Mattrey RF, Mitten RM, Peterson T (1990b) The physiologic basis of the radiodense renal medulla after the administration of blood pool contrast agent, PFOB. Invest Radiol 25:1287–1293

Coley BD, Trambert MA, Mattrey RF (1994) Perfluorocarbon enhanced sonography: value in detecting acute venous thrombosis in rabbits. AJR 163:961–964

Correas JM, Quay SD (1996) EchoGen emulsion : a new ultrasound contrast agent based on phase shift colloids. Clin Radiol 51(Suppl 1):11–14

Deichert U, Schleif R, van de Sandt M, Juhnke I (1989) Transvaginal hysterosalpingo-contrast-sonography (Hy-Co-Sy) compared with conventional tubal diagnostics. Hum Reprod 4:418–424

Feinstein SB, Ten Cate FJ, Zwehl W, et al. (1984) Two-dimensional contrast echocardiography. I. In vitro development and quantitative analysis of echo contrast agents. J Am Coll Cardiol 3:14–20

Feinstein SB, Cheirif J, Ten Cate FJ, et al. (1990) Safety and efficacy of a new transpulmonary ultrasound contrast agent: initial multicenter clinical results. J Am Coll Cardiol 16:316–324

Giuliano AE, Jones RC, Brennan M, Statman R (1997) Sentinel lymphadenectomy in breast cancer. J Clin Oncol 15:2345–2350

Gramiak R, Shah PM (1968) Echocardiography of the aortic root. Invest Radiol 3:356–366

Hanna G, Saewert D, Shorr J, Flaim K, Leese P, Kopperman M, Wolf G (1994) Preclinical and clinical studies on lymph node imaging using perflubron emulsion. Art Cells, Blood Subst Immob Biotech 22:1429–1439

Hauff P, Fritzsch T, Reinhardt M, Weitschies W, Luders F, Uhlendorf V, Heldmann D (1997) Delineation of experimental liver tumors in rabbits by a new ultrasound contrast agent and stimulated acoustic emission. Invest Radiol 32:94–99

Hilpert PL, Mattrey RF, Mitten RM, Peterson T (1989) IV injection of air-filled human albumin microspheres to enhance arterial Doppler signal: a preliminary study in rabbits. AJR Am J Roentgenol 153:613–616

Holte J, Rasmussen C, Morris H (1995) First clinical experience with sonicated human serum albumin (Albunex) as an intrafallopian ultrasound contrast medium. Ultrasound Obstet Gynecol 6:62–65

Holz K, Becker R, Schurmann R (1997) Ultrasound in the investigation of tubal patency. A meta-analysis of three comparative studies of Echovist-200 including 1007 women. Zentralbl Gynakol 119:366–373

Ikomi F, Hanna G, Schmid Schonbein GW (1994) Intracellular and extracellular transport of perfluoro carbon emulsion from subcutaneous tissue to regional lymphatics. Art Cells Blood Subst Immob Biotech 22:1441–1447

Keller MW, Feinstein SB, Briller RA, Powsner SM (1986) Automated production and analysis of echo contrast agents. J Ultrasound Med 5:493–498

Kelley MC, Ollila DW, Morton DL (1998) Lymphatic mapping and sentinel lymphadenectomy for melanoma. Semin Surg Oncol 14:283–290

Kremkau FW, Gramiak R, Carstensen EL, Shah PM, Kramer DH (1970) Ultrasonic detection of cavitation at catheter tips. Am J Roentgenol Radium Ther Nucl Med 110:177–183

Lund PJ, Fritz TA, Unger EC, Hunt RK, Fuller E (1992) Cellulose as a gastrointestinal US contrast agent. Radiology 185:783–788

Mattrey RF, Scheible FW, Gosink BB, Leopold GR, Long DM, Higgins CB (1982) Perfluoroctylbromide: a liver/spleen-specific and a tumor-imaging ultrasound contrast material. Radiology 145:759–762

Mattrey RF, Leopold GR, vanSonnenberg E, Gosink BB, Scheible FW, Long DM (1983) Perfluorochemicals as liver and spleen seeking ultrasound contrast agents. J Ultrasound Med 2:173–176

Mattrey RF, Strich G, Shelton RE, Gosink BB, Leopold GR, Lee T, Forsythe J (1987a) Perfluorochemicals as US contrast agents for tumor imaging and hepatosplenography: preliminary clinical results. Radiology 163:339–343

Mattrey RF, Mitten R, Peterson T, Long DC (1987b) Vascular ultrasonic enhancement of tissues with perfluoroctylbromide for renal tumor detection. Radiology 165(P):76

Mattrey RF (1989) Perfluorooctyl bromide: a new contrast agent for CT, sonography, and MR imaging. Am J Roentgenol 152:247–252

Mattrey RF, Andre MP (1984) Ultrasonic enhancement of myocardial infarction with perfluorocarbon compounds in dogs. Am J Cardiol 54:206–210

Mattrey RF, Steinbach GC (1991) Ultrasound contrast agents. State of the art. Invest Radiol 26(Suppl 1):S5–S11

Mattrey RF, Wrigley R, Steinbach GC, Schutt EG, Evitts DP (1994a) Gas emulsion as ultrasound contrast agents: preliminary results in rabbits and dogs. Invest Radiol 29:S139–S141

Mattrey RF, Steinbach GC, Peterson T, Hall LA (1994b) Echogenic enhancement of the perfused myocardium following the intravenous administration of PFC microbubbles. Radiology 193(P):367

Mattrey RF, Baker K, Hall LA, Steinbach GC, Peterson T (19••) Placental enhancement with Imagent® US (AF0145), a perfluorochemical (PFC) stabilized microbubble ultrasound contrast agent. Contrast Media Research Symposium 6/95, Turku, Finland

Meyer-Schwickerath M, Fritzsch T (1986) Sonographic imaging of the kidney cavity system using an ultrasonic contrast medium. Ultraschall Med 7:34–36

Mobley J, Marsh JN, Hall CS, Hughes MS, Brandenburger GH, Miller JG (1998) Broadband measurements of phase velocity in Albunes suspensions. J Acoust Soc Am 103:2145–2153

Moriyasu F, Kono Y, Kamiyama N, et al. (1998) Flash echo imaging of liver tumors using ultrasound contrast agent and intermittent color Doppler scanning. J Ultrasound Med 17:S63

Munzing D, Mattrey RF, Reznik VM, Mitten RM, Peterson T (1990) The potential role of PFOB enhanced sonography of the kidney. Part I. Detection of renal function and acute tubular necrosis. Kidney Int 39:733–739

Muradali D, Burns PN, Pron G, Hope-Simpson D, Wilson S (1998) Improved retroperitoneal and gastrointestinal sonography using oral contrast agents in a porcine model. AJR 17:475–481

Ophir J, Parker KJ (1989) Contrast agents in diagnostic ultrasound. J Ultrasound Med Biol 15:319–333

Ophir J, McWhirt RE, Maklad NF (1979) Aqueous solutions as potential ultrasonic contrast agents. Ultrason Imaging 1:265–279

Parker KJ, Tuthill TA, Lerner RM, Violante MR (1987) A particulate contrast agent with potential for ultrasound imaging of liver. Ultrasound Med Biol 13:555–566

Phillips D, Chen X, Baggs R, Rubens D, Violante M, Parker KJ (1998) Acoustic backscatter properties of the particle/bubble ultrasound contrast agent. Ultrasonics 36:883–892

Robbin ML, Eisenfeld AJ (1998) Perflenapent emulsion: a US contrast agent for diagnostic radiology – multicenter, double-blind comparison with a placebo. EchoGen Contrast Ultrasound Study Group. Radiology 207:717–722

Satterfield R, Tarter M, Schumacher D, Tran P, Mattrey RF (1993) Comparison of different perfluorocarbons as ultrasound contrast agents. Invest Radiol 28:325–331

Schutt EG, Pelura TJ, Hopkins RM (1996) Osmotically stabilized microbubble sonographic contrast agents. Acad Radiol 3(Suppl 2):S188–190

Sehgal CM, Arger PH, Pugh CR (1995) Sonographic enhancement of renal cortex by contrast media. J Ultrasound Med 14:741–748

Sisler WJ, Tilcock C (1995) Effect of cellulose concentration on the efficacy of a cellulose-based oral contrast agent for gastrointestinal ultrasonography. J Ultrasound Med 14:267–272

Slinn DSL, Green SW (1982) Fluorocarbon fluids for use in the electronics industry. In: Banks RE (ed) Preparation, properties, and industrial applications of organofluorine compounds. Ellis Horwood, Chichester, UK, pp 45–82

Smith MD, Kwan OL, Reiser HJ, DeMaria AN (1984) Superior intensity and reproducibility of SHU-454, a new right heart contrast agent. J Am Coll Cardiol 3(4):992–998

Smith MD, Elion JL, McClure RR, Kwan OL, DeMaria AN (1989) Left heart opacification with peripheral venous injection of a new saccharide echo contrast agent in dogs. J Am Coll Cardiol 13:1622–1628

Swart P, Mol BW, van der Veen F, van Beurden M, Redekop WK, Bossuyt PM (1995) The accuracy of hysterosalpingography in the diagnosis of tubal pathology: a meta-analysis. Fertil Steril 64:486–491

Tyler TD, Ophir J, Maklad NF, Gobuty A (1981) In vivo enhancement of ultrasonic image luminance by aqueous solutions with high speed of sound. Ultrason Imaging 3:323–329

Unger EC, Lund P, Shen D, Fritz T, Fuller L, Yellowhair D (1991) Aerosomes as blood pool and cardiovascular contrast agent for US: in vivo studies (abstract). Radiology 181(P):225

Violante MR, Dean PB, Fischer HW, Mahoney JA (1980) Particulate contrast media for computed tomographic scanning of the liver. Invest Radiol 15(6 Suppl):S171–S175

Violante MR, Baggs RB, Tuthill T, Dentinger P, Parker KJ (1991) Particle-stabilized bubbles for enhanced organ ultrasound imaging. Invest Radiol 26(Suppl 1):S194–S197

Wolf GL, Rogowska J, Hanna GK, Halpern EF (1994) Percutaneous CT lymphography with perflubron: imaging efficacy in rabbits and monkeys. Radiology 191:501–505

Wrigley RW, Saunders HB, Lim G, Arellano RA, Mattrey RF (1993) Indirect ultrasonographic lymphography with perflubron emulsion. Radiology 189(P):285

26 Interaction of Ultrasound and Contrast Agents

P.P. Chang and K.K. Shung

CONTENTS

26.1 Introduction

There has been an increasing interest in recent years in the development of ultrasonic contrast agents, primarily because of the advent of technology that allows the production of contrast agents capable of traversing pulmonary circulation and persisting in the bloodstream for more than a few seconds, and the many clinical applications that these agents possess (Ophir and Parker 1989; Goldberg et al. 1994; de Jong 1996). The most important function that an ultrasound contrast agent performs is to enhance the backscattered signal of a certain anatomical structure that contains the agent, turning what is obscure in an ultrasonic image into a more recognizable structure. Contrast agents that contain gas are most effective due to the mismatch in acoustic impedance between the gas and soft tissues.

To better understand how these agents enhance signet, and what and how ultrasound propagation parameters affect the performance of these agents, this chapter presents the physical basis of the interaction between the impinging ultrasonic wave and the contrast agent, including the effect of the agent on the attenuation and scattering of ultrasound. A brief review of the theoretical development and some of the experimental results will also be included.

Harmonic imaging and Doppler involving a gaseous contrast agent came about because a serious problem may arise in contrast imaging and Doppler. When the backscattered signals from the contrast agents are comparable to those from structures surrounding the target, the application of a contrast agent may actually reduce the image contrast between the target and the surrounding tissues. This problem occurs, for example, when imaging flow in blood vessels at frequencies higher than 50 MHz.

Certain properties of contrast agents may be exploited to discriminate the echoes from the contrast agent and the non-contrast-containing structures. Harmonic imaging and Doppler measurements that utilize the resonance properties of gas-containing agents, first investigated by Schrope and co-workers (Schrope et al. 1992; Schrope and Newhouse 1993) have generated considerable interest. The feasibility of using 2nd harmonic signal produced by gas-containing agents such as Albunex and Levovist for imaging and Doppler measurements has been demonstrated (Burns et al. 1994; de Jong et al. 1994a,b; Chang et al. 1995, 1996; Forsberg et al. 1996).

26.2 Ultrasonic Propagation in a Distribution of Encapsulated Gaseous Microspheres

The ultrasonic beam generated by a transducer or array is fairly complicated (Shung and Zipparo 1996; Zagzebski 1996). Many factors must be considered when attempting to do a quantitative

P.P. Chang, PhD, Research Scientist, Applied Physics Laboratory, University of Washington, 1013 NE 40th St., Seattle, WA 98105-6698, USA
K.K. Shung, PhD, Professor of Bioengineering, Bioengineering Program, 31 Hallowell Bldg., The Pennsylvania State University, University Park, PA 16802, USA

measurement or interpretation of the image or data. However, for a qualitative assessment, sometimes approximations can be made to simplify the interpretation. Here it is assumed that the wave generated by an ultrasonic probe is a plane wave, i.e., the wave front is planar. As it penetrates a distribution of scatterers, the wave amplitude represented by pressure P_z and intensity I_z decreases according to the following equations (SHUNG et al. 1992; ZAGZEBSKI 1996):

$$I_z = I_0 e^{-2\beta z} \tag{26.1}$$

$$P_z = P_0 e^{-\beta z}, \tag{26.2}$$

where z = distance traveled, I_0 = intensity at $z = 0$, P_0 = pressure at $z = 0$, and β = pressure attenuation coefficient in np/cm (= 8.686 × β dB/cm) of the medium.

For a distribution of low bubble concentration, the attenuation coefficient is given by:

$$\beta = \frac{n\sigma_e}{2}, \tag{26.3}$$

where n = scatterer or bubble concentration or number of scatterers per unit volume, and σ_e = extinction cross-section or total scattering cross-section (ISHIMARU 1978; SHUNG et al. 1992; DE JONG et al. 1992).

26.2.1 Extinction Cross-section

The extinction cross-section σ_e, with a unit of cm^2, is frequency dependent and represents the total energy loss for an ultrasonic wave resulting from the presence of one scatterer in a unit volume, e.g., cm^3. It is the sum of the absorption cross-section σ_a and the scattering cross-section σ_s (ISHIMARU 1978; SHUNG et al. 1992; DE JONG et al. 1992):

$$\sigma_e = \sigma_a + \sigma_s. \tag{26.4}$$

Both σ_a and σ_s have the dimension cm^2 and represent the energy absorbed and scattered, respectively, due to the presence of one scatterer in a unit volume. The question that often arises is the relative contribution of each of these terms to the total attenuation. The attenuation, if accurately estimated, can sometimes give information about the properties of the tissue, but in general it is not desirable, especially the absorption component. To achieve optimal ultrasonic contrast, the absorption of the contrast agent should be made as low as possible to avoid losing energy and shadowing biological structures, while the scattering is maximized.

26.2.2 Scattering Cross-section

The scattering properties of biological tissues and blood have long been an area of intensive investigation because these signals are used to form an ultrasonic image (SHUNG and THIEME 1993). Several investigators have also studied the acoustic properties of liquids containing gas bubbles (DEVIN 1959; MEDWIN 1977; ANDERSON and HAMPTON 1980). Their principal motivation has involved underwater acoustics. Nevertheless, these theories can be readily applied to the present case, in which gaseous contrast agents are suspended in a liquid medium.

MEDWIN (1977) has shown that the total scattering cross-section of a single bubble can be expressed as:

$$\sigma_s = \frac{4\pi R^2}{\left(\frac{f_r^2}{f^2} - 1\right)^2 + \delta^2}, \tag{26.5}$$

where R = radius of the bubble, f_r = resonance frequency of the bubble, f = frequency of the incident ultrasonic wave, and δ = total damping constant.

26.2.2.1 Resonance Frequency of a Bubble

The resonance frequency of a bubble can be determined, assuming the following: the wavelength of the ultrasonic wave is much larger than the bubble diameter; the radial displacement of the bubble is small compared to its radius; and the surrounding fluid is incompressible. These conditions are easily fulfilled for the majority of ultrasound contrast agents. Also, water and blood can virtually be considered incompressible.

The simplest equation of resonance frequency for a bubble in water was given by MINNAERT (1933):

$$f_r = \frac{1}{2\pi R}\sqrt{\frac{3\gamma P_0}{\varrho_w}} \tag{26.6}$$

or:

$$f_r = \frac{1}{2\pi}\sqrt{\frac{S_a}{m}}, \tag{26.7}$$

where γ = ratio of specific heats of the gas (≈ 1.4), P_0 = hydrostatic ambient pressure (= 1.013×10^6 dyne/cm^2), ϱ_w = density of the water (= 1.03 g/cm^3), S_a = adiabatic stiffness (= $12\pi\gamma P_0 R$), and m = effective mass of the system (= $4\pi R^3 \varrho_w$). Here, an adiabatic equation of state was assumed. However, for bubbles of small radii, surface tension becomes a significant additional restoring force and needs to be considered. The oscillation in this case is closer to an isothermal process. When these points are considered, the equation for resonance frequency changes. P_0 in Eq. 26.6 is replaced by the average *interior* pressure including surface tension, ζP_0, and γ is replaced by the *effective* ratio of specific heats in the presence of thermal conductivity, γb (MEDWIN 1977; DE JONG et al. 1992; DE JONG 1996):

$$f_r = \frac{1}{2\pi R}\sqrt{\frac{3\gamma b \zeta P_0}{\varrho_\omega}}, \tag{26.8}$$

where:

$$B = 3(\gamma - 1)\left[\frac{X(\sinh X + \sin X) - 2(\cosh X - \cos X)}{X^2(\cosh X - \cos X) + 3(\gamma - 1)X(\sinh X - \sin X)}\right] \tag{26.9}$$

$$b = \left(1 + B^2\right)^{-1}\left[1 + \frac{3(\gamma - 1)}{X}\left(\frac{\sinh X - \sin X}{\cosh X - \cos X}\right)\right]^{-1} \tag{26.10}$$

$$\zeta = 1 + \frac{2\sigma}{P_0 R}\left(1 - \frac{1}{3\gamma b}\right) \tag{26.11}$$

$$X = R\left(2\omega\varrho_g C_{pg} / K_g\right)^{1/2}. \tag{26.12}$$

In these equations, K_g = thermal conductivity of gas (= 5.6×10^{-5} cal/cm-s°C); ϱ_g = density of free gas at sea level (= 1.29×10^{-3} g/cm^3); σ = surface tension (= 75 dyn/cm); C_{pg} = specific heat at constant pressure for air (= 0.24 cal/g), γ = ratio of specific heats, and ω = angular frequency.

The parameters b and ζ are plotted in Fig. 26.1 as a function of bubble radius at sea level. Figure 26.2 shows how the resonance frequency varies with the size of the bubbles. Note that small bubbles have very high resonance frequencies.

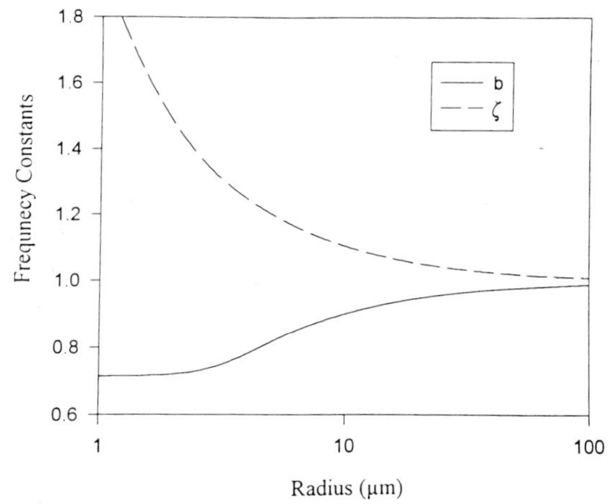

Fig. 26.1. Frequency constants for resonance frequency of air bubbles.

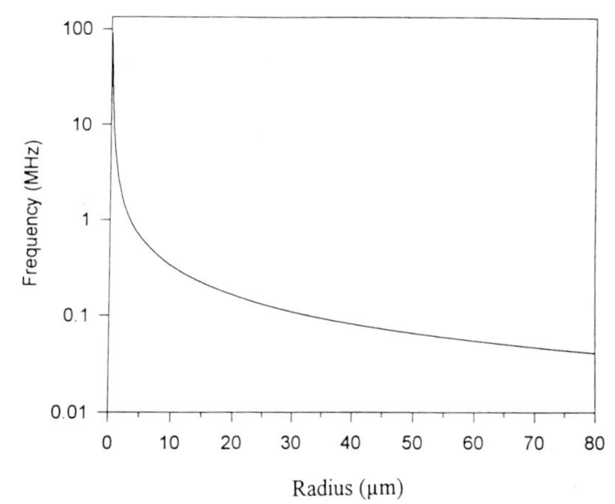

Fig. 26.2. Resonance frequency versus radius of the bubble.

26.2.2.2 Damping Constant

In Eq. 26.5 the damping constant δ can be written as the sum of three components (DEVIN 1959):

$$\delta = \delta_r + \delta_t + \delta_v, \tag{26.13}$$

where $\delta_r = kR$ = damping constant due to reradiation, k = wave number, $\delta_t = B(f_r/f)^2$ = damping constant due to thermal conductivity, $\delta_v = 4\eta/(\varrho_w \omega R^2)$ = damping constant due to shear viscosity, and η is the shear viscosity of the surrounding liquid (= 0.01 g/cm-s).

Using Eqs. 26.5–26.13, the scattering cross-section of a bubble can be calculated using the numerical values of parameters given above. The scattering cross-section of a bubble of 1.7 μm radius at an ambient pressure of 1 atm is shown in Fig. 26.3.

26.2.3 Absorption Cross-section

The portion of the energy absorbed or converted into heat by a scatterer from an ultrasonic wave is

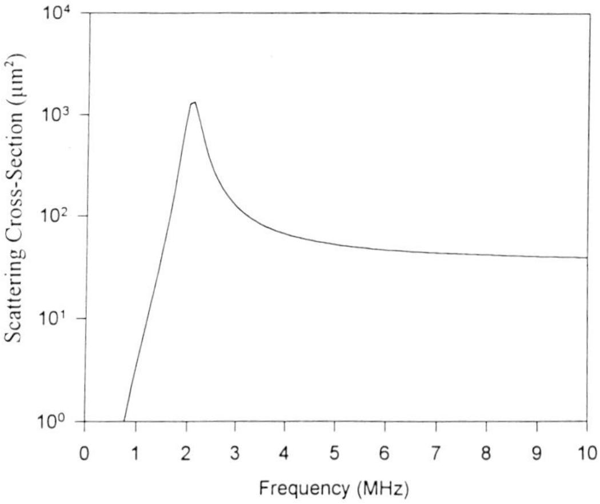

Fig. 26.3. Scattering cross-section for a 1.7 μm bubble

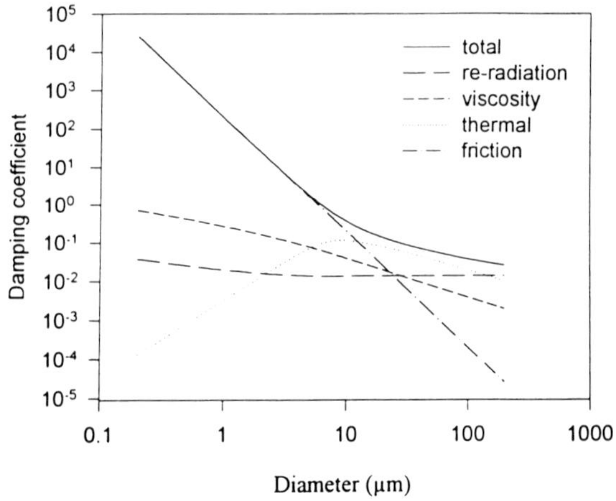

Fig. 26.4. Resonance damping constants for a 3 μm encapsulated air bubble at one atmosphere

referred as the absorption cross-section, and it is related to scattering cross-section by the following equation (MEDWIN 1977; DE JONG et al. 1992):

$$\sigma_a = \sigma_s\left(\frac{\delta}{\delta_r} - 1\right). \tag{26.14}$$

26.2.4 Bubbles with an Elastic Shell

So far, only the acoustic properties of a free bubble have been discussed, and the elastic shell of the gaseous contrast agents has not been considered. In fact, there have been very few theoretical studies on encapsulated gaseous microspheres. An early work by FOX and HERZFIELD (1954) discussed the issue that gas bubbles acting as cavitation nuclei are stabilized by an organic monomolecular skin. The organic skin would act as an elastic shell and as a mechanical barrier to diffusion. The organic skin provides rigidity and, therefore, would increase the resonance frequency of the bubbles. The stabilization of bubbles by an organic skin is essential for ultrasound contrast agents in order to increase their persistence in the bloodstream. One significant contribution to the development of theoretical models, describing ultrasonic propagation in a distribution of bubbles with an encapsulated shell, was made by DE JONG et al. (1992), who considered the shell surrounding Albunex bubbles as layers of elastic solids. Recently, CHURCH (1995) treated the surface layers by including numerical values for such parameters as modulus of elasticity, density, viscosity, and thickness.

DE JONG et al. (1992) hypothesized that the shell causes an additional restoring force to the system which tends to increase the resonance frequency and decrease the scattering cross-section. The contribution of the shell to the bubble stiffness is given by the following equation:

$$S_{\text{shell}} = 8\pi\frac{Et}{1-\nu} = 8\pi\cdot S_p, \tag{26.15}$$

where E = shell elasticity, t = wall thickness, ν = Poisson ratio, and $S_p = Et/(1-\nu)$ = the shell parameter given in dynes/cm. Although the shell elasticity, the wall thickness, and the Poisson ratio are unknown, the shell parameter can be estimated by matching the experimental results of attenuation coefficient to the theory. The model has shown better agreement for larger microspheres (lower resonant frequencies) than for small ones. In order to improve the agreement between theory and measurements, DE JONG and HOFF (1993) added an additional damping term, referred to as shell friction parameter (S_f), which accounts for the internal friction or viscosity within the shell. The damping coefficient due to the shell friction introduces an additional term to the total damping coefficient:

$$\delta_{\text{tot}} = \delta_r + \delta_t + \delta_v + \delta_f, \tag{26.16}$$

where:

$$\delta_f = \frac{S_f}{m\omega}. \tag{26.17}$$

Figure 26.4 shows how each term of Eq. 26.16 varies with the diameter of the bubble. Calculations were made at resonance for a 3-μm air bubble at one atmosphere. S_f was assumed equal to 0.004 g/s (or dyn·s/cm). DE JONG and HOFF (1993) found the optimum values for S_p and S_f to be 8×10^3 dyn/cm and 0.004 g/s respectively.

The resonance frequency, taking the shell stiffness into account, is given by:

$$f_{rs} = \frac{1}{2\pi}\sqrt{\frac{S_a b\zeta + S_{\text{shell}}}{m}}. \qquad (26.18)$$

26.3 Cloud of Bubbles

The dynamics of individual bubbles are of limited importance when considering the response of ultrasound contrast agents to an acoustic wave. A method for determining the effects of a cloud of bubbles is needed. When the concentration of the scatterers is low, the scattered power is proportional to the concentration of the scatterers (MORSE and INGARD 1968). For a distribution of bubbles of different sizes, the mean attenuation or scattering property at a single frequency ϕ_t can be calculated by considering the contribution of each bubble divided by the total concentration:

$$\phi_t(f) = \frac{\int_0^\infty \phi(R,f)n(R)dR}{N}, \qquad (26.19)$$

where R = radius of the scatterer, f = ultrasound frequency, $n(R)dR$ = number of bubbles of radius between R and $R + dR$ per unit volume of scattering medium, $\phi(R,f)$ = the attenuation or scattering property of a scatterer with radius R, and N = total concentration of scatterers.

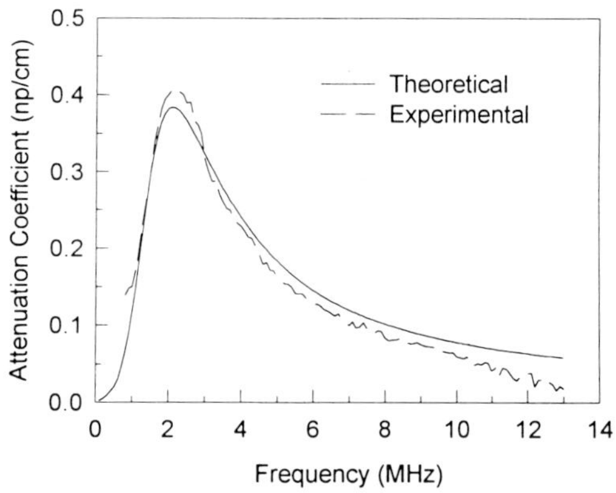

Fig. 26.5. Experimental and theoretical curves of attenuation coefficient as a function of the frequency. Example for Albunex (mean diameter = 3.15 μm, volume concentration = 8.8×10^4 spheres/ml)

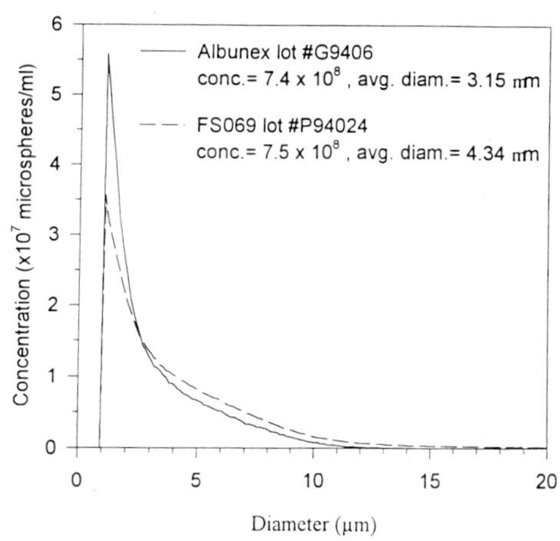

Fig. 26.6. Size distributions of Albunex and FS069

26.4 Attenuation Coefficient of Albunex

Figure 26.5 shows typical results of attenuation coefficient as a function of the frequency for Albunex. The experimental results obtained using a broadband approach (BLEEKER et al. 1990; DE JONG et al. 1992; CHANG et al. 1995, 1996) agree well with the theory developed for encapsulated gas microspheres discussed above, especially in the vicinity of the resonance of the bubbles. The size distribution of Albunex shown in Fig. 26.6 was used to calculate the theoretical curve. The attenuation coefficient peaks at 2.1 MHz and the values of S_p and S_f were assumed to be 5500 dyn/cm and 0.004 g/s, respectively. Attenuation coefficients of other contrast agents and Albunex at different concentrations have also been measured (HOFF et al. 1996; MARSH et al. 1997).

26.5 Nonlinear Interactions Between Ultrasound and Bubbles

When a bubble is excited by a pulse of ultrasound, it resonates as previously discussed. A resonant frequency can be derived by assuming a linear relationship between the exciting force and the response, in this case the variation of the bubble radius. Given this assumption, the response of the bubble is linearly proportional to the change of the excitation ultrasound amplitude (Minnaert 1993; Leighton 1994). This, however, is not the case in reality. The bubble is a nonlinear oscillator. This means that, when there is a change in the excitation amplitude, the elicited response will not merely include a corresponding change in the bubble radius proportional to the amplitude change. Other modes of oscillation will occur (Leighton 1994). The bubble will oscillate at frequencies of $1/3f_r$, $1/2f_r$, f_r, $2f_r$, $3f_r$, . . . where $1/3f_r$, $1/2f_r$ are called subharmonics and $2f_r$, $3f_r$, higher harmonics. Here, the term $2f_r$ is called the second harmonic because f_r, the fundamental frequency, is conventionally labeled the first harmonic (Leighton 1994).

In the past 25 years there has been a considerable interest in the nonlinear aspects of bubble oscillations. Welsby and Safar (1969) described the changes in the effective acoustic nonlinearity of a liquid brought about by the presence of a tiny amount of bubbles. They developed an analytical method for describing the first and second harmonic bubble vibrations.

Because of the highly nonlinear nature of even the simplest bubble models, analytical investigations have been found to be extremely difficult unless further approximations are made. Lauterborn in 1976 used fast digital computers (for that time) to survey the response of a bubble to a sound field when parameters such as frequency, pressure amplitudes, and bubble radii were varied.

Experimental works have paralleled the development of theories. Initially, the interest was motivated by the established connection between subharmonic emissions and the presence of cavitation (Neppiras 1969; Coakley and Nyborg 1978). Ultrasonic detection of bubbles at higher harmonics has been reported by Miller (1981). They showed that, by monitoring the second harmonic responses of resonant bubbles, 4.2-μm-diameter resonant bubbles can produce signals 40 times larger than 500-μm-diameter bubbles. It is, therefore, a much better technique than the first harmonic in discriminating nonresonant bubbles or other inhomogeneities. Crum and Prosperetti (1983) measured the harmonic activity of an individual bubble and adapted pertinent theories to account for their experimental conditions. Eatock and Nishi (1985), using a numerical approach, studied the magnitude of the nonlinear effect in the scattering of ultrasound by nitrogen bubbles in water for ultrasonic frequencies and amplitudes typical of diagnostic medical devices, to determine its effect on the detection of bubbles in blood or tissue.

These earlier works employed air bubbles without a shell. However, ultrasound contrast agents are generally stabilized against dissolution by the presence of a surface active layer of molecules at the gas-liquid interface, which supports strain that counters surface tension, thus stabilizing the bubbles.

26.5.1 The Rayleigh-Plesset Equation

The Rayleigh-Plesset equation is a nonlinear equation that describes the response of a spherical bubble to a time-varying pressure field in an incompressible liquid. It is also called the RPNNP equation, named after its developers, Rayleigh (1917), Plesset (1949), Neppiras and Noltingk (1951), and Poritsky (1952). The equation assumes that the motion of the bubble is symmetric; the wavelength of ultrasound is much larger than the radius of the bubble; the bubble contains gas and vapor; there is no rectified diffusion; and the gas in the bubble is compressed and expanded according to the gas law with the polytropic constant. The derivation of this equation can be found in Leighton (1994), and only the result is given below:

$$\varrho R\ddot{R} + \frac{3}{2}\varrho\dot{R}^2 = P_g\left(\frac{R_0}{R}\right)^{3\kappa} + P_v - P_0 - \frac{2\sigma}{R} - \delta\omega\varrho R\dot{R} - P_a\cos(\omega t), \qquad (26.20)$$

where a dot denotes time derivative, R_0 = initial bubble radius, ϱ = density of a Newtonian liquid, P_0 = ambient pressure, P_v = vapor pressure, σ = surface tension, κ = polytropic exponent of the gas, δ = damping coefficient, P_a = amplitude of the incident acoustic pressure with angular frequency ω, and P_g = gas pressure inside the bubble (= $P_0 - P_v + 2\sigma/R_0$). The term $2\sigma/R_0$ is the surface tension pressure, P_σ.

The internal pressure within the bubble, P_i, is given by the sum of the internal gas pressure and vapor pressure ($P_i = P_g + P_v$). The pressure within a bubble at rest is greater than the pressure in the liquid immediately outside the bubble as a result of surface tension forces. Therefore, the internal pressure of a bubble can also be written as $P_i = P_0 + P_\sigma$, with the result $P_g = P_0 + P_\sigma - P_v$.

The polytropic exponent of gas, κ, evaluates to γ for the adiabatic condition, and to 1 for the isothermal condition, where γ is the ratio of heat capacity at constant pressure and constant volume. The value of $\kappa = \gamma b$ can be calculated from Eq. 26.10. Figure 26.7 shows the simulation result for κ as a function of the

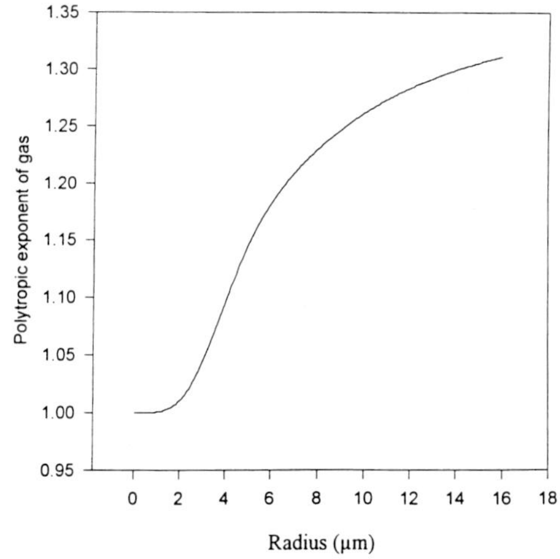

Fig. 26.7. The polytropic exponent of gas contained within air bubbles pulsating in a liquid

size of the bubble. When the bubble radius becomes small, the gas compression and expansion are more isothermal, and the surface tension will exert a significant pressure $2\sigma/R$ on the gas. CRUM (1983) measured the polytropic exponent for three different gases (argon, air, and carbon dioxide). The values for the ratio of specific heats in this case varied approximately from 5/3 (monoatomic) to 7/5 (diatomic) to 4/3 (triatomic).

For an air bubble in water, the physical constants in Eq. 26.20 may be assumed to have the following values: $\varrho = 0.998\,\text{g/cm}^3$, $\sigma = 72.75\,\text{dyn/cm}$, $c = 1.5 \times 10^5\,\text{cm/s}$, $P_v = 2.33 \times 10^4\,\text{dyn/cm}^2$, $P_0 = 1.013 \times 10^6\,\text{dyn/cm}^2$, and $\gamma = 1.4$.

26.5.2 Modified Rayleigh-Plesset Equation

For encapsulated contrast agents like Albunex there is an additional loss term due to the internal friction inside the shell and an additional restoring force due to the shell stiffness. Equation 26.20 has been modified by DE JONG et al. (1994a) in order to take into account the values of shell friction parameter, S_f (included in δ_{tot}), and shell elasticity parameter, S_p:

$$\varrho R\ddot{R} + \frac{3}{2}\varrho\dot{R}^2 = P_g\left(\frac{R_0}{R}\right)^{3\kappa} + P_v - P_0 - \frac{2\sigma}{R} - 2S_p\left(\frac{1}{R_0} - \frac{1}{R}\right) - \delta_{\text{tot}}\omega\varrho R\dot{R} - P_a\cos(\omega t). \quad (26.21)$$

The total damping coefficient is $\delta_{\text{tot}} = \delta + \delta_f$, where $\delta_f = S_f/m\omega$ (m is the effective mass of the bubble-liquid system $= 4\pi R^3\varrho$). S_f was assumed equal to 0.004 g/s. S_p can be found using the method described by CHANG et al. (1996).

DE JONG and HOFF (1993) considered S_p to be a constant equal to 8×10^3 dyn/cm. However, recent results obtained by CHANG et al. (1996) indicate that S_p may vary from 4.5×10^3 to 14×10^3 dyn/cm depending on the mean diameter of the batch of contrast agent. The shell stiffness of FS069 was found to be smaller than that of Albunex. This may explain the higher values of second harmonic signal obtained for FS069, as these bubbles can vibrate more intensely. DE JONG et al. (1992) have found a theoretical expression for the shell elasticity parameter, $S_p = Et/(1 - \nu)$, where E is the Young's modulus of elasticity, t is the shell thickness, and ν is the Poisson ratio. The shell elasticity parameter was assumed to be independent of the radius of the bubbles, which disagrees with the present experimental results. This discrepancy may be reconciled by considering the effect of the increasing radius on E and ν if the change in t is assumed to be negligible.

26.5.3 Solutions to Rayleigh-Plesset Equation

The Rayleigh-Plesset Equation can be solved either analytically or numerically (MILLER 1981; DE JONG et al. 1994a). Figure 26.8 shows the change in radius and velocity of an air bubble in water at 20°C in the time domain and frequency domain, driven at its resonance frequency and calculated numerically. The driving source was a 2-MHz sinusoidal wave of 30 cycles with an amplitude of 40 kPa. The initial conditions were those of a resting bubble. Only the results of the last ten cycles, a time when the system reaches a steady-state response, are shown. For calculating these results, the bubble radius was assumed to be 1.7 μm, which resulted in a resonance frequency of 2 MHz. The bottom figure shows the Fourier transform of the change in radius waveform. As expected, at either the maximum or the minimum of the radius variation of the bubble, the velocity is zero.

Figure 26.9 shows the response for an Albunex microbubble driven at its resonance frequency. There are two major differences between its response and the response of an air bubble. First, the resonance frequency of Albunex is higher due to the stiffness of the bubble's shell. In order to excite the bubbles at 2 MHz, the radius of Albunex should be

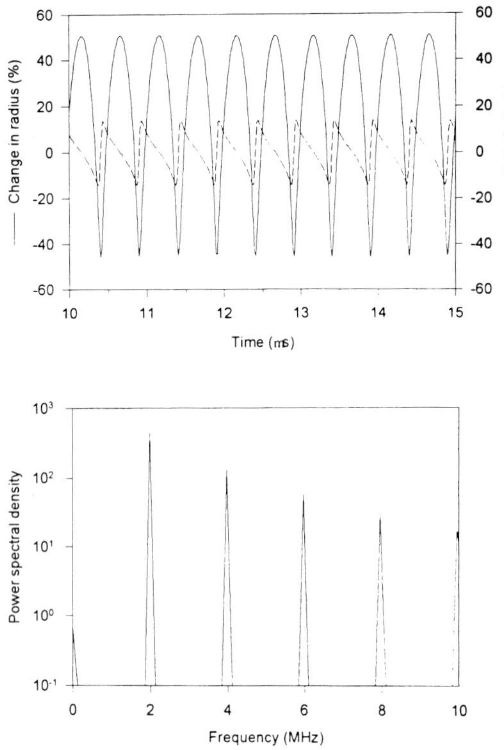

Fig. 26.8. Response of an air bubble driven at its resonance frequency by an acoustic wave of 40 kPa: (top) changes in radius and velocity of the bubble's wall, and (bottom) corresponding Fourier transform

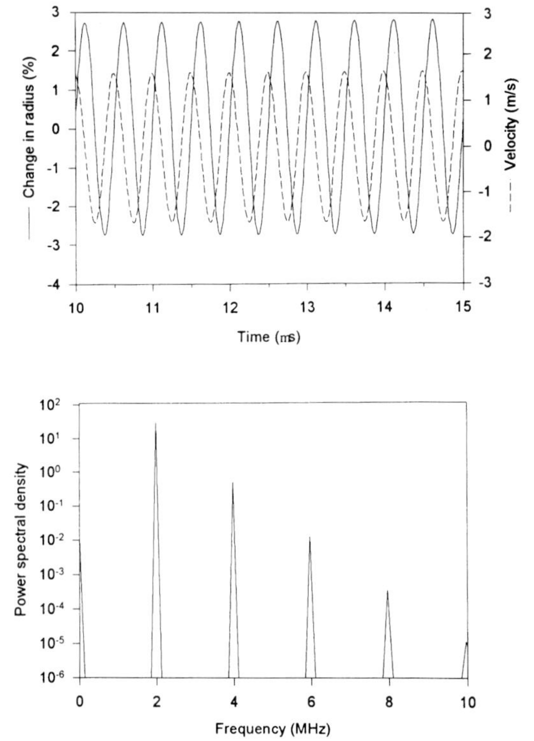

Fig. 26.9. Response of Albunex driven at its resonance frequency by an acoustic wave of 40 kPa: (top) changes in radius and velocity of the bubble's wall, and (bottom) corresponding Fourier transform

4.8 μm. These values were used, with the values of shell elasticity parameter S_p = 8000 dyn/cm and shell friction parameter S_f = 0.004 g/s. The second difference is that the magnitude of the variation is smaller for Albunex than for the air bubble.

Figure 26.10 shows the calculated scattering cross-section of a gas bubble and Albunex at first and second harmonic as a function of the transmitted frequency, following the approach taken by DE JONG et al. (1994a). Both the first and the second harmonic peak at 2 MHz. Above this frequency, the scattering cross-section equals the physical scattering cross-section ($4\pi R^2$). Note that the second harmonic is prominent only in the vicinity of the resonance frequency. For the air bubble, there is a secondary maximum at half the resonance frequency, which is not noticeable for Albunex.

Figure 26.11 shows the calculated scattered power for a distribution of Albunex microbubbles, where the size distribution of the agent depicted by Fig. 26.6 is considered. The transmitted frequency was 2 MHz, which yields bubbles with a resonance size of 4.8 μm radius. Both the first and the second harmonic peak at the same radius size, but the second harmonic curve drops faster for bubbles bigger than the resonance size.

Figure 26.12 shows the simulated results of normalized scattering signals at the first and second harmonic as a function of the frequency. The peak value of scattering cross-section is at 1.4 MHz for the second harmonic. For the first harmonic, the scattering cross-section is approximately independent of the frequency above 2.7 MHz.

Figure 26.13 shows the ratio of the second harmonic to first harmonic RMS Doppler amplitude (R_2/R_1), as a function of the transmitted frequency (CHANG et al. 1996). The theoretical results were calculated from Eq. 26.21. While experimental results show a decrease of R_2/R_1 at a rate of approximately 7 dB/MHz for both agents, simulation for Albunex (dashed line) shows a slope of −5 dB/MHz. The theoretical curve agrees better with the experimental data at lower frequencies than at higher frequencies (above 3.5 MHz).

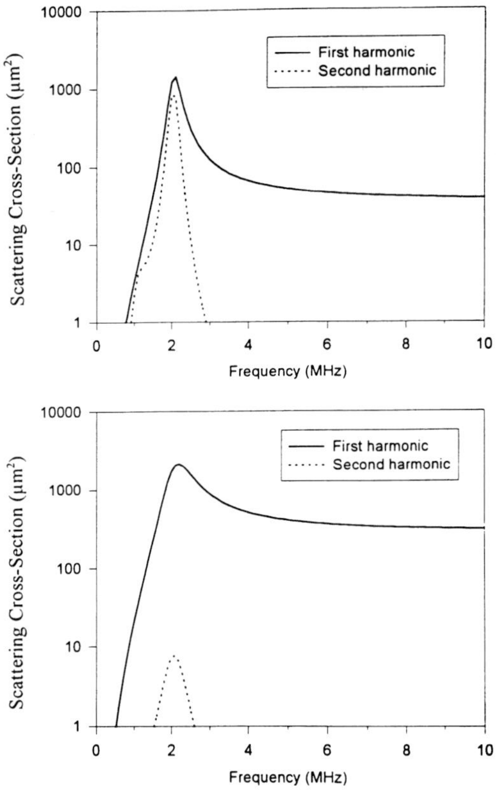

Fig. 26.10. Scattering cross-section as a function of the transmitted frequency at a driving presure of 40 kPa: (top) air bubble of 1.7 μm radius, and (bottom) Albunex of 4.8 μm radius

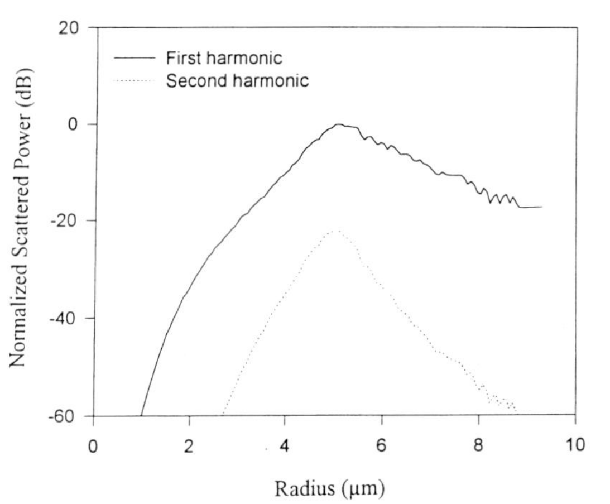

Fig. 26.11. Scattered power at first and second harmonic as a function of the radius Albunex micropheres. The size distribution of Albunex shown in Fig. 26.6 was used. The transmitted frequency and pressure were 2 MHz and 40 kPa respectively

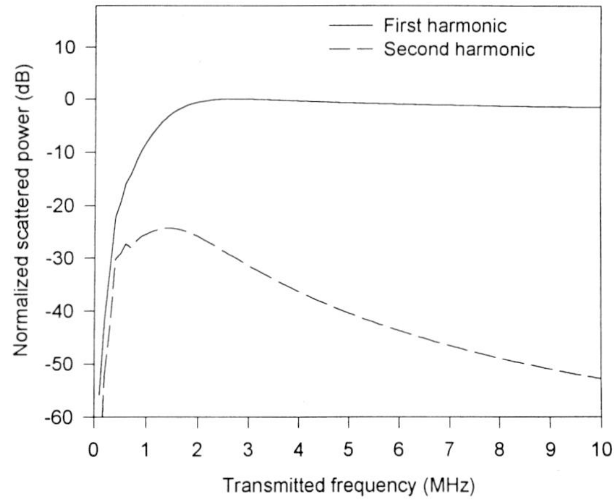

Fig. 26.12. Simulated results of normalized scattered power as a function of the transmitted frequency at a pressure amplitude of kPa, S_p = 5500 dyn/cm, and S_f = 0.004 g/s.

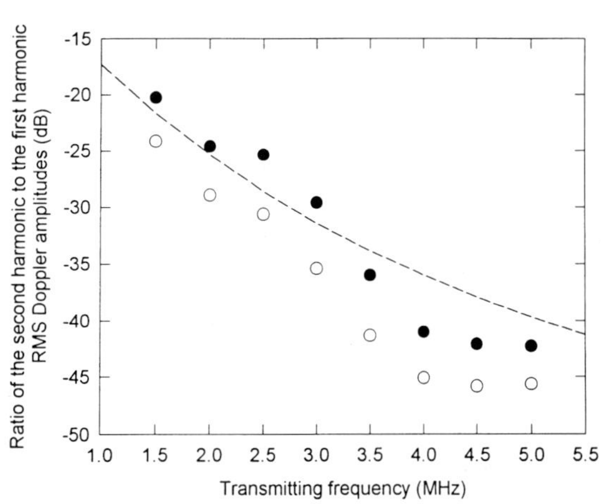

Fig. 26.13. Ratio of the second harmonic RMS Doppler amplitude to the first harmonic amplitude versus transmitting frequency (● FS069, ○ Albunex, and --- Theory)

26.6 Ultrasound Beam Characteristics

In preceding discussions, the ultrasound wave impinging upon the contrast agents was assumed to be a plane wave, but in actuality, the ultrasonic beam generated by a transducer or array is far from a plane wave (SHUNG and ZIPPARO 1996; ZAGZEBSKI 1996). For a single-element transducer, the beam diverges beyond the focal point. From the focal point forward, beam intensity decreases as a function of $1/z^2$. In the near field, the intensity distribution is so complicated that this region is seldom used in quantitative measurements. These factors must be taken into consideration when performing quantitative measurements and when a theoretical model is used for interpreting the experimental data.

Although linear arrays that use dynamic focusing allow for extended focusing of the beam in the azimuthal plane, the slice thickness or focusing in the elevational plane is still controlled by fixed focusing via a lens. This makes a quantitative interpretation of the results obtained directly from an imaging scanner quite difficult, if not impossible.

References

Anderson AL, Hampton LD (1980) Acoustics of gas-bearing sediments: I. Background. J Acoust Soc Am 67:1865–1889

Bleeker HJ, Shung KK, Barnhart JL (1990) Ultrasonic characterization of Albunex, a new contrast agent. J Acoust Soc Am 87:1792–1797

Burns PN, Powers JE, Simpson DH, et al. (1994) Harmonic power mode Doppler using microbubble contrast agents: an improved method for small vessel flow imaging. IEEE Ultras Symp Proc 1547–1550

Chang PH, Shung KK, Levene H (1995) Second harmonic imaging and harmonic Doppler measurements with Albunex. IEEE Trans Ultrasonics, Ferroelect Freq Cont 42: 1020–1027

Chang PH, Shung KK, Levene H (1996) Quantitative measurements of second harmonic Doppler using ultrasound contrast agents. Ultrasound Med Biol 22:1205–1214

Church CC (1995) The effects of an elastic solid surface layer on the radial pulsations of gas bubbles. J Acoust Soc Am 97:1510–1521

Coakley WT, Nyborg WL (1978) Cavitation; dynamics of gas bubbles; applications. In: Fry FJ (ed) Ultrasound: its applications in medicine and biology. Part I. Elsevier Scientific, New York, pp 77–159

Crum LA (1983) The polytropic exponent of gas contained within air bubbles pulsating in a liquid. J Acoust Soc Am 73:116–120

Crum LA, Prosperetti A (1983) Nonlinear oscillations of gas bubbles in liquids: an interpretation of some experimental results. J Acoust Soc Am 73:121–127

de Jong N (1996) Improvements in ultrasound contrast agents. IEEE Eng Med Biol Mag 15:72–82

de Jong N, Hoff L (1993) Ultrasound scattering properties of Albunex microspheres. Ultrasonics 31:175–181

de Jong N, Hoff L, Skotland T, Bom N (1992) Absorption and scatter of encapsulated gas filled microspheres: theoretical considerations and some measurements. Ultrasonics 30: 95–103

de Jong N, Cornet R, Lancée CT (1994a) Higher harmonics of vibrating gas-filled microspheres. Part 1. Simulations. Ultrasonics 32:447–453

de Jong N, Cornet R, Lancée CT (1994b) Higher harmonics of vibrating gas-filled microspheres. Part 2. Measurements. Ultrasonics 32:455–459

Devin C (1959) Survey of thermal, radiation, and viscous damping of pulsating air bubbles in water. J Acoust Soc Am 31:1654–1667

Eatock BC, Nishi RY (1985) Numerical studies of the spectrum of low-intensity ultrasound scattered by bubbles. J Acoust Soc Am 77:1692–1701

Forsberg F, Goldberg BB, Liu JB, Merton DA, Rawool NM (1996) On the feasibility of real-time, in vivo harmonic imaging with proteinaceous microspheres. J Ultrasound Med 15:853–860

Fox FE, Herzfield KF (1954) Gas bubbles with organic skin as cavitation nuclei. J Acoust Soc Am 26:984–989

Goldberg BB, Liu JB, Forsberg F (1994) Ultrasound contrast agents: a review. Ultrasound Med Biol 20:319–333

Hoff L, Sontum PC, Hoff B (1996) Acoustic properties of shell-encapsulated gas-filled contrast agents. 1996 IEEE Ultras Symp Proc 1441–1444

Ishimaru A (1978) Wave propagation and scattering in random media. Academic Press, New York

Lauterborn W (1976) Numerical investigation of nonlinear oscillations of gas bubbles in liquids. J Acoust Soc Am 59: 283–293

Leighton TG (1994) The acoustic bubble. Academic Press, San Diego

Marsh JN, Hall CS, Hughes MS, Mobley J, Miller JG, Brandenburger (1997) Broadband through transmission signal loss measurements of Albunex at concentrations approaching in vivo doses. J Acoust Soc Am 101:1155–1161

Medwin H (1977) Counting bubbles acoustically: a review. Ultrasonics 15:7–13

Miller DL (1981) Ultrasonic detection of resonant cavitation bubbles in a flow tube by their second harmonic emissions. Ultrasonics 19:217–224

Minnaert M (1933) On musical air bubbles and sounds of running water. Phil Mag 10:235–248

Morse PM, Ingard KU (1968) Theoretical acoustics. McGraw Hill, New York

Neppiras EA (1969) Subharmonic and other low-frequency emissions from bubbles in sound-irradiated liquids. J Acoust Soc Am 46:587–601

Neppiras EA, Noltingk BE (1951) Cavitation produced by ultrasonics: theoretical conditions for the onset of cavitation. Proc Phys Soc B64:1032–1038

Ophir J, Parker KJ (1989) Contrast agents in diagnostic ultrasound. Ultrasound Med Biol 15:319–325

Plesset MS (1949) The dynamics of cavitation bubbles. J Appl Mech 16:277–282

Poritsky H (1952) The collapse or growth of a spherical bubble or cavity in a viscous fluid. Proceed First U.S. National Congress on Appl Mech 813–821

Rayleigh Lord (1917) On the pressure developed in a liquid during the collapse of a spherical cavity. Phil Mag 34:94–98

Schrope B, Newhouse VL (1993) Second harmonic ultrasonic blood perfusion measurement. Ultrasound Med Biol 19: 567–579

Schrope B, Newhouse VL, Uhlendorf V (1992) Simulated capillary blood flow measurement using a nonlinear contrast agent. Ultrason Imaging 14:134–158

Shung KK, Thieme GA (1993) Ultrasonic scattering in biological tissue. CRC Press, Boca Raton, Fl.

Shung KK, Zipparo M (1996) Ultrasonic transducers and arrays. IEEE Eng Med Biol Mag 15:20–30

Shung KK, Smith MB, Tsui BMW (1992) Principles of medical imaging. Academic Press, San Diego

Welsby VG, Safar MH (1969) Acoustic nonlinearity due to microbubbles in water. Acoustica 22:177–182

Zagzebski JA (1996) Essentials of ultrasound physics. Mosby, St Louis

27 Contrast-Specific Instrumentation and Its Potential Applications

G.C. STEINBACH

CONTENTS

27.1 Introduction

Microbubble-based contrast materials have shown great promise in enhancement of backscattered ultrasound signals from blood and tissues (MATTREY and STEINBACH 1991; MATTREY et al. 1994). The scattering properties of the contrast media are dependent upon the characteristics of the agent, particularly the size and the compressibility of the microbubble (ANDERSON and HAMPTON 1980; OPHIR and PARKER 1989). Furthermore, the scattering properties are also dependent on the frequency and amplitude of the interrogating acoustic wave (DE JONG et al. 1991). The complex relationship between transmitted frequency, transmitted acoustic pressure, and received frequency for image creation are the keys in development of instrumentation specifically designed to benefit from the presence of contrast media.

Ultrasound imaging, as compared with x-ray computed tomography and magnetic resonance imaging, is uniquely suited to take advantage of the physical differences between microbubbles and surrounding tissues to maximize image contrast. Some of these differences are the nonlinear behavior of bubbles and the loss of bubbles when exposed to ultrasound. The increased computing power, decreased space requirement, and cost have significantly influenced the design of ultrasound machinery. As a result, more signal and real-time processing capabilities have become possible. Digital beamforming techniques have been developed that provide for programming flexibility and larger dynamic range of RF signal as compared with conventional analog beamformers (KRISTOFFERSEN 1996). These advances, as well as progress in transducer design that allows for greater bandwidth and customized frequency characteristics, are critical for development of instrumentation that takes advantage of the benefits provided by contrast materials.

27.2 Background

27.2.1 Resonance Behavior of Microbubbles

A bubble exposed to an acoustic (oscillating) pressure field oscillates with the field at the transmitted frequency. The bubble size changes instantaneously with the pressure change of the acoustic field. As the wavelength of the sound wave approaches the effective cross-sectional area of the bubble, bubbles begin to resonate (DE JONG et al. 1991). It is fortunate that the resonance frequency of small bubbles, able to pass through the capillary bed, falls in the ultrasonic frequency band used by diagnostic instruments. When a bubble oscillates at resonance, the effective cross-sectional area is increased and the scattered

G.C. STEINBACH, MSBE, Department of Radiology, UCSD Medical Center, 200 W. Arbor Drive, San Diego, CA 92103-8756, USA energy is significantly greater than that scattered at nonresonant frequencies. Therefore, by exciting a population of bubbles at their resonant frequency, further enhancement is possible due to the presence of the contrast material. However, at resonance, greater stress is placed on the shell of the contrast material, leading to more rapid bubble loss. The resonant frequency of a bubble is dependent on both physical and material properties of the bubble. Of particular importance are the size of the bubble, the encapsulated gas, and the elastic properties of the shell.

In a given contrast agent that contains a mixture of microbubbles with approximately the same material properties, the most important physical property is bubble size. As the size of the bubble decreases, its resonance frequency increases (DE JONG et al. 1991). In practice, the administered contrast material has a gaussian distribution of particle sizes and the interrogating ultrasonic beam has a distribution of frequencies within its effective bandwidth. Taking advantage of the size-dependent resonant frequency, as well as the nonlinear scattering characteristics of bubbles, forms the foundation for many contrast-specific imaging techniques.

27.2.2
Influence of Acoustic Pressure

As bubbles oscillate, their radius changes with the cyclic intensity oscillations of the insonating acoustic wave (Fig. 27.1a,b). The degree of oscillation, or degree of change in bubble size, is dependent upon the intensity of the acoustic energy. Low acoustic pressure will create smaller oscillations or size reductions and larger acoustic pressures will create larger oscillations or size modifications (Fig. 27.1b,c). High acoustic pressure eventually leads to bubble deflation; the magnitude of pressure required for disruption depends upon the physical characteristics of the bubble and the insonating frequency (Fig. 27.1d). As a further complication, the scattering mechanism of the bubble is dependent on the applied acoustic pressure. At low acoustic pressures, microbubbles scatter the ultrasonic wave in a linear manner (UHLENDORF and HOFFMANN 1994). At higher pressure amplitudes, the bubble response becomes nonlinear as more energy is deposited into the higher harmonics (multiples of the fundamental or excitation frequency). At even higher amplitudes, it has been hypothesized that the microbubble shell is

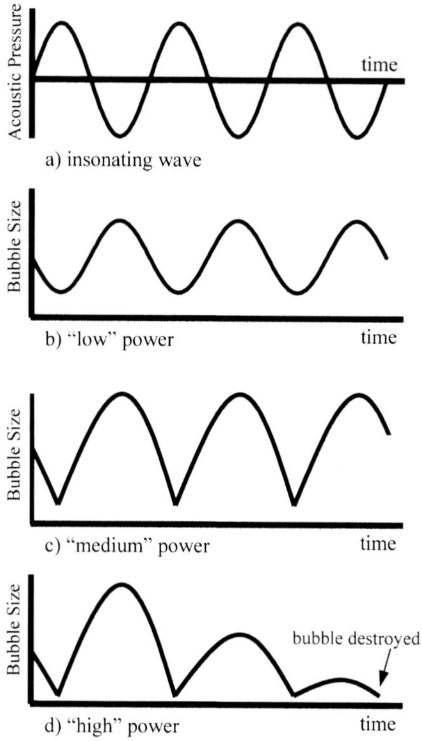

Fig. 27.1. As a bubble is exposed to the oscillations of the insonating acoustical wave (**a**) the radius of the bubble changes with the cyclic acoustic intensity. The degree of change in bubble size is dependent on the intensity of the acoustic energy. Low intensity creates small, linear size oscillations (**b**). Medium intensity creates larger, nonlinear size oscillations (**c**). High intensity creates highly nonlinear size oscillations and rapid bubble disruption (**d**). The intensity required to disrupt the bubble depends upon the physical characteristics of the bubble and the insonating frequency

disrupted, producing a naked bubble that is short-lived, and a transient nonlinear acoustic emission is generated (BURNS et al. 1995) (Fig. 27.1). Each of these response regimes can be manipulated in unique ways to generate images highlighting regions containing contrast material (DE JONG and TEN CATE 1996; KAUL 1997).

Bubble disruption rates are dependent upon both the physical properties of the contrast material and the intensity and duration of exposure to ultrasound (DAYTON et al. 1996; MORGAN et al. 1996). An agent will experience greater disruption, and therefore reduced levels of backscatter from insonified tissues, as transmit power or exposure time is increased (SIRLIN et al. 1997, 1998). As acoustic intensity is reduced, based on the attenuation of the beam through the tissue, contrast material close to the transducer will experience higher intensities and greater disruption than contrast material in the far field. The duration of exposure to acoustic energy is primarily dependent upon the transit time of the contrast material through the tissue. Areas of slow flow will experience greater disruption, and therefore less enhancement, as compared with areas of fast flow (SIRLIN et al. 1998). These characteristics can be used by the clinician in various ways. Overlying attenuation due to the presence of contrast can be eliminated by using higher transmit powers to disrupt some of the bubbles in the imaging field. Vascular imaging can be improved by selection of acoustic parameters such that significant bubble loss is taking place in tissues (region of slow flow) while vasculature (region of fast flow) is clearly visualized (SIRLIN et al. 1998). Bubble destruction can be used in tissue imaging to identify perfusion anomalies based on the loss of reflectivity in poorly perfused (slow flow) regions as compared with normally perfused (fast flow) regions (PORTER et al. 1996; FIRSCHKE et al. 1997).

27.3 Potential Contrast-Induced Artifacts

The introduction of contrast material can produce artifacts that occur as a result of the presence of the bubbles and the dramatic increase in backscattered signal strength. The majority of artifacts occur during Doppler examinations. Color Doppler imaging is impacted by color blooming, whereas spectral Doppler imaging is impacted by modifications of the Doppler spectrum (FORSBERG et al. 1994).

27.3.1 Phase Aberrations

Phase aberrations in the sound beam result when the sound wave travels through a mixture of materials with different acoustic velocities (O'DONNELL and FLAX 1988). The speed of sound in gas is significantly less than that of tissues. Therefore, when bubbles are distributed in tissues, geographic heterogeneity of acoustic velocities is generated. When sound is transmitted through a tissue containing contrast, the beam front is no longer in phase as part of the beam travelling through the bubbles is slowed. The ultimate result of phase aberrations is constructive and destructive interference and signal loss (MILLER et al. 1998).

27.3.2 Doppler Spectral Effects

The presence of contrast material enhances the received Doppler signal in a dose-dependent fashion (ANDRE et al. 1992; SCHWARTZ et al. 1993). The contrast-enhanced Doppler spectrum may exhibit some very large noise patterns, often heard as "crackling" and seen as aliased "spikes" in the spectrum. The frequency content of the spectrum contains a frequency response similar to that of the precontrast spectrum, with the addition of some spectral broadening and a significant increase in signal amplitude at all frequencies. This effect can result in an increase in the measured Doppler velocity, depending on the measurement technique employed by the manufacturer of the ultrasound scanner (SPONHEIM and MYHRUM 1995). If the velocity estimation is based on absolute amplitude thresholds, the velocity indicated after contrast will likely be higher than that observed prior to the administration of contrast material (ABILDGAARD et al. 1996). This effect would also occur prior to contrast if the gain settings were increased so that the amplitude of the signals was similar. Conversely, if the velocity estimation is based on relative amplitude as compared to the maximum amplitude of the received signal, the velocity measurements will be similar before and after contrast administration. The measurement discrepancy can be countered by reducing the gain such that the postcontrast signal amplitude is similar to the amplitude received prior to the contrast injection (ABILDGAARD et al. 1996; SPONHEIM and MYHRUM 1996; MELANY et al. 1998; FORSBERG et al. 1998).

27.3.3 Color Blooming

The presence of the contrast material significantly increases the backscattered signal strength. Following the administration of contrast material, color (flow) is often observed on large portions of the image where clearly flow is not present. This effect is easily observed clinically and is a result of the amplitude thresholding technique that is used to identify pixels to be displayed in color (FORSBERG et al. 1994). Similar to the Doppler spectrum effects, this phenomenon has some dependence on the color Doppler implementation by each scanner manufacturer and can generally be reduced or eliminated by reducing overall color gain. Decreasing the bolus dose or using slow infusion of a large dose can also help reduce these artifacts by decreasing contrast concentration and signal strength (Albrecht et al. 1998).

27.4 Contrast-Specific Imaging Techniques

27.4.1 Standard (Linear) Imaging

At low acoustic pressures, microbubble-based contrast media perform as linear scatterers. The contrast material scatters sound much more intensely than an equivalent size liquid or solid particle, owing to the significant acoustic impedance mismatch created by the presence of the gas within the shell of the bubble. In addition, the effective scatterer cross-section is significantly larger for a membrane filled with gas (i.e., a microbubble contrast agent) than for one filled with liquid (i.e., an erythrocyte or liquid-filled contrast agent) (Ophir and Parker 1989). The significant difference in acoustic impedance between the contrast material and the surrounding tissue or blood permits significant enhancement to be achieved from a relatively small number of microbubbles. The degree of image enhancement is dependent upon the dose of the contrast media administered and bubble characteristics (size, density, elasticity) (Steinbach et al. 1998).

Conventional ultrasound scanners, those that transmit and receive at the same frequency, will experience significant image enhancement with contrast materials, based on the increased reflectivity generated by the introduction of the gaseous material. This effect will be observed in all Doppler as well as B-mode and M-mode imaging techniques. The increased reflectivity from blood containing contrast results in significant increases in the received Doppler amplitude, as well as opportunities to use signal-processing algorithms that benefit from greater signal amplitudes and increased signal-to-noise ratio (Andre et al. 1992).

27.4.2 Correlation Techniques

The presence of contrast material allows the use of correlation techniques to enhance the visualization of areas containing moving contrast material. The regions where bubbles are flowing have greater temporal variations than those of surrounding stationary or slow-moving structures. By analyzing the decorrelation rates in subsequent image frames or A-lines, images can be created which emphasize regions of differing decorrelation rates. The rapid decorrelation rates produced by flowing contrast media can be separated from the slower decorrelation rates found in the surrounding tissue, enhancing the visualization of regions that contain flowing blood with contrast materials (Ostensen et al. 1997; Olstad 1996). A similar technique has been used to suppress scatter from blood cells in intravascular ultrasound (Li et al. 1996). These techniques, which can be applied at any interrogating frequency, are potentially applicable in standard or harmonic imaging systems and are being refined for applications such as perfusion, velocity, blood flow, and velocity profile estimation. However, other decorrelation imaging techniques can also be used, which utilize the Doppler circuitry and postprocessing available on all equipment, and are described in Sect. 27.4.4.

27.4.3 Intermittent Imaging

Due to the pressure sensitivity of most microbubble-based contrast materials, intermittent or gated imaging techniques have proven useful. By using intermittent imaging, the acoustic exposure can be reduced by the ratio of gated to continuous frequency. For example, if the continuous imaging frequency is 30 Hz and a gating routine is employed to reduce the frame rate to 3 Hz, the acoustic exposure is reduced by a factor of 10. Since transit time is related to the ratio of blood volume to blood flow rate, intermittent imaging produces tissue enhancement that is inversely related to exposure time and transit time: the greater the exposure and the greater the transit time, the less the enhancement.

Another benefit of intermittent imaging is the filling of the vascular space with bubbles during the off-cycle. The number of accumulated bubbles affects tissue echogenicity observed on the first frame following the delay. The degree of filling produces enhancement that is directly related to blood volume and blood flow. The higher the flow rate, the greater the number of bubbles that will enter the region of interest; the greater the fractional blood volume, the greater the number of bubbles per voxel will be.

There are two techniques of intermittent imaging: single frame acquisition, gated to either an internal or an external pulse such as the electrocardiogram R wave, or multiple consecutive pulses separated by a delay period. The former has been used to increase image contrast between regions with different blood flow rates (PORTER 1996). As slow-moving contrast material is insonified for a longer period, it experiences greater acoustic pressure per unit time than does fast-moving contrast materials. As a result, contrast enhancement in slow-flow regions can be reduced due to the reduction in the number of bubbles in the sample volume (PORTER et al. 1996). Further, during the off-cycle, regions of higher flow rate accumulate more bubbles, resulting in greater enhancement. The resultant image contrast in the single-frame technique, assuming that bubble concentration in the feeding artery is at a steady state, is an equilibrium between bubble destruction when the ultrasound beam is on and number of bubbles delivered when the ultrasound beam is off.

The intermittent technique that delivers multiple pulses separated by delay is used to measure fractional blood volume and flow rate. By properly adjusting ultrasound exposure, it is possible to ensure that all bubbles in tissues are destroyed during the exposure period. Since all bubbles are destroyed, the number of bubbles in a region when the first frame is acquired is then strictly related to bubble delivery during the off-cycle. By gradually increasing the off-cycle period, a curve can be drawn that will increase exponentially as a larger portion of the tissue blood volume is filled with bubbles. The growth rate of the curve is related to blood flow rate and the plateau is related to fractional blood volume. This technique has been successfully used to measure myocardial blood flow (WEI et al. 1998).

For the purpose of enhancing tissues, the reduction of acoustic exposure improves contrast enhancement in perfused tissues, such as myocardium and liver parenchyma. When studying the myocardium, it was noted that intermittent imaging produced 3 times the anterior myocardial contrast intensity as compared with continuous imaging (PORTER and XIE 1995). When assessing the effect of intermittent imaging on liver enhancement, it was noted that contrast between normal and infarcted liver increased by 44% when the frame rate was reduced from 28 to 1 frame/s (SIRLIN et al. 1998).

Flash echo imaging is one of the terms given to intermittent imaging where the first frame following delay is either stored in a cine loop or shown on the screen alongside real-time scans acquired at very low power to minimize bubble destruction (KONO et al. 1997). Flash echo can be used with any imaging technique. Its only requirement is that it is intermittent in nature to allow bubble delivery to influence image contrast. The intermittent acquisition has been successfully used to alter contrast between liver and lesions as delay times were increased to help in lesion detection as well as lesion characterization (MORIYASU et al. 1998).

27.4.4
Transient Response Imaging

Another imaging technique that utilizes the pressure sensitivity of microbubble-based contrast media is known as transient response imaging or stimulated acoustic emission. It typically involves color Doppler with or without intermittent imaging schemes along with modifications in transmit power, which is typically set high to assure bubble disruption with the first pulse. Using phase-insensitive detection of two consecutive pulses and differentiation of the pulses allows the detection of microbubble destruction. Beamformer timing adjustments for aberration corrections may also be applied, based on signals generated during the disruption of the contrast material (JOHNSON and POWERS 1995).

When used following a brief pause in imaging, a color mosaic image is generated, based on signals received from the hypothesized acoustic emission that results when the bubble is destroyed by the insonating beam (UHLENDORF and HOFFMANN 1994). As tissue motion and flash artifacts can contaminate the region of interest, such techniques are best utilized in combination with harmonic imaging to maximize contrast between regions with and regions without bubbles. The technique, particularly when used with harmonic imaging, appears to have the potential to identify regions with significantly different perfusion rates (MORIYASU et al. 1998). When used with real-time acquisition, regions with the highest flow rates (typically blood vessels) are visible as the delay time between acquisitions is minimal. During real-time acquisition, this technique is analogous to color or power Doppler imaging but rather than strictly relying on motion to detect flow, it also relies on bubble loss to detect the regions containing bubbles.

A unique agent designed specifically for transient response imaging (SHU563, Schering AG, Germany) (HAUFF et al. 1997) is currently in clinical trials. After an initial blood pool phase, the stiff-shell microbubbles accumulate in the reticuloendothelial cells of the liver and spleen or regions of bleeding.

The bubbles act as scatterers when insonated at low pressure but are hypothesized to emit sound when the bubble is disrupted at high pressure. The emitted sound is broad band, which is uniquely suited for harmonic imaging (Burns et al. 1995). The agent is used to detect its location as a target in the setting of hemorrhage (Goldberg et al. 1996) or as background to detect filling defects in the liver and spleen (Hauff et al. 1997).

27.4.5 Harmonic Imaging

In the harmonic imaging technique, detection of the contrast material is improved based on the differences in the acoustic frequency signatures received from the tissue and from bubbles. Although the frequency spectrum received from bubbles contains subharmonic and harmonic peaks of the transmitted frequency, the technique generates images based on the signal at twice the fundamental frequency and is called 2nd harmonic imaging. The reason for the generation of harmonics from bubbles is related to their elasticity and the fact that they expand and compress to different degrees when exposed to alternating ultrasound pressure. Although tissues are capable of generating harmonics at high pressure, the nonlinear behavior of the contrast material induces backscattered energy at the harmonic frequency with much greater strength than tissues. The resulting image created from the received harmonic frequency has high contrast as it shows strong signal from bubble-containing regions and suppressed signal from surrounding tissues that contain little or no contrast material (Fig. 27.2). The magnitude of the received harmonic echo is dependent upon the characteristics of the contrast agent and the acoustic pressure and frequency of the insonating beam.

Due to the relatively broad bandwidth on both the transmit and receive frequency bands, overlap of the transmit and receive frequencies occurs, contaminating the harmonic image with fundamental frequency. Also, tissues can reflect some harmonic frequency components, especially at high transmit powers. These result in degradation of the quality of the harmonic image by displaying regions that do not contain significant amounts of contrast material. The harmonic imaging technique relies on a narrow bandwidth to help prevent contamination from the fundamental response. To achieve a narrow bandwidth, the pulse length is typically increased and/or the signal is significantly filtered. The longer pulse length decreases spatial resolution, but achieves a higher quality harmonic image (Powers et al. 1997).

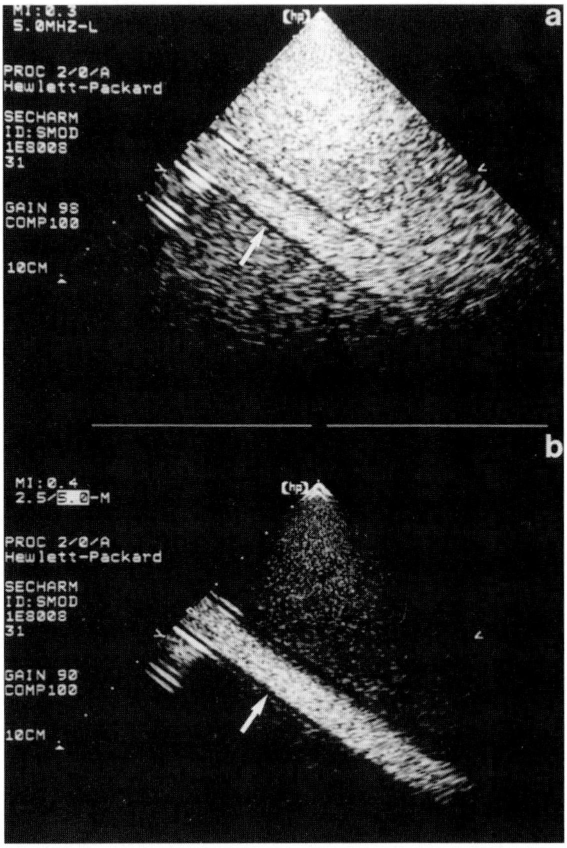

Fig. 27.2. Fundamental (**a**) and 2nd harmonic (**b**) images of a tissue-mimicking flow phantom circulating contrast material show an enhanced vessel that has echogenicity similar to the tissue-mimicking background in **a**, but that is markedly suppressed in **b** because it only contains linear scatterers

One implementation of a harmonic or nonlinear imaging technique uses multiple excitation levels and signal subtractions to generate the image. By analyzing the gain-corrected response from different excitation levels and subtracting, the linear response can be reduced while the sensitivity to the nonlinear responses is increased. The resulting image emphasizes the nonlinear or second harmonic response, which will be most pronounced in areas containing contrast materials (Brock-Fisher et al. 1996).

Detection of Pressure. The resonance frequency of a given bubble is highly dependent upon the size of the bubble. Furthermore, the size of the bubble will depend on the local pressure to which the bubbles are exposed. Using these concepts in tandem, it has been proposed that monitoring the resonant frequency may be a way to determine pressure noninvasively (HORTON 1972; FAIRBANK and SCULLY 1977; TICKNER 1981). Several groups have evaluated this technique by looking at the resonant frequency, harmonic response, and subharmonic response from contrast materials. Recent research has suggested that the subharmonic peak is most sensitive to pressure changes (SHI et al. 1998).

27.4.6 Dual-Pulse/Wideband Harmonic Imaging

Another imaging technique that relies on the nonlinearity of contrast material uses a wide bandwidth and delivers two ultrasound pulses, where the second pulse is inverted and slightly delayed relative to the first. Signal-processing algorithms that utilize the combination of the received response from the two pulses are used to generate an image that highlights regions containing nonlinear scattering material (KRISHNAN and O'DONNELL 1996; CHAPMAN and LAZENBY 1997; HWANG and SIMPSON 1998).

There are several instrument and physiological factors that contribute to image contrast between bubble-containing and non-bubble-containing regions with this technique (Table 27.1) (STEINBACH et al. 1998). The dominant effect is due to the presence of nonlinear scatterers such as microbubbles. Linear scatterers, such as tissues without bubbles, are significantly suppressed. The image echogenicity is dependent on both bubble concentration and velocity. Because there is delay between the two pulses, any bubble displacements will add additional signal, resulting in velocity-dependent enhancement. There is also additional enhancement due to bubble destruction that occurs with the first pulse. Since the image enhancement is based on relationships between the first and second pulses, bubbles disrupted with the first pulse will add additional signal.

Regions containing bubbles, and particularly bubbles in motion, dominate the echogenicity on the final image. Vascular anatomy is particularly enhanced, where arteries (high velocity) are the brightest structures and are brighter than neighboring veins (low velocity), which are brighter than enhanced tissues (Fig. 27.3). Areas with no contrast are essentially anechoic. Arterial enhancement is pulsatile as the systolic and diastolic velocities generate different levels of enhancement (Fig. 27.4) (STEINBACH et al. 1998). Veins enhance less than arteries, but their enhancement is also due to both the presence and the motion of the contrast agent. Perfused tissues also show enhancement, but to a lesser degree as both bubble concentration and velocity are reduced. In tissues, the nonlinearity of the contrast material becomes the significant mechanism of enhancement. Optimization of the ultrasound technique, in terms of transmit power and pulse delay, is important to maximize vascular contrast and arterial-venous discrimination (STEINBACH et al. 1998).

The dual-pulse, nonlinear imaging techniques are able to utilize shorter pulse lengths, resulting in wider bandwidth. This is possible because contamination from the fundamental frequency is no longer an issue. As a result, the spatial resolution of the images is not compromised as described with the 2nd harmonic imaging techniques. The ability to use high transmit frequencies also adds to the greater spatial resolution of this technique as compared with 2nd harmonic imaging.

The main limitation of this approach is the significant reduction in linear tissue reflectivity, resulting

Table 27.1. Machine and physiological parameters that contribute to image contrast between bubble-containing and non-bubble-containing regions

Machine parameters	Physiological parameters
Pulse repetition interval	Contrast concentration
Transmit power	Scatterer velocity
Transmit frequency	
Receive gain	

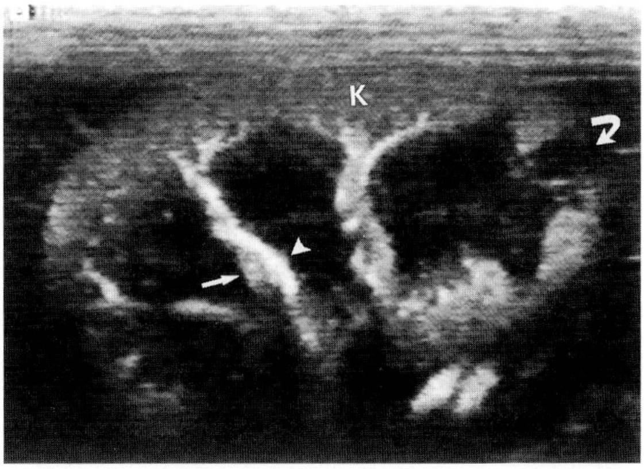

Fig. 27.3. A longitudinal view of a rabbit kidney with a focal infarction (*curved arrow*) acquired with the wideband harmonic technique at 7 MHz using the Siemens Elegra scanner following the bolus injection of 0.5 ml AF0150 (Alliance Pharmaceutical Corp., San Diego) shows the artery (*arrowhead*) brighter than vein (*arrow*) and also shows the normally perfused kidney parenchyma (*K*) to be slightly less echogenic than vein but more echogenic than the infarction (*curved arrow*)

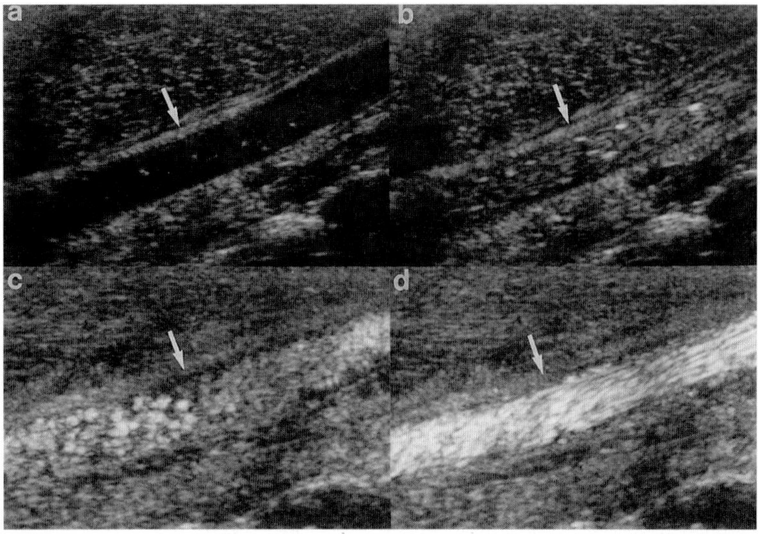

Fig. 27.4. Vascular images obtained at 7 MHz using the Siemens Elegra scannerwith the wideband harmonic technique during diastole (**a** and **c**) and systole (**b** and **d**). **a** and **b** were obtained before and **c** and **d** after the administration of AF0150. First note that the aortic lumen fills with weak echoes in systole precontrast due to the increased velocity of the linear scatterers (*arrow* in **b**). Second, the aorta (*arrow*) enhances postcontrast in both diastole and systole compared with precontrast, and the brightness of the lumen postcontrast is greater in systole (**d**) than in diastole (**c**)

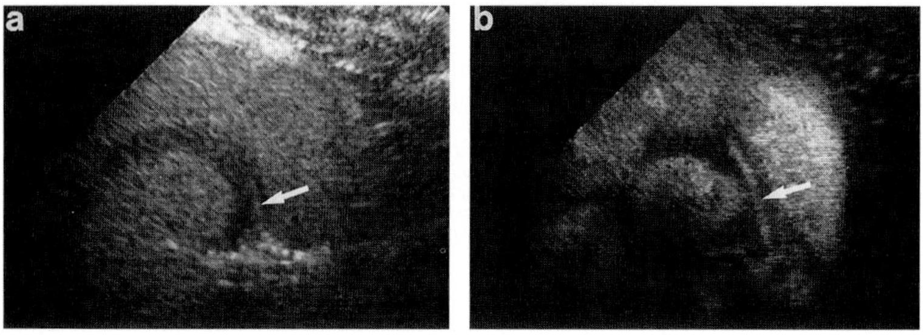

Fig. 27.5. Fundamental (**a**) and wideband harmonic (**b**) images of a rabbit heart at 7 MHz using the Siemens Elegra scannerafter contrast administration (0.5ml AF0150). In both images, enhancement of the cardiac chambers is observed. The wideband harmonic image (**b**) provides greater sensitivity to contrast-containing regions because of the reduction in echogenicity of less contrast-containing tissue. Note that the decreased echogenicity of the septum allowed better visualization of a septal coronary artery (*arrow*) in the rapidly beating rabbit heart. Tissue motion does not significantly interfere with this imaging technique

in difficulty in locating the anatomy of interest prior to the introduction of contrast material. Although this limitation can be overcome by increasing transmit power, the efficient tissue subtraction is beneficial, as it provides a significant amount of contrast between tissues with and tissues without contrast materials. Although blood flow can be visualized without contrast because of motion (Fig. 27.4), cardiac motion is not detrimental to the technique, as the myocardium is effectively suppressed. When contrast is introduced, enhancement of the cardiac chambers and the myocardium occurs. However, the septal coronary arteries are well visualized in rabbits and dogs because of the sensitivity of the technique to moving bubbles and the effective suppression of tissues, despite the rapidly beating heart of the rabbit (Fig. 27.5). Although tissue motion is an issue in theory, it has not been a significant problem in practice, likely because of the overwhelming dependence of enhancement on the presence of bubbles. Further, tissue motion problems are reduced when the pulse delay is minimized such that the displacements are very small during the pulse interval.

With this technique it is possible to manipulate image contrast based on the presence of bubbles. Adjusting power increases the nonlinear behavior of bubbles but also increases bubble disruption. This also increases contrast between vessels and tissues, as less bubbles are delivered to tissues and those that are delivered are quickly disrupted (Sirlin et al. 1997). Increasing the pulse delay increases general image brightness as subtraction of linear reflectors becomes less efficient. However, arterial to venous differentiation diminishes because of the weakening influence of velocity (Fig. 27.6). By proper optimization of the machine settings, enhancement of vascu-

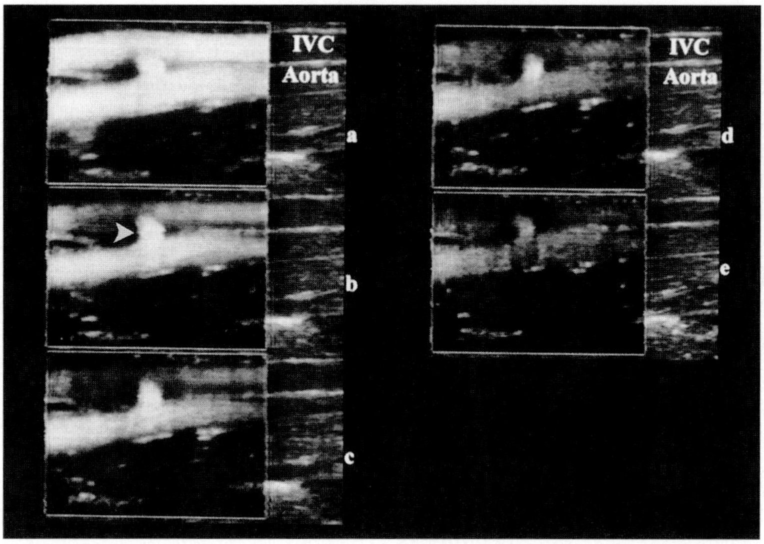

Fig. 27.6 a–e. Images of the inferior vena cava (*IVC*: top vessel) and the aorta (lower vessel) at the level of the renal artery branch (*arrowhead* in **b**) were acquired with the wideband harmonic technique at 7 MHz using the Siemens Elegra scanner in a normal rabbit given 0.5 ml of AF0150. Each image shows the wideband harmonic region as an overlay on a standard B-mode image, similar to a color Doppler display. The images are a sequence of gradually decreasing pulse delay (**a**: longest; **e**: shortest). Note that as the pulse delay is decreased from **a** to **e** there is an overall decrease in enhancement. There is also greater contrast between the rapid-flow region (aorta) and the slow-flow region (IVC). Also note that the renal artery branch is brighter than IVC, and as the delay decreases becomes brighter than aorta because its bubbles did not receive the first pulse

larity, high-resolution tissue imaging, and visual differentiation of arterial and venous flow can be achieved.

27.5 Current Contrast-Specific Instrumentation

27.5.1 Overview

Commercial production of contrast-specific ultrasound instrumentation is in its infancy but has gained momentum in the past few years as contrast media development has entered clinical testing. Prototype scanners have been developed by many companies, including Acuson, ATL, General Electric, Hewlett-Packard, Siemens, and Toshiba, demonstrating significant investment in instrumentation development. Images from these systems are of varying states of development and quality. This is a good indication of corporate research and development efforts, and suggests that more products will soon become commercially available that not only improve image contrast but also provide quantitative capabilities.

27.5.2 Products and Manufacturers

During the second quarter of 1996, two manufacturers announced the availability of a contrast-specific ultrasound scanner. Hewlett-Packard (Andover, Mass.) announced the release of a contrast-specific scanner built on the SONOS 2500 platform, and ATL (Bothell, Wash.) announced a contrast-specific package as an option/upgrade on the HDI 3000 platform. Acuson originally developed harmonic imaging on the XP platform and is currently shipping its Native Tissue Harmonic Imaging as an application/upgrade on the Sequoia platform. This package is designed to perform harmonic imaging on native tissues and could likely be used effectively with contrast materials as designed or with slight modifications. Toshiba, Siemens, and many other manufacturers have multifrequency transducers and prototype contrast-specific scanners in research environments and are likely to offer commercially available products between 1998 and 2000.

The initial trend to develop contrast-specific ultrasound scanners was through software upgrades on existing platforms. These scanners used the same transducers and excitation hardware as conventional scanners, with software changes installed to allow nonlinear imaging capabilities. Other companies have redesigned the software as well as the hardware and have developed specialized equipment to handle nonlinear imaging tasks. For efficient contrast-specific imaging, it is important that the transducers are designed with appropriate transmit and receive efficiencies at the required frequencies. Future advances in transducer design and in computer power are likely to significantly influence the development of high-quality, contrast-specific ultrasound scanners.

27.5.3 Useful Features

Several important features would be especially useful in ultrasound machinery that is to be used with contrast materials. The scanner needs the capability to offer a nonlinear imaging technique. It would be most useful if this feature was available in all imaging modes and with all transducers. Gating would be a critical factor and would need to be a bit more complex than that generally available on ultrasound units today. A cardiac gating input would be important, as would the ability to input a gating signal from another source and the ability to set an internal trigger source to adjust a gating speed of any duration. Further, it would be beneficial to provide a feature allowing the acquisition of a specified number of frames at a specified time interval.

As contrast materials are sensitive to acoustic pressure and insonating frequency, it would be valuable to have fine control over transmit power, transmit frequency, and receive frequency. Control of the pulse interval is also important on machines incorporating dual-pulse imaging techniques. Many machines incorporate some rough control over these parameters, but providing a control that divides the dynamic range of the setting into at least ten steps would provide the user with much better ability to tune the system to the patient and contrast material used. With the adjustment of transmit power, it would be useful to have a standardized power output display at all times, so that a clinician could use different machines but expect similar contrast agent performance when the frequency and power were adjusted similarly.

The complexity of performing nonlinear imaging in various imaging modes often results in a reduction of the imaging frame rate. It would be important to maintain a frame rate of at least 30 Hz, with some potential ultrasound contrast agent applications benefiting from significantly higher frame rates (Lee et al. 1998). Therefore, it would be useful to provide controls over frame rate speed, a feature already present on some clinical scanners. Finally, pseudo-quantitation may be possible if time-intensity curves could be generated over a region of interest (ROI) selected by the user. A possible incorporation of this feature could be a lengthy cine save followed by a calculation package, which allows the ROI selection and subsequent graphical display of the intensity-time relationship.

References

Abildgaard A, Egge TS, Klow NE, Jakobsen JA (1996) Use of sonicated albumin (Infoson) to enhance arterial spectral and color Doppler imaging. Cardiovasc Intervent Radiol 19:265–271

Albrecht T, Urbank A, Mahler M, et al. (1998) Prolongation and optimization of Doppler enhancement with a microbubble US contrast agent by using continuous infusion: preliminary experience. Radiology 207:339–347

Anderson AL, Hampton LD (1980) Acoustics of gas-bearing sediments. J Acoust Soc Am 67:1865–1903

Andre MP, Steinbach GC, Mattrey RF (1992) Sensitivity of pulsed-wave and Color Doppler to flowing blood and its enhancement with perflubron. Med Phys 19:1139 (abstract)

Brock-Fisher GA, Poland MD, Rafter PG (1996) (To Hewlett-Packard Company), "Means for increasing sensitivity in non-linear ultrasound imaging systems." U.S. Patent 5,577,505, November 26, 1996

Burns PN, Fritzsch T, Weitschies W, Uhlendorf V, Hope-Simpson D, Powers JE (1995) Pseudo-Doppler shifts from stationary tissues due to the stimulated emission of ultrasound from a new microsphere contrast agent. Radiology 197(P):402

Chapman C, Lazenby J (1997) (To Siemens Medical Systems, Inc.), "Ultrasound imaging system employing phase inversion subtraction to enhance the image." U.S. Patent 5,632,277, May 27, 1997

Dayton P, Goode A, Morgan K, Klibanov S, Brandenburger G, Ferrara K (1996) Action of microbubbles when insonified: experimental evidence. In: Levy M, Schneider SC, McAvoy BR (eds) IEEE Ultrasonics Symposium Proceedings 2:1131–1134. 3–6 November 1996, San Antonio, Tex., USA

de Jong N, Ten Cate FJ, Lancee CT, Roelandt J, Bom N (1991) Principles and recent developments in ultrasound contrast agents. Ultrasonics 29:324–330

de Jong N, Ten Cate FJ (1996) New ultrasound contrast agents and technological innovations. Ultrasonics 34:587–590

Fairbank WM, Scully MO (1977) A new noninvasive technique for cardiac pressure measurement: resonant scattering of ultrasound from bubbles. IEEE Trans Biomed Eng 24:107–110

Firschke C, Lindner JR, Wei K, Goodman NC, Skyba DM, Kaul S (1997) Myocardial perfusion imaging in the setting of coronary artery stenosis and acute myocardial infarction using venous injection of a second-generation echocardiographic contrast agent. Circulation 96:959–967

Forsberg F, Liu JB, Burns PN, Merton DA, Goldberg BB (1994) Artifacts in ultrasonic contrast agent studies. J Ultrasound Med 13:357–365

Forsberg F, Merton DA, Schultz SM, Goldberg BB, Needleman L, Rawool NM (1998) Contrast induced Doppler waveform changes in women with breast lesions. J Ultrasound Med 17:S97 (abstract)

Goldberg BB, Forsberg F, Merton DA, Rawool NM, Liu J (1996) Sonographic detection of bleeding sites and other structures with use of a contrast agent. Radiology 201(P): 197

Hauff P, Fritzsch T, Reinhardt M, Weitschies W, Luders F, Uhlendorf V, Heldmann D (1997) Delineation of experimental liver tumors in rabbits by a new ultrasound contrast agent and stimulated acoustic emission. Invest Radiol 32:94–99

Horton JW (1972) (To International Business Machines Corporation), "Blood flow pressure measurement technique employing injected bubbles and ultrasonic frequency scanning." U.S. Patent 3,640,271, February 8, 1972

Hwang JJ, Simpson DH (1998) (To Advanced Technology Laboratories, Inc.), "Ultrasonic diagnostic imaging with harmonic contrast agents." U.S. Patent 5,706,819, Jan. 13, 1998

Johnson KW, Powers JE (1995) (To Advanced Technology Laboratories, Inc.), "Ultrasonic detection of contrast agents." U.S. Patent 5,456,257, October 10, 1995

Kaul S (1997) New developments in ultrasound systems for contrast echocardiography. Clin Cardiol 20(10 Suppl 1): I27–I30

Kono Y, Moriyasu F, Nada T, et al. (1997) Flash echo imaging of the liver with galactosed-based microbubbles. J Ultrasound Med 16:S71 (abstract)

Krishnan S, O'Donnell M (1996) Transmit aperture processing for nonlinear contrast agent imaging. Ultrason Imaging 18:77–105

Kristoffersen K (1996) Future machinery and ultrasound contrast agents. First European Symposium on Ultrasound Contrast Imaging, 25–26 January 1996, Rotterdam, The Netherlands (abstract, p 40)

Lee YZ, Steinbach GC, Mattrey RF (1998) Flow velocity profile estimation using B-mode ultrasound and contrast agents. J Ultrasound Med 17:S98 (abstract)

Li W, van der Steen AF, Lancee CT, Honkoop J, Gussenhoven EJ, Bom N (1996) Temporal correlation of blood scattering signals in vivo from radiofrequency intravascular ultrasound. Ultrasound Med Biol 22:583–590

Mattrey RF, Steinbach GC (1991) Ultrasound contrast agents: state of the art. Invest Radiol 26(S1):S5–S11

Mattrey RF, Wrigley R, Steinbach GC, Schutt EG, Evitts DP (1994) Gas emulsions as ultrasound contrast agents. Preliminary results in rabbits and dogs. Invest Radiol 29:S139–S41

Melany M, Grant E, McElroy D, Kimme-Smith C (1998) Effect of contrast agents on spectral velocities: an in vitro evaluation of several agents. J Ultrasound Med 17:S56 (abstract)

Miller JG, Mobley J, Hall CS, Marsh JN, Hughes MS, Brandenburger GH (1998) Potential effects on ultrasonic images of concentration dependent velocity of sound in Albunex. UCSD Ultrasound Contrast Research Symposium, 6–8 February 1998, San Diego, California (abstract #24)

Morgan K, Dayton P, Klibanov S, Brandenburger G, Kaul S, Wei K, Ferrara K (1996) Properties of contrast agents insonified at frequencies above 10 MHz. In: Levy M, Schneider SC, McAvoy BR (eds) IEEE Ultrasonics Symposium Proceedings 2:1127–1130. 3–6 November 1996, San Antonio, Tex., USA

Moriyasu F, Kono Y, Kamiyama N, et al. (1998) Flash echo imaging of liver tumors using ultrasound contrast agent and intermittent color doppler scanning. J Ultrasound Med 17:S63 (abstract)

O'Donnell M, Flax SW (1988) Phase aberration measurements in medical ultrasound: human studies. Ultrason Imaging 10:1–11

Olstad B (1996) (To Vingmed Sound A/S), "Method for motion encoding of tissue structures in ultrasonic imaging." U.S. Patent 5,568,811, October 29, 1996

Ophir J, Parker KJ (1989) Contrast agents in diagnostic ultrasound. Ultrasound Med Biol 15:319–333

Ostensen J, Eriksen M, Hoff L, Frigstad S, Sponheim N, Dyrstad K (1997) (To Nycomed Imaging AS), "Ultrasound Imaging," U.S. Patent 5,601,085, February 11, 1997

Porter TR (1996) (To The Board of Regents of the University of Nebraska), "Suspended ultra-sound induced microbubble cavitation imaging." U.S. Patent 5,560,364, October 1, 1996

Porter TR, Xie F (1995) Transient myocardial contrast after initial exposure to diagnostic ultrasound pressures with minute doses of intravenously injected microbubbles. Demonstration and potential mechanisms. Circulation 92:2391–2395

Porter TR, Xie F, Li Li S, D'Sa A, Rafter P (1996) Increased ultrasound contrast and decreased microbubble destruction rates with triggered ultrasound imaging. J Am Soc Echocardiogr 9:599–605

Powers JE, Burns PN, Souquet J (1997) Imaging instrumentation for ultrasound contrast agents. In: Nanda NC, Schlief R, Goldberg BB (eds) Advances in echo imaging using contrast enhancement. Kluwer Academic, Dordrecht, pp 139–170

Schwartz KQ, Bezante GP, Chen X, Schlief R (1993) Quantitative echo contrast concentration measurement by Doppler sonography. Ultrasound Med Biol 19:289–297

Shi WT, Raichlen JS, Forsberg F, Goldberg BB (1998) Effect of ambient pressure changes on subharmonic response of microbubbles. J Ultrasound Med 17:S55 (abstract)

Sirlin CB, Girard MS, Steinbach GC, Baker KG, Broderdorf SK, Hall LA, Mattrey RF (1997) Effect of ultrasound transmit power on liver enhancement with Imagent US, a PFC-stabilized microbubble contrast agent. Int J Imaging Sys Tech 8:82–88

Sirlin CB, Girard MS, Baker KG, Steinbach GC, Deiranieh LH, Mattrey RF (1998) Effect of Acquisition Rate on Liver and Portal Vein Enhancement with Microbubble Contrast. Submitted to Jour of Ultr in Med and Bio

Sponheim N, Myhrum M (1995) An ultrasound contrast agent's influence on the measured Doppler signal. In: Levy M, Schneider SC, McAvoy BR (eds) IEEE Ultrasonics Symposium Proceedings 2:1133–1136. 7–10 November 1995, Seattle, Wash., USA

Sponheim N, Myhrum M (1996) An in vitro study on the influence of limited frequency resolution on contrast agent-enhanced Doppler signals. Ultrasonics 34:599–601

Steinbach GC, Lee YZ, Lazenby JC, Peterson TM, Mattrey RF (1998) Vascular echogenicity on B-mode high resolution harmonic imaging as a function of velocity and contrast concentration. J Ultrasound Med 17:S55 (abstract)

Tickner EG (1981) (To Rasor Associates, Inc.), "Method of determining pressure within liquid containing vessel." U.S. Patent 4,265,251, May 5, 1981

Uhlendorf V, Hoffmann C (1994) Nonlinear acoustical response of coated microbubbles in diagnostic ultrasound. In: Levy M, Schneider SC, McAvoy BR (eds) IEEE Ultrasonics Symposium Proceedings 3:1559–1562. 1–4 November 1994, Cannes, France

Wei K, Jayaweera AR, Firoozan S, Linka A, Skyba DM, Kaul S (1998) Quantification of myocardial blood flow with ultrasound-induced destruction of microbubbles administered as a constant venous infusion. Circulation 97:473–483

28 Bubble Destruction

C.B. SIRLIN, T. PELURA, and R.F. MATTREY

CONTENTS

28.1 Introduction

Microbubbles are promising ultrasound contrast agents with potentially important clinical applications in cardiovascular and body imaging. Although other ultrasound contrast agents have been proposed (MATTREY et al. 1982; VIOLANTE et al. 1988), microbubbles are most promising because of their high effectiveness at very small dosages (MATTREY et al. 1996). They typically consist of a free gas bubble, or gas contained within an elastic, semirigid, or rigid shell. Microbubbles are effective scatterers owing to the large impedance difference between the surrounding fluid (e.g., blood) and the encapsulated gas, as well as their resonance in the ultrasound beam. The amplitude of the reflected signal is linearly related to bubble concentration and to the bubble's radius raised to the sixth power (POWSNER et al. 1986; MORSE and INGARD 1968; VUILLE et al. 1994; VANDENBERG and MELTON 1994; WIENCEK et al. 1993). The bubbles in plasma have similar rheology as red blood cells and can traverse the pulmonary and systemic circulation (GOLDBERG et al. 1994; POWSNER et al. 1986; WIENCEK et al. 1993).

In addition to withstanding ambient pressures, microbubbles must also withstand the surface tension (La Place pressure) exerted by plasma, which increases with decreasing bubble diameter. Therefore, the small size required to allow transpulmonary passage makes the bubble inherently unstable in vivo, as the exerted pressure promotes rapid diffusion of the plasma-soluble air out of the bubble (SHAPIRO et al. 1990; VUILLE et al. 1994; CHEN et al. 1994; MOTTLEY et al. 1990; GOTTLIEB et al. 1990; MOR-AVI et al. 1994). Gas loss further decreases bubble diameter, ultimately leading to rapid collapse and loss of reflectivity (PORTER and XIE 1995; VUILLE et al. 1994; PADIAL et al. 1995).

To increase microbubble longevity in plasma, three approaches have been pursued in the following order of effectiveness: (1) increasing the stiffness of the protective shell, (2) addition of surfactant to decrease surface tension, and (3) addition of less plasma-soluble gas to the microbubble. The addition of a protective shell, such as denatured protein, increases bubble longevity to one or two circulation times (PORTER and XIE 1995; HILPERT et al. 1988; TERASAWA et al. 1993; VON BIBRA et al. 1993; UNGER et al. 1991), but also decreases reflectivity (CHURCH 1995). Despite the more rigid shell, such microbubbles remain susceptible to pressure, as shown by in vivo (SHAPIRO et al. 1990) and numerous in vitro (VUILLE et al. 1994; CHEN et al. 1994; MOTTLEY et al. 1990; GOTTLIEB et al. 1990) and isolated heart (MOR-AVI et al. 1994) experiments. The addition of surfactant, such as palmitic acid, increases plasma longevity to a few minutes (ALBRECHT et al. 1998). By far the most effective improvement was achieved by the addition of perfluorocarbon (PFC) vapor to the microbubble, which not only increased bubble longevity to several minutes but also allowed a sufficient number of bubbles to reach the circulation to produce gray-scale enhancement of vessels and tissues (MATTREY et al. 1994a; SCHUTT et al. 1996).

Although formulation differences affect vascular half-life, all PFC-containing agents provide several

C.B. SIRLIN, MD, C/O R.F. MATTREY, Department of Radiology, University of California, San Diego Medical Center, 200 W. Arbor Drive, San Diego, CA 92109-8756, USA
T. PELURA, PhD, Alliance Pharmaceutical Corp., 3040 Science Park Road, San Diego, CA 92121, USA
R.F. MATTREY, MD, Department of Radiology, University of California, San Diego Medical Center, 200 W. Arbor Drive, San Diego, CA 92109-8756, USA

minutes of imaging (Mattrey et al. 1994a, 1996). Owing to osmotic pressure, a bubble made with pure PFC gas will expand when injected intravenously by drawing nitrogen and oxygen out of solution. The bubble will ultimately get trapped in the lung or tissues, or its growth will stop when the sum of the partial pressures of the air and PFC vapor inside the microbubble equals the sum of the partial pressure of air in plasma and La Place and ambient hydrostatic pressures. Conversely, microbubble preparations containing insufficient PFC concentrations will decrease in size until a threshold radius is reached (the collapsing radius), at which the collapsing forces exceed the vapor pressure of the PFC, converting the highly scattering gas bubble into a much lower scattering PFC liquid droplet. Formulations in which the osmotic pressure differentials across the membrane are balanced exhibit marked stability under physiologic conditions and limit the potential for bubble size growth in vivo. Schutt et al. (1996) found that a perfluorohexane concentration of 2.2 mg/ml in the filling gas, for example, was able to counteract 190 torr of ambient pressure.

Although these late-generation agents may be optimally designed to withstand the ambient pressures experienced in the cardiovascular system, they suffer the effects of the positive and negative pressures of an ultrasound beam, which exceed physiologic pressures by orders of magnitude (3800–11 400 mmHg) (Vandenberg and Melton 1994). Moreover, the high-frequency oscillation between compression and expansion caused by the ultrasound beam produces bubble resonance at diagnostic frequencies of 2–5 MHz. This rapid change in bubble size promotes bubble destruction (Vandenberg and Melton 1994; Neppiras et al. 1983; Vandenberg 1990; Shandas et al. 1990; Wray et al. 1991).

28.2 Evidence of Bubble Destruction in Tissues

While testing the liver-enhancing potential of several formulations, we empirically observed that liver enhancement outside the field most recently scanned was consistently greater than enhancement of the recently scanned region. This suggested that microbubbles have greater persistence in the liver when not exposed to ultrasound. Moreover, at microbubble contrast doses that induce excessive attenuation and shadowing, the echogenicity of the far field increased as the near field became less echogenic during the course of insonation, indicating that bubbles in more intense sound fields have shorter survival. In order to explain this observation, we conducted two experiments using the rabbit liver. In the first, we varied the transmit power and insonation time (Sirlin et al. 1997). In the second, we varied the delay time between frames acquired at a fixed transmit power (Sirlin et al. 1998).

In both experiments we used a region of infarcted liver as an internal standard against which liver and portal vein enhancement was compared. The infarction was produced by injecting 1 ml of ethyl alcohol directly into the liver under ultrasound guidance. The assessment of liver and vascular enhancement was accomplished by videodensitometry.

In the first experiment we used eight rabbits. Each rabbit had four separate scans: two continuous scanning sessions, one at maximum power and one at 9 dB less than maximum, and two sessions where 5 s of continuous scanning was performed at 9 dB below maximum power either every 15 s or every 60 s. Each scan session had a separate contrast injection (AF0150, Alliance Pharmaceutical Corp., San Diego). For the second experiment, we used seven rabbits and five different scanning sessions, where the ultrasound instrument was gated with an external pulse. Each session had a different acquisition rate at a fixed transmit power (6 dB less than maximum): one frame every 30 s, one frame every 5 s, one frame every second, four frames per second, and 28 frames per second. Scanning for both experiments was performed at 7 MHz using an XP10 Acuson scanner.

In both experiments, the liver parenchyma became subjectively more echogenic after each contrast injection, as compared with its precontrast appearance, irrespective of transmit power, insonation time, or acquisition frequency.

Liver enhancement at minimum power and minimum insonation time was significantly greater ($P < 0.001$) than that achieved with the three other imaging protocols (Fig. 28.1). Enhancement at maximum power and continuous scanning was significantly less ($P < 0.01$) than the enhancement achieved with the three other protocols. There was no statistical difference between minimum power transmitted either continuously or for 5 s every 15 s.

When the same transmit power was used per frame but the delay time between frames was increased from 1/28 to 1/4 to 1, 5, and 30 s, liver contrast increased in a stepwise fashion (Fig. 28.2) ($P < 0.001$). In fact, the time–enhancement curve achieved with each imaging protocol was statistically different from all other acquisition protocols

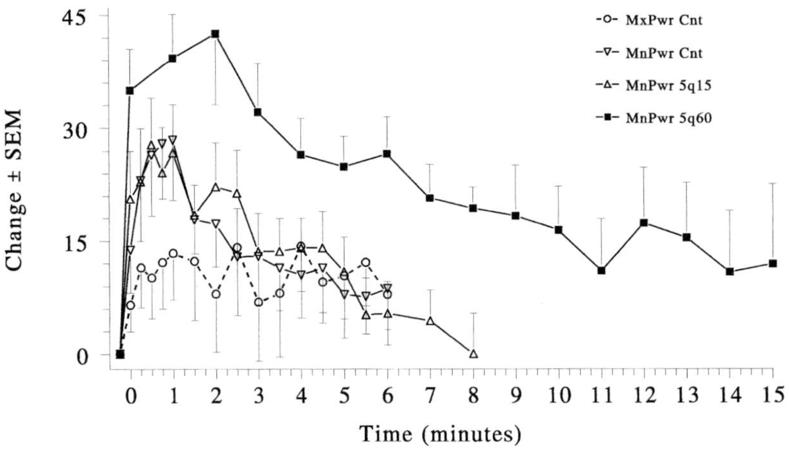

Fig. 28.1. Mean change ± standard error of the mean in liver-to-lesion contrast (intensity difference) over time as a function of the insonation protocol. *MxPwr Cnt*, Continuous maximum power; *MnPwr Cnt*, continuous minimum power; *MnPwr 5q15*, minimum power for 5 s every 15 s; *MnPwr 5q60*, minimum power for 5 s every 60 s. Liver enhancement during real-time imaging at maximum power was statistically different from all three other imaging protocols. (From SIRLIN et al. 1997)

a

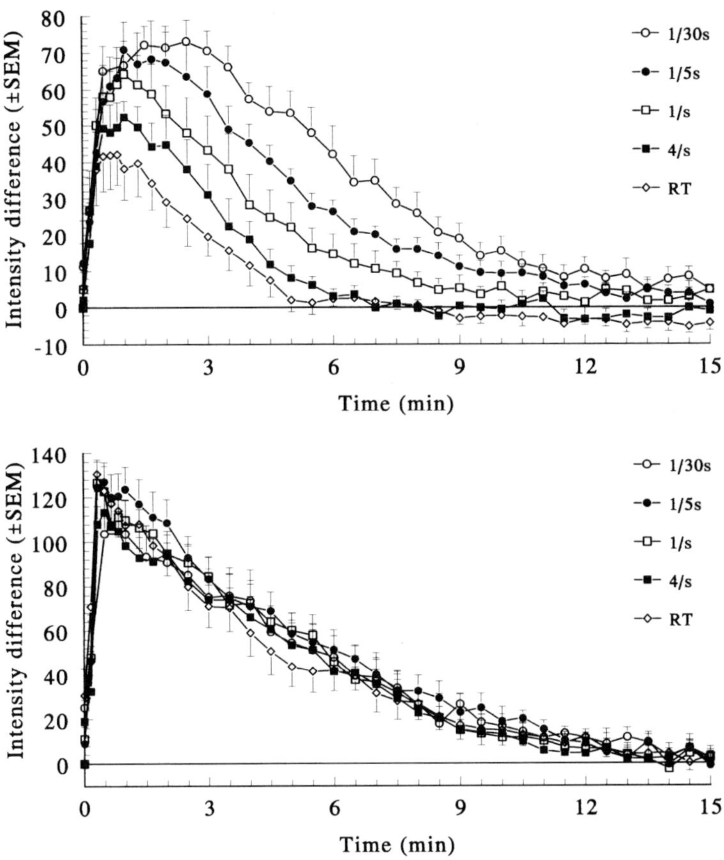

b

Fig. 28.2. Baseline corrected liver-to-lesion (**a**) and portal vein-to-lesion (**b**) videointensity difference for each imaging protocol: 1 frame every 30 s (1 fr/30 s), 1 fr/5 s, 1 fr/s, 4 fr/s, and real-time (RT) acquired at 28 fr/s shown as mean difference ± SEM. All liver time-intensity curves were statistically significant as a function of time and imaging protocol and were statistically different from each other. All portal vein time-intensity curves were statistically similar. Note that while the acquisition rate affected liver enhancement, it had no effect on vascular enhancement. (From SIRLIN et al. 1998)

($P < 0.05$). In contradistinction to liver time-intensity behavior, portal vein enhancement was unaffected by acquisition rate. All delay times, including the real-time acquisition, were similar (Fig. 28.2). The difference between the liver and portal vein videointensity is shown in Fig. 28.3. The portal vein enhanced more than liver for all frame rates except for the 1 fr/30 s acquisition. Note that for the real-time acquisition, the portal vein was brighter than liver for over 3 min. Figure 28.4 is an example of a rabbit with liver ablation showing the effect of frame rate on liver and portal vein enhancement relative to the infarcted region. Although we did not measure vascular enhancement in the first experiment, we would expect that power and exposure would also have no effect.

Bubble destruction has been demonstrated both in vitro (PORTER et al. 1997; WALKER et al. 1997) and

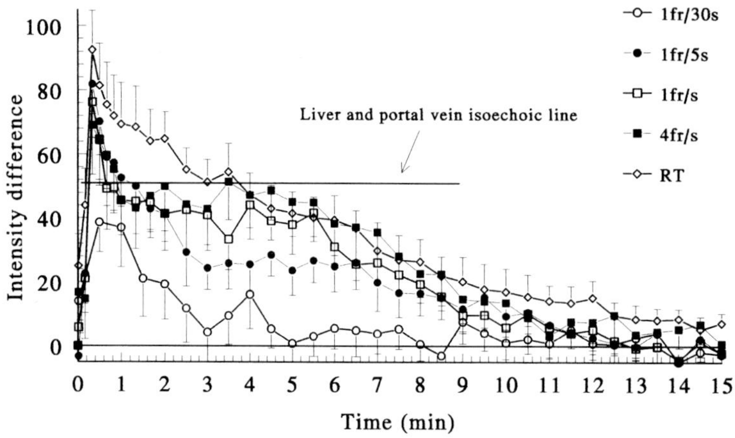

Fig. 28.3. Baseline corrected portal vein to liver videointensity difference for each imaging protocol: 1 frame every 30 s (1 fr/30 s), 1 fr/5 s, 1 fr/s, 4 fr/s, and real-time (RT) acquired at 28 fr/s shown as mean difference ± SEM. When the curve is above the liver and portal vein isoechoic line, the portal vein is more echogenic than the enhanced liver. Note that the portal vein was more echogenic than liver for approximately 3.5 min at real time. Except for the first minute after injection, it was nearly isoechoic with liver with intermittent imaging. (From Sirlin et al. 1998)

a

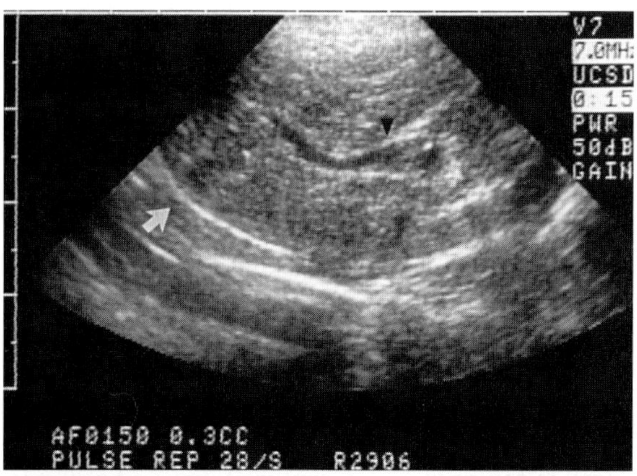

b

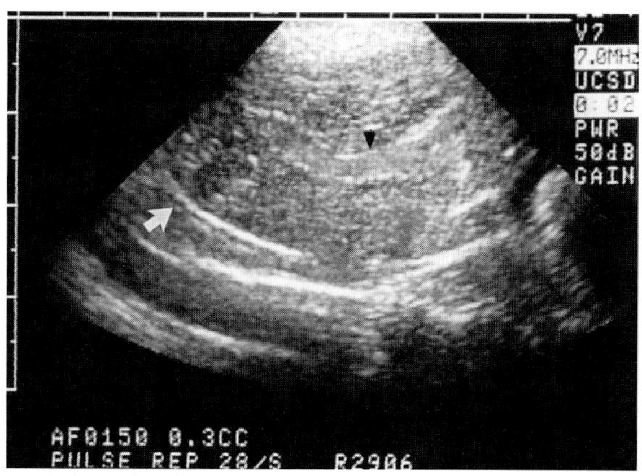

c

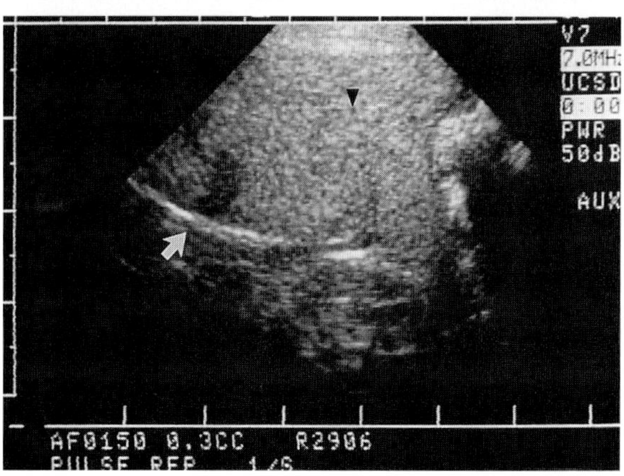

Fig. 28.4. Images obtained over the portal vein (*arrowhead*) and alcohol ablation lesion (*arrow*) precontrast (**a**) and 2 min following 0.3 ml of AF0150 (Alliance Pharmaceutical Corp., San Diego) while imaging at 28 frames/s (**b**) or 1 frame/s (**c**). Note that the portal vein is hyperechoic relative to liver in **b** and isoechoic to liver in **c**. (From Sirlin et al. 1998)

in vivo (Villarraga et al. 1997). Although it is difficult to extrapolate in vitro data to in vivo in ultrasound contrast experiments, the studies clearly showed the effect of bubble exposure to ultrasound. The in vivo experiment showed that variation in power and delay time during intermittent imaging affected left ventricular opacification or intravascular dwell time.

Studies have not elucidated the process that leads to bubble destruction under acoustic pressure. There are three possible mechanisms. The first is that microbubbles temporarily decrease in size under the influence of external pressure, with transient loss of reflectivity, but rebound to steady-state size and reflectivity when the pressure has been removed (Mor-Avi et al. 1994; Shandas et al. 1990). The second is that microbubbles collapse under the influence of external pressure, with permanent loss of reflectivity due to accelerated diffusion of gas out of the bubble or conversion of gas to liquid (SCHUTT et al. 1998; VUILLE et al. 1994; PADIAL et al. 1995). The third is that microbubbles expand during the negative pressure wave, exceeding the capability of the shell or surfactant to maintain its integrity. The expansion causes fractures, fragmentation, and weakening of the shell, leaving a naked bubble that is short lived. In the case of the elastic shell of surfactant bubbles, the surface area of the bubble that must be covered by surfactant increases 100-fold as the radius increases by as much as tenfold during the expansion phase. This increase leads to loss of some surfactant, resulting in a smaller bubble when the expansion force is removed. The smaller bubble experiences greater surface tension, increasing the PFC vapor pressure, which accelerates the loss of bubble contents to either plasma or an adjacent larger bubble with less PFC partial pressure. While several plausible hypotheses exist, the likely mechanism is a combination of multiple factors. The available data indicate that bubbles disappear by shrinking as visualized under high-speed video microscopy rather than by explosion (DAYTON et al. 1997).

Although in vitro work with albumin-coated microbubbles and microbubbles made from hand-agitated saline and diatrizoate solutions suggests that cyclic hydrostatic pressure causes at least somewhat reversible changes in echogenicity (MOR-AVI et al. 1994; PADIAL et al. 1995), constant hydrostatic pressure (DE JONG et al. 1993; VUILLE et al. 1994; GOTTLIEB et al. 1990) and the acoustic pressure produced by commercial ultrasound systems cause permanent bubble destruction (VILLARRAGA et al. 1997; VANDENBERG and MELTON 1994; WRAY et al. 1991; SIRLIN et al. 1997, 1998).

28.3 Significance of Bubble Destruction

Microbubbles show great promise in numerous experimental models, including the detection of perfusion abnormalities in solid organs such as liver (GIRARD et al. 1998a), spleen, and kidney (MATTREY et al. 1995; FORSBERG et al. 1995), the visualization and assessment of blood vessels for intrinsic disease (COLEY et al. 1994), and the assessment of the left ventricular chamber and myocardial perfusion (MATTREY et al. 1994b). However, it appears that all agents are susceptible to acoustic pressure (WALKER et al. 1997), with some agents being more susceptible than others, depending on their collapsing radius and shell stiffness. Therefore, it is beneficial to develop imaging protocols to prolong the enhancement effect in tissues and to allow the detection of perfusion abnormalities.

28.3.1 Disadvantages

The only disadvantage of bubble destruction is the more transient contrast effect and shorter intravascular dwell time. Regions of slow flow are poorly enhanced as bubbles are lost before sufficient concentrations can be achieved to affect tissue enhancement. Cine mode capture and intermittent imaging have been used to overcome the transient effect and inability to enhance tissues with slow flow.

Cine mode capture has allowed the visualization of bubbles as they are destroyed from one frame to the next. The technique was described as flash-echo imaging (MORIYASU et al. 1996). With this technique, the ultrasound is turned off for a period of time and then turned on. It shows dramatic enhancement on the first frame that fades on subsequent frames as bubbles are destroyed during the preceding frame. The first frame is the most revealing diagnostically, as it depicts the bubbles that accumulate in the field when the sound is turned off. If the first frame is the only frame captured, the technique is then called intermittent or gated imaging.

With intermittent imaging, it is possible to dial in the desired effect of the contrast agent, as shown in Fig. 28.5. Note that during real-time imaging, the kidney and the vessels are hyperechoic relative to liver because of their rapid blood flow. However, with increasing delay time, the liver becomes more echogenic because of its greater fractional blood volume. Therefore, when intraparenchymal blood vessels need to be seen, high frame rates and/or high transmit power is needed. If, on the other hand, greater tissue contrast is needed to visualize tumors or areas of necrosis or infarction, intermittent imaging with 1-s or longer delay time is needed (Fig. 28.6). It should be clear that blood vessels are unaffected by frame rate because they are continuously and rapidly replenished with fresh unexposed bubbles, and because the bubbles in vessels have rapid transit through the scanning field, decreasing bubble exposure to ultrasound energy.

Gated imaging in radiologic application is complicated by the great variability of relevant anatomy, which requires the sonographer to view a near-continuous flow of images to maintain anatomic

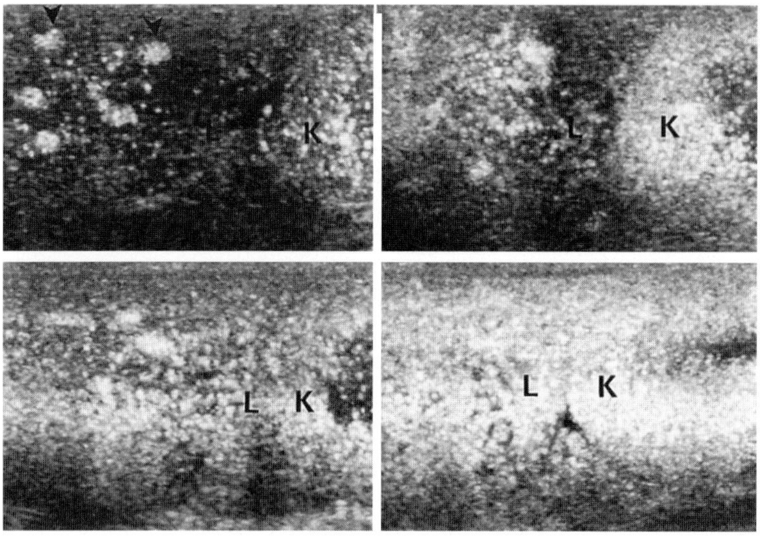

Fig. 28.5. Standard B-mode images obtained over the kidney and liver of a normal rabbit at 7 MHZ using a Siemens Elegra scanner show the effect of intermittent imaging on image contrast when frames were acquired in real time (*upper left*), 5 frames/second (*upper right*), 1 frame/second (*lower left*), and 1 frame/5 s (*lower right*). With real-time imaging, the kidney (*K*) is more echogenic than liver (*L*) because of the rapid delivery of bubbles to the kidney and the slower and delayed delivery of bubbles to the liver. Also, vessels (*arrowheads*) are bright because their bubbles are replenished between frames. With greater delay, the liver begins to fill with bubbles, increasing its echogenicity relative to kidney until the liver and kidney become isoechoic

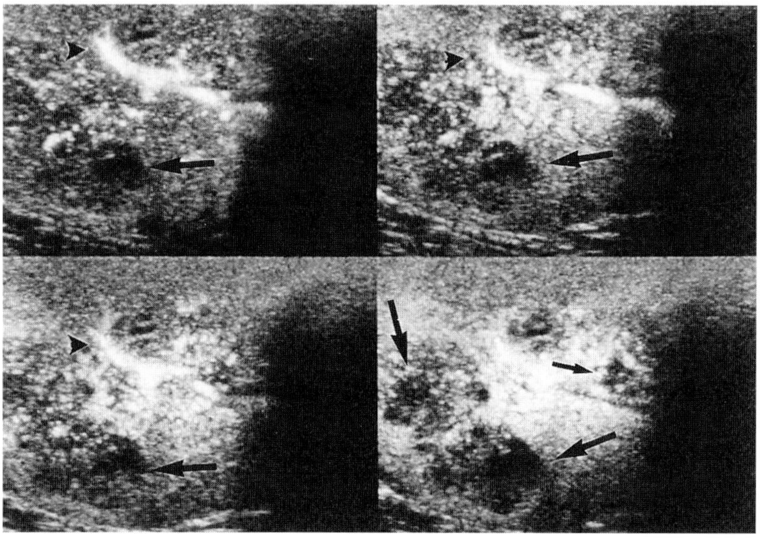

Fig. 28.6. Wideband harmonic images obtained over a Vx2 tumor of a rabbit at 7 MHZ using a Siemens Elegra scanner show the effect of intermittent imaging on tumor depiction when frames were acquired in real time (*upper left*), 1 frame/2 s (*upper right*), 1 frame/5 s (*lower left*), and 1 frame/10 s (*lower right*). With real-time imaging, vessels are most echogenic (*arrowhead*) and necrotic regions (*arrows*) least echogenic. With increasing delay, note that the liver begins to increase in echogenicity to become isoechoic with vessel and markedly more echogenic than the nonnecrotic tumor. Note on the 1 frame/10 s image (*lower right*) multiple tumor nodules (*arrows*) become visible that were less apparent on real-time

orientation. In triggered ultrasound, the near-continuous flow of images is replaced by a series of static, distinct images, making anatomic orientation difficult to maintain. In the study conducted with triggered acquisition, we found that at 1 frame/s it was relatively easy to maintain anatomic orientation, so long as the transducer was moved slowly. At 1 frame/s, image contrast increased by 44% and contrast duration was doubled, as compared with real-time acquisition (Sirlin et al. 1998).

Intermittent imaging is a powerful technique that allows the visualization of bubbles in vascular beds with slow flow such as capillaries. The acquired frame following a certain delay time demonstrates enhancement that is dependent upon fractional blood volume, blood flow, and delay time between frames (Sirlin et al. 1997, 1998; Ohmori et al. 1997; Wei et al. 1998). With short delay times, the number of bubbles in each voxel is mostly dependent upon flow rate, or the number of bubbles delivered per unit time. With long delay times, the number of bubbles in each voxel is dependent upon fractional blood volume, as the blood that has been insonated is totally replaced by new blood with unexposed bubbles. This capability is particularly useful, as it provides a visual index of blood volume and blood flow by merely altering the delay time, unlike Doppler, which strictly reflects velocity. For a more detailed discussion, please refer to Chap. 32.

If bubbles are not destroyed, then image contrast is strictly dependent upon fractional blood volume during the vascular phase of the product. Blood flow data are available only during the arrival of the agent (initial rise time) as it circulates for the first time. Further, because increased backscatter is accompanied by attenuation, imaging the attenuated far field is not possible until bubbles are eliminated pharmacologically (Behan et al. 1993). This is a significant disadvantage as contrast elimination would occur simultaneously from the near-field as well as far field.

To use intermittent imaging to estimate relative blood flow requires the total destruction of bubbles, as any remaining bubbles would contribute to the next triggered frame. To accomplish this result, multiple frames are acquired rapidly, followed by a delay time that is gradually incremented to determine the rise time and to define the plateau. Such data provide not only relative flow rates between two regions, but also relative blood volume.

28.3.2 Advantages

Several advantages are associated with bubble destruction. The most obvious is the ability to gradually image from the near-field to the far field while tissues are maximally enhanced. This is possible because the near-field bubbles shield the far-field bubbles from the sound beam. As bubbles are destroyed from the near field, the sound can reach deeper into the tissue to allow its assessment. The greater penetration of the less attenuated beam destroys the deeper bubbles and so on.

As discussed in the above section, it is not necessary to destroy all bubbles with intermittent imaging to assess relative blood volume; however, to assess relative blood flow, all bubbles must be eliminated from the scan field. If total bubble destruction is achieved, then the number of bubbles, or image contrast, present following a predetermined delay is related to blood flow.

Bubble destruction has prompted the development of multipulse imaging techniques, in which brightness on the image is related to the difference between the signals detected by the second pulse and the first pulse. The presence of bubbles in a voxel returns a strong signal when the first pulse is transmitted. The second pulse returns a relatively weak signal from the same voxel, as the first pulse has destroyed the bubbles present within it. Voxels with no or few bubbles, or if bubbles have not been destroyed by the first pulse, return nearly comparable signals on both pulses, resulting in little or no difference in signal. The correlation between two consecutive pulses is the process used for color Doppler imaging, which has been adapted for contrast media. This technique is called transient response imaging (Bauer et al. 1997; Hauff et al. 1997). The disadvantage of this technique is that the first pulse must destroy the bubble, which is difficult to accomplish in large organs, such as the liver. Further, unless bubbles are replenished, which is possible with the late-generation agents or with contrast infusion, the technique can only be used once. For this purpose, bubble design would be optimized if bubbles were made more sensitive to ultrasound pressure, to increase the opportunity for their destruction with one pulse.

Bubble destruction is exploited in the field of drug delivery. Although bubbles can be made nontargeted, they can be made to deliver their load in any region of interest, simply by insonating that region following bubble administration. As the greatest bubble destruction will occur in the insonated region, specific drug delivery can be achieved. For further discussion of this topic, please refer to Chap. 34.

Acknowledgements. This work was supported in part by a grant from NIH, RSNA, and Alliance Pharmaceutical Corp.

References

Albrecht T, Urbank A, Mahler M, et al. (1998) Prolongation and optimization of Doppler enhancement with a microbubble US contrast agent by using continuous infusion: preliminary experience. Radiology 207:339–347

Bauer A, Schlief R, Zomack M, Urbank A, Niendorf H-P (1997) Acoustically stimulated microbubbles in diagnostic ultrasound: properties and implications for diagnostic use. In: Nanda N, Schlief R, Goldberg BB (eds) Advances in echo imaging using contrast enhancement, 2nd edn. Kluwer Academic, Lancaster, pp 669–684

Behan M, O'Connell D, Mattrey RF, Carney DN (1993) Perfluorooctyl bromide as a contrast agent for sono-graphy and computed tomography. Am J Roentgenol 160:399–405

Chen MH, Padial LR, Vuille C, Guerrero JL, Weyman AE, Picard MH (1994) Effect of pulsatile pressure on echocardiographic contrast persistence: Is it due to peak or duration of pressure? (abstract). J Am Coll Cardiol 23:25A

Church CC (1995) The effects of an elastic solid surface layer on the radial pulsations of gas bubbles. J Acoust Soc Am 97:1510–1521

Coley BD, Trambert MA, Mattrey RF (1994) Perflurorcarbon enhanced sonography: value in detecting acute venous thrombosis in rabbits. Am J Roentgenol 163:961–964

Dayton PA, Morgan KE, Klibanov AL, Brandenburger G, Nightingale KR, Ferrara KW (1997) A preliminary evaluation of the effects of primary and secondary radiation forces on acoustic contrast agents. IEEE Trans Ultrason

Ferroelectr Freq Control 44:1264–1277
de Jong N, Cate FJT, Vletter WB, Roelandt JRTC (1993) Quantification of transpulmonary echocontrast effects. Ultrasound Med Biol 19:279–288
Forsberg F, Liu JB, Merton DA, Rawool NM, Goldberg BB (1995) Parenchymal enhancement and tumor visualization using a new sonographic contrast agent. J Ultrasound Med 14:949–957
Girard MS, Baker KG, Steinbach GC, Deiranieh LH, Peterson TM, Mattrey RF (1998a) Assessment of liver and kidney enhancement using perflurocarbon vapor-stabilized ultrasound contrast agent. Acad Radiol (in press)
Girard MS, Sirlin CB, Healey K, Mattrey RF (1998b) Liver tumor detection with ultrasound contrast, a blinded prospective animal study. Acad Radiol 5(Suppl 1):S189–S191
Goldberg BB, Liu J-B, Forsberg F (1994) Ultrasound contrast agents: a review. Ultrasound Med Biol 20:319–333
Gottlieb S, Ernst A, Litt L, Schwarz KQ, Meltzer RS (1990) Effect of pressure on echocardiographic videodensity from sonicated albumin: an in-vivo model (abstract). J Am Soc Echocardiogr 3:238
Hauff P, Fritzsch T, Reinhardt M, Weitschies W, Luders F, Uhlendorf V, Heldmann D (1997) Delineation of experimental liver tumors in rabbits by a new ultrasound contrast agent and stimulated acoustic emission. Invest Radiol 32:94–99
Hilpert PA, Mattrey RF, Mitten RM, Peterson T (1988) Injection of air-filled human albumin microspheres to enhance arterial Dopplar signal: a preliminary study in rabbits. Am J Roentgenol 153:613–616
Mattrey RF, Scheible FW, Gosink BB, Leopold GR, Long DM, Higgins CB (1982) Perfluoroctylbromide: a liver/spleen-specific and tumor-imaging ultrasound contrast material. Radiology 145:759–762
Mattrey RF, Wrigley R, Steinbach GC, Schutt EG, Evitts DP (1994a) Gas emulsion as ultrasound contrast agents: preliminary results in rabbits and dogs. Invest Radiol 29:S139–S141
Mattrey RF, Steinbach GC, Peterson T, Hall LA (1994b) Echogenic enhancement of the perfused myocardium following the intravenous administration of PFC microbubbles (abstract). Radiology 193(P):367
Mattrey RF, Girard MS, Steinbach GC, Peterson T (1995) Improvement in tissue contrast enhancement at the second harmonic frequency in a renal infarct model following the intravenous injection of a perfluorochemical-stabilized microbubble contrast agent. Radiology 197(P):403
Mattrey RF, Manspeaker P, Pelura TJ, Batra S, Leese PT (1996) Safety and preliminary efficacy of AF0150, a phase I clinical trial in healthy volunteers. Radiology 201(P):158
Mor-Avi V, Shroff SG, Robinson KA, Ng AF, Cholley BP, Marcus RH, Lang RM (1994) Effect of left ventricular pressure on sonicated albumin microbubbles: evaluation using an isolated rabbit heart model. J Am Coll Cardiol 24:1779–1785
Moriyasu F, Kono Y, Nada T, Matsumara T, Suginoshita Y, Kobayashi K (1996) Flash echo (passive cavitation) imaging of the liver by using US contrast and intermittent scanning sequence. Radiology 201(P):196
Morse PM, Ingard KV (1968) Theoretical acoustics. McGraw-Hill, New York
Mottley J, Everbach EC, Schwarz KQ, Schlief R, Meltzer RS (1990) Decay of ultrasound integrated backscatter from a saccharide contrast agent is accelerated by increased pressure (abstract). Circulation 82(Suppl III):III-28
Neppiras EA, Nyborg WL, Miller DL (1983) Non-linear behaviour and stability of trapped micron-sized cylindrical gas bubbles in an ultrasonic field. Ultrasonics 21:109–115
Ohmori K, Cotter B, Kwan OL, Mizushige K, DeMaria AN (1997) Relation of contrast echo intensity and flow velocity to the amplification of contrast opacification produced by intermittent ultrasound transmission. Am Heart J 134:1066–1074
Ophir J, Parker KJ (1989) Contrast agents in diagnostic ultrasound. Ultrasound Med Biol 15:319–333
Padial LR, Chen MH, Vuille C, Guerrero JL, Weyman AE, Picard MH (1995) Pulsatile pressure affects the disappearance of echocardiographic contrast agents. J Am Soc Echocardiogr 8:285–292
Porter TR, Xie F (1995) Visually discernible myocardial echocardiographic contrast after intravenous injection of sonicated dextrose albumin microbubbles containing high molecular weight, less soluble gases. J Am Coll Cardiol 25:509–515
Porter TR, Kricsfeld D, Cheatham S, Li S (1997) The effect of ultrasound frame rate on perfluorocarbon-exposed sonicated dextrose albumin microbubble size and concentration when insonifying at different flow rates, transducer frequencies, and acoustic outputs. J Am Soc Echocardiogr 10:593–601
Powsner SM, Keller MW, Saniie J, Feinstein SB (1986) Quantitation of echo-contrast effects. Am J Physiol Imaging 1:124–128
Rayleigh JWS (1945) The theory of sound, 2nd edn. Dover Publishers, New York
Schlief R (1991) Ultrasound contrast agents. Curr Opin Radiol 3:198–207
Schlief R, Schurman R, Niendorf HP (1993) Basic properties and results of clinical trials of ultrasound contrast agents based on galactose. Ann Acad Med 22:762–767
Schutt EG, Pelura TJ, Hopkins RM (1996) Osmotically stabilized microbubble ultrasound contrast agents. Acad Rad 3(Suppl 2):S188–S190
Shandas R, Sahn DJ, Bales G, Elkadi T, Yau K-K, Charib M (1990) Persistence of Albunex (Alb) ultrasound contrast agent: in-vitro study of the effects of pressure and acoustic power on particle size, and the duration of contrast and Doppler enhancement (abstract). Circulation 82(Suppl III):III-95
Shapiro JR, Reisner SA, Lichtenberg GS, Meltzer RS (1990) Intravenous contrast echocardiography with use of sonicated albumin in humans: systolic disappearance of left ventricular contrast after transpulmonary transmission. J Am Coll Cardiol 16:1603–1607
Sirlin CB, Girard MS, Steinbach GC, Baker KG, Broderdorf SK, Hall LA, Mattrey RF (1997) Effect of ultrasound transmit power on liver enhancement with Imagent US, a PFC-stabilized microbubble contrast agent. Int J Imaging Systems Technol 8:82–88
Sirlin CB, Girard MS, Baker KG, Steinbach GC, Deiranieh LH, Mattrey RF (1998) Effect of acquisition rate on liver and portal vein enhancement with microbubble contrast. J Ultrasound Med Biol (in press)
Terasawa A, Miyatake K, Nakatani S, Yamagishi M, Matsuda H, Beppu S (1993) Enhancement of Doppler flow signals in the left heart chambers by intravenous injection of sonicated albumin. J Am Coll Cardiol 21:737–742
Unger EC, Lund P, Shen D, Fritz T, Fuller L, Yellowhair D (1991) Aerosomes as blood pool and cardiovascular contrast agents for US: in vivo studies (abstract). Radiology 181(P):225

Vandenberg BF (1990) Reproducibility of albumin microbubble backscatter measurement: influence of acoustic output (abstract). Clin Res 38:887A

Vandenberg BF, Melton HE (1994) Acoustic lability of albumin microspheres. J Am Soc Echocardiogr 7:582–589

Villarraga HR, Foley DA, Aeschbacher BC, Klarich KW, Mulvagh SL (1997) Destruction of contrast microbubbles during ultrasound imaging at conventional power output. J Am Soc Echocardiogr 10:783–791

Violante MR, Parker KJ, Fischer HW (1988) Particulate suspensions as ultrasonic contrast agents for liver and spleen. Invest Radiol 23(Suppl 1):S294–S297

von Bibra H, Becher H, Firschke C, Schlief R, Emslander HP, Schomig A (1993) Enhancement of mitral regurgitation and normal left atrial color Doppler flow signals with peripheral venous injection of a saccharide-based contrast agent. J Am Coll Cardiol 22:521–528

Vuille C, Nidorf M, Morrissey RL, Newell JB, Weyman AE, Picard MH (1994) Effect of static pressure on the disappearance rate of specific echocardiographic contrast agents. J Am Soc Echocardiogr 7:347–354

Walker KW, Pantely GA, Sahn DJ (1997) Ultrasound-mediated destruction of contrast agents. Effect of ultrasound intensity, exposure, and frequency. Invest Radiol 32:728–734

Wei K, Jayaweera AR, Firoozan S, Linka A, Skyba DM, Kaul S (1998) Quantification of myocardial blood flow with ultrasound-induced destruction of microbubbles administered as a constant venous infusion. Circulation 97:473–483

Wiencek JG, Feinstein SB, Walker R, Aronson S (1993) Pitfalls in quantitative contrast echocardiography: the steps to quantitation of perfusion. J Am Soc Echocardiogr 6:395–416

Wray RA, Quiñones MA, Zoghbi WA, Cheirif JC (1991) Relation of mean pixel intensity to concentration of sonicated albumin microspheres: Effects of ultrasound system settings. Clin Cardiol 14(Suppl V):V-23–V-28

29 Potential for Quantification

M.J.K. Blomley, R.J. Eckersley, and D.O. Cosgrove

CONTENTS

29.1 Why Quantify Echo Enhancement?

In this chapter, we will first discuss why we should want to quantify echo enhancement, before describing how we might set about doing this, and then discussing some mathematical approaches to analyze resultant data.

Perhaps the most obvious application is in pharmacological research, where quantification may offer considerable advantages over subjective assessment. For example, there is often a need for objective comparison of different agents or delivery regimes (e.g., infusion versus bolus). In a recent phase I study, an analysis of the intensity of the femoral artery spectral Doppler signal was used to demonstrate the effectiveness of Levovist (Schering AG, Berlin, Germany) infusions (Albrecht et al. 1998a). This was also found to be the case in a recent phase I study of the contrast agent Sonovue (Bracco SpA, Milan, Italy), where quantitative techniques showed an excellent dose-response relationship and proved much more consistent than a subjective evaluation (Blomley et al. 1997a).

More importantly, there are strong grounds for believing that quantitative echo enhancement could, in itself, be an important diagnostic tool. In recent years, the cross-sectional imaging techniques have been increasingly appreciated as ways of imaging function as well as anatomy. By observing the changes produced by an injection of a contrast agent through vessels and tissues, much useful physiological information can be obtained and correlated with anatomy. Magnetic resonance (MR) and computed tomography (CT) have shown great promise as noninvasive techniques for assessing the microcirculation (Hawighorst et al. 1996; Müller-Schlimpfle et al. 1993; Miles et al. 1993). By comparison, ultrasound has lagged behind other modalities, owing to the lack (until recently) of effective contrast agents and the difficulties of quantifying ultrasound displays. This situation is unfortunate, as ultrasound compares favorably with these other techniques in terms of cost-effectiveness, safety, and availability. Moreover, ultrasound complements the other modalities in that blood pool agents are not widely available in CT and MR, and microbubbles do not generally reach the interstitial spaces of the body. Ultrasound would thus lend itself particularly well to the measurement of such indices as fractional vascular volume and perfusion (flow per unit volume), whereas MR and CT may be best for the measurement of permeability.

Quantitative echo enhancement may prove of great value in the myocardium or kidney, where the measurement of tissue perfusion would have an immediate and obvious value. As discussed elsewhere in this book, the measurement of such indices may also be important in other applications, especially in tumor imaging. It is important to emphasize, however, as the title of this chapter suggests, that this is a

M.J.K. Blomley, MB, FRCR, Hammersmith Hospital and Imperial College School of Medicine, du Cane Road, London W12 OH5, UK
R.J. Eckersley, PhD, Hammersmith Hospital and Imperial College School of Medicine, du Cane Road, London W12 OH5, UK
D.O. Cosgrove, BM, FRCR, Hammersmith Hospital and Imperial College School of Medicine, du Cane Road, London W12 OH5, UK

young subject. The material covered in this chapter is therefore best seen as a pointer to future applications, rather than as a didactic guide.

Ultrasound equipment manufacturers are responding to the growing interest in this subject by providing on-line quantification facilities, but at present these are rudimentary, with some notable exceptions as discussed below. It is, therefore, necessary for investigators in this area to have a reasonable understanding of the underlying principles of quantification and to be prepared to perform some of the steps involved.

Several distinct stages are involved in the quantification of an ultrasound contrast study, i.e., (1) the scanning process, (2) the transfer of the data from the scanner to a suitable analysis platform, and (3) the actual processing of the data to generate the required results. The remainder of this chapter addresses each of these stages in some detail.

29.2 Choice of Scanner Mode and Settings

Any ultrasound imaging mode can be used to perform some degree of quantitative assessment, but some important principles need to be understood first. The first of these is the complexity of the interaction between the ultrasound beam and microbubbles. Somewhat simplistically (the interested reader is referred to De Jong 1997), a division will be drawn in this chapter between "passive" and "active" enhancement mechanisms for most microbubbles. At lower sound pressures, the dominant enhancement mechanism is a relatively simple resonance phenomenon, which is "linear" in the sense that a proportionate relationship can be expected between relative microbubble concentration and the increase in the intensity of the backscattered signal. At higher sound pressures, however, microbubble disruption occurs, associated with the production of various nonlinear or transient signals. These signals form the basis of many recent imaging techniques that rely on microbubble disruption or destruction, such as transient response imaging (Porter et al. 1997), related intermittent harmonic gray-scale techniques (Kamiyama et al. 1996; Moriyasu et al. 1996), and stimulated acoustic emission imaging with Doppler (Tieman et al. 1997; Blomley et al. 1998b). These techniques offer many potential advantages, including increased sensitivity and specificity to the presence of microbubbles and the ability to detect very slowly moving or stationary microbubbles. They may also offer the potential for a unique type of physiological measurement as refilling of a tissue bed can be observed and measured after a destructive pulse of ultrasound. Their destructive nature, however, may create severe problems for accurate quantitation as the imaging process may destroy what it is trying to detect: a microbubble "uncertainty principle."

As hinted above, the division between these "active" and "passive" mechanisms is actually somewhat blurred. For example, microbubble destruction may still occur at low sound energies. The important point to grasp, however, is that there are two alternative approaches to quantitative imaging with microbubbles: aiming deliberately to disrupt microbubbles with sound, and striving to minimize such effects. These approaches lead to different considerations in the choices of scanner mode and machine settings.

For passive modes, the aim is to detect microbubbles in the tissue bed of interest while keeping disruption to a minimum. In general, therefore, low transmit power settings should be used. Both B-mode and Doppler techniques are useful, although B-mode imaging has the advantage of generally requiring lower sound pressures. This advantage may be outweighed, however, by the much greater sensitivity of Doppler techniques, particularly in radiology, where motion artifacts are less of a problem. Such artifacts can make the use of Doppler modes difficult in some situations such as the rapidly beating heart. Of the two two-dimensional (2D) color imaging modes, conventional (velocity) color Doppler and power (or energy) color Doppler, hereafter referred to as color Doppler and power Doppler, respectively, the latter is the more logical choice, as the relationship between the color intensity and microbubble concentration is much closer. From a mathematical point of view, the power Doppler map approximates to a log-compressed map of the number of moving reflectors. Thus, in principle, regional microbubble concentration can be estimated after appropriate corrections, as discussed later in this chapter.

In a conventional color Doppler mode, by contrast, the relationship between microbubble concentration and color display is much more complex and less intuitive. Here, microbubbles produce enhancement by augmenting low-amplitude Doppler signals, which were previously below the noise floor of the system, causing them to be displayed. If only a small sample volume (such as a single vessel) needs to be studied, spectral Doppler may offer advantages, as very high temporal sampling rates are possible, whereas color modes are more appropriate for larger regions of interest.

Separate considerations apply to the use of active modes. Here, in general, high sound pressures should be used, although still within the limits permitted for diagnostic imaging. 2D Doppler techniques may have special advantages here, as the autocorrelation systems used in almost all Doppler systems rely on comparisons between pulses sent and received. The sudden disappearance of a reflector is interpreted as a random frequency Doppler signal (BURNS et al. 1995; BAUER et al. 1997a,b). Autocorrelation-based color Doppler systems are known to be particularly sensitive to stimulated acoustic emission (FORSBERG et al. 1997). If B-mode imaging is used, harmonic techniques such as second harmonic imaging and pulse inversion (wideband harmonic imaging) techniques should be considered, as they are more microbubble-specific and microbubble disruption is known to be associated with the production of harmonic signals (DE JONG 1997).

There is one final and most important issue relating to the scanning techniques required for accurate quantification. If different studies are to be compared, then the scanner settings, such as the B-mode/color map, dynamic range, gain, transmit power, and pulse repetition frequency and wall filters, should all be kept constant to the extent possible to ensure a comparable baseline.

29.3 Data Acquisition

This section deals with the process of acquiring, or extracting, the data from the scanner so that quantification may be performed.

One potential approach that would bypass some of the machine-dependent aspects affecting quantification is to use the unprocessed radiofrequency (RF) data of the ultrasound system. Unfortunately, access to RF data is not usually available, although certain manufacturers may provide adaptations to their scanners to facilitate this approach, which requires specialized hardware and software. As a result, this method is unlikely to be appropriate for the great majority of clinical researchers and users, but has been used successfully by some investigators (BURNS 1995).

Until recently, few manufacturers have provided quantitation packages, but this situation is rapidly changing. Several companies now either provide or are developing quantitation systems. One manufacturer has provided an on-line gray-scale quantitation system, developed over several years, which can correct for log-compression and other nonlinear machine processing to provide time-enhancement data for different regions of interest. This works from stored cine loop data, and has proved encouraging in cardiological research (GOENS and MARTIN 1996; DITTRICH et al. 1995). Another manufacturer offers some specialist users dedicated software that will run on a PC, thus enabling them to acquire and quantitate color or power Doppler cine loops offline, again with the potential to draw multiple regions of interest and correct for nonlinear machine processing (Powers, personal communication).

At the time of writing, however, these systems are not universally available and even where available may be limited in the length of study that can be analyzed or the modes that can be quantified. For many users, the best solution is to try to exploit the machine-processed data provided by the manufacturers. There are several ways to do this, including the use of spectral Doppler audio data, digital ultrasound images, direct transfer of video data to a computer, and the use of videotape. These methods are considered below.

Spectral Doppler signals can provide an accurate means of measuring relative microbubble concentration. Changes in the intensity or "loudness" (measured in units of or proportional to volts squared) of the audio signal can be used to measure the relative concentration of microbubbles. This has been demonstrated with Levovist in a phantom model by SCHWARZ et al. (1993). The technique has also been used to understand the behavior of infusions of Levovist (ALBRECHT et al. 1998a), to show an accurate dose-response relationship with Sonovue in man (BLOMLEY 1997a), and to show an accurate dose-response relationship with Albunex in a canine model (HARTLEY et al. 1993). This type of signal may be acquired using a personal computer with an analog/digital (A/D) converter. With such a system, the sound signal can be digitized at very high rates (up to compact disc audio quality) and the intensity calculated as often as required. Alternatively, the audio signal may be stored on good-quality tape, such as DAT (digital audio tape) or the soundtrack of an SVHS videotape, and processed offline.

Quantification using spectral Doppler is limited to a single restricted area; thus, it is hard to analyze multiple vessels, and the analysis as a result can be affected by movement. For some studies, however, where only a single relatively static vessel (such as a femoral artery) is involved, this may not be a problem. Even where considerable respiratory excursions occur, good data can be obtained with a little temporal smoothing.

Two-dimensional imaging, both B-mode and Doppler, enables the analysis of a larger area or of multiple regions. It is important to remember, however, that the increased volume of data may significantly affect the temporal resolution with which quantification measurements can be made. As indicated above, it is also strongly dependent on the processing and settings of the scanner. 2D images can be acquired via the video output, or as digital ultrasound images that can be stored during a study and extracted via removable storage devices. The latter technique is especially useful for active modes of imaging where a single image may suffice. In practice, however, the acquisition of a sequence of digital images during a contrast study on patients can be inconvenient and impractical (primarily due to the length of around 5–10 min for a typical study), and the use of video signal is often more convenient.

It is also likely that in the near future it will be convenient and economical to record the video signals from the scanner directly onto a computer in digital form.

For practical reasons it is thus generally necessary to use intermediate storage of the video signal from the scanner (e.g., on digital video, Betacam or SVHS videotape). The recorded data can then be analyzed in a manner similar to that for audio data; a video frame grabber card is needed for analysis of video data. With current technology, the temporal sampling rates for this approach are far below those for audio signals. Typically a full color frame will take at least 1 s to acquire, whereas smaller regions of the image or B-mode images may be grabbed at higher frame rates. The reduced temporal sampling means that effects of pulsatility over the cardiac cycle should not be ignored, and an increased frame-to-frame persistence setting on the scanner may be used to smooth the data over time. In our experience, the use of manual selection of systolic images is helpful, but this is not feasible for a long study. There is one additional drawback of this approach: in addition to the nonlinearity introduced by the ultrasound scanner processing, the video stage and A/D processing both introduce further noise, both spatial and particularly color, which needs to be corrected for. Drawbacks aside, such a system (Bell et al. 1995) has been used successfully to acquire and analyze both conventional color Doppler and power Doppler data, as discussed below.

29.4 Data Processing

This section describes the issues surrounding the conversion of the digitized audio or video ultrasound data into the required quantitative result, for both active and passive modes of scanning.

Two points need to be emphasized: First, it is important to remember that ultrasound is inherently nonlinear, primarily as a result of tissue attenuation, which produces an exponential falloff in signal with depth. Although attenuation will not significantly affect temporal indices (e.g., duration of enhancement), it does affect other indices that increase directly with signal strength (e.g., peak enhancement or area under the time enhancement curve). Comparison between tissues at different depths will then be difficult. It may be possible to correct for this using various techniques (e.g., assuming tissue attenuates sound at a given rate, such as 1 dB/cm/MHz), but this remains a major limitation in quantitative ultrasound.

Second, all manufacturers rely heavily on nonlinear processing to produce their displayed images. This is partly aesthetic – to produce a visually acceptable and appealing image – but is mostly for practical reasons. In particular, the range of backscatter and color intensity values that we need to be able to display is so vast that logarithmic compression of both the B-mode and color display is essential. Without correction for this, meaningful quantification can be problematic, as described below.

29.4.1 Quantification of Audio Data

In the case of audio data, the intensity of the sound is generally calculated over fixed intervals (e.g., 1 s) as a moving average. This result can be achieved with some simple programming. The intensity of a sound file, in units of (or proportional to) volts-squared, can be baseline-subtracted and plotted against time. This technique essentially results in a time-intensity profile, which measures relative concentration of microbubbles as a function of time, for the region sampled by the spectral gate.

29.4.2 Quantification of Video Data

Having reduced our study to a series of digital images, the next step is to try to correct for nonlinear machine and display processing. The logarithmic compression applied to gray-scale images must be reversed. For example, in an image with a 50-dB dynamic range, the difference between "white" and "black" areas is as high as a factor of 10^5. Without such corrections, attempts to quantify enhancement changes can be misleading. For example, suppose a renal study was performed, and peak cortical and medullary echogenicity were recorded as 25 and 20 dB, respectively, after a bolus of a microbubble at approximately the same tissue depth (so that attenuation effects were minimized). On a linear scale, these values correspond to backscatter measurements of $10^{2.5}$ and 10^2 or 316 and 100, respectively. If we assume that the ratio between peak cortical and medullary backscatter is a measure of relative perfusion, this gives a perfusion ratio of 3 times as high for cortex compared with medulla, in line with expectations. If, however, we use the log compressed numbers, we might estimate relative perfusion as 25/20 or 25% higher for cortex, which is a very different estimate.

Such corrections can be applied using user-written programs or macros written within image-processing software - for example NIH Image, a freeware program available on the Internet.

If color images are to be quantified, the color must first be segmented from the black-and-white pixels. This, too, is possible, using image-processing software, but can be difficult. Videotaped data can be especially problematic, as image noise can create spurious color pixels or remove existing ones.

A dedicated software package has been developed for the analysis of color Doppler and power Doppler images (Bell et al. 1995). This program segments out color pixels from the gray-scale background and quantifies the color data, using the colors within the displayed color bar to generate a lookup table that can be used to correct for nonlinear processing. This system, originally described for conventional color Doppler, has been adapted for power Doppler and includes the necessary correction for log-compression. It has been successfully employed to measure relative microbubble numbers in vitro and in vivo, even when videotaped data are used (Blomley et al. 1996).

29.5 Mathematical Aspects

Assuming we have now obtained numerical data, various approaches can be used to quantify it. Here, very different considerations apply to the use of active and passive modes of scanning.

29.5.1 Passive Modes

In passive modes, typically, a time-enhancement profile will have been constructed for one or more vessels or tissue regions of interest (Figs. 29.1, 29.2). What use can we make of this?

First, we can look for a particular shape, or compare the shape to a model distribution to obtain a numerical index. Although simple, this can be a powerful technique. For example, some malignant tumors appear to be associated with an abnormal, delayed, irregular washout (Albrecht et al. 1998b). Second, we can calculate simple indices, such the area under the curve (AUC). AUC, following elementary indicator-dilution theory, is proportionate to dose and is a good measure of the degree of enhancement. A strong dose-response relationship in man with a microbubble agent has been shown using

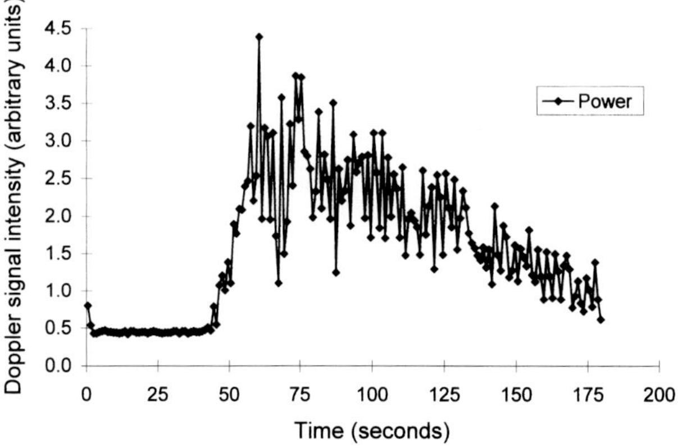

Fig. 29.1. A real time signal curve for a portal vein (spectral Doppler) with Sonovue. The intensity of the spectral Doppler signal is plotted as a function of time, in seconds, after an injection

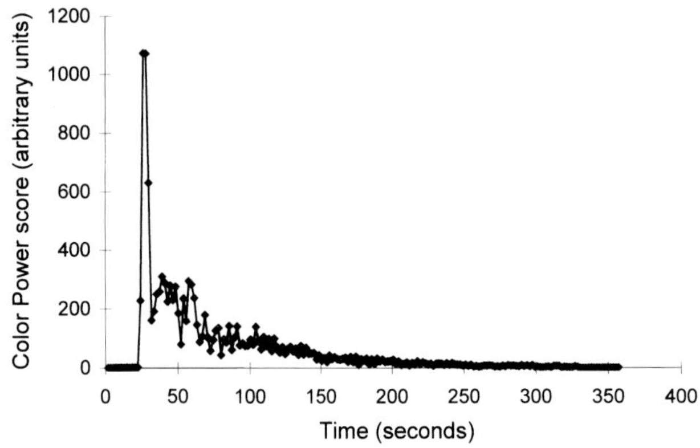

Fig. 29.2. A real time signal curve for a prostate (power Doppler) with Sonovue using two separate injections. The intensity of the power Doppler signal was calculated against time (in seconds) after segmentation of the color data, videodensitometry with respect to the color bar, and conversion from a log-compressed to a linear scale

power Doppler (BLOMLEY et al. 1997a) and spectral Doppler (HARTLEY et al. 1993).

A group from MGH/Harvard has performed a number of studies in which relatively straightforward quantitation of contrast-enhanced power Doppler displays have been used to good effect. Using either mean pixel intensity increases or the areas under the time-enhancement curve, they have shown a good correlation between calculated indices and expectations in cerebral and renal blood flow in animal models, even without correction for the log-compression and nonlinear machine processing in power Doppler displays (GREENBERG et al. 1996; TAYLOR et al. 1996, 1998).

Can we improve further on this approach and calculate indices that have a closer relationship to direct physiological markers?

In principle, three main types of indeces might be extracted: purely temporal indices of transit or enhancement times, fractional vascular volume, and perfusion (i.e., flow per unit volume). Note that these indices are all related: for an intravascular agent, when mean transit time is calculated as described in the next section, perfusion is precisely the ratio of fractional vascular volume to mean transit time (the "Central Volume Theorem") (MAIER and ZIERLER 1954; AXEL 1980). Active modes may offer an alternative way of measuring these indices, as described in the next section.

29.5.2 Temporal Indices Using Passive Modes

The time-enhancement curve of a contrast agent can be quantified in several ways in the time domain. The width of the curve is easy to calculate using indices such as full-width, half-maximum (the time interval between rising to half the maximum and falling to half-maximum). Another index which is relatively easy to calculate is the rise time or the time to peak enhancement. A further technique is to calculate the "centroid" of the curve. The centroid, or weighted first moment of a function or curve $f(t)$, is the ratio $\int tf(t)dt/\int f(t)dt$.

It may be helpful to visualize this expression as the same one a physicist would use to calculate the center of gravity of an object described by a curve $f(t)$. In other words, if a time-enhancement curve is calculated for a parenchymal region of interest, the centroid of this curve represents the "average" enhancement time in that area. Note that this value should not be called the "mean transit time" of an organ, as is sometimes done. Strictly speaking, the true mean transit time (MTT) of an organ is a slightly different value, referring to the average time to pass from the inflow to the outflow of an organ. MTT cannot be directly calculated from parenchymal data. It can, however, be calculated from data on input and output vessels, and this is best done by subtracting the difference in the centroid values of the vein and the artery supplying it. For example, if the centroid of a renal vein time-signal curve was 15 s and that of a renal artery 10 s, the renal MTT would be 5 s. This type of approach was attempted in the dog heart with Albunex, but self-shadowing artifact limited its application (GALANTI et al. 1993).

In many organs, input and output vessels cannot be studied simultaneously, and we must make do with curves for a single vessel and tissue. An example would be the study of cardiac blood flow using data for the myocardium with data for the left ventricle as an input function. Unfortunately, estimates of MTT based on tissue (or "residue function") data are prone to errors of up to 100%. The interested reader is referred elsewhere for a fuller discussion of these issues (AXEL 1980; GOBBEL et al. 1991). Nevertheless, this index is still a very useful and objective way of estimating the "average" enhancement time of an organ.

Useful information may also be obtained from the "shape" or regularity/irregularity of the time-concentration curve. There is some evidence that this may be especially helpful in tumor imaging and data using subjective assessments suggest that cancers enhance longer than benign lesions (KEDAR et al. 1996) Recent work, using quantitative power Doppler imaging of breast tumors with EchoGen, suggests that cancers may have a particularly irregular washout phase (ALBRECHT et al. 1998b). Abnormal flow profiles could be characterized by a variety of indices, such as the difference between the centroid of the curve and arrival time, the curve "duration" (e.g., time at which the curve is above 10% of baseline), or the skewness or kurtosis.

Another technique is to smooth the time signal curves and correct for recirculation using a "gammavariate" curve fit. In practice vascular time-attenuation curves after a bolus of contrast have an initial maximum, followed by a series of smaller peaks representing recirculation. The first-pass phase is easily modeled by a gamma-variate fit, that is, by a curve of the form:

$$a(t) = k(t - t_0)^a e^{-(t-t_0)/b},$$

where $a(t)$ is the enhancement from baseline at time t, t_0 is the arrival time of contrast at the vascular ROI, and k, a, and b are constants, which are parameters of the fit. The gamma-variate curve fit is a widely accepted method of extracting the initial (first-pass) phase from the time-concentration curve of a tracer. The mean transit time of such a curve can be calculated as the arrival time plus $b(a + 1)$ (THOMPSON et al. 1963). WU et al. (1997) used a modified version of this relationship in myocardial contrast echocardiography with Albunex. They calculated an index of myocardial transit time and multiplied this by myocardial perfusion obtained from microsphere measurements to obtain an estimate of intramyocardial blood volume.

A relatively simple technique, which may turn out to be extremely powerful, has recently been described (BLOMLEY et al. 1997b, 1998a; ALBRECHT et al. 1997). This method is to analyze the time-intensity curve of a hepatic vein after a bolus injection of Levovist. In a normal subject this will increase relatively late, typically 30 s or more from injection. In cirrhosis and many malignancies, however, the increase occurs much earlier. A simple analysis of the rise time has proved both sensitive and specific in pilot studies for cirrhosis and malignancy, although it is likely that more sophisticated temporal indices will be developed as the technique evolves.

A number of temporal indices can thus be calculated. These all have the dimension of time only, and thus are, to a certain extent, independent of the means used to measure microbubble concentration. Thus, even if an indirect means of estimating microbubble concentration is used, such as quantification of conventional color Doppler, the indices retain some validity. This is not true of other indices of fractional vascular volume or perfusion, which will be considered next.

29.5.3 Fractional Vascular Volume

Fractional vascular volume and perfusion are relatively easy concepts to understand. They are the proportion of tissue occupied by blood and the blood flow per unit volume (or mass), respectively. The practical importance of these indices is that they are measures the physiological "vascularity" of a region.

In principle, these indices could be measured without the use of echo-enhancing agents. For example, power Doppler imaging, in which the signal reflects the number of moving reflectors, should give a map of regional red cell concentration and thus of fractional vascular volume. A simple approach is to correct a power Doppler image from a log-compressed to a linear scale, and calculate the ratio of parenchymal to purely vascular Doppler intensity (RUBIN et al. 1995, 1997). Difficulties include the problem of obtaining a sufficiently good signal-to-noise ratio and the effects of erythrocyte clumping. Another problem, often glossed over in the physiological imaging literature, is that of hematocrit differences. The hematocrit of capillary blood is 2–5 times that in the systemic circulation, probably mainly due to the Fahreus effect, where red cells in small vessels travel faster than mean flow rate (DESJARDINES and DULING 1987; SECOMB and GROSS 1984). Estimates of fractional vascular volume based on erythrocyte differences will need to be corrected for this factor.

If an echo-enhancing agent is used with power Doppler, the estimates should be much better, as the signal-to-noise ratio is improved. However, it is not yet clear whether the Fahreus effect also affects microbubble agents.

The fractional vascular volume can be calculated in other ways that are likely to be more cumbersome but less prone to such errors. For example, the ratio of the areas under the time-concentration curve for a parenchymal and a vascular region of interest will estimate fractional vascular volume (MOR-AVI et al. 1993).

29.5.4 Perfusion

Perfusion, whether measured as flow per unit volume or mass, is a fundamental measure of blood flow at the level of the microcirculation. Essentially, it is blood flow normalized to the amount of tissue under consideration. For convenience, we will define perfusion as flow per unit volume, rather than mass, as the specific gravity of the solid organs of the body is close to 1. There are two techniques for its calculation, of which the first can be derived from the preceding discussion. For an intravascular tracer, such as a microbubble, perfusion can be found simply by dividing the fractional vascular volume by the mean transit time, if this is calculated using the central volume theorem.

This approach has been used with Albunex, both in a phantom (HEIDENREICH et al. 1993) and in the canine kidney and heart using gray-scale imaging (MOR-AVI et al. 1993; ARONSEN et al. 1993). By analogy with the central volume theorem, flow across an organ bed can be calculated from the ratio of blood volume and blood flow. Cardiac output is thus proportional to the reciprocal of pulmonary transit time, as has been shown using Albunex (GALANTI et al. 1993).

There is, however, an alternative strategy: per fusion may be calculated directly if the time-concentration curves for parenchymal and vascular regions of interest can be defined. If the parenchymal microbubble concentration at time t is $p(t)$ and that in a supply artery is $a(t)$ (after correction for recirculation), then, provided the input bolus is fast compared with parenchymal transit and venous washout is reasonably slow, perfusion may be calculated as the ratio between the peak value of $p(t)$ and the area under the arterial time enhancement curve, or $\int a(t)$.

Alternatively, perfusion may be calculated as the peak gradient of $p(t)$ divided by the peak value of $a(t)$, that is:

$$\frac{dp(t)/dt|_{\max}}{a(t)|_{\max}}.$$

The second, "gradient" relationship is slightly less sensitive to errors from venous washout, but, as it involves a differentiation process, it is more sensitive to noise. These two relationships do not seem to have been applied to contrast-enhanced ultrasound, but have been usefully used with ultrafast CT studies of the myocardium, liver, and kidney, and in some tumor applications. The interested reader is referred elsewhere for a fuller discussion (BLOMLEY et al. 1993, 1997c).

29.5.5 Active Modes

Two types of approach have been made to the use of active or transient mode. In the first approach, varying scanning parameters are used to alter the amount of microbubble destruction during an infusion, and physiological measurements are made from this. The second approach uses active methods to image static microbubbles in tissue-specific phases and to attempt tissue characterization.

The first method is based on in vitro observations made with microbubbles while they are being infused in phantom models. Microbubble destruction, observed as reductions in reflectivity, can be shown with a variety of agents. It is more marked with higher sound energies and is not seen at very low energies. When flow is slowed, microbubble destruction increases because microbubbles are exposed to sound for longer periods (WALKER et al. 1997; OHMORI et al. 1997). Thus, in principle, flow velocity in the microcirculation could be measured by using pulsed ultrasound and varying the pulsing interval. The relationship between echogenicity and pulsing interval should be a measure of tissue flow.

This principle was extended to the measurement of myocardial blood flow in a dog model by WEI et al. (1998). They infused the microbubble MRX-115 while scanning in an intermittent mode, and observed the relationship between pulsing interval and echogenicity in a phantom and then in a dog model. They observed an exponential relationship between pulsing interval PI and video intensity VI:

$$\mathrm{VI} = \mathrm{VI}_{\max}\left(1 - e^{-\beta.\mathrm{PI}}\right),$$

where $\mathrm{VI}_{\max}$ is the maximal video intensity, seen at longer pulsing intervals. The initial upslope of this curve will be proportional to microbubble velocity in the area being insonated. Wei and colleagues observed a good correlation between changing flow rates and this value, both in vitro and in vivo.

These exciting results suggest that regional flow can be measured in the microcirculation directly, although it is not clear how easy the technique would be to perform in clinical practice, particularly in rapidly moving tissues such as the myocardium.

A second, quite different type of quantitation attempts to make static measurements of microbubble numbers in different regions of tissue using nonlinear imaging modes. In an early published description of the stimulated acoustic emission (SAE) effect, whereby microbubble disruption is associated with a sudden transient acoustic response, using the polymeric agent SH563A, UHLENDORF and HOFFMAN (1994) suggested that the effect could be used to count individual microbubbles. As each microbubble is disrupted, a signal is produced that, in principle, could be detected and counted. SAE does not rely on reflector motion and instead detects the presence of microbubbles. The principle is thus similar to radionuclide scintigraphy; indeed, the term "sonoscintigraphy" has been proposed (BLOMLEY et al. 1998c). One way of attempting to count the number of SAE effects would be to scan in color Doppler mode, in which SAE characteristically produces a mosaic-like effect. At low concentrations, and if all color Doppler signals are due to SAE (e.g., if a high pulse repetition prefrequency and low color gain are used), the number of color pixels in principle counts microbubble concentration. In early work using SAE, an attempt has been made to use this effect to study the late liver phase of the agent Levovist. Color pixel densities were compared within and without metastases, to show that the effect increases the conspicuity of metastatic lesions (which show reduced SAE) (BLOMLEY et al. 1998d). In another study, an attempt was made to demonstrate the liver uptake of Levovist quantifiably. The same method was also used to see whether differences in late-phase Levovist uptake could distinguish between patients with and patients without cirrhosis, although no difference was seen (BLOMLEY et al. 1998e). It is likely that this type of quantitation will become very important in clinical trials with the newer agents, such as SHU563, which have both strong liver-specific and SAE effects.

29.6 Displaying Data

Most of the work described above has been done using a region of interest analysis. A natural extension of this technique is the production of true parametric or functional images, where an index such as fractional vascular volume, transit time, or arrival time is overlayed on a pixel-by-pixel basis over an

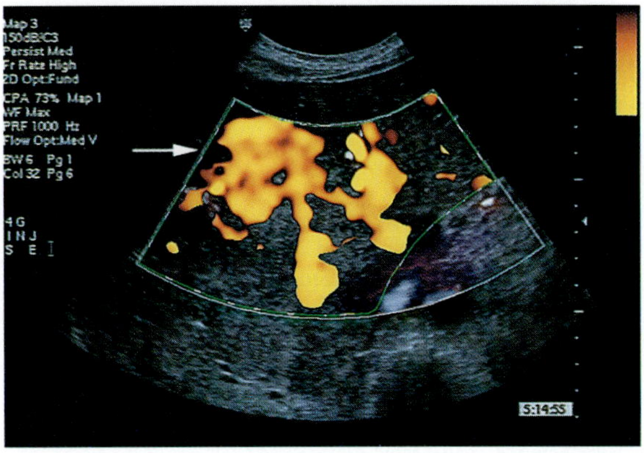

Fig. 29.3. A parametric map of the rise time (defined as the time to reach 50% of maximum) of a contrast bolus in the liver. A transverse section has been scanned using harmonic power Doppler on a breath-hold after injection of a bolus Levovist; the right lobe of the liver was heavily involved with metastatic carcinoid tumor, while the left lobe was not. Color pixels have been displayed for pixels where the arrival time of the contrast bolus was less than 25 s after injection; earlier enhancement in shown as brighter color. Note that most of the early enhancement is seen on the *right-hand side* of the image, particularly over one of the larger metastases (*arrow*), corresponding with the location of the disease

anatomical image. This technique is likely to be particularly well suited to heterogeneous tissues, such as tumors, which may contain both necrotic and relatively highly vascularized areas.

In very preliminary work, liver imaging might turn out to be a promising application. The logic behind this is that a contrast bolus might be expected to enhance a tumor (which is mainly arterially supplied) rather than the surrounding liver parenchyma (which is mainly supplied by the portal vein.) Thus a parametric map of arrival time might give useful information. An example is shown in Fig. 29.3, in which a parametric map of the rise time (defined as the time required to reach 50% of maximum) of a contrast bolus in the liver is shown.

29.7 Summary

Quantification of echo-enhancement is helpful in pharmacological research, and may provide new indices for use in the clinic. It is possible to quantify all ultrasound scanning modes, although it is critical to understand the enhancement mechanism of interest and the details of any nonlinear machine processing. Where appropriate, corrections can be applied to overcome these limitations. The extraction of clinically useful indices and meaningful physiological values from the time-intensity curves obtained is the subject of much interest and ongoing research.

References

Albrecht TA, Blomley MJK, Jayaram V, et al. (1997) Functional assessment of hepatic blood supply in diffuse liver disease using microbubble enhanced Doppler US of the hepatic veins. Radiology 205(P):197

Albrecht T, Urbank A, Mahler M, Doré C, Blomley MJK, Cosgrove DO, Schlief R (1998a) Prolongation and optimization of Doppler enhancement with the ultrasound contrast agent Levovist by continuous infusion: preliminary experience. Radiology 207:339–347

Albrecht T, Patel N, Cosgrove DO, Jayaram V, Blomley MJK, Eckersley R (1998b) Enhancement of power Doppler signals from breast masses with the ultrasound contrast agent EchoGen - subjective and quantitative assessment. Acad Radiol 5(Suppl 1):S195–S198

Aronsen S, Wiencek JG, Feinstein SB, Heidenreich PA, Zaroff JG, Walker R, Roizen MF (1993) Assessment of renal blood flow with contrast ultrasonography. Anesth Analg 76:964–970

Axel L (1980) Brain blood flow determination by rapid sequence computed tomography. Radiology 137:679–686

Bauer A, Zomack M, Lohse D, Hilgenfeldt S, Urbank A, Schlief R (1997a) Acoustic response of microbubbles - acoustic emission and localization imaging. Radiology 205(P):278

Bauer A, Schlief R, Zomack M, Urbank A, Niendorf H-P (1997b) Acoustically stimulated microbubbles in diagnostic ultrasound: properties and implications for diagnostic use. In: Nanda N, Schlief R, Goldberg BB (eds) Advances in echo imaging using contrast enhancement, 2nd edn. Kluwer Academic, Lancaster, UK, pp 669–684

Bell DS, Bamber JC, Eckersley RJ (1995) Segmentation and analysis of colour Doppler images of tumour vascularity. Ultrasound Med Biol 21:635–647

Blomley MJ, Coulden R, Bufkin C, Lipton MJ, Dawson P (1993) Contrast bolus dynamic computed tomography for the measurement of solid organ perfusion. Invest Radiol 28(Suppl 5):S72–S77

Blomley MJK, Cosgrove DO, Albrecht T, Powers JE, Urbank A, Bell D, Bamber JC (1996) Quantification of microbubble concentration using color power Doppler ultrasound. Radiology RSNA supplement 158

Blomley M, Jayaram V, Cosgrove DO, Patel N, Albrecht T, Llull J-B, Eckersley R, Bell D, Bamber JC (1997a) Linear dose response relationship with the US contrast agent BR1; a quantitative study in normal volunteers. Eur Radiol 7(Suppl):S69

Blomley MJK, Albrecht TA, Jayaram V, Cosgrove DO, et al. (1997b) The hepatic venous response to bolus injections of the echo-enhancing agent Levovist: a novel functional imaging technique for assessing liver malignancy. Radiology 205(P):337

Blomley MJK, Coulden RA, Lim-Dunham JE, Kormano MJ, Dawson P, Lipton MJ (1997c) Splenic perfusion studied with UFCT. Acad Radiol 4:13–24

Blomley MJK, Albrecht T, Cosgrove DO, et al. (1998a) Liver vascular transit analyzed using bolus injections of ultrasound contrast: early experience in seven patients with metastases. Radiology (in press)

Blomley MJK, Albrecht T, Cosgrove DO, Jayaram V, Butler-Barnes J, Eckersley RJ (1998b) Stimulated acoustic emission in liver parenchyma with Levovist. Lancet 351:568

Blomley MJK, Albrecht T, Cosgrove DO, et al. (1998c) Stimulated acoustic emission imaging ("sonoscintigraphy") in the liver with Levovist; a reproducible effect with potential clinical utility. Acad Radiol 5(Suppl 1):S236–S239

Blomley MJK, Albrecht T, Cosgrove DO, et al. (1998d) Improved imaging of liver metastases using stimulated acoustic emission in the late enhancement phase of the ultrasound contrast agent Levovist, early experience. Radiology (in press)

Blomley MJK, Albrecht T, Cosgrove DO, et al. (1998e) The use of stimulated acoustic emission to image a late liver-specific phase of Levovist: an investigation in normal volunteers and in patients with and without liver disease. Ultrasound Med Biol (in press)

Burns PN (1995) Contrast agents for Doppler ultrasound. In: Taylor KJ, Burns PN, Wells PNT (eds) Clinical applications of Doppler ultrasound, 2nd edn. Raven Press, New York, pp 367–380

Burns PN, Fritzsch T, Weitschies W, Uhlendorf V, Hope-Simpson D, Powers JE (1995) Pseudo-Doppler shifts from stationary tissue due to the stimulated emission of ultrasound from a new microsphere contrast agent. Radiology 197(P):402

De Jong N (1997) Physics of microbubble scattering. In: Nanda N, Schlief R, Goldberg BB (eds) Advances in echo imaging using contrast enhancement, 2nd edn. Kluwer Academic, Dordrecht, The Netherlands, pp 39–64

Desjardines C, Duling BR (1987) Microvessel hematocrit: measurement and implications for capillary oxygen transport. Am J Physiol 252:H494–H503

Dittrich HC, Bales GL, Kuvelas T, Hunt RM, McFerran BA, Greener Y (1995) Myocardial contrast echocardiography in experimental coronary artery occlusion with a new intravenously administered contrast agent. J Am Soc Echocardiogr 8:465–474

Forsberg F, Shi WT, Liu J, Merton DA, Wu Y, Goldberg BB (1997) On the detection of US contrast induced acoustic emission signals. Radiology 205:278

Galanti G, Jayaweera AR, Villeneuva FS, Glasheen WP, Kaul S (1993) Transpulmonary transit of microbubbles during contrast echocardiography: implications for estimating cardiac output and pulmonary blood volume. J Am Soc Echocardiogr 6:272–278

Gobbel GT, Cann CE, Fike JR (1991) Measurement of regional cerebral blood flow using ultrafast computed tomography; theoretical aspects. Stroke 22:768–771

Goens MB, Martin GR (1996) Acoustic quantification: a new tool for diagnostic echocardiography. Curr Opin Cardiol 11:522–560

Greenberg RS, Taylor GA, Stapleton JC, Hillseley CA, Spinak D (1996) Analysis of regional cerebral blood flow in dogs with an experimental microbubble based US contrast agent. Radiology 201:119–123

Hartley CJ, Cheirif J, Collier KR, Bravenec JS, Mickelson JK (1993) Doppler quantification of echo-contrast injections in vivo. Ultrasound Med Biol 19:269–278

Hawighorst H, Knapstein PG, Schaeffer U, et al. (1996) Pelvic lesions in patients with recurrent cervical carcinoma: efficacy of pharmacokinetic analyses in distinguishing recurrent tumors from benign conditions. AJR 166:401–408

Heidenreich PA, Wiencek JG, Zaroff JG, Aronsen S, Segil LJ, Harper PV, Feinstein SB (1993) In vitro calculation of flow by use of contrast ultrasonography. Am Soc Echocardiogr 6:51–61

Kamiyama N, Moriyasu F, Kono Y, Mine Y, Nada T, Yamazaki N (1996) Investigation of the "flash echo" signal associated with an ultrasound contrast agent. Radiology 201(P):158

Kedar RP, Cosgrove DO, McCready VR, Bamber JC, Carter EC (1996) Microbubble contrast agent for color Doppler US: effect on breast masses. Radiology 198:679–686
Maier P, Zierler KL (1954) On the theory of indicator dilution method for the measurement of blood flow and volume. J Appl Physiol 4:308–314
Miles KA, Hayball MP, Dixon AK (1993) Functional images of hepatic perfusion obtained with dynamic CT. Radiology 188:405–1127
Mor-Avi V, David D, Akselrod S, Bitton Y, Choshniak I (1993) Myocardial regional blood flow: quantitative measurement by computer analysis of contrast enhanced echocardiographic images. Ultrasound Med Biol 19:619–633
Moriyasu F, Kono Y, Nada T, Matsumura ••, Suginoshita Y, Kobayashi K (1996) Flash Echo (passive cavitation) imaging of the liver by using US contrast agents and intermittent scanning sequence. Radiology 201(P):196
Müller-Schlimpfle M, Brix G, Layer G, et al. (1993) Recurrent rectal carcinoma: diagnosis with dynamic MR imaging. Radiology 189:881–894
Ohmori K, Cotter B, Kwan OL, Mizushige K, deMaria AN (1997) Relation of contrast echo intensity and flow velocity to the amplification of contrast opacification produced by intermittent ultrasound transmission. Am Heart J 134: 1066–1074
Porter TR, Li S, Kricsfeld D, Armbruster RW (1997) Detection of myocardial perfusion in multiple echocardiographic windows with one intravenous injection of microbubbles using transient response second harmonic imaging. J Am Coll Cardiol 29:791–796
Rubin JM, Adler RS, Fowlkes JB, et al. (1995) Fractional blood volume: estimation with power Doppler US. Radiology 197:183–190
Rubin JM, Bude RO, Fowlkes JB, Spratt RS, Carson RL, Adler RS (1997) Normalizing fractional moving blood volume estimates with power Doppler US: defining a stable intravascular point with the cumulative power distribution. Radiology 205:757–765
Schwarz KQ, Bezante GP, Chen X, et al. (1993) Quantitative echo-contrast concentration measurement by Doppler sonography. Ultrasound Med Biol 129:289–297
Secomb TW, Gross JF (1984) Theory of microvascular hematocrit fluctuations. In: Courtice FC, Garlick DG, Perry MA (eds) Progress in microcirculatory research II. Committee in Postgraduate Medical Education, University of New South Wales, Sydney, Australia
Taylor GA, Ecklund K, Dunning PS (1996) Renal cortical perfusion in rabbits: visualization with color amplitude imaging and an experimental microbubble based US contrast gent. Radiology 201:125–129
Taylor GA, Barenwolt CE, Adler BA, Dunning PS (1998) Renal cortical ischaemia in rabbits revealed by contrast enhanced power Doppler sonography. AJR 170:417–422
Thompson HK, Starmer CF, Whalen RE, McIntosh HD (1963) Indicator transit time considered as a gamma variate. Circ Res 14:502–515
Tieman K, Becher H, Bimmel D, Schlief R, Nanda N (1997) Stimulated acoustic emission. Non backscatter contrast effect of microbubbles seen with harmonic power Doppler imaging. Echocardiography 14:65–69
Uhlendorf V, Hoffman C (1994) Non-linear acoustic response of coated microbubbles in diagnostic ultrasound. Proc IEEE Ultrason Symp 1559–1562
Walker KW, Pantely GA, Sahn DJ (1997) Ultrasound mediated destruction of contrast agents: effects of ultrasound intensity, exposure and frequency. Invest Radiol 32:728–734
Wei K, Jayaweera AR, Firoozan S, Linka A, Skyba DM, Kaul S (1998) Quantification of myocardial blood flow with ultrasound induced destruction of microbubbles administered as a constant venous infusion. Circulation 97:73–83
Wu CS, Feldman MD, Mills JD, et al. (1997) Myocardial contrast echocardiography can be used to quantify intramyocardial blood volume. Circulation 96:1004–1011

30 The Vascular Space

C.B. Sirlin, B. Coley, and R.F. Mattrey

CONTENTS

30.1 Introduction

Ultrasound contrast agents capable of adequately increasing backscatter are particulates or microbubbles of a size sufficient to limit their distribution to the intravascular space. While the many proposed agents vary in structure and formulation, they serve to enhance the backscatter of blood (André et al. 1993; Schwarz et al. 1994).

The first agents allowed visualization of flowing blood within the cardiac chambers of the right heart, but did not survive passage through the pulmonary circulation to allow evaluation of the left ventricle or other vascular spaces in the body (Schurmann and Schlief 1994). Improvements in formulation led to the development of three different agents: a protein encapsulated air microbubble (Albunex, Molecular Biosystems, San Diego) (Keller et al. 1987), a galactose-based palmitic acid-containing formulation (Levovist, Schering AG, Berlin), and the phase-shift liquid fluorocarbon emulsion that becomes gaseous at body temperature (Echogen, Sonus Pharmaceuticals, Bothell, Wash). These agents are visible on gray-scale in the heart. The first agent produces Doppler enhancement of the systemic circulation on the first pass, the second produces enhancement for 1–3 min, and the third produces enhancement for several minutes.

The first two agents do not achieve sufficient concentration, or do not produce sufficient backscatter, to be visible on gray-scale in the systemic circulation (Hilpert et al. 1989; Goldberg et al. 1990; Bauer et al. 1997). The phase-shift agent, although capable of producing gray-scale enhancement of the vascular space following a 0.4 ml/kg dose (Sehgal et al. 1995), has been tested in man at a 0.05 ml/kg dose, which has been limited to Doppler enhancement (Robbin and Eisenfeld 1998).

Clinical experience with the Doppler-enhancing agents is increasing since Levovist has been available in Europe. The dominant application of such agents is to identify vascular signal when no color Doppler is detected in a region of interest. If no flow is detected following contrast administration, then it can be assumed that the region is not vascularized.

For the purpose of vascular imaging, the goals of the sonographic test are: to determine vascular patency; to ascertain the presence of atherosclerosis and its effect on luminal diameter; to assess the direction of flow and the flow velocity profile; and to visualize the vascular tree. It should be clear that, if the vessel is well seen and the Doppler signal is adequate, all the required data that can be collected from the Doppler technique are available. In such a setting, further increase in Doppler signal will likely not improve the results, add new data, or eliminate the limitation of Doppler imaging. In fact, enhancing signal will likely lead to blooming artifact and worsening of imaging data. Further, if subtle differences in vascularity exist between two perfused regions, the addition of contrast will likely hide this difference, as enhancement will lead both regions to signal saturation (O'Hara et al. 1996).

When vessels or the vascular lumen are poorly visualized, or flow is too slow to be detected with the lowest filter that must be used, contrast media are of significant benefit. In such a setting, contrast admin-

C.B. Sirlin, MD, c/o R.F. Mattrey, MD, Department of Radiology, University of California, San Diego Medical Center, 200 W. Arbor Drive, San Diego, CA 92109-8756, USA
B. Coley, MD, 4370 Limerick Lane, Dublin, OH 43017, USA
R.F. Mattrey, MD, Department of Radiology, University of California, San Diego Medical Center, 200 W. Arbor Drive, San Diego, CA 92109-8756, USA

istration will allow the assessment of the vascular bed, and in fact salvage what would have been an inadequate examination (Robin and Eisenfeld 1998). Further, the use of contrast in suboptimal imaging situations will shorten the examination time, as less time is spent locating the vessels of interest.

Thus, Doppler-enhancing agents should be used for the purpose of vascular imaging when any region requiring Doppler assessment is inadequately evaluated. The expected result of the contrast Doppler study is what would have been achieved had the precontrast study been adequate. Rather than enumerating the various vascular systems that can be assessed, this chapter will address the concept of vascular imaging with contrast media, and the potential of harmonic techniques to achieve complete visualization of the arterial or venous lumen.

30.2 Is Filling the Vascular Lumen with Signal Needed?

Although the vascular lumen is generally anechoic and well seen, acute thrombi are typically difficult to detect, as they are generally isoechoic with blood (Cronan et al. 1988; Vogel et al. 1987). The high sensitivity and specificity of duplex real-time sonography with compression have made this noninvasive technique the primary study for evaluating venous thrombosis in the lower extremity (Cronan 1993). Its limitations arise when the recognition of the veins is inadequate, or when compression is difficult, as in the inferior vena cava, iliac and calf veins, and the lower extremities in patients after surgery or trauma (Cronan 1993; White et al. 1989; Rubens et al. 1991; Ginsberg et al. 1991). Color Doppler aids in recognizing nonocclusive thrombi and speeds the localization of vessels. However, despite the improvement in calf vein identification (Foley et al. 1989; Polak et al. 1989), sonography remains less sensitive in this region than in the thigh (Lensing et al. 1989; Rubens et al. 1991; Aitken and Godden 1987). Therefore, color Doppler imaging is insufficient to exclude thrombi, mostly because of blooming of color pixels and the insensitivity to slow flow.

The ability to distinguish acute from chronic thrombosis remains important for proper patient management. This characterization is inconsistent when duplex sonography is used with compression (Murphy and Cronan 1990). Color Doppler aids in distinguishing acute from chronic thrombi but the ability to adequately fill the vessel with color to demonstrate recanalization, webbing, wall irregularities, and valve incompetence is inconsistent (Lewis et al. 1994). With contrast venography, where the lumen is filled with radiopaque material, it is possible to characterize clots, as their architecture becomes apparent. As color Doppler has fallen short in filling the lumen reliably, because of slow flow or blooming or poor signal-to-noise ratio, we believe that filling the lumen with contrast on gray-scale real-time imaging should provide detail similar to that of standard contrast venography (Coley et al. 1994). This technique overcomes the two limitations of color Doppler. The entire lumen is filled, independent of flow velocity, and the spatial resolution is comparable to that of standard gray-scale imaging.

The need to fill the arteries with signal is even more critical than filling the veins. The discussion here focuses on the carotid arteries, as they are the most commonly examined vessels and the most ideal to image. The consequences of atherosclerotic disease in any artery are stenosis, limiting blood delivery, and embolization from plaque rupture or from clots that develop on the ulcerated surface. Therefore, ideal evaluation of carotid disease requires accurate estimation of lumen stenosis (ECACAS 1995), precise assessment of plaque size (Arbeille et al. 1995; Delcker and Diener 1994), and reliable delineation of luminal surface characteristics, including irregularities and ulceration (Widder et al. 1990; Arbeille et al. 1995; Belcaro et al. 1993; ECPSG 1995; Iannuzzi et al. 1995).

Duplex ultrasound is currently the most widely used technique in the evaluation and follow-up of carotid disease. It is readily accessible, noninvasive, and relatively inexpensive compared with alternative imaging methods. Gray-scale imaging does permit reasonably accurate determination of plaque composition (Gray-Weale et al. 1988; van Damme and Vivario 1993; Widder et al. 1990; Iannuzzi et al. 1995). Despite its sufficient spatial resolution, it has several limitations, the most important of which are: the difficulty of identifying echolucent plaques and ulcerations (O'Donnell et al. 1985; Widder et al. 1990; Barry et al. 1990; Young et al. 1992; Iannuzzi et al. 1995; Delcker and Diener 1994; Arbeille et al. 1995; O'Leary et al. 1987a,b), imprecise estimation of luminal stenosis (Widder et al. 1990; Meairs et al. 1995; Sitzer et al. 1994; ECACAS 1995), and unreliable differentiation of critical stenosis from complete occlusion.

It was hoped that color Doppler would fill the arterial lumen with color to highlight the inner arterial wall and plaques analogous to a color angiogram. Although color Doppler did not reliably achieve this expectation, it did aid significantly in the rapid identification of flow and in guiding the sonographer to the most optimal location and angle correction to acquire reliable spectral data. The inability of color Doppler to adequately fill the lumen is in part due to its dependence on the angle of incidence, which may be suboptimal in diseased vessels, poor spatial resolution and signal-to-noise ratio, blooming and other artifacts, and regions within the lumen with velocities below the detection limit, particularly in diseased vessels. Because of these limitations, the angiographic effect of color Doppler did not provide sufficient or reliable endovascular detail for direct measurement of luminal narrowing (Widder et al. 1990; Meairs et al. 1995; Sitzer et al. 1994) or identification of surface irregularities.

Spectral Doppler is utilized to measure flow velocity as a surrogate for stenosis. The link between velocity and stenosis is through the relationship (flow = pressure gradient/resistance), where the gradient and resistance are measured across the vascular segment of interest. In turn, velocity is equal to flow divided by the cross-sectional area of the vessel of interest. Since flow (ml/min) across the vessel is constant, as the cross-sectional area decreases because of plaque formation, velocity increases. However, because velocity can be influenced by many hemodynamic factors – such as systemic pressure, the presence or absence of one or more upstream or downstream stenoses, or the integrity of the contralateral carotid system and the ipsilateral external carotid artery (Lee et al. 1997) – it remains a rough estimate of stenosis that is used to group patients into broad categories of disease severity. Further, when luminal stenosis becomes severe enough to impede volumetric flow, blood velocity decreases, potentially leading to overestimation of lumen diameter and underestimation of disease. When the stenoses are sufficiently severe to limit the amount of blood crossing the lesion, both duplex and color Doppler signals become weak, and the ability to reliably distinguish subcritical stenosis from total occlusion is impaired.

X-ray angiography is considered the gold standard because it displays the inner margin of the carotid artery in high resolution, by filling its lumen with radiopaque contrast. Because angiography is a projection technique, it can only detect disease when the affected surface is seen in profile. Also, because the outer surface of the artery cannot be seen, plaque thickness and length are determined by subjectively estimating the position of the normal outer wall. As estimation can be difficult at the level of the carotid bulb, poor sensitivity and specificity may result (Eikelboom et al. 1983).

Detail similar to angiography can be achieved with gray-scale sonography if moving blood within the vascular lumen is filled with echoes (Sirlin et al. 1996, 1997). Because sonography is a cross-sectional technique, it displays both the inner and outer margins of the vessel, allowing a more complete assessment of the vessel wall. This should accurately reveal plaque size and extent, and whether the plaque surface is smooth or irregular due to ulceration. Although not yet evaluated in that setting, it is anticipated that flow through a severely stenotic lumen should be visible particularly when aided with harmonic imaging. Coupled with the high frame rate that is possible with sonography, contrast-enhanced gray-scale imaging of the carotid system should become a powerful technique.

30.3 Venous Disease

Although Doppler enhancement is easily accomplished in veins (Hilpert et al. 1989) and can improve the accuracy of detecting lower extremity venous thrombosis (Schweizer et al. 1993), gray-scale filling of the vein should improve venous assessment. This is because gray-scale signal is independent of flow velocity, angle of incidence, or motion-related artifacts. Given the knowledge that a liquid fluorocarbon emulsion fills veins with echoes on gray-scale (Mattrey et al. 1987), Coley et al. studied the impact of this capability in an animal model with venous thrombosis (Coley et al. 1990, 1994). They showed that, although unenhanced sonography correctly identified nine of ten animals with thrombus, the boundaries of the clot were poorly defined, and clot extent was both over- and underestimated. Contrast-enhanced sonography allowed gray-scale visualization of the hypoechoic boundaries of the clot against the more echogenic flowing blood (Fig. 30.1). The extent of thrombosis correlated closely with venography. By being able to directly visualize moving reflectors in flowing blood, contrast-enhanced sonography allowed differentiation of completely occlusive from nonocclusive thrombus (Fig. 30.2). As the vena cava and portal vein were found to be enhanced on gray-scale in human subjects (Mattrey et al. 1996), we would expect thrombosis of the portal and deep veins to be better assessed with contrast media, whether or not compression is possible.

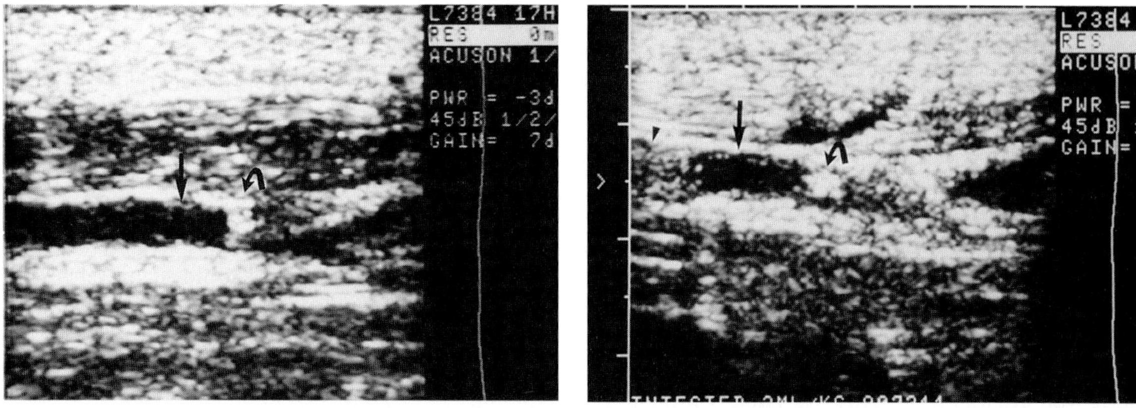

a b

Fig. 30.1. Longitudinal view of the inferior vena cava shows a totally occlusive echogenic clot produced by Gelfoam embolization pre- (**a**) and postcontrast (**b**) administration. Note the clot is echogenic precontrast (*curved arrow*) but the superior echolucent clot is isoechoic with blood. Postcontrast the vena cava fills with echoes (*arrowhead*) highlighting the clot (*arrow*) superior to the Gelfoam. (From Coley et al. 1994)

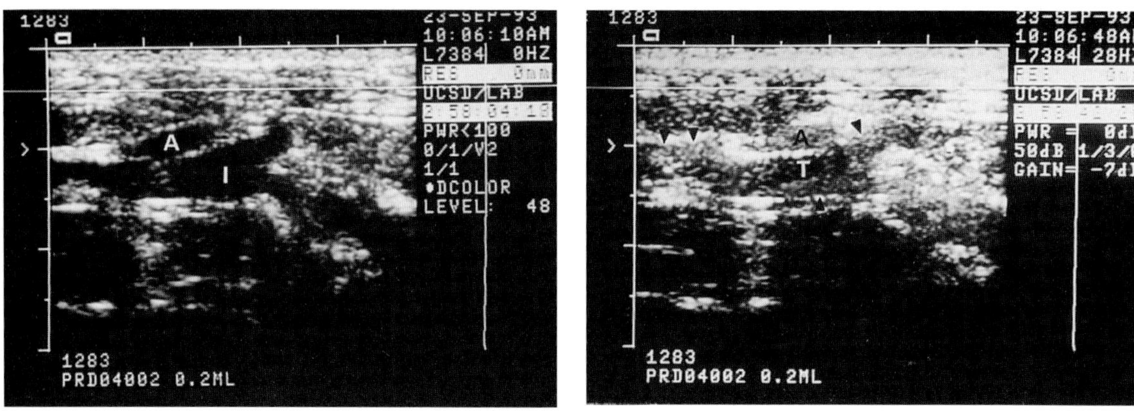

a b

Fig. 30.2. Coronal view of the inferior vena cava (I) at the level of the bifurcation shows a clot produced by a sclerosing agent. No flow could be detected in the vena cava precontrast, either on gray-scale (**a**) or on color (not shown). Postcontrast (**b**), the aorta (*A*) and vena cava (*I*) fill with contrast (*arrowheads*), highlighting a partially occluding thrombus (*T*) not seen precontrast. (From Coley et al. 1994)

30.4 Arterial Disease

The late generation agents have been visible in arteries on gray-scale in animals (Mattrey et al. 1994) and in man (Mattrey et al. 1996), providing up to several minutes of subjectively effective arterial enhancement. Motivated by the observation that filling veins with echoes on gray-scale improved the evaluation of intraluminal venous disease (Coley et al. 1994), Sirlin et al. performed two experiments to determine whether filling arteries with echoes would also improve the evaluation of arterial disease (Sirlin et al. 1996, 1997).

The first experiment used an atherosclerotic rabbit model (Saso et al. 1992). It consisted of injuring the rabbits' infrarenal aortic endothelium with a J-wire or a balloon catheter and then maintaining the rabbits on a high-fat, high-cholesterol diet. The rabbits developed a spectrum of atherosclerotic aortic disease, including fusiform aneurysms, intimal thickening, and focal plaques within 10–20 weeks. The second experiment used silicone replicas of actual human diseased carotid artery bifurcations that were imaged in a tissue phantom. The transparent elastic models duplicated the lumen of the diseased carotids and accurately reproduced lesion characteristics such as surface irregularities, ulcerations, and various degrees of lumen stenoses (Kerber and Heilman 1992). They were imaged as whole porcine blood was pumped through at physiologic flow rates. Postcontrast standard gray-scale

B-mode was compared with noncontrast color Doppler in both models, and with power Doppler in vitro, using a 7-MHz linear transducer. Postcontrast color and power Doppler were suboptimal, as extensive blooming artifacts occurred.

Both models confirmed numerous benefits for contrast-enhanced gray-scale imaging of arteries over precontrast gray-scale, color, or power Doppler imaging. Scanning the vessel of interest on gray-scale was technically challenging prior to contrast administration in both experiments. In vitro, attenuation and reverberation artifacts made it difficult to locate the vessel lumen to delineate its internal anatomy (Fig. 30.3b). By demonstrating regions of flow, color and power Doppler allowed rapid localization of the lumen. However, filling the lumen completely without blooming with color and power Doppler required meticulous and time-consuming optimization of instrumentation settings and insonation angle without consistently achieving adequate results (Fig. 30.3c,d). After contrast, echoes filled the lumen of the vessel on gray-scale in its entirety, allowing the vessels to stand out from surrounding tissues (Fig. 30.3e). Moreover, as the echoes precisely defined the boundaries of the lumen irrespective of instrumentation settings, confusion due to reverberation artifacts was resolved and inspection of the luminal surface became expeditious. In vivo, aneurysms and intimal thickening could be observed precontrast; however, the latter was interrupted, and the luminal margin was not consistently seen (Fig. 30.4a). When color Doppler was used, filling the lumen completely without blooming again required meticulous and time-consuming optimization without consistently achieving adequate results (Fig. 30.4b). Contrast-enhanced gray-scale required only the adjustment of the focal zone and gain. It showed the lumen in detail, allowed the recognition of the luminal margin, and demonstrated intimal thickening and plaques with precision (Fig. 30.4c).

More important than its technical facility, contrast-enhanced gray-scale showed greater accuracy than the other modalities in the assessment of intraluminal disease. In general, luminal abnormali-

a

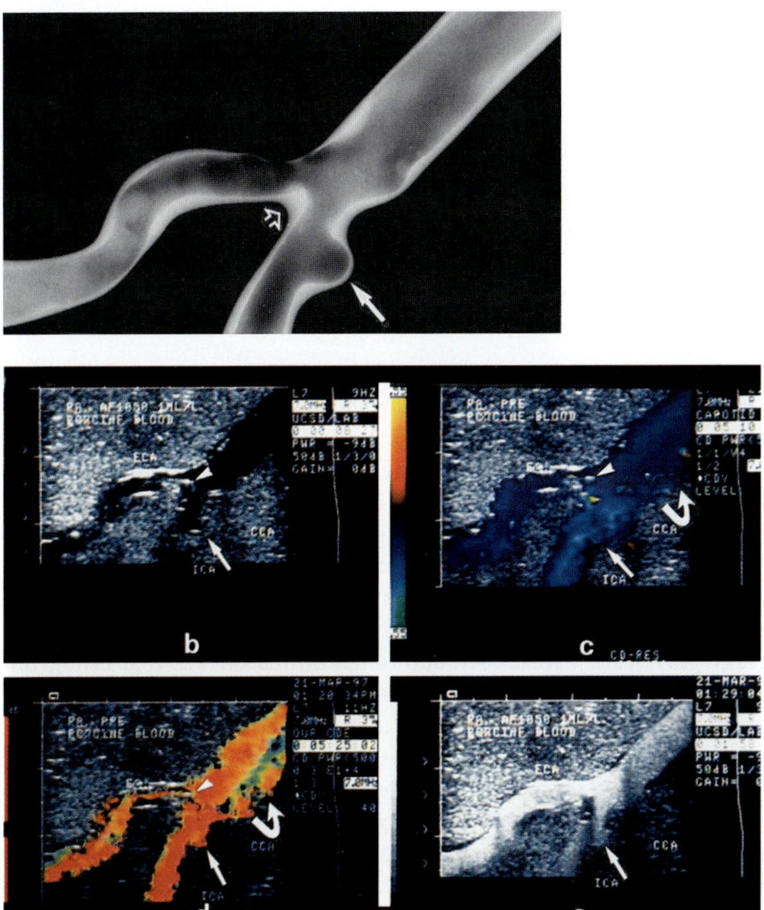

Fig. 30.3. An x-ray of a carotid replica (**a**) shows the ulceration (*arrow*) along the posterior wall of the internal carotid artery and a clump of silicone at the bifurcation (*open arrow*). The replica was imaged in a tissue-mimicking phantom precontrast with gray-scale (**b**), color Doppler (**c**), and power Doppler (**d**). All three precontrast images suggest a posterior irregularity (*arrows*). A reverberation prevented the accurate assessment of the origin of the external carotid artery (*arrowhead* in **b**). When color gain was adjusted to show the anterior wall, blooming was seen posteriorly (*curved arrows*), and when the gain was decreased to eliminate blooming, the vessel did not fill completely (not shown). **e** After contrast administration, flowing echoes sharply outline the luminal surface on gray-scale, allowing immediate identification and assessment of the ulcer (*arrow*). Also, as echoes fill the lumen completely, the accurate assessment of the external carotid (*arrowhead* in **d**) became possible. Although shadowing from the bifurcation (*open arrow*) decreases the quality of the posterior vessel on the frozen image, the recognition of the lumen was clear on real-time. (From Sirlin et al. 1997)

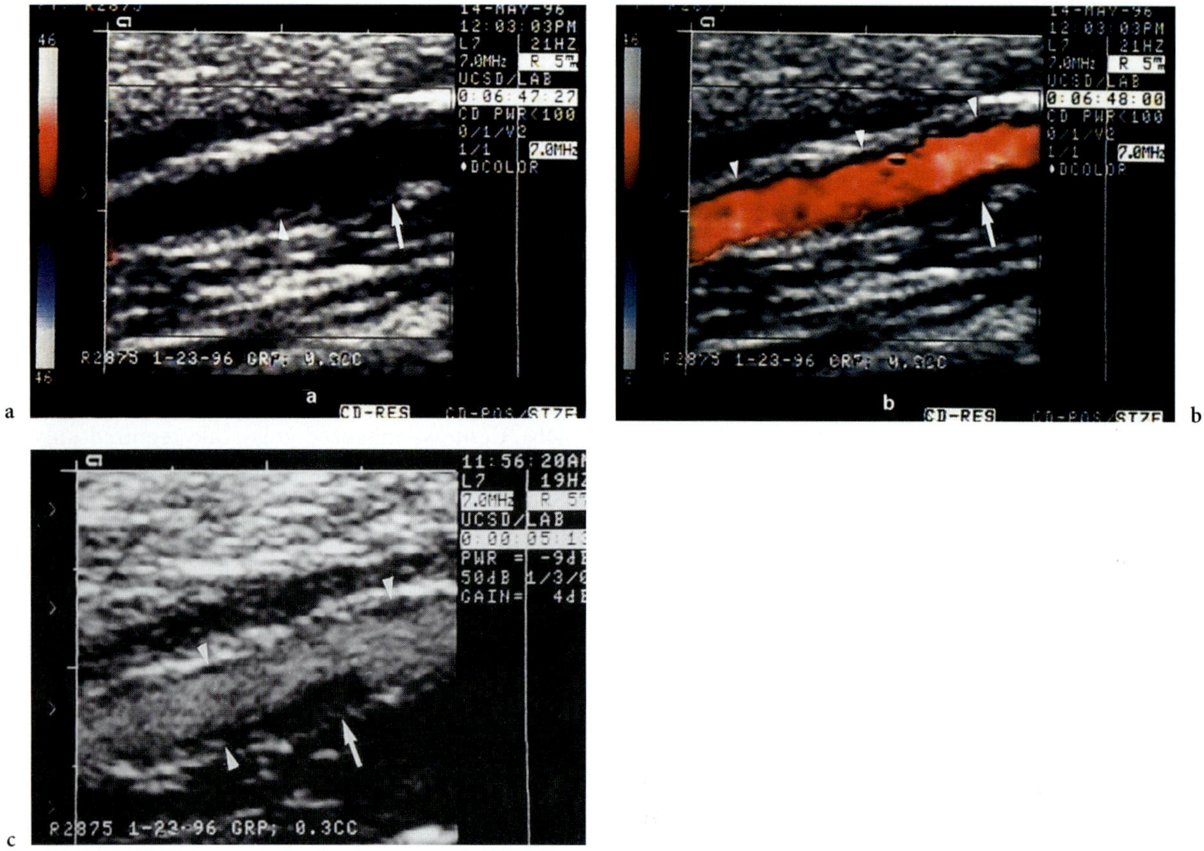

Fig. 30.4. Longitudinal views of the abdominal aorta of an atherosclerotic rabbit is shown precontrast (**a** and **b**) and following (**c**) the bolus injection of 0.5ml of AF0150 (Imagent, Alliance Pharmaceutical Corp., San Diego, Calif.). Precontrast, intimal thickening and irregularity (*arrowheads*) could be recognized; however, no plaque was seen. Postcontrast, the plaque (*arrow*) was easily seen as it was highlighted by the flow stream of echoes. Areas of intimal thickening (*arrowheads*) appeared as dark bands separating the contrast column from the wall. Once the plaque was localized, a noncontrast color Doppler image was obtained over the plaque. It is shown with the color overlay off (**a**) and on (**c**). Note that the plaque is subtly perceptible on gray-scale without contrast (*arrow* in **a**) and is overlayed with color (*arrow* in **b**). Intimal thickening was partially seen with color off (*arrowheads* in **a**). However, with color gain optimized to show the plaque region, a black band is seen along the anterior wall (*arrowheads* in **b**) that is an artifact or a region with slow flow. (From Sirlin et al. 1996)

ties such as diffuse intimal thickening, plaques, and ulcerations were either invisible or not recognized precontrast with any technique. These were readily apparent postcontrast on gray-scale as well-demarcated wall abnormalities at the margin of the contrast column. Contrast-enhanced gray-scale also improved the evaluation of the lumen in a region attenuated by an anterior plaque. Finally, contrast-enhanced gray-scale permitted confident identification of normal vessels. The advantages of gray-scale after contrast administration were most obvious during real-time imaging, as the flow of echoes within the lumen contributed to the visual discrimination of lumen from wall.

Imaging with contrast had a few disadvantages, however. As the scattering of the ultrasound beam by microbubbles is independent of flow velocity (Steinbach et al. 1997), the entire bubble-filled lumen was homogeneously enhanced without regard to local variations in velocity caused by turbulence. Identification of turbulence required visualization of discrepancies in the velocity of individual flowing echoes. Although such discrepancies could be appreciated on real-time imaging, they were not as obvious as on precontrast color Doppler, and they could not be appreciated on static images (Fig. 30.3e, 30.4c). An additional limitation was that echogenic lesions became isoechoic to the lumen after contrast administration, they were however apparent on real time as immobile reflectors distinct from the flowing echoes within the flow stream. These two limitations were overcome when wideband harmonic imaging was employed (Lee et al. 1997). The plaque signal was suppressed and became less echogenic than the lumen, and because wideband harmonic imaging is sensitive to flow velocity, turbulence was readily apparent.

30.5 Contrast-Specific Imaging

The advent of second harmonic techniques has improved Doppler imaging by decreasing the flash artifacts generated from non-contrast-containing pulsatile perivascular tissues and by limiting color to regions filled with bubbles (Burns et al. 1992). However, these techniques do not overcome the limitations of Doppler, such as unreliable filling of vessels, poor spatial resolution of color, and poor temporal resolution of power Doppler. Second harmonic imaging with gray-scale improves upon standard gray-scale imaging by increasing contrast between the lumen and surrounding tissues.

As compared to second harmonic imaging, wideband harmonic imaging is a superior technique because of its higher spatial resolution, more effective tissue suppression, and greater signal from microbubbles (Mattrey et al. 1998). The greater signal from bubbles results from the added effect of bubble destruction and the dependence of wideband imaging on velocity. These factors confer a very high sensitivity to small amounts of contrast media, thus producing dramatic image contrast between the flowing arterial or venous blood and the surrounding tissue, where arteries are more echogenic than veins and the latter more echogenic than tissues (Fig. 30.5).

Using the same replicas used by Sirlin et al. (1997), Lee et al. (1997) showed that, following contrast administration, high-resolution harmonic imaging was superior to standard gray-scale imaging in recognizing the luminal interface and assessing luminal narrowing, particularly when anterior plaque shadowed the vessel (Fig. 30.6). This was because of the greater sensitivity to bubbles and suppression of the vessel wall signal. They also showed that the direct measurement of the vessel on contrast-enhanced gray-scale imaging correlated well with the replicas, and that this measurement was not susceptible to flow alterations caused by concomitant systemic factors, ipsilateral or contralateral stenoses. Finally, because of the sensitivity of wideband imaging to flow velocity – and likely because of the detection of bubble destruction – turbulence, particularly in areas of low velocity, was more easily appreciated.

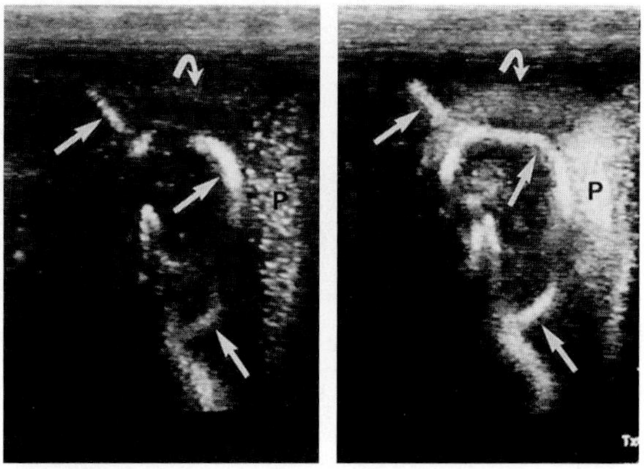

a,b

Fig. 30.5. Oblique view obtained with wideband harmonic imaging with a Siemens Elegra at 7.2 MHz shows a branch of the hepatic artery (*arrows*) alongside a branch of the portal vein (*curved arrow*) during the early arrival (**a**) of a 0.5-ml contrast bolus of AF0150 (Imagent, Alliance Pharmaceutical Corp., San Diego, Calif.) and during equilibrium 2 min later (**b**). Note that when the bolus has reached the hepatic artery, the branch of the portal vein has not yet filled with contrast (*curved arrow* in **a**). The main portal vein (*P*) has echoes from a few bubbles remaining from a prior injection and from the sensitivity of wideband harmonic imaging to velocity. The arterial branch remains brighter than the portal vein branch several minutes later (**b**). (From Mattrey et al. 1998)

Filling of the vessel in a human subject was easily achieved at miniscule doses and allowed the visualization of turbulence (Fig. 30.7). The wideband harmonic technique allowed the assessment of the lumen deeper to a shadowing small calcification in the anterior wall (Fig. 30.8). It showed the thickness between the calcification and the lumen to be minimal, indicating absence of significant plaque formation. This information should prove useful in the assessment and monitoring of atherosclerotic changes, to better define the severity of carotid disease, and to provide more accurate surrogate data to assess risk for stroke and cardiac events (Wofford et al. 1991).

Because of the dependence of wideband harmonic imaging on velocity, intraparenchymal vessels are readily apparent relative to background tissues. When observing the arrival of a bolus to a region of interest, such as the kidney (Fig. 30.9), the arteries are visualized first, followed by capillary blush, with no additional vessels becoming apparent thereafter except for the larger veins. This suggests that the visualized small vessels within tissues are arteries. This observation was confirmed when the coronary arteries were imaged in a normal dog, where all echogenic structures within the septum could be seen emanating from a major coronary

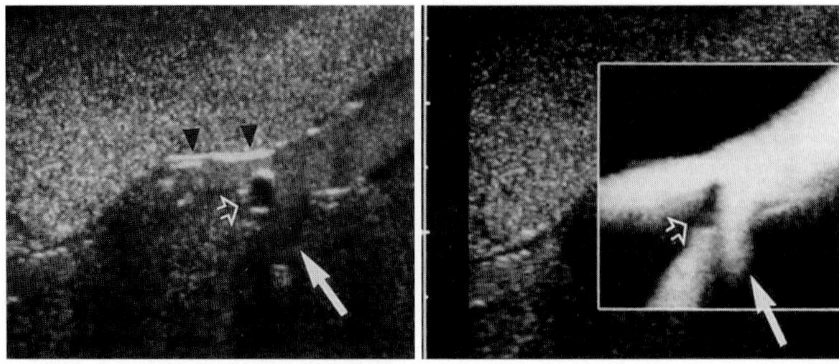

Fig. 30.6. Standard gray-scale (**a**) and wideband harmonic image (**b**) obtained with a Siemens Elegra at 7.2 MHz show the same replica shown in Fig. 30.3 after AF0150 had been added to the porcine blood. Note that the echogenic vessel wall is clearly seen on standard gray-scale (*arrowheads* in **a**). In addition, the thick plastic at the bifurcation (*open arrow*) shadows the posterior wall, decreasing the visibility of the ulceration (*arrow*). The wideband harmonic image (**b**) is shown as an overlay on the standard gray-scale image. It shows only the contrast column within the overlay. Note that the background is completely suppressed and so is the vessel wall, allowing the clear visualization of the ulcer (*arrow*). (From LEE et al. 1997)

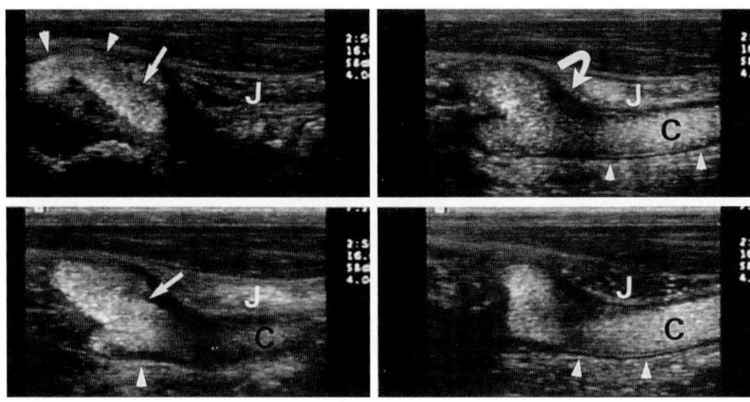

Fig. 30.7 a–d. Longitudinal scans obtained with wideband harmonic imaging with a Siemens Elegra at 7.2 MHz over the carotid bifurcation (*C*) and the jugular vein (*J*) of a human subject imaged following flushing the needle 30 min after the bolus injection of 3.6 ml AF0150 (Imagent, Alliance Pharmaceutical Corp., San Diego, Calif.) used to image the liver. Note the clear depiction of the vessel wall (*arrowheads*). Hypoechoic flow stream (*arrow*) within the solid contrast column on the internal carotid artery is blood with different flow velocity and/or fewer bubbles that had been destroyed when located in a region of eddy current adjacent to an area of wall thickening (*curved arrow*)

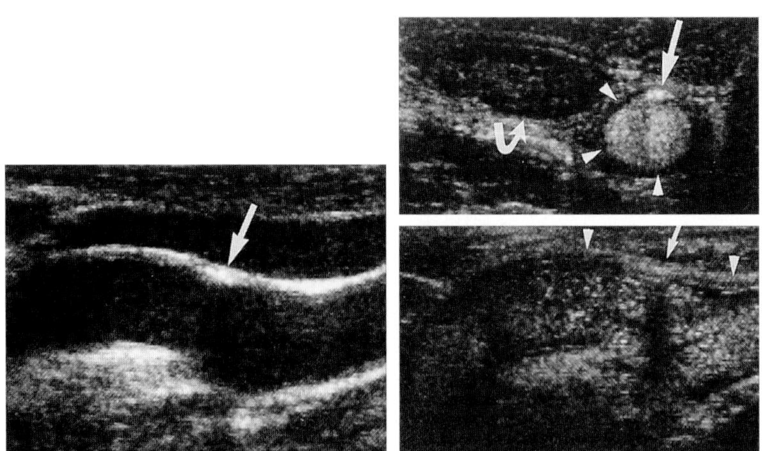

Fig. 30.8. Longitudinal standard gray-scale scan at 7.2 MHz of the carotid bulb (**a**) shows a small calcification along the anterior wall with shadowing (*arrow*). Thirty minutes after the administration of a 3.6-ml bolus injection of AF0150 (Imagent, Alliance Pharmaceutical Corp., San Diego, Calif.) used to image the liver, wideband harmonic imaging (Siemens Ultrasound, Issaquah, Wash.) at 7.2 MHz of the carotid shows near-complete filling of the lumen with contrast. The transverse (**b**) and longitudinal (**c**) scans obtained at the level of the calcified plaque show the exact thickness of the vessel wall (*arrowheads*) and the proximity of the flow stream to the inner margin of the calcification (*arrow*), excluding the presence of significant plaquing. An enlarged lymph node is seen on the transverse view (*curved arrow* in **b**) from this patient's known lymphoma

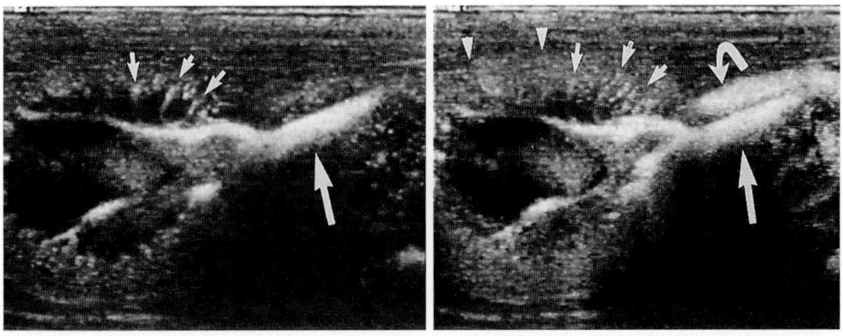

a b

Fig. 30.9 a,b. Transverse views of the right kidney obtained with wideband harmonic imaging with a Siemens Elegra at 7.2 MHz over the renal artery and vein of a rabbit, during the arrival of a 0.5-ml bolus of AF0150 (Imagent, Alliance Pharmaceutical Corp., San Diego, Calif.). The contrast bolus fills the artery (*arrow*) and small vascular branches (*small arrows*) radiating within the cortex (**a**). A few seconds later (**b**), there is capillary blush (*arrowheads*) enhancing the renal cortex, and filling of the main renal vein (*curved arrow*). Note that, although the contrast column has reached the renal vein, the same small vessels are still seen within the cortex (*small arrows*) with no additional small vessels seen. This suggests that the only small intraparenchymal vessels visible with this technique are arteries, owing to their higher velocity. (From Mattrey et al. 1998)

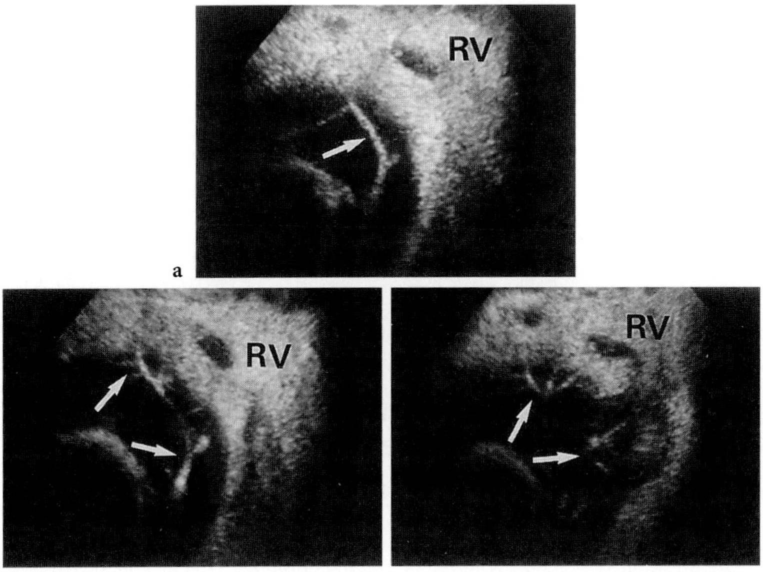

a b,c

Fig. 30.10. Contiguous parasternal transverse views obtained from superior (**a**) to inferior (**c**) at the base of the heart following the bolus injection of 0.5 ml of AF0150 (Imagent, Alliance Pharmaceutical Corp., San Diego, Calif.) using a Siemens Elegra scanner at 7.2 MHz. The images are of the superior aspect of the interventricular septum just posterior and inferior to the right ventricular outflow tract (*RV*). Note the clear depiction of the first septal coronary artery (*arrows*) seen from near its origin (**b**) and branching into multiple smaller arteries. (From Mattrey et al. 1998)

branch (Fig. 30.10). The coronary example also demonstrates that, although this is sensitive to motion, myocardial suppression is effective despite cardiac activity.

30.6 Conclusions

Analogous to angiography or venography with radiopaque contrast media, filling vessels with echoes on gray-scale highlights endovascular lesions, such as plaques or thrombi, as filling defects within the echo-filled lumen of the vessel of interest. Small channels that would otherwise be missed because of slow flow or small quantity of blood flowing through them become visible. The ability to see the inner and outer wall of arteries should make the assessment of plaque size simpler and possibly more accurate than with angiography. This should allow more accurate monitoring of disease regression or progression. The degree of stenosis will be directly measured, rather than estimated by the indirect evidence of increased velocity. These hypotheses, however, remain to be proven in clinical practice.

Although duplex ultrasound with compression is highly accurate and effective in the assessment of thigh veins, the addition of contrast will expand this accuracy to regions where compression is difficult to perform and where veins are difficult to see. Contrast-aided sonography will therefore improve the assessment of pelvic and abdominal veins and the veins in patients at high risk from thrombosis following trauma or surgery.

Contrast-specific imaging techniques, particularly wideband harmonic imaging, should prove highly effective in localizing and evaluating vessels. This will be true in large as well as small intraparenchymal vessels. Such techniques will further expand the role of contrast-enhanced vascular sonography.

Acknowledgement. Work reported herein was supported in part by a grant from NIH, RSNA, and Alliance Pharmaceutical Corp.

References

Aitken AGF, Godden DJ (1987) Real-time ultrasound diagnosis of deep vein thrombosis: a comparison with venography. Clin Radiol 38:309–311

André M, Steinbach G, Mattrey RF (1993) Enhancement of the echogenicity of flowing blood by the contrast agent Perflubron. Invest Radiol 28:502–506

Arbeille P, Desombre C, Aesh B, Philippot M, Lapierre F (1995) Quantification and assessment of carotid artery lesions: degree of stenosis and plaque volume. J Clin Ultrasound 23:113–124

Barry R, Pienaar C, Nel CJC (1990) Accuracy of B-mode ultrasonography in detecting carotid artery plaque hemorrhage and ulceration. Ann Vasc Surg 4:466–470

Bauer A, Becker G, Henz P, Jachimczak P, Schwarz KQ, Haase A, Bogdahn U (1997) Transcranial duplex ultrasound: experience with contrast enhancing agents. Int Angiol 16:216–221

Belcaro G, Laurora G, Cesarone MR, et al. (1993) Ultrasonic classification of carotid plaques causing less than 60% stenosis according to ultrasound morphology and events. J Cardiovasc Surg 34:287–294

Burns PN (1997) Overview of echo-enhanced vascular ultrasound imaging for clinical diagnosis in neurosonology. J Neuroimaging 7(Suppl 1):S2–S14

Burns PN, Powers JE, Fritzsch T (1992) Harmonic imaging: new imaging and Doppler method for contrast-enhanced ultrasound. Radiology 185(P):142

Coley BD, Trambert MA, Heiberg E, Mattrey RF (1990) Sonographic detection of deep venous thrombosis with PFOB "sonographic venography" (abstract). Radiology 177(P)(Suppl):215

Coley BD, Trambert MA, Mattrey RF (1994) Perfluorocarbon-enhanced sonography: value in detecting acute venous thrombosis in rabbits. AJR 163:961–964

Cronan JJ (1993) Venous thromboembolic disease: the role of US. Radiology 186:619–630

Cronan JJ, Dorfman GS, Grusmark J (1988) Lower-extremity deep venous thrombosis: further experience with refinements US assessment. Radiology 168:101–107

Delcker A, Diener HC (1994) 3D ultrasound measurement of atherosclerotic plaque volume in carotid arteries. Bildgebung 61:116–121

ECACAS (Executive Committee for the Asymptomatic Carotid Atherosclerosis Study) (1995) Endarterectomy for asymptomatic carotid artery stenosis. JAMA 273:1421–1428

ECPSG (European Carotid Plaque Study Group) (1995) Carotid artery composition – relationship to clinical presentation and ultrasound B-mode imaging. Eur J Endovasc Surg 10:23–30

Eikelboom BC, Riles TR, Mintzer R, Baumann FG, DeFillip G, Lin J, Imparato AM (1983) Inaccuracy of angiography in the diagnosis of carotid ulceration. Stroke 14:882–885

Foley WD, Middleton WD, Lawson TL, Erickson S, Quiroz FA, Macrander S (1989) Color Doppler ultrasound imaging of lower-extremity venous disease. AJR 152:371–376

Ginsberg JS, Caco CC, Brill-Edwards PA, et al. (1991) Venous thrombosis in patients who have undergone major hip or knee surgery: detection with compression US and impedance plethysmography. Radiology 181:651–654

Goldberg BB, Hilpert PL, Burns PN, Liu JB, Newman LM, Merton DA, Witlin LA (1990) Hepatic tumors: signal enhancement at Doppler US after intravenous injection of a contrast agent. Radiology 177:713–717

Gray-Weale AC, Graham JC, Burnett JR, Byrne K, Lusby RJ (1988) Carotid artery atheroma: comparison of preoperative B-mode ultrasound appearance with carotid endarterectomy specimen pathology. J Cardiovasc Surg (Torino) 29:676–681

Hilpert PL, Mattrey RF, Mitten RM, Peterson T (1989) IV injection of air-filled human albumin microspheres to enhance arterial Doppler signal: a preliminary study in rabbits. AJR 153:613–616

Iannuzzi A, Wilcosky T, Mercuri M, Ruba P, Bryan FA, Bond MG (1995) Ultrasonographic correlates of carotid atherosclerosis in transient ischemic attack and stroke. Stroke 26:614–619

Keller MW, Feinstein SB, Watson DD (1987) Successful left ventricular opacification following peripheral venous injection of sonicated contrast agent: an experimental evaluation. Am Heart J 114:570–575

Kerber CW, Heilman CB (1992) Flow dynamics in the human carotid artery. I. Preliminary observations using a transparent elastic model. AJNR 13:173–180

Lee YZ, Sirlin CB, Steinbach GC, Mattrey RF (1997) High resolution harmonic imaging (HRH) versus duplex sonography for the evaluation of carotid artery stenosis (abstract). Radiology 205(P):419

Lensing AWA, Prandoni P, Brandles D, et al. (1989) Detection of deep-vein thrombosis by real time B-mode ultrasonography. N Engl J Med 320:342–345

Lewis BD, James EM, Welch TJ, Joyce JW, Hallett JW, Weaver AL (1994) Diagnosis of acute deep venous thrombosis of the lower extremities: prospective evaluation of color Doppler flow imaging versus venography. Radiology 192:651–655

Mattrey RF, Mitten R, Peterson T, Long DC (1987) Vascular ultrasonic enhancement of tissues with perfluorooctyl bromide for renal tumor detection. Radiology 165(P):76

Mattrey RF, Wrigley R, Steinbach GC, Schutt EG, Evitts DP (1994) Gas emulsions as ultrasound contrast agents: preliminary results in rabbits and dogs. Invest Radiol 29 (Suppl 2):S139–S141

Mattrey RF, Girard MS, Steinbach GC, Peterson T (1995) Improvement in tissue contrast enhancement at the second harmonic frequency in a renal infarct model following the intravenous injection of a perfluorochemical-stabilized microbubble contrast agent. Radiology 197:403

Mattrey RF, Manspeaker P, Pelura TJ, Batra S, Leese PT (1996) Safety and preliminary efficacy of AF0150, a phase I clinical trial in normal volunteers. RSNA. December 1996. Chicago, Illinois

Mattrey RF, Steinbach G, Lee Y, Wilkening W, Lazenby J (1998) High-resolution harmonic gray-scale imaging of normal and abnormal vessels and tissues in animals. Acad Radiol 5(Suppl 1):S63–S65

Meairs S, Rother J, Nef W, Hennerici M (1995) New and future developments in cerebrovascular ultrsound, magnetic resonance angiography and related techniques. J Clin Ultrasound 23:139–149

Murphy TP, Cronan JJ (1990) Evolution of deep venous thrombosis: a prospective evaluation with US. Radiology 177:543–548

O'Donnell TF, Erdoes L, Mackay WC, et al. (1985) Correlation of B-mode ultrasound imaging with pathologic findings at carotid endarterectomy. Arch Surg 120:443

O'Hara SM, Frush DP, Babcock DS, et al. (1996) Doppler contrast sonography for detecting reduced perfusion in experimental ischemia of prepubertal rabbit testes. Acad Radiol 3:319–324

O'Leary DH, Holen J, Ricotta JJ, Roe S, Schenk EA (1987a) Carotid bifurcation disease: prediction of ulceration with B-mode US. Radiology 162:523–525

O'Leary DH, Bryan FA, Goodison MW, et al. (1987b) Measurement variability of carotid atherosclerosis: real-time (B-mode) ultrasonography and angiography. Stroke 18:1011–1017

Polak JF, Culter SS, O'Leary DH (1989) Deep veins of the calf: assessment with color Doppler flow imaging. Radiology 171:481–485

Robbin ML, Eisenfeld AJ (1998) Perflenapent emulsion: a US contrast agent for diagnostic radiology - multicenter, double-blind comparison with a placebo. EchoGen Contrast Ultrasound Study Group. Radiology 207:717–722

Rubens DJ, Holen J, Blebia JS, Tofferman SM, Frances CW, Pelligrina YD Jr (1991) Color flow Doppler US: an insensitive screening examination for asymptomatic deep venous thrombosis (abstract). Radiology 181:(P)134

Saso Y, Kitamura K, Yasoshima A, Iwasaki HO, Takashima K, Doi K, Morita T (1992) Rapid induction of atherosclerosis in rabbits. Histology Histopathol 7:315–320

Schurmann R, Schlief R (1994) Saccharide-based contrast agents. Characteristics and diagnostic potential. Radiol Med (Torino) 87(5 Suppl 1):15–23

Schwarz KQ, Becher H, Schimpfky C, Vorwerk D, Bodgahn U, Schlief R (1994) Doppler enhancement with SHU 508A in multiple vascular regions. Radiology 193:195–201

Schweizer J, Oehmichen F, Brandl HG, Altmann E (1993) Color-coded duplex ultrasound and contrast medium enhanced duplex ultrasound in deep venous thrombosis. Vasa 22:22–25

Sehgal CM, Arger PH, Pugh CR (1995) Influence of post-processing curves on contrast-echographic imaging: preliminary studies. J Ultrasound Med 14:735–740

Sirlin CB, Girard M, Peterson TM, Baker K, Hall LA, Steinbach G, Mattrey RF (1996) Improved sonographic delineation of atherosclerotic plaque after intravenous administration of a perfluorochemical-stabilized microbubble (abstract). Radiology 201(P):265

Sirlin CB, Steinbach GC, Girard MS, Casola G, Mattrey RF (1997) Improved visualization of the arterial luminal surface in replicas of diseased human carotids using ultrasound contrast media (abstract). J Ultrasound Med 16:S62

Sitzer M, Furst G, Siebler M, Steinmetz H (1994) Usefulness of an intravenous contrast medium in the characterization of high-grade internal carotid stenosis with color Doppler-assisted duplex imaging. Stroke 25:385–389

Steinbach GC, Sirlin CB, Peterson TM, Baker KG, Hall LA, Mattrey RF (1997) Effect of ultrasound system settings on enhancement of the pulsed-wave Doppler signal with ultrasound contrast media. J Ultrasound Med 16: S36

van Damme H, Vivario M (1993) Pathologic aspects of carotid plaques: surgical and clinical significance. Int Angiol 12:299–311

Vogel P, Laing FC, Jeffrey RB, Wing VW (1987) Deep venous thrombosis of the lower extremity: US evaluation. Radiology 163:747–751

White RH, McGahan JP, Daschbach MM, Hartling RP (1989) Diagnosis of deep-vein thrombosis using duplex ultrasound. Ann Intern Med 111:297–304

Widder B, Paulat K, Hackspacher J, et al. (1990) Morphological characterization of carotid artery stenoses by ultrasound duplex scanning. J Ultrasound Med Biol 16:349–354

Wofford JL, Kahl FR, Howard GR, McKinney WM, Toole JF, Crouse JR 3d (1991) Relation of extent of extracranial carotid artery atherosclerosis as measured by B-mode ultrasound to the extent of coronary atherosclerosis. Arterioscler Thromb 1991;11:1786–1794

Young N, Soo YS, Fischer P (1992) Comparison of duplex ultrasound with angiography in assessment of carotid bifurcation disease. Australas Radiol 36:54–58

31 Tumor Imaging with Ultrasound Contrast

T. ALBRECHT and R.F. MATTREY

CONTENTS

31.1 Introduction

Computed tomography (CT) and magnetic resonance imaging (MRI) are currently considered the standards for detection, characterization, and staging of tumors, particularly those in the liver. Their superiority is due in large part to the availability of intravenous contrast agents, which promote lesion visualization and characterization. The increase in tissue contrast is due to the differences in the wash-in and wash-out rates of the agent through normal and abnormal tissues, requiring fast infusion rates and rapid multiphasic imaging (MITSUZAKI et al. 1996). Except in the breast, where there is a need to know whether lesions are cystic or solid, and the scrotum, where there is a need to know whether masses are intra- or extratesticular, sonography plays a limited role in oncologic disease. The main limitation of sonography is its inability to fully assess tumor vascularity and perfusion.

The high prevalence of primary and metastatic liver tumors demands improved liver lesion detection, particularly outside North America and Western Europe, in countries where sonography serves a more primary role in liver imaging than CT and MRI. Further, because of the low cost and availability of sonography, any improvement in lesion detection would have a greater impact on health care and cost. The need to detect and size all liver lesions is heightened by the proof that lesion resection increases survivorship, and that resection is limited to those patients with a few small lesions with specific distribution.

It is not a surprise that tumor imaging is one of the most promising applications of ultrasound contrast agents. Most of the ongoing work, however, is still considered experimental (either in animals or in clinical trials). With the recent availability of Levovist (Schering AG, Berlin, Germany) for routine clinical use in many countries around the world, contrast applications are now entering radiological practice. Given that Levovist is a Doppler rather than a gray-scale enhancing agent, most studies have focused on the enhancement of tumor Doppler signals, with some very encouraging results. With the advent of the late-generation perfluorocarbon (PFC) stabilized agents, which have a longer intravascular dwell time and are capable of enhancing vessels and tissues on gray-scale, a new dimension for sonographic imaging of tumors is on the horizon. These agents are in early to late stages of clinical development. Also on the horizon are a series of contrast specific ultrasound imaging techniques such as transient response, second harmonic, and wideband harmonic imaging that promise to increase image contrast and contrast agent efficacy. Furthermore some microbubble agents have liver- and spleen-specific properties that will be particularly useful in tumor detection.

T. ALBRECHT, MD, FRCR, Department of Radiology and Nuclear Medicine, Universitätsklinikum Benjamin Franklin, Freie Universität Berlin, Hindenburgdamm 30, D-12205 Berlin, Germany
R.F. MATTREY, MD, Department of Radiology, University of California, San Diego Medical Center, 200 W. Arbor Drive, San Diego, CA 92109-8756, USA

In this chapter we will discuss tumor blood flow physiology, the different classes of agents, and imaging modalities used to detect and characterize tumors.

31.2 Vascular Morphology

The aggressive behavior of malignant tumors is critically dependent on vascular supply. In the early stages of development of a clone of tumor cells, oxygen and nutrient supply are achieved by diffusion; however, for further growth and eventual formation of metastatic nodules, an autonomous vascular supply is a prerequisite. This is achieved by the expression of tumor angiogenesis factors that stimulate neovascular development from host vessels (Folkman et al. 1971). Vascular buds and sprouts grow out from the host venules and soon develop a lumen. They fuse randomly with arterioles and with one another to commence perfusion. The newly formed vascular network is sometimes both supplied and drained by venules (Vaupel 1994).

Neovascularity of some highly differentiated tumors can have a fairly mature architecture. Conversely, the hastily formed new vessels in rapidly growing tumors show a series of severe morphological abnormalities. Although malignant tumors are often hypervascular relative to their host tissue, they may also be hypovascular. Further, blood flow to tumors shows considerable temporal and spatial heterogeneity, with a mixture of hypo- and hyperperfused areas. As tumors enlarge and their growth outstrips their blood supply, their centers become hypoperfused. Because of poor lymphatic drainage, tumors have high water content and interstitial pressure.

Anatomically, there is loss of normal vascular hierarchy. Trifurcations, vascular loops, arteriovenous shunts, sinusoidal vessels ("venous convolutes or lakes") arising from and ending in veins, and blind-ending vessels (including capillary sprouts) are commonly found. Tumor vessels, and in particular venules, are typically tortuous, elongated, and dilated. They often show contour irregularities that contribute to marked caliber changes, particularly at branching points. These wall irregularities are due to incomplete or missing endothelial lining where tumor cell cords often line the blood channels. Furthermore, the wall usually lacks smooth muscle, leading to abnormal or absent contractile function. The result of all these features is a highly irregular, tangled, and chaotic vascular pattern, with leaky capillaries that allow the passage of submicron-sized particles (Jain 1988; Less et al. 1991; Vaupel 1994; Brasch et al. 1998).

The described changes in vascular morphology involve the entire vascular tree, from the feeding arterioles (luminal diameter 200–250 μm) down the branching generations to the capillaries (luminal diameter 10–50 μm) and extending to the postcapillary venules and small veins. The often dilated veins contain most of the blood volume in tumors. The luminal diameter of venules in a mammary tumor model was reported by Less et al. (1991) to exceed 3 times that of the arterioles.

Although the classic imaging modality for demonstrating tumor neovascularity is angiography (Strickland 1959; Gammill et al. 1976; Maeda 1979), its use is limited by its invasiveness, and it is therefore reserved for patients in whom therapeutic intervention is needed. Many of the features of tumor neovascularity can be imaged noninvasively with color or power Doppler sonography and wideband harmonic imaging. Doppler features have been used to aid in tumor characterization of the breast, liver, ovary, and other organs. However, because the changes described occur in small vessels where flow is usually slow, it is necessary to use contrast agents to overcome the limitations of tumor Doppler signal. As the minimum diameter of vessels from which flow can be detected with contrast-enhanced Doppler imaging is on the order of 30–60 μm, several of the larger branching generations of tumor neovascularity can be displayed. Detail is limited because of the poor spatial resolution of color Doppler sonography, which often produces a "vascular blush" following contrast administration. Even with these limitations, contrast-enhanced color and power Doppler ultrasound are currently the only noninvasive imaging techniques that allow the study of the morphology of small tumor vessels. Standard gray-scale imaging shows a blush of the perfused portion of the tumor following contrast administration (Girard et al. 1998a). However, when aided with contrast specific instrumentation this technique has the potential to demonstrate flow in small submillimeter vessels (Mattrey et al. 1998).

Contrast enhancement of tumors in CT and MRI also makes use of tumor neovascularity, but the limited spatial and temporal resolution does not allow the display of small tumor vessels. Furthermore, the diffuse contrast blush seen in tumors with these modalities is partly due to hypervascularity, but mostly due to the diffusion of nonspecific CT and

MR agents through leaky tumor vessels into the interstitium. This is a fundamental difference between CT and MR agents, as the 2- to 3-μm microbubbles remain confined to the intravascular space, giving sonography the ability to exclusively study vascular morphology and flow. Although blood pool agents for CT and MRI remain intravascular, they are either protein or polymer based, or are submicron-sized particles that typically leak through the capillaries, thus decreasing vascular conspicuity (MATTREY 1989).

31.3 Hemodynamic Changes

Blood flow in tumor neovascularity differs considerably from that of normal vascular beds. The flow rate of blood, Q, in any tissue, whether normal or neoplastic, is given by:

$$Q = \delta p / FR$$

where δp, the driving pressure – the pressure difference between arterial and venous ends – is dependent on the microvascular pressures within the tissue, and FR is the flow resistance, a complex function of vascular morphology and the rheological properties of blood. The three major factors that influence blood flow, morphology, microvascular pressure, and rheology, are different in tumors than in normal tissue (JAIN 1988).

The blindly ending, dilated, and irregular vessels and "venous lakes" reduce regional blood flow, whereas arteriovenous shunts increase blood flow. Although pressure in arteries feeding tumors is comparable to that in those feeding normal tissues, venous pressure is substantially lower, resulting in a larger pressure gradient and, therefore, increased blood flow (JAIN 1988). However, the impaired lymphatic drainage increases interstitial pressure and microvascular resistance (BOUCHER et al. 1996). These pressure changes in tumors result in reduction or even stasis of blood flow on the venous side, whose volume constitutes most of the vascular volume of tumors (JAIN 1988).

In addition to the hemodynamic effects, the less-understood rheology and blood viscosity in tumor patients further influence blood flow. Although the low hematocrit that is commonly encountered in cancer patients decreases viscosity, there are many local and systemic factors that increase viscosity. Some of these factors are: (a) increased red cell aggregation due to the low shear rate caused by slow flow in relatively large vessels; (b) increased red cell aggregation and rigidity caused by the frequently elevated fibrinogen and globulin concentrations (RILEY 1976, TIETJEN et al. 1977); and (c) increased hemoconcentration due to the fluid loss across the leaky capillaries, as has been shown in breast cancer (SEVICK and JAIN 1988; VAUPEL et al. 1987).

While it is obvious that such factors influence tumor blood flow, it is difficult to predict which of these competing factors dominates regional flow. However, it is more likely that the overall effect is in favor of increased viscosity and resistance, and thus a reduction in tumor blood flow (JAIN 1988; VAUPEL 1994). Flow data from multiple sites of measurement have shown up to a 55-fold difference in perfusion within individual tumors (ACKER et al. 1990). Tumor flow is dynamic, with marked temporal and spatial variation; regions with slow flow can become regions of high flow and visa versa.

These hemodynamic properties of tumors are relevant for contrast-enhanced ultrasound, as microbubble agents can be used not only to display the morphology of tumor vessels but also to study blood flow kinetics. Bolus injections of microbubble agents can be used as intravascular tracers, allowing the quantitation of the wash-in and wash-out kinetic profile when frames are sampled and analyzed at regular intervals (for example, every second). Although an obvious parallel to dynamic MRI of the breast exists, microbubbles are blood pool rather than interstitial agents. Their dynamic behavior is, therefore, independent of capillary leak and diffusion abnormalities.

A prerequisite for quantitative functional studies is the ability to obtain meaningful microbubble concentration measurements from ultrasound data, a complex task due to the nonlinear image processing algorithms of ultrasound scanners. However, when variables and conditions are accounted for, accurate in vivo quantification of relative microbubble concentrations is possible using spectral Doppler (ALBRECHT et al. 1997a) or power Doppler (BLOMLEY et al. 1997a). Quantification of ultrasound signals is covered in detail elsewhere in this book.

Once time-enhancement curves of a tumor have been obtained, they can be analyzed for a number of indices, such as rise time, time to peak enhancement, duration of enhancement, mean transit time, area under the enhancement curve, and many more. The morphological abnormality of tumor vessels and, more importantly, the functional abnormalities of tumor blood flow are expected to influence the shape and indices of the time-intensity curve. Arteriovenous shunts increase flow and shorten the arrival time of the bolus and the time to peak enhancement. Increased vascular resistance, increased viscosity, and the low venous pressure gradient prolong the washout, the duration of enhancement, and the mean transit time. The hypervascularity of the rim of many malignant lesions should result in a higher peak enhancement. When greater peak enhancement is combined with rapid rise time and prolonged washout, the area under the curve increases.

The relative differences in some of these indices between normal and abnormal regions can be recognized with specialized imaging techniques. With the knowledge that bubbles are destroyed by ultrasound, intermittent imaging provides an imaging index of the rise time. Once bubbles are destroyed, image contrast on the next frame is dependent upon the number of bubbles that enter, which in turn is dependent upon differences in blood flow and fractional blood volume. Intermittent imaging is discussed in more detail later in this chapter.

31.4 Clinical Potential of Doppler Agents

Although unenhanced Doppler studies can provide information regarding the pattern and degree of vascularity when lesions are well seen, contrast-enhanced Doppler studies ensure that such data can be acquired from all lesions. Except for the added ability to assess contrast wash-in and wash-out rates, it is not expected that contrast media would add significantly to a high-quality unenhanced Doppler study.

The pattern and degree of vascularity of the primary tumor aid in patient management as predictors for the development of metastases and as prognostic indicators (Srivastava et al. 1988; Weidner et al. 1991). From a diagnostic point of view, the morphological and functional information obtained from contrast-enhanced Doppler studies of tumor vascularity can be used in several ways. The most important, but probably also the most ambitious, is the differential diagnosis of tumors. The differentiation of tumors from scar tissue, complex cysts, or focal fatty infiltration of the liver based on vascularity is relatively straightforward and often useful in a clinical situation. The differentiation of benign or inflammatory lesions from malignant tumors is a more difficult task, as benign lesions have neovascularization, albeit less marked and more orderly. With this potentially significant overlap of features, we await further improvements in spatial resolution and clinical experience to uncover additional signs that could aid in this differentiation.

Another promising clinical application of contrast-enhanced Doppler ultrasound of tumor vascularity is medical, interventional, or radiotherapy treatment monitoring. The vascular bed is an early response site in chemo- and radiotherapy (Moore and West 1991), and unenhanced Doppler studies have been reported to demonstrate an early reduction of vascularity during medical treatment that often antedates tumor shrinkage (Kedar et al. 1994). Furthermore, antiangiogenic drugs are being developed that directly target tumor angiogenesis (Baillie et al. 1995). Because contrast-enhanced Doppler allows better visualization of tumor vessels, greater sensitivity to tumor response would be expected, thus positioning enhanced Doppler studies as the primary modality to monitor therapeutic effectiveness. The assessment of viable tumor tissue is critical to the complete eradication of tumors in image-guided therapy; in this setting, enhanced Doppler has been shown to aid in the management of lesion therapy by providing real-time control of where and how much to treat (Solbiati et al. 1996).

The specific clinical applications that have been evaluated will be discussed separately for different organs in the following sections.

31.4.1 Liver

Focal liver lesions have been studied with ultrasound contrast agents by several investigators (Angeli et al. 1994; Campani et al. 1994; Leen et al. 1994; Maresca et al. 1994; Hosten et al. 1997; Strunk et al. 1998). Because of the large variety of focal benign and malignant liver lesions, the dual blood supply of the liver, the liver's large size, and the difficulty in visualizing the entire liver, assessment of liver lesions is by far the most challenging, both before and after the administration of contrast media. Clinical experience with contrast-enhanced Doppler studies as reported in the literature is limited, and what is available is contradictory. However, some typical features of several pathologic entities are emerging that could aid in lesion characterization.

Hepatocellular carcinomas are vascularized throughout and show peripheral more than central enhancement after contrast administration. However, similar features have been described for some benign lesions, such as focal nodular hyperplasia and adenomas. Focal fatty infiltration and scarring are good examples of benign lesions that, by their very definition, will not display abnormal vascularity; contrast agents are helpful in confirming their diagnosis. We have recently studied several hemangiomas, using various contrast agents, and have found that demonstration of vessels in smaller lesions (<3 cm) is rare, although larger hemangiomas usually display peripheral vessels after contrast administration. Most metastases of common tumors, such as colorectal or pancreatic carcinomas, typically show only a mild degree of peripheral vascularity, whereas "hypervascular metastases" (e.g., from neuroendocrine tumors or renal cell carcinomas) often display vascularity throughout the lesion after contrast. In one recent series, however, 7 of 15 metastases showed no flow signals after Levovist, thus underscoring the limitations of contrast-enhanced Doppler ultrasound in the differentiation of liver lesions. Although there are certain vascular characteristics brought out with contrast agents that could aid in focal liver lesion characterization, current Doppler techniques are not useful due to overlap between lesions.

The improved visualization of flow in tumor vessels with contrast-enhanced Doppler ultrasound has been successfully used to guide and monitor percutaneous ablation procedures (SOLBIATI et al. 1996). Areas of perfused residual or recurrent tumor tissue can be identified with sensitivity similar to that of contrast-enhanced spiral CT.

No data have so far been published on quantitative and/or dynamic studies of contrast enhancement of hepatic tumor vascularity. Our group has recently taken a slightly different approach to the dynamic assessment of liver malignancy (BLOMLEY et al. 1997b). In a small pilot study, we measured the time-intensity curves of a Levovist bolus with spectral Doppler intensitometry of hepatic veins. We found striking differences in the shapes of the curves, and thus in hepatic blood flow, in patients with metastases as compared to controls. Although five of the seven patients with metastases had an early peak (before 45 s), all six control subjects had a late peak (after 45 s). In one of the two patients with metastases with a late peak, the sampled hepatic vein drained the non-tumor-bearing lobe; the other patient had only a small subcapsular metastasis. These early results suggest that analyzing liver transit time of a microbubble bolus may increase the sensitivity of ultrasound in suspected liver metastases.

31.4.2 Kidney

Few data are available in the literature on the assessment of renal tumors with contrast-enhanced Doppler ultrasound (FILLIPONE et al. 1994; WESKOTT and BRANDS 1997). Most renal cell carcinomas are hypervascular (22 of 28 in the study by Fillipone et al. using Levovist). Although some benign lesions, such as angiomyolipomas, may show vascularity on enhanced Doppler studies, the presence of vessels increases the risk for malignancy. So far, no patterns have been identified which offer improvement in tumor characterization with Doppler agents.

Contrast-enhanced Doppler ultrasound can be very helpful in differentiating complex (e.g., hemorrhagic) cysts, which are completely avascular, from hypovascular tumors, which usually display at least some vascularity (CORREAS et al. 1997). Similarly, it is very useful in confirming a prominent column of Bertin by demonstrating normal vascular architecture and density, thus ruling out the presence of tumor.

31.4.3 Breast

The breast is the most suitable organ for the clinical evaluation of contrast-enhanced Doppler ultrasound of tumor vascularity. Breast tumors are common, and histology is often available for correlation. The number of common solid pathologic entities (carcinoma, fibroadenoma, benign change, scarring) is limited in comparison to other organs such as the liver. Breast cancers are usually well vascularized, which is not necessarily the case for other primary sites. Lastly, scanning is optimal because high-frequency probes can be used, providing high spatial resolution, and tissues can be stabilized, minimizing motion artifacts.

Several studies have looked at contrast-enhanced color Doppler ultrasound of breast lesions. Most of these studies have suffered from small patient numbers. Generally, malignant lesions are more vascular than their benign counterparts, but most authors have observed some overlap between the two groups. Therefore, a simple subjective assessment of degree of vascularity is not sufficient for the successful characterization of breast masses.

Kedar and colleagues took a more ambitious semiquantitative approach in their study of 36 patients with breast masses, of which 18 were cancers

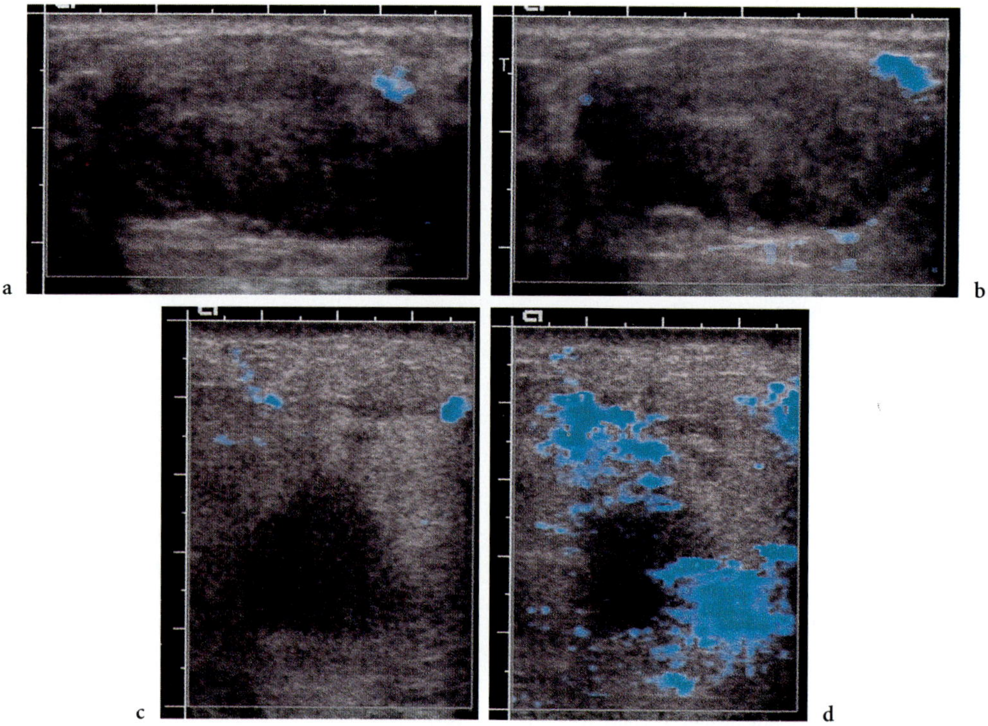

Fig. 31.1. Example of typical vascular architecture of benign (**a**, **b**) and malignant (**c**, **d**) breast lesions. Power Doppler scan of a fibroadenoma before contrast (**a**) shows only a single small vessel at the edge of the tumor. Identical section of the fibroadenoma after contrast (EchoGen) administration (**b**) shows only mild enhancement in the same vessel, and no additional vessels are visible. Power Doppler scan of a carcinoma of the breast (**c**) shows three small feeding vessels at the periphery of the hyperechoic and centrally necrotic (echo-free) tumor. After contrast (EchoGen) (**d**), many more and highly irregular vessels are seen within the solid parts of the cancer. Note the marked difference in vascularity displayed after contrast between the fibroadenoma and the carcinoma

(Kedar et al. 1996). They subjectively scored the number and complexity of the vessels of the lesions on color Doppler ultrasound after Levovist injection. They also looked at the dynamic indices of contrast enhancement by subjectively determining the time to peak and duration of enhancement. The results showed a significantly larger number of vessels in cancers; in addition, the vessels of malignant lesions were more tortuous and took a predominantly radial penetrating course, in contrast to the peripheral and circumferential vessels in fibroadenomas. Furthermore, the authors found large knot-like apparent interconnections between vessels in all cancers, but in none of the benign lesions – these were called shunts. The dynamic indices showed cancers to have significantly longer enhancement duration (5 min 40 s vs 3 min) and shorter time to peak (45 s vs 1 min 5 s) as compared to benign masses. Using all discussed criteria in combination, the sensitivity and specificity for malignancy was improved from 89% and 88% before Levovist administration to 100% and 100%, respectively, post Levovist, with four correct changes of diagnosis.

Inspired by these very promising results, we have recently completed a small study of 20 patients with breast lesions (11 of them cancers) using power Doppler ultrasound after the administration of EchoGen (Sonus Pharmaceuticals, Bothell, Wash., USA) (Albrecht et al. 1998) (Fig. 31.1). In addition to subjective evaluation according to the criteria of Kedar et al. (1996), we took a truly quantitative approach. We produced time-intensity curves from a single level scan and analyzed them for a number of variables. The results showed two main differences between benign and malignant lesions. First, the duration of enhancement was longer in carcinomas (6 min 3 s vs 4 min 43 s). Second, the shape of the wash-out limb of the time-intensity curve was simple and monophasic in six of nine benign lesions, but complex and multiphasic in 8 of 11 malignant lesions (Fig. 31.2). This intriguing feature may be a reflection of the temporal, and probably also the spatial, heterogeneity of the flow in malignant tumor vessels (assuming some unavoidable movement of the ultrasound transducer during the scan).

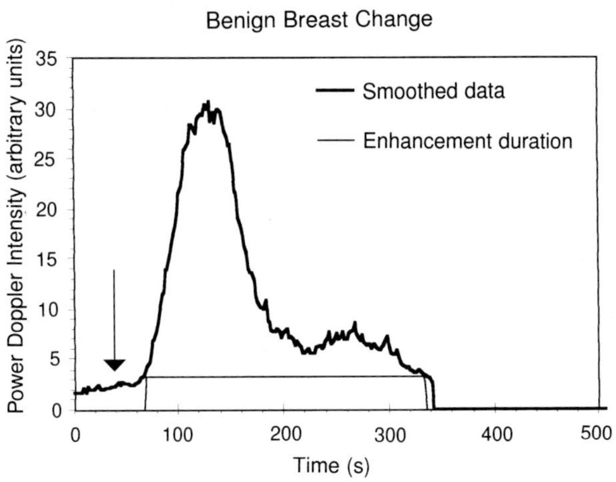

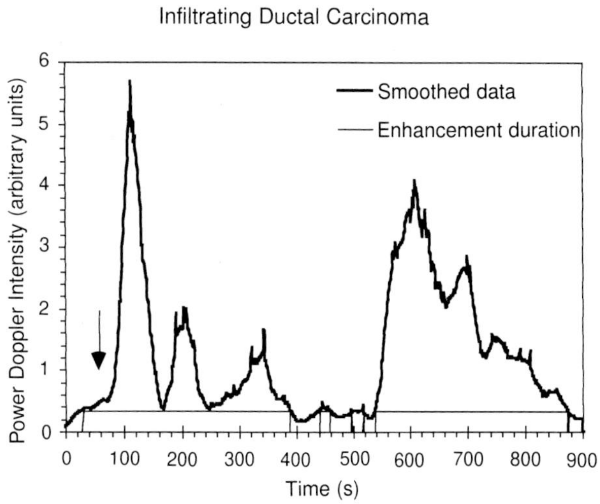

Fig. 31.2. Comparison of typical time-enhancement curves of a benign (**a**) and a malignant lesion (**b**) of the power Doppler signal after EchoGen injection (*arrow* = time of injection). The benign lesion (**a**) shows regular, monophasic wash-out after peak enhancement. The overall enhancement duration is relatively short (4 min 22 s). In contrast, the time-enhancement curve of the breast carcinoma shows irregular, multiphasic wash-out after peak enhancement with several smaller later peaks. The overall enhancement duration is longer than in the case of the benign lesion (11 min 56 s).

Using subjective criteria, all 11 cancers in our study were correctly classified as malignant after contrast enhancement. Two of these were misdiagnosed as benign on the unenhanced scan. The sensitivity was thus improved from 82% precontrast to 100% postcontrast. Specificity, however, decreased from 89% precontrast to 56% postcontrast, as four of the nine benign lesions (three benign breast changes and one fibroadenoma) also showed several suspicious vessels within the lesion after contrast. It appears, therefore, that a combination of morphologic and quantitative data may provide the best discrimination of benign from malignant breast lesions.

One situation where contrast-enhanced Doppler ultrasound of the breast appears particularly useful is the differentiation of scar tissue from local recurrence. Scar tissue is invariably avascular on contrast-enhanced Doppler ultrasound, whereas local recurrences are hypervascular. In a recent series of 20 patients studied with Levovist, local recurrences were discriminated from scar tissue with an accuracy of 100% (B.J. Hackelöer, personal communication, 1997).

31.4.4 Prostate

A few small series with Levovist have highlighted the potential of contrast-enhanced color Doppler ultrasound of the prostate. Allen and colleagues studied 20 patients (ten with carcinomas) and correctly diagnosed all cases after contrast, based on the increased vascularity in cancers. Three patients with carcinomas were thought to have benign disease on the unenhanced scans but showed hypervascularity after Levovist (Balen et al. 1993). These findings were recently confirmed by Rifkin and colleagues, who found two additional hypervascular cancers in 13 patients with prostate carcinoma after enhancement with EchoGen emulsion (Rifkin et al. 1997).

In another series of 20 patients with prostatic carcinoma – seven of them undergoing hormone treatment – marked hypervascularity was seen in all untreated cases, often with intervascular communications, presumably representing shunts. Conversely, six of the seven treated cases were strikingly less vascular, and some of them even appeared avascular on contrast-enhanced color Doppler. The one treated case in which the prostate was hypervascular had a rising prostate-specific antigen level, suggesting treatment failure (Cosgrove 1994). These results underscore the potential for treatment monitoring in the prostate. A European multicenter study of serial contrast-enhanced scans before and during medical treatment is currently under way.

In a recent pilot study, Blomley and colleagues used a dynamic, quantitative approach to examine 16 patients (ten with untreated cancers, three with treated cancers, and three with benign prostate hyperplasia) with power Doppler after the administration of Sonovue (BR1, Bracco SPA, Milan, Italy). Untreated cancers showed a substantially larger area under the curve than benign lesions and treated cancers. No difference in the area under the curve was observed between the benign lesions and the treated cancers. The untreated cancers also showed considerably longer enhancement duration, with a mean transit time almost twice that of the benign cases. The mean transit time of the treated cancers was between that of benign lesions and untreated cancers (Blomley et al. 1997c).

31.4.5 Brain

The low frequency that is required for transcranial Doppler and the attenuated signal have limited color Doppler to the assessment of main intracranial vessels. Contrast-aided ultrasound displays far more intracranial vessels, including those of brain tumors, than can be displayed precontrast. The potential of contrast-enhanced transcranial Doppler to display tumor vessels was assessed in a pilot study by Bogdahn et al. (1994). They found that, after Levovist administration in 28 patients with brain tumors, flow signals were detected in 9 of 14 low-grade lesions and in all 14 high-grade lesions. Vascularity of high-grade lesions was generally more marked than that of low-grade lesions and the former had atypical arterial and venous Doppler spectra.

31.5 Standard and Contrast-Specific B-Mode Imaging

Perfluorocarbon-stabilized microbubble agents provide gray-scale enhancement of vessels and tissues with standard B-mode imaging, including those of the liver. While imaging liver tumors, a triple-phase enhancement pattern was observed (Fig. 31.3) (Mattrey et al. 1995; Girard et al. 1998a). The initial arterial phase was shimmering enhancement of the tumor's vascular portions that were hyperechoic relative to the surrounding liver and the tumor center; this corresponded with the arrival of the contrast agent through the hepatic arterial system. When the contrast agent reached the portal vein 10–20 s later, the liver parenchyma enhanced. During this phase, although tumor rim enhancement and shimmering were still observed, the progressive enhancement of the surrounding liver caused the echogenicity differential between the liver and the vascularized portion of the tumor to fade, and the differential between the liver and the nonvascularized portion to increase. During the final enhancement phase, the liver parenchyma continued to enhance, surpassing all regions of the tumor and converting the entire tumor into a hypoechoic focus. The parenchymal enhancement phase continued for several minutes.

The dynamic nature of contrast sonography, where bubble delivery, distribution, and elimination can be observed in real time, is a powerful capability that is unique to sonography and is the only technique applicable at the patient's bedside. The ability to observe the ultrasound contrast agent on B-mode imaging as it traverses the hepatic circulation has the potential to improve lesion characterization. This would be a significant advance, given that the sonographic appearance of most entities is nonspecific. Kudo et al. (1992) and Veltri et al. (1994) showed that lesion characterization was possible with intra-arterial injection of carbon dioxide. Data are not yet available to determine whether similar results can be obtained from intravenous injections. Using intermittent imaging and flash echo techniques, Moriyasu et al. (1998) suggested that it was possible to distinguish hemangiomas from hepatocellular carcinomas.

It should be noted, however, that imaging the liver and spleen with contrast will be the most challenging application of contrast sonography. This is due to entrapment of microbubbles in the liver, causing significant attenuation. Although bubbles will be first destroyed from the near field, allowing the gradual assessment of the liver from the near to the far field, the imaging time window will likely be agent-specific and short. The solution to this problem may be the use of contrast-specific imaging techniques that increase image contrast, allowing the use of smaller doses to avoid potential attenuation. These techniques are discussed in more detail elsewhere in this book. They will be presented in this chapter briefly and specifically, as they relate to tumor imaging.

31.5.1 Transient Response Imaging

Transient response imaging, also called stimulated acoustic emission (SAE) transient scattering, loss of correlation (LOC) imaging, or sono-scintigraphy, is a microbubble-specific effect that utilizes the standard Doppler circuitry and software on commercially available units. As the Doppler technique is a multipulse sequence that aims to detect a difference in backscatter from each voxel between two consecutive pulses, and as many bubbles are destroyed by the first pulse, a difference in backscatter

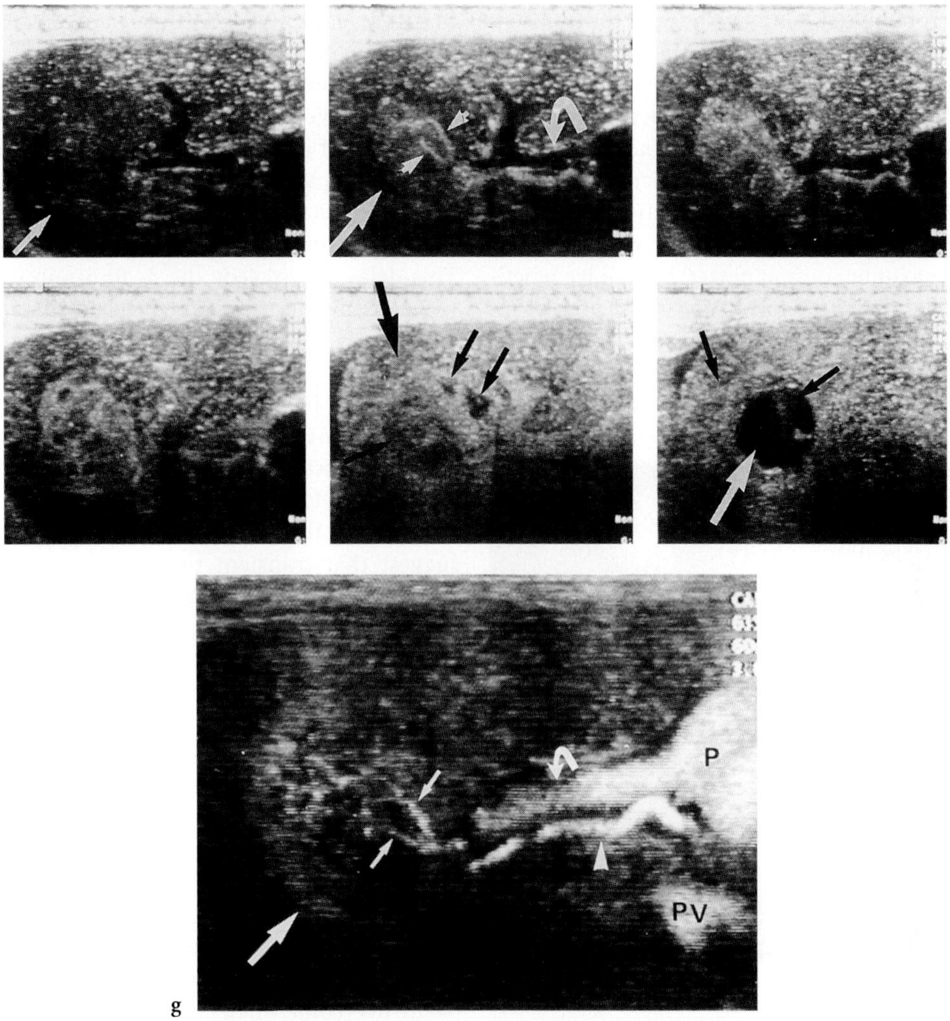

a,b c
d,e f
g

Fig. 31.3. Several frames from a real-time series were acquired following 0.5-ml bolus of AF0150 (Imagent, Alliance Pharmaceutical Corp., San Diego, Calif., USA) while imaging a moderate size V × 2 tumor in a rabbit liver. Precontrast (**a**), the tumor (*arrow*) was slightly hypoechoic to liver. During the early arterial phase (**b**), the hepatic artery (*arrowhead*) fills with contrast while the portal vein (*curved arrow*) remains anechoic. Tumor vessels become visible (*small arrows*) and the tumor (*arrow*) becomes slightly hyperechoic. Several frames later (**c**), while the portal vein (*curved arrow*) remains anechoic, the tumor (*arrow*) becomes hyperechoic and the tumor vessels are no longer visible. When contrast reaches the portal vein (*curved arrow*) (**d**), the liver enhances. During the late portal phase (**e**), the vascular portion of the lesion (*arrows*) is isoechoic with liver; however, areas of necrosis or hypoperfusion (*small arrows*) become hypoechoic. During the parenchymal phase, 2–3 min later (**f**), the liver is more echogenic than tumor, including both the necrotic (*arrow*) and solid regions (*small arrow*). With wideband imaging (**g**) acquired during the portal and equilibrium phases, the tortuous feeding hepatic artery (*arrowhead*) is again visible and is more echogenic than the portal vein (*curved arrow*), and the latter is more echogenic than liver. Tumor vessels (*small arrows*) are again visible within the tumor. *P*, Main portal vein; i = inferior vena cava

is detected from voxels containing bubbles, whether or not they are in motion. This difference, related to bubble loss rather than motion, has a characteristic mosaic-like color overlay when color maps are used (Fig. 31.4), and a bright overlay when gray-scale maps are used (Fig. 31.5).

Transient response imaging has been best demonstrated with SHU563 (Schering AG, Berlin, Germany) (Hauff et al. 1997), a novel encapsulated agent that is now in clinical trials. After an initial blood pool phase, the stiff-shell microbubbles accumulate in the reticuloendothelial cells of the liver and spleen. As tumors lack such cells, lesions of the liver or spleen stand out as focal color voids against a background of diffuse polychromatic color. In animal trials, very small lesions a few millimeters in diameter could be visualized under ideal imaging conditions (Bauer et al. 1997).

All microbubble systems can be used for transient response imaging; however, they are less effective than SHU563 at filling the entire liver with color, probably because they achieve lesser concentration in the liver, and are more elastic and resistant to destruction. Levovist and other microbubble systems have been shown to have a reasonable, albeit transient, effect if appropriate scanner parameters are used: maximum output power, high pulse repetition frequency, and the focal zone at the area of interest (Albrecht et al. 1997b; Forsberg et al. 1997; Blomley et al. 1998a; Moriyasu et al. 1998). Work with Levovist has shown that it accumulates in the liver and spleen of dogs and humans 3 min after injection, given that these organs are not insonated (Blomley et al. 1998a). In their study of more than 100 patients, signal generated from Levovist showed that the effect persists for up to 30 min after contrast administration, so long as no imaging is performed. This delay far exceeds the 3- to 5-min duration of vascular enhancement. The mechanism of this accumulation is as yet unknown. The two possible explanations are uptake by the reticuloendothelial cells or entrapment in the sinusoids. Using the transient response generated from Levovist, detection of new lesions not seen on B-mode was possible (Blomley et al. 1998b) (Fig. 31.6).

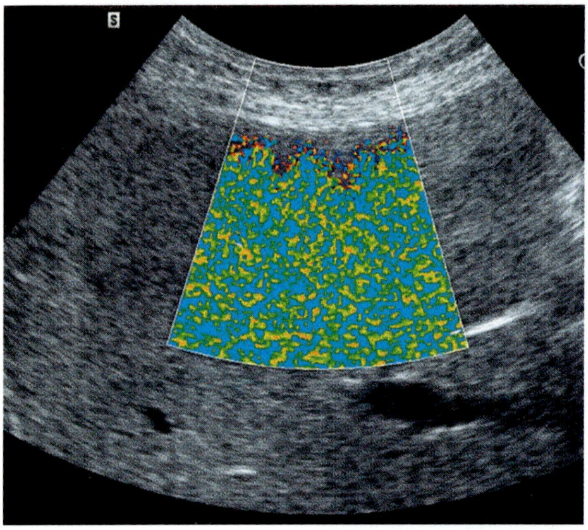

Fig. 31.4. Characteristic mosaic-like pattern of the stimulated acoustic emission signals of liver parenchyma displayed in color Doppler mode after Levovist injection

Although these early results are encouraging and suggest that transient response imaging may improve the detection of metastases, the technique has some limitations. First, there is a depth limitation, in that sufficient power must be deposited to destroy bubbles with the first pulse. This has not proved possible deeper than 12–13 cm. Second, the effect is highly dependent on the position of the focal zone, and therefore hardly ever covers the entire field of view. Multiple focal zones for color Doppler may overcome this limitation. Third, with Levovist, the effect is transient and fades after two or three frames, requiring the use of cine loop to review the frozen images. However, scanning the entire liver is hardly feasible with this approach. The latter limitation is partly overcome when late-generation microbubbles are infused (Moriyasu et al. 1998).

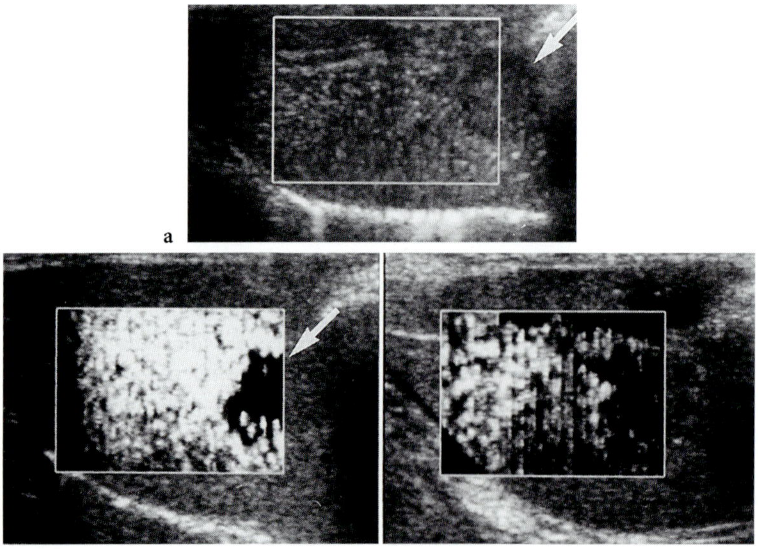

a

b,c

Fig. 31.5. Transverse views of a small V × 2 tumor (*arrow*) placed half within and half outside the "burst-mode" overlay box while scanning at very low power (**a**) following the bolus injection of 0.5 ml AF0150 (Imagent). When the "burst-mode" is applied (high-power double pulse), the tumor (*arrow*) within the overlay is essentially anechoic relative to the signal-filled liver because of the high bubble content of the liver (**b**). The second burst (**c**), applied 1 s later, shows less contrast in the liver, as an insufficient number of bubbles have replenished the vascular spaces within the liver

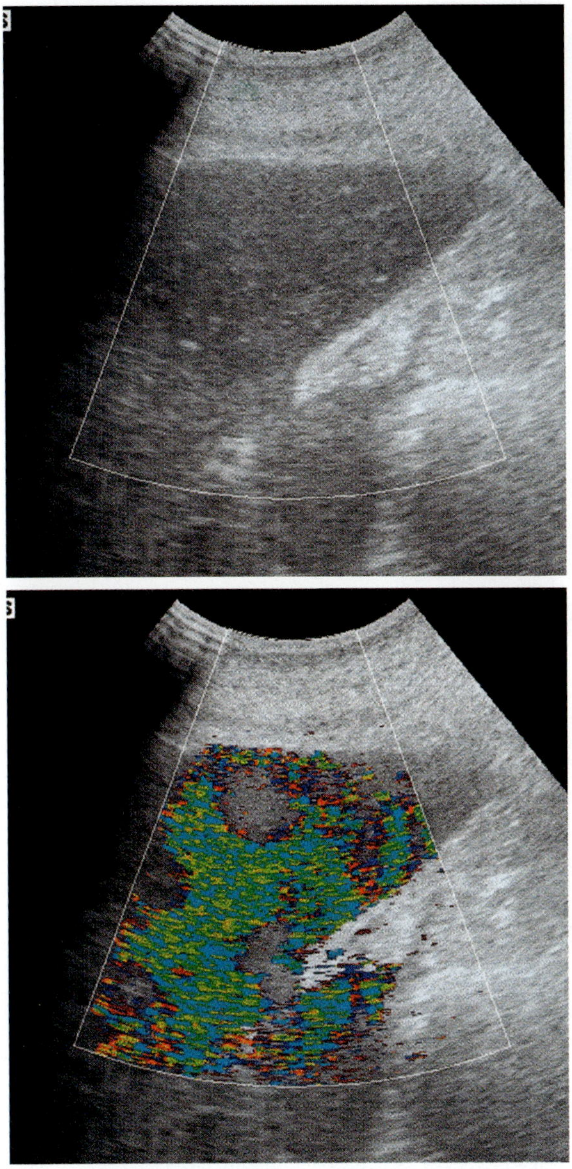

a

b

Fig. 31.6 a,b. Improved detection of liver metastases with stimulated acoustic emission in a patient with histologically proved extensive cholangiocarcinoma metastases. The B-mode image (**a**) of the left lobe of the liver shows a somewhat heterogeneous parenchyma but no definite focal lesions. The stimulated acoustic emission image (**b**) obtained in the identical position after Levovist shows multiple metastases

31.5.2 Second Harmonic Imaging

Similar to transient response imaging, second harmonic imaging highlights the voxels containing bubbles; however, it does so by suppressing signal from non-bubble-containing voxels, and requires minor modification of the unit. This technique relies on the fact that bubbles generate harmonics of the transmitted frequency, whereas tissues do not. By creating images from the signal received at twice the transmitted frequency, high image contrast is achieved between regions with and without bubbles (Burns et al. 1992). With the second harmonic technique, vessels are hyperechoic to surrounding perfused tissues, and the latter, hyperechoic relative to less perfused or nonperfused tissues such as tumors and regions of necrosis or infarction (Girard et al. 1998b). Second harmonic imaging has been used in B-mode imaging to increase tumor detection (Kono et al. 1997). When the second harmonic technique was combined with intermittent imaging, Moriyasu et al. (1998), using FS069 (Optison, Molecular Biosystems, San Diego, Calif., USA), showed that image contrast became dependent upon blood flow and blood volume differences. This added capability improved the detection and characterization of hepatocellular carcinoma.

31.5.3 Wideband Harmonic Imaging

Because second harmonic imaging relies on narrow bandwidth transmission, it suffers from lower spatial resolution than standard imaging. A new harmonic imaging technique that utilizes broadband transmission delivers two pulses, the second pulse 180° out of phase with the first. As tissue scatterers behave similarly during the high- and low-pressure phases of the pulse, the reflections from the first and second pulses are equal and opposite. The slight delay between the two pulses results in near-complete cancellation and a weak signal. Bubbles, on the other hand, behave differently during the high- and low-pressure phases of the pulse, generate harmonics, and can be destroyed by the first pulse. Therefore, reflections from voxels containing bubbles with the first and second pulses are different, resulting in a strong signal (Fig. 31.7). Further, scatterers entering the field after the first pulse is delivered, and those with sufficient velocity, do not subtract efficiently, thus providing signal that is greater when the scatterer is a microbubble. The resultant image has high contrast between regions with and regions without microbubbles. More importantly, because of the dependence on velocity, arteries are brighter than veins, veins brighter than perfused tissues, and perfused tissues brighter than less perfused or nonperfused tissues (Fig. 31.8). This capability has allowed the visualization of small submillimeter

a,b

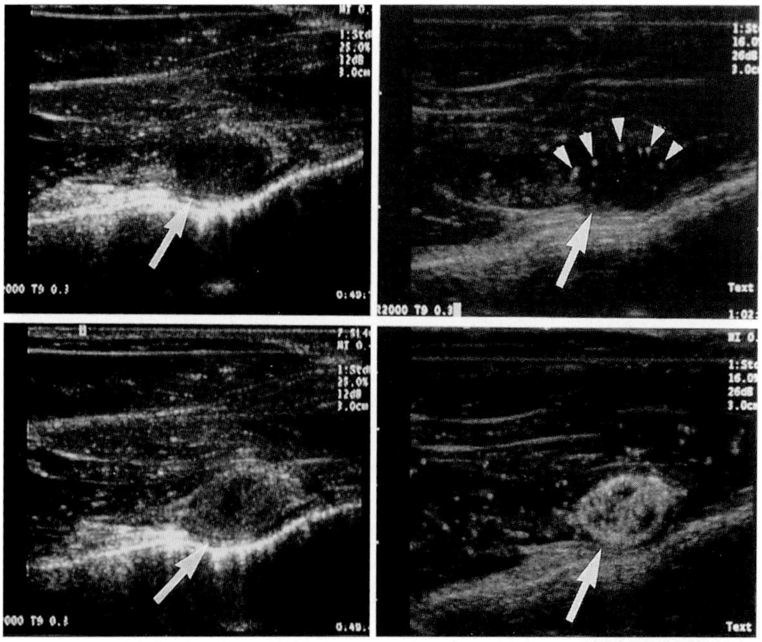

c,d

Fig. 31.7. Small V × 2 tumor implanted in the rabbit leg (*arrow*) is shown precontrast (**a**, **b**) and following 0.5 ml bolus of AF0150 (Imagent) (**c**, **d**) while imaging in standard (**a**, **c**) and wideband harmonic (**b**, **d**) imaging. Note the near-complete suppression of tissues with wideband harmonic imaging, allowing the visualization of a few persistent bubbles at the tumor periphery from an earlier injection (*arrowheads* in **b**). Although tumor enhancement is evident on standard B-mode (**c**), the poorly perfused muscle remains anechoic post contrast, allowing clear depiction of the vascular tumor (**d**)

a,b c

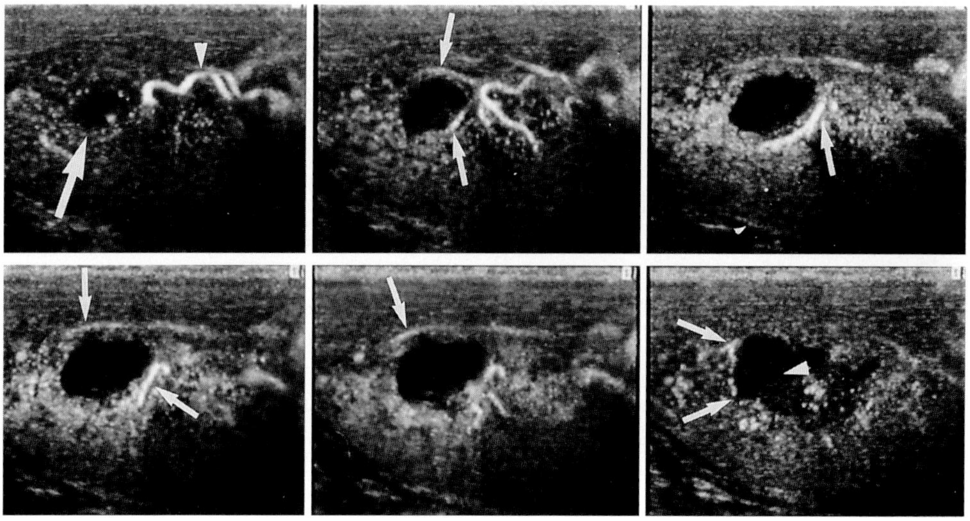

d,e f

Fig. 31.8 a–f. Several frames from a real time series was acquired in the parenchymal phase, following 0.5-ml bolus of AF0150 (Imagent) as the transducer was swept across a V × 2 tumor in a rabbit liver. Note the feeding tortuous artery (*arrowhead* in **a**) leading to the tumor (*arrow*) and coursing through the liver and branching into multiple small peripheral (*small arrows*) and deep tumor vessels (*arrowhead* in **f**)

intraparenchymal arteries and tumor neovascularity (Fig. 31.8).

Arterial visualization lasts for several minutes, and when the instrument is switched back and forth between the two techniques, vessels can only be discriminated from the enhanced background tissue with the wideband technique (Fig. 31.3). This capability is ultimately very powerful, as it highlights the feeding arteries and the abnormal tumor vessels. Improved lesion characterization is anticipated, and monitoring tumor response to therapy will be possible at high resolution.

31.5.4 Intermittent Imaging

Intermittent imaging is a technique that compensates for and capitalizes on the fact that microbubbles are destroyed by acoustic pressure. Bubble loss affects

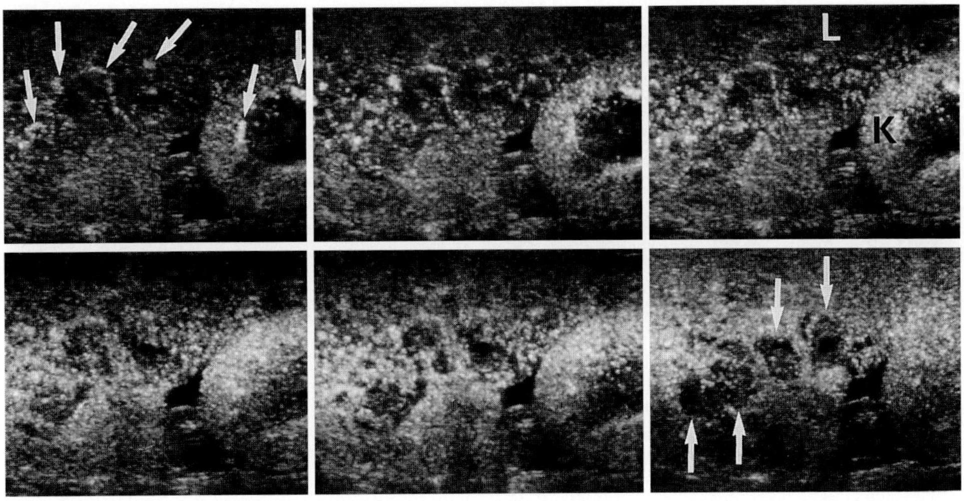

Fig. 31.9 a–f. The effect of intermittent imaging on tumor visualization is shown as a multinodular V × 2 tumor in a rabbit liver, scanned during the infusion of AF0150 (Imagent). Scanning was performed over the identical plane slice in real time (0 s delay) (**a**) and with 0.2-(**b**), 0.4-(**c**), 1-(**d**), 5-(**e**), and 10-s (**f**) delays. Note that, as the delay increases from 0 to 10 s, there is improved definition of tumor nodules and tumor margins (*arrows* in **f**). As the delay decreases, there is improved depiction of liver, kidney, and tumor vessels (*arrows* in **a**). Because short delay times increase contrast between tissues with different blood flow rates, liver (*L*) to kidney (*K*) contrast is optimal at 0.4-s delay (**c**)

not only the duration but also the degree of contrast enhancement. Intermittent imaging decreases the exposure of bubbles to the sound beam and allows fresh, unexposed bubbles to accumulate in tissues when sound is turned off (Ohmori et al. 1997). It can be accomplished by gating the acquisition to an internal pulse or to an external pulse, such as the R-wave of an electrocardiogram (Porter et al. 1997).

Because real-time scanning is necessary in radiologic applications to maintain anatomic orientation, intermittent imaging can be difficult during survey scanning. In a study using alcohol ablation as an internal standard, 1 frame/second was fast enough to allow for anatomic orientation, and slow enough to increase liver enhancement by 44% and enhancement duration by 100% relative to real-time scanning (Sirlin et al. 1998).

Because of the rapid replenishment of vessels by fresh, unexposed bubbles, and because of the faster transit rate of bubbles through the scanned plane as compared to tissues, tissue echogenicity, with intermittent imaging, is dependent upon frame rate, whereas vascular echogenicity is not (Sirlin et al. 1998). It should, therefore, be possible to image intermittently at 1 frame/second to maximize liver-to-lesion contrast, which will not permit adequate vascular delineation, and then revert to real time, to decrease tissue enhancement and promote parenchymal vascular visualization. This capability is also relevant for other tissues, such as the kidney (Figs. 31.9, 31.10).

Intermittent imaging has the potential to estimate regional flow differences. If bubbles are destroyed during the imaging phase, echogenicity on the first frame after the delay period will be dependent upon the delay time, blood flow, and fractional blood volume of the region. Contrast on images with short delay times reflects blood flow differences, whereas that of long delay times reflects blood volume differences. Although it is important to ultimately measure blood flow, in most clinical settings it is sufficient to know where regions of high or low blood flow exist.

The adjustment of the delay time was used with transient response imaging to successfully distinguish hepatocellular carcinoma from hemangioma in the liver. During FS069 infusion, the hepatocellular cancer was hyperechoic relative to liver during short delay times because of its faster arterial flow. With long delay times, the liver was hyperechoic to tumor because of its larger fractional blood volume. Hemangiomas were hypoechoic during short delay time and increased their echogenicity as the delay time was increased (Moriyasu et al. 1998).

31.6 Conclusion

In this chapter we have given an overview of the current state of contrast-enhanced sonography of tumors. Several different approaches with promising

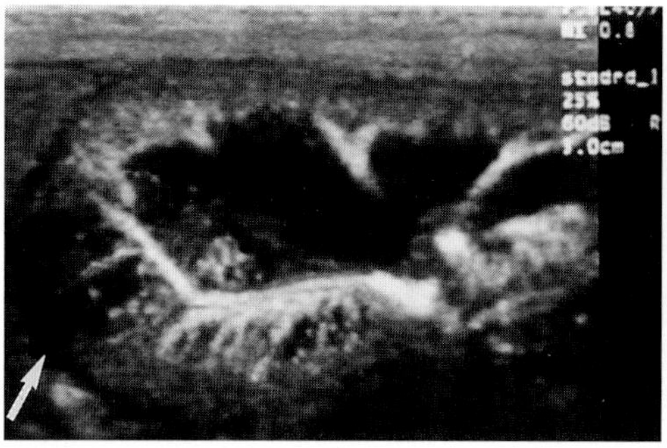

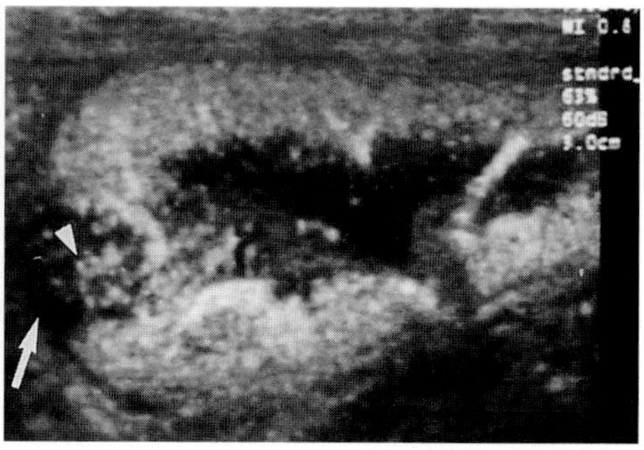

a b

Fig. 31.10. Small cortical V × 2 tumor (*arrow*) implanted in the kidney is shown during real time (**a**) and at 1 frame/second intermittent acquisition (**b**) following 0.5-ml bolus of AF0150 (Imagent). Note that normal parenchymal and tumor vessels are well seen during real-time imaging (**a**). Although vessels are not as clearly depicted with intermittent imaging (**b**), the tumor margin and contrast with normal cortex are improved, and the perfused portion of the tumor center is enhanced (*arrowhead* in **b**)

potential for the future are being explored, and some of the results are encouraging. To date, however, most studies have involved small patient numbers and, therefore, no firm conclusions can be drawn.

The introduction of several contrast-specific imaging techniques and specialized contrast media could aid in liver and spleen imaging, the most challenging applications. Although the clinical role of contrast-aided sonography of tumors has yet to be defined, the preclinical and early clinical data provide encouraging evidence that contrast media will have a significant impact on lesion detection, characterization, and monitoring.

References

Acker JC, Dewhirst MW, Honore GM, Samulski TV, Tucker JA, Oleson JR (1990) Blood perfusion measurements in human tumors: evaluation of laser Doppler methods. Int J Hyperthermia 6:287–304

Albrecht T, Blomley MJ, Urbank A, Jayaram V, Cosgrove DO, Schlief R (1997a) Doppler quantification with Levovist Infusions in vivo – a linear dose response relationship. Radiology 205(P):337

Albrecht T, Blomley MJK, Cosgrove DO, et al. (1997b) Stimulated Acoustic Emission (SAE) mit Levovist – ein leberspezifischer Kontrasteffekt. Ultraschall in der Medizin 18(Suppl):S39

Albrecht T, Patel N, Cosgrove DO, Jayaram V, Blomley MB, Eckersley R (1998) Enhancement of power Doppler signals from breast lesions with the ultrasound contrast agent EchoGen emulsion: subjective and quantitative assessment. Acad Radiol 5(Suppl 1):S195–S198

Angeli E, Carpanelli R, Crespi G, Zanello A, Sironi S, Del Maschio A (1994) Efficacy of SHU 508 A (Levovist) in color Doppler ultrasonography of hepatocellular carcinoma vascularization. Radiol Med (Torino) 87(Suppl):24–31

Baillie CT, Winslet MC, Bradley NJ (1995) Tumor vasculature – a potential diagnostic target. Br J Cancer 72:257–267

Balen FG, Allen CM, Gardener JE, Kelly I, Rickards D, Lees WR (1993) Three-dimensional imaging of blood flow in benign and malignant conditions of the prostate. Proceedings of the 51st Annual Congress of the British Institute of Radiology, p 91

Bauer A, Schlief R, Zomack M, Urbank A, Niendorf H-P (1997) Acoustically stimulated microbubbles in diagnostic ultrasound: properties and implications for diagnostic use. In: Nanda N, Schlief R, Goldberg BB (eds) Advances in echo imaging using contrast enhancement, 2nd edn. Kluwer Academic, Lancaster, pp 669–684

Blomley MJ, Albrecht T, Jayaram V, Cosgrove DO, Bell D, Bamber JC (1997a) Quantitative contrast-enhanced power Doppler ultrasound: accuracy in vivo. Radiology 205(P): 418

Blomley MJ, Albrecht T, Jayaram V, Cosgrove DO, Patel N, Urbank A (1997b) The hepatic venous response to bolus injections of the echo-enhancing agent Levovist: a novel functional imaging technique for assessing liver malignancy. Radiology 205(P):337

Blomley MJ, Cosgrove DO, Jayaram V, Eckersley R, Albrecht T, DeSouza NM, Butler-Barnes J (1997c) Quantitation of enhanced transrectal ultrasound of the prostate: work in progress using the echo-enhancing agent BR1. Radiology 205(P):280

Blomley M, Albrecht T, Cosgrove D, et al. (1998a) Stimulated acoustic emission imaging ("sono-scintigraphy") with the ultrasound contrast agent Levovist: a reproducible Doppler ultrasound effect with potential clinical utility. Acad Radiol 5(Suppl 1):S236–S239

Blomley M, Albrecht T, Cosgrove DO, et al. (1998b) Improved imaging of liver metastases using stimulated acoustic emission in the late enhancement phase of the ultrasound contrast agent Levovist. Radiology (in press)

Bogdahn U, Fröhlich T, Becker G, et al. (1994) Vascularization of primary central nervous system tumors: detection with contrast-enhanced color-coded real-time sonography. Radiology 192:141–148

Boucher Y, Leunig M, Jain RK (1996) Tumor angiogenesis and interstitial hypertension. Cancer Res 56:4264–4266

Brasch RC, Daldrup H, Shames D, Wendland M, Okuhata Y, Rosenau W (1998) Macromolecular contrast media-enhanced MRI estimates of microvascular permeability correlate with histopathologic tumor grade. Acad Radiol 5(Suppl 1):S2–S5

Burns PN, Powers JE, Fritzsch T (1992) Harmonic imaging: new imaging and Doppler method for contrast-enhanced ultrasound. Radiology 185(P):142

Campani R, Bozzini A, Calliada F, Botenelli O, Anguissola R, Conti MP, Corsi G (1994) Color Doppler imaging of liver metastases. The value phase III of a ultrasound contrast agent: SHU 508A (Levovist) Schering. Radiol Med (Torino) 87(Suppl):32–40

Correas JM, Hélénon O, Menassa L, Moreau JF (1997) Renal ultrasonography: the additional value of ultrasound contrast agents. Eur J Ultrasound 6(Suppl 2):S27

Cosgrove DO (1995) TRUS with contrast agents in carcinoma of the prostate. In: Muphy G, Khoury S, Chatelain C, Denis L (eds) Proceedings of the fourth international symposium on recent advances in urological cancer, 1994. Scientific Communications International, Jersey, pp 131–141

Fillipone A, Muzi M, Basilico R, Di Giandomenico V, Trapani AR, Bonomo L (1994) Color flow imaging of renal disease. Value of a new intravenous contrast agent: SH U 508 H (Levovist). Radiol Med (Torino) 87(Suppl):50–58

Folkman J, Merler E, Abernathy C, Williams G (1971) Isolation of a tumor factor responsible for angiogenesis. J Exp Med 133:275–288

Forsberg F, Goldberg BB, Liu JB, Merton DA, Rawool NM (1996) On the feasibility of real-time, in vivo harmonic imaging with proteinaceous microspheres. J Ultrasound Med 15:853–860

Forsberg F, Goldberg BB, Liu J, Merton DA, Fujimoto M, Johnson DK (1997) Detection of hepatic VX-2 tumors in rabbits with ultrasound contrast and induced acoustic emission. Radiology 205(P):280

Gammill SL, Shipkey FH, Himmelfarb EH, Parvey LS, Rabinowitz JG (1976) Roentgenology-pathology correlative study of neovascularity. AJR 126:376–385

Girard MS, Sirlin CB, Baker KG, Deiranieh LH, Mattrey RF (1998a) B-mode enhancement of the liver with microbubble contrast: a blinded study in rabbits with VX2 tumors. Acad Radiol 5 (Suppl 1):S189–S191

Girard MS, Mattrey RF, Baker KG, Peterson T, Deiranieh LH, Steinbach GC (1998b) Comparison of standard and second harmonic b-mode sonography in the detection of renal infarction with ultrasound contrast in a rabbit model. J Ultrasound Med (in press)

Hauff P, Fritzsch T, Reinhardt M, Weitschies W, Luders F, Uhlendorf V, Heldmann D (1997) Delineation of experimental liver tumors in rabbits by a new ultrasound contrast agent and stimulated acoustic emission. Invest Radiol 32:94–99

Hosten N, Steger W, Bechstein WO, et al. (1997) Vaskularisationsmuster in fokalen Leberläsionen: Vergleich der nativen und signalverstärkten amplitudenmodulierten Farbduplexsonographie. Fortschr Röntgenstr 166:507–513

Jain RK (1988) Determinants of tumor blood flow: a review. Cancer Res 48:2641–2658

Kedar RP, Cosgrove DO, Smith IE, Mansi JL, Bamber JC (1994) Breast carcinoma: measurement of tumor response to primary medical therapy with color Doppler flow imaging. Radiology 190:825–830

Kedar RP, Cosgrove DO, McCready VR, Bamber JC, Carter ER (1996) Microbubble contrast agent for color Doppler ultrasound: effect on breast masses. Work in progress. Radiology 198:679–686

Kono Y, Moriyasu F, Mine Y, et al. (1997) Gray-scale second harmonic imaging of the liver with galactose-based microbubbles. Invest Radiol 32:120–125

Kudo M, Tomita S, Tochio H, et al. (1992) Sonography with intraarterial infusion of carbon dioxide microbubbles (sonographic angiography): value in differential diagnosis of tumors. AJR 158:65–74

Leen E, Angerson WJ, Warren HW, O'Gorman, Moule B, Carter EC, McArdle CS (1994) Improved sensitivity of colour Doppler flow imaging of colorectal hepatic metastases using galactose microparticals: a preliminary report. Br J Surg 81:252–254

Less JR, Skalak TC, Sevick EM, Jain RK (1991) Microvascular architechture in a mammary carcinoma. Cancer Res 51:265–273

Maeda M (1979) Die weibliche Brust – neue angiographische Kenntnisse. Fortschr Röntgenstr 130:711–715

Maresca G, Barbaro B, Summaria V, De Gaetano AM, Salcuni M, Mirk P, Marano P (1994) Color Doppler ultrasonography in the differential diagnosis of focal hepatic lesions. The SHU 508A (Levovist) experience. Radiol Med 87(Suppl):41–49

Mattrey RF (1989) Perfluorooctylbromide: a new contrast agent for CT, sonography, and MR imaging. AJR Am J Roentgenol 152:247–252

Mattrey RF, Baker KG, Hall LA, Peterson T, Steinbach GC (1995) Liver lesion detection using a perfluorocarbon gas based ultrasound contrast agent. AIUM, San Francisco J Ultrasound Med 14:S21

Mattrey RF, Steinbach G, Lee Y, Wilkening W, Lazenby J (1998) High-resolution harmonic gray-scale imaging of normal and abnormal vessels and tissues in animals. Acad Radiol 5(Suppl 1):S63–S65

Mitsuzaki K, Yamashita Y, Ogata I, Nishiharu T, Urata J, Takahashi M (1996) Multiple-phase helical CT of the liver for detecting small hepatomas in patients with liver cirrhosis: contrast-injection protocol and optimal timing. AJR 167:753–757

Moore JV, West DC (1991) Vasculature as a target for anticancer therapy, 1st edn. Taylor and Francis, London

Moriyasu F, Kono Y, Kamiyama N, et al. (1998) Flash echo imaging of liver tumors using ultrasound contrast agent and intermittent color Doppler scanning. J Ultrasound Med 17:S63

Ohmori K, Cotter B, Kwan OL, Mizushige K, DeMaria AN (1997) Relation of contrast echo intensity and flow velocity to the amplification of contrast opacification produced by intermittent ultrasound transmission. Am Heart J 134:1066–1074

Porter TR, Li S, Kricsfeld D, Armbruster RW (1997) Detection of myocardial perfusion in multiple echocardiographic windows with one intravenous injection of microbubbles using transient response second harmonic imaging. J Am Coll Cardiol 29:791–799

Rifkin MD, Albany NY, Tublin ME, Chjeruvu SK, Li S, Ross J (1997) Ultrasound contrast enhanced color Doppler: initial results in the evaluation of the prostate. Radiology 205(P):280

Riley V (1976) Erythrocyte sedimentation rate in breast cancer. Science 191:86–88

Sevick EM, Jain RK (1988) Blood flow and venous pH of tissue isolated Walker 256 carcinoma during hyperglycemia. Cancer Res 48:1201–1207

Sirlin CB, Girard MS, Baker KG, Steinbach GC, Deiranieh LH, Mattrey RF (1998) Effect of acquisition rate on liver and portal vein enhancement with microbubble contrast. J Ultrasound Med Biol (in press)

Solbiati L, Lerace T, Crespi L, Rizato G (1996) Three-dimensional power Doppler with an intravascular echo enhancement agent and second harmonic imaging in radiofrequency ablation of liver metastases. Radiology 201(P):196

Srivastava A, Laidler P, Davies R, Horgan K, Hughes LE (1988) The prognostic significance of tumor vascularity in intermediate thickness (0.76–4 mm thick) skin melanoma. Am J Pathol 133:419–423

Strickland B (1959) The value of arteriography in the diagnosis of bone tumors. Br J Radiol 32:705–713

Strunk HM, Textor J, Hortling N, Schild HH (1998) Native and signal-enhanced power Doppler sonography for characterization of liver lesions (in German). Rofo Fortschr Geb Rontgenstr Neuen Bildgeb Verfahr 168:344–351

Tietjen GW, Chien S, Scholtz P, Gump FE, Kinney JM (1977) Changes in blood viscosity and plasma proteins in carcinoma. J Surg Oncol 9:53–59

Vaupel PW (1994) Blood flow, oxygenation, tissue pH distribution, and bioenergetic status of tumors, 1st edn. Ernst Schering Foundation, Berlin, pp 7–14

Vaupel P, Fortmeyer HP, Runkel S, Kallinowski F (1987) Blood flow, oxygen consumption and tissue oxygenation of human breast cancer xenografts in nude rats. Cancer Res 47:3496–3503

Veltri A, Capello S, Faissola B, Spalluto F, Farinet S, Grosso M (1994) Dynamic contrast-enhanced ultrasound with carbon dioxide microbubbles as adjunct to arteriography of liver tumors. Cardiovasc Intervent Radiol 17:133–137

Weidner N, Semple JP, Welch WR, Folkman J (1991) Tumor angiogenesis and metastasis – correlation in invasive breast carcinoma. N Engl J Med 324:1–8

Weskott HP, Brands A (1997) Transpulmonary ultrasound contrast agent helps to characterize small renal masses. Radiology 205(P):242

32 Tissue Perfusion and Enhancement on Gray-scale

R.F. Mattrey and M.S. Girard

CONTENTS

32.1 Introduction

The availability of contrast agents has conferred upon computed tomography (CT) and magnetic resonance imaging (MRI) the ability to expand beyond anatomic depiction of normal and diseased tissues. Using intravenous contrast, which is common practice with CT and MR, these modalities provide information on the relative vascularity of a suspect lesion and, with repeated observations, the wash-in and wash-out patterns of the agent to allow for lesion characterization (Barentsz et al. 1996).

The common thinking to date, driven by the limited capabilities of the Doppler enhancing agents, has been that ultrasound contrast agents are of value to enhance vessels and Doppler signal. However, the new generation of microbubbles has the potential to enhance tissues on standard gray-scale sonography, thus conferring the capabilities of CT and MR agents on sonography. The ability to distinguish tissues, based on differing degrees and characteristics of vascularity, stands to broaden the scope of ultrasound's diagnostic potential while maintaining its many advantages, including lack of ionizing radiation, wide availability, portability, and lesser cost. Further, ultrasound offers real-time imaging at very high frame rates when compared with CT and MRI, thereby providing an additional parameter with which to assess the malignant potential of lesions (Barentsz et al. 1996).

Although Doppler signal is easily enhanced by contrast media, Doppler techniques are suboptimal for solid organ imaging postcontrast because of blooming and flash artifacts, poor spatial resolution of color Doppler, and poor temporal resolution of power Doppler. B-mode imaging has been optimized to allow real-time scanning at sufficiently high frame rates while maximizing contrast and spatial resolution.

Concomitant with the increased backscatter induced by contrast agents, there is increased attenuation, as less sound energy remains to propagate forward. Because the backscatter from contrast is at the high end of the dynamic range, standard B-mode imaging has poor resolution to differences in contrast concentration. This property requires the administration of a relatively large number of microbubbles to achieve visible B-mode contrast between the target and background tissue. The high dose worsens attenuation. Although an optimal dose could potentially exist that maximizes contrast at acceptable attenuation, the dose range would likely be narrow and agent-specific. Contrast-specific imaging techniques may provide the opportunity to maximize image contrast at a lesser dose to minimize attenuation.

This chapter will describe the tissue-enhancing properties of contrast media and their potential clinical application. Contrast-specific imaging and the ability to quantitate perfusion will also be presented.

32.2 Tissue-Enhancing Properties and Their Assessment

Although it is sufficient to accept that a region is vascular by demonstrating the existence of any vas-

R.F. Mattrey, MD, Department of Radiology, University of California, San Diego Medical Center, 200 W. Arbor Drive, San Diego, CA 92109-8756, USA
M.S. Girard, MD, c/o R.F. Mattrey, MD, Department of Radiology University of California, San Diego Medical Center, 200 W. Arbor Drive, San Diego, CA 92109-8756, USA

cular flow within it, such an approach does not allow an objective assessment of the degree of vascularity or vascularity relative to background tissue. Further, when assessing tissue perfusion with Doppler, there is a limit to resolution, as the frequency of the returned signal is filtered to eliminate signal from moving tissues. It is estimated that the minimum diameter of vessels from which flow can be detected with contrast-enhanced Doppler imaging is on the order of 50 μm, which limits visualization to arterioles and venules with sufficiently high flow to be detected. Since most of the blood volume is in capillaries, Doppler techniques are severely handicapped.

Gray-scale imaging makes no assumptions relating to flow or motion. It strictly displays the location and intensity of the received signal. This characteristic places B-mode techniques at a significant advantage, as the received signal is influenced by contrast located in all tissue spaces. Further, gray-scale imaging has been optimized for maximum contrast and spatial and temporal resolution that exceed those of color or power Doppler techniques.

Numerous agents are under development that in the animal model have demonstrated accentuated echogenicity differences between adjacent normal and abnormal tissues (FORSBERG et al. 1995, 1997; MATTREY et al. 1994; SCHNEIDER et al. 1994; SEHGAL et al. 1995a; UNGER et al. 1997). The ability to affect tissue enhancement will allow the observer to assess the amount of contrast delivered to one region relative to another by assessing relative echogenicity.

The increase in echogenicity from contrast media is multifactorial. Backscatter signal is linearly related to the number of scatterers in the field, assuming the scatterers are of equal size. It is also related to bubble size and/or their aggregates, and the distance between them. Therefore, in regions where aggregation can occur – such as vessels of sufficiently large size and low shear rate – reflectivity would be different from that in regions where aggregation is impeded, as in small vessels or vessels with a high shear rate. Further, the relationship between backscattered signals and echogenicity is nonlinear. Echogenicity is affected by pre- and postprocessing routines and lookup tables, dynamic range, video conversion, and other factors. It should be clear that resultant echogenicity is related to contrast concentration in a complex and nonlinear fashion that is affected by anatomical, physiological, pharmacological, and instrumentation factors. Despite this, analyzing videointensity to assess tissue enhancement is a reasonable approach, short of directly measuring backscattered signal (SCHWARZ et al. 1998). After all, the relative difference in videointensity reflects what is observed on the image. However, this should be done with an internal standard and the postprocessing lookup table should be linear, as nonlinear lookup tables could over- or underemphasize the change in videointensity (SEHGAL et al. 1995b). It should be noted that, even with the availability of instruments that allow a linear display of echogenicity relative to integrated backscatter, attention to technical settings is still important (SCHWARZ et al. 1998).

Traditionally, CT, a quantitative tool, was ideally suited to assess the biodistribution and elimination of radiopaque contrast agents because of the linear relationship of attenuation to contrast concentration (MATTREY et al. 1990). With MR, the varied signals assigned to tissues based on the pulsing sequences used, and the nonlinear relationship of intensity to contrast concentration, required the use of external standards. These were easily incorporated in the scan field without interfering with the tissue response to the agent. Further, so long as the scanner was not recalibrated and the same sequence was employed, signals remained stable and reproducible over time.

Because sonography is qualitative rather than quantitative, and because the backscattered signal is dependent upon many variables other than the contrast concentration in the tissue of interest, it is difficult to objectively assess the echogenic effect of an agent on tissues. It is also not possible to incorporate an external standard, as is done with MRI, because of the difficulty in maintaining proper contact and because backscatter is in part dependent upon depth and intervening tissues. Because the sonographic agent can attenuate sound, it can interfere with the intervening tissues, thus affecting the echogenicity of the deeper region of interest (BAHR and WRIGLEY 1997). Therefore, an internal standard, located at the same depth and with the same intervening tissues as the tissue of interest, is needed to properly assess the alteration in echogenicity caused by the contrast agent.

We have described a simple method to produce an internal standard for the sonographic assessment of time-dependent changes in echogenicity (GIRARD et al. 1998a). Briefly, an alcohol injection is given to produce focal infarction in the tissue of interest under ultrasound guidance (FUJITA et al. 1996). We showed that the infarcted region was not affected by the contrast injection, except for a decrease in echogenicity at peak effect following the highest dose, likely due to attenuation (Fig. 32.1) (Girard et al. 1998a). Alternatively, any infarction – such as that produced by radiofrequency ablation, or by any other tissue destruction technique – can serve as an internal standard against which tissue echogenicity changes can be compared, thereby eliminating the influence of depth and some of the instrumentation effects.

32.3 Enhancement of Perfused Tissues

Using alcohol ablation in the liver of rabbits, we showed liver, kidney, and tumor rim enhancement with small doses of microbubble contrast (Girard et al. 1998a). Increasing dose increased the degree of enhancement and enhancement duration (Fig. 32.2).

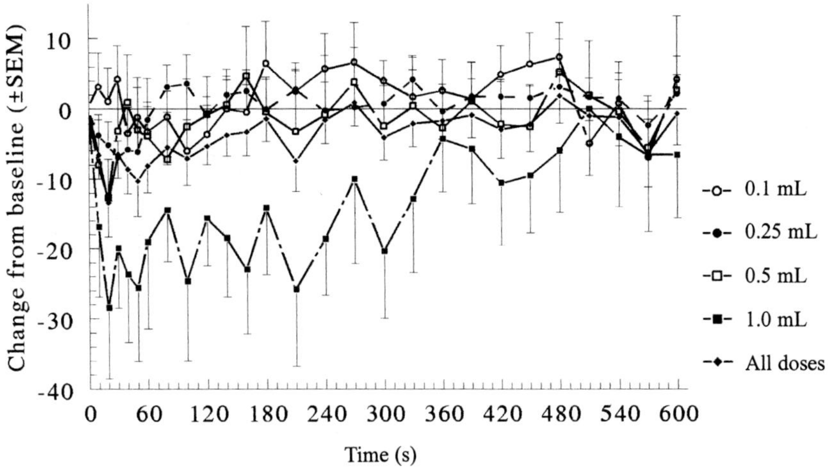

Fig. 32.1. Baseline-correctd change in videointensity of the ablated region over time for each dose. All doses show lack of enhancement with a decrease in intensity corresponding to the time period of peak enhancement in the surrounding tissues, which is pronounced after the 1.0-ml dose of AF0145 (Imagent, Alliance Pharmaceutical Corp., San Diego). Although the decrease observed following the 1.0-ml dose was not significantly different from baseline, it was significantly different from other doses. (From Girard et al. 1998a)

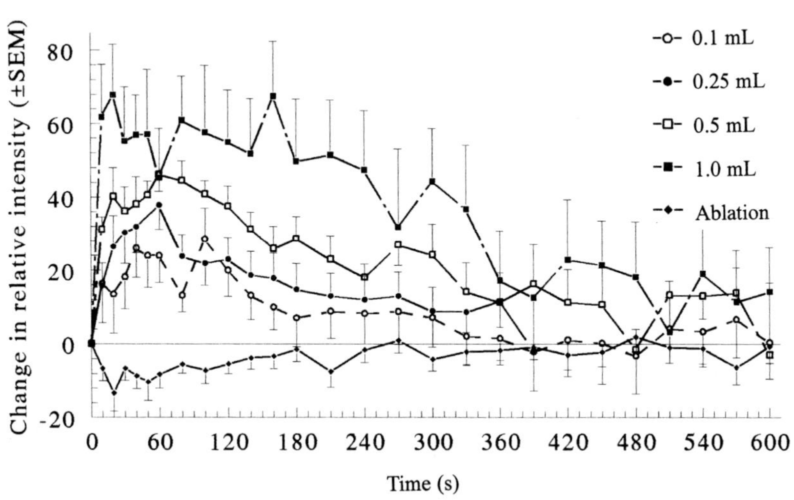

Fig. 32.2. Baseline-corrected change in videointensity of liver relative to ablated region over time for each dose of AF0150 [Imagent, Alliance Pharmaceutical Corp., San Diego, Calif. USA]. Also plotted is the average videointensity of the ablated region for all doses. The baseline-corrected liver echogenicity increased 70 gray levels postcontrast and peaked between 20 s and 1 min after the end of the saline flush; thereafter it slowly decayed, reaching baseline at 6.5 min. The decrease in videointensity of the ablated regions after the 1.0-ml dose was most likely due to increased attenuation of the intervening liver. (From Girard et al. 1998a)

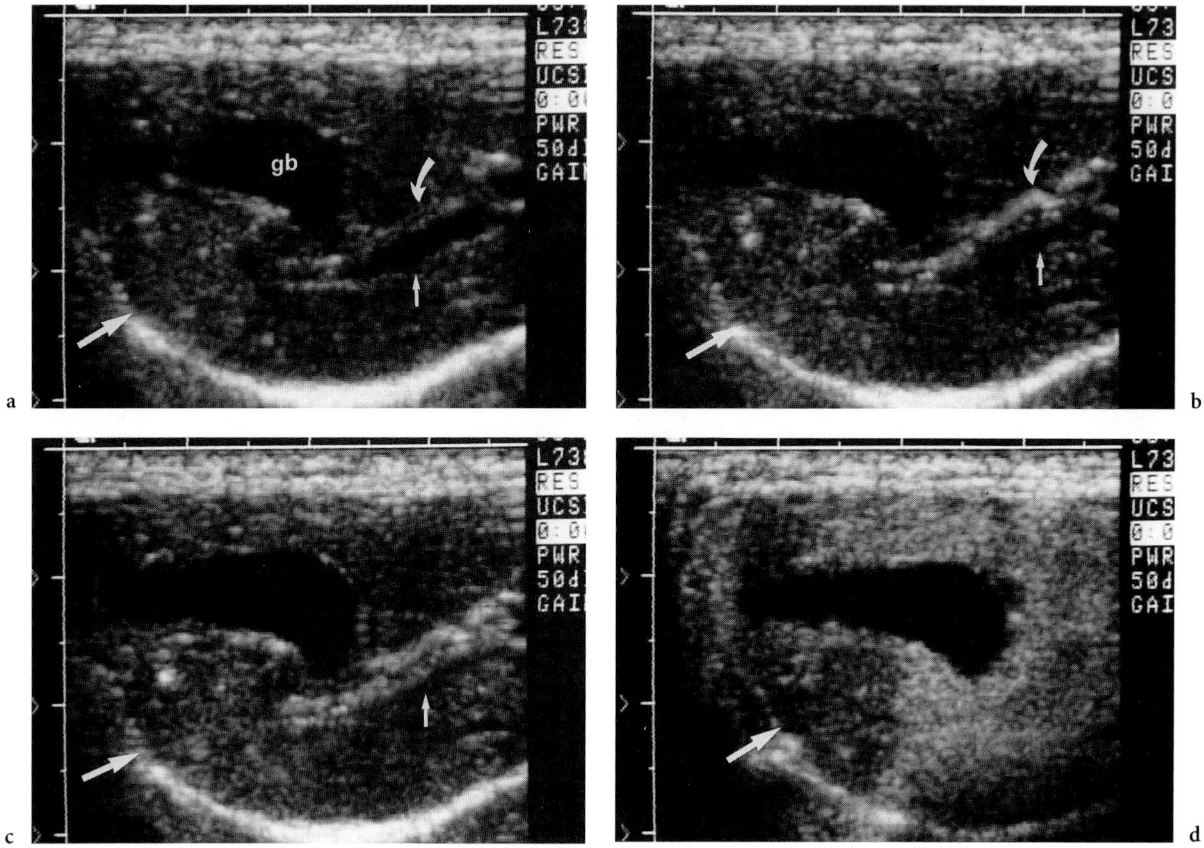

Fig. 32.3 a–d. Images from a typical rabbit with a 7-day-old alcohol lesion demonstrating liver contrast enhancement after a 0.5-ml dose of AF0150 [Imagent]. **a** Precontrast the lesion (*arrow*) is located posterior to the gallbladder (*gb*) and is echogenic relative to liver. An intrahepatic portal vein (*small arrow*) and an accompanying hepatic arterial branch (*curved arrow*) can be seen. **b** During the arterial phase, filling of the hepatic arterial branch (*curved arrow*) but not the portal vein (*small arrow*) is evident. Note that the liver is now nearly isoechoic with the lesion (*arrow*). **c** The portal vein fills with echoes (*small arrow*) early in the portal venous phase. The lesion (*arrow*) is clearly isoechoic with liver. **d** During the parenchymal phase, the liver is now more echogenic than the lesion (*arrow*). (From Girard et al. 1998a)

The baseline-corrected liver echogenicity increased significantly postcontrast, peaking between 10 and 60 s after the end of the saline flush, and slowly decayed to baseline over the following 10 min. Peak change for liver after the 1.0-ml dose (highest dose given) was approximately 70 gray levels. That translates to approximately a 14-dB increase, as we used a 50-dB dynamic range and a linear postprocessing curve. The peak of the curve at the highest dose was flat and likely underestimated true enhancement due to intervening increased attenuation.

Liver enhancement relative to the ablated region was multiphasic because of the liver's dual vascular supply. It was possible to observe the early arrival of the contrast agent through the hepatic artery and then through the portal vein. Later, during the parenchymal phase, the liver became more echogenic than the ablated area. A typical example demonstrating the change in liver echogenicity relative to an ablated region, following the injection of a 0.5-ml dose, is shown in Fig. 32.3.

Contrast administration produced prolonged enhancement of the liver in comparison to kidney and tumors, indicating hepatic entrapment. The exact mechanism for this is as yet unclear but there are two possibilities: (a) uptake of microbubbles by the reticuloendothelial cells and (b) slow microbubble transit through the sinusoids, where flow is sluggish and where the microbubbles remain until they return to the circulation or are eliminated. The latter mechanism is more likely, as bubbles tend to float when flow is slowed, as is the case in the sinusoids of the liver and spleen.

The kidney, like the liver, enhanced significantly postcontrast, but returned to baseline earlier than liver (Fig. 32.4). The maximum intensity and time to

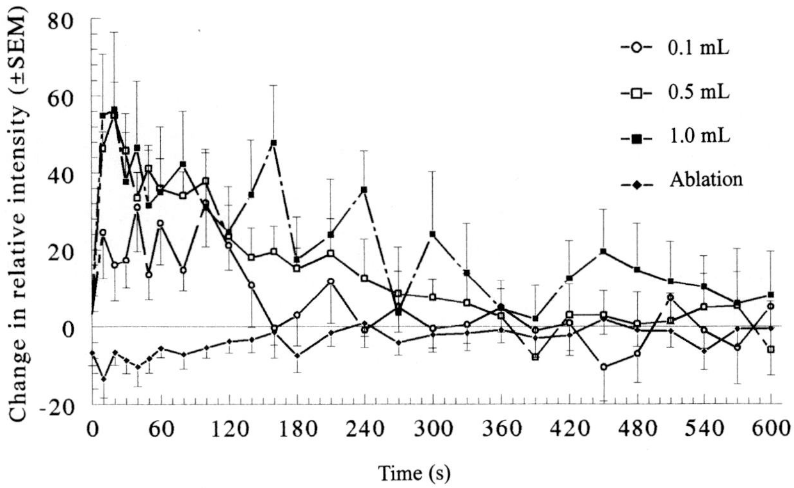

Fig. 32.4. Baseline-corrected change in videointensity of kidney relative to ablated region over time for each dose. Also plotted is the average videointensity of the ablated region for all doses. Renal cortex echogenicity increased significantly postcontrast. The change in echogenicity following the 0.1-ml dose was not significantly different from baseline. The 0.5- and 1.0-ml doses were not statistically different from each other but were both different from baseline. Peak occurred between 20–60 s after the end of the saline flush, with a return to baseline by approximately 4 min (From GIRARD et al. 1998a)

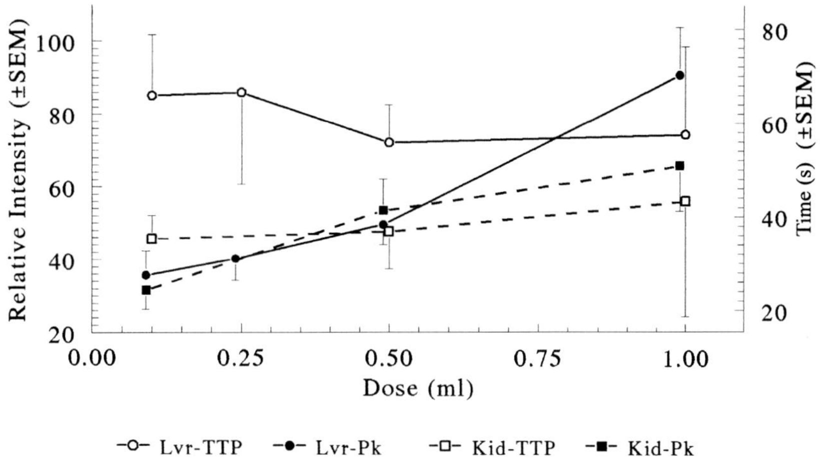

Fig. 32.5. Peak baseline-corrected intensity level (*Pk*) reached by the liver (*Lvr*) and kidney (*Kid*) are plotted along the left y-axis and the time to peak enhancement (*TTP*) is plotted along the right y-axis. Peak enhancement was statistically significant from baseline at all doses and followed a linear relationship with dose. Time to peak enhancement was unaffected by dose. (From GIRARD et al. 1998a)

peak for both liver and kidney at each dose are plotted in Fig. 32.5. Note that the peak intensity of liver and kidney had a linear response with dose. However, the time to peak enhancement for both tissues was unaffected by dose. Also note that peak liver enhancement occurred approximately 20 s later than that of kidney, as would be expected, given that 70% of liver perfusion is through the portal vein, which receives its blood from the splenic and mesenteric veins.

When the lesion in the liver is vascular, such as a Vx2 tumor, liver and tumor enhancement had a characteristic pattern because of the arterial supply of tumors. The vascular portion of the tumor enhanced early and to a greater degree than liver. As contrast reached the portal vein, liver enhancement increased to become nearly isoechoic with the vascular portion of the tumor. The liver then continued to enhance until the entire tumor became hypoechoic relative to liver. Figure 32.6 shows an example of a

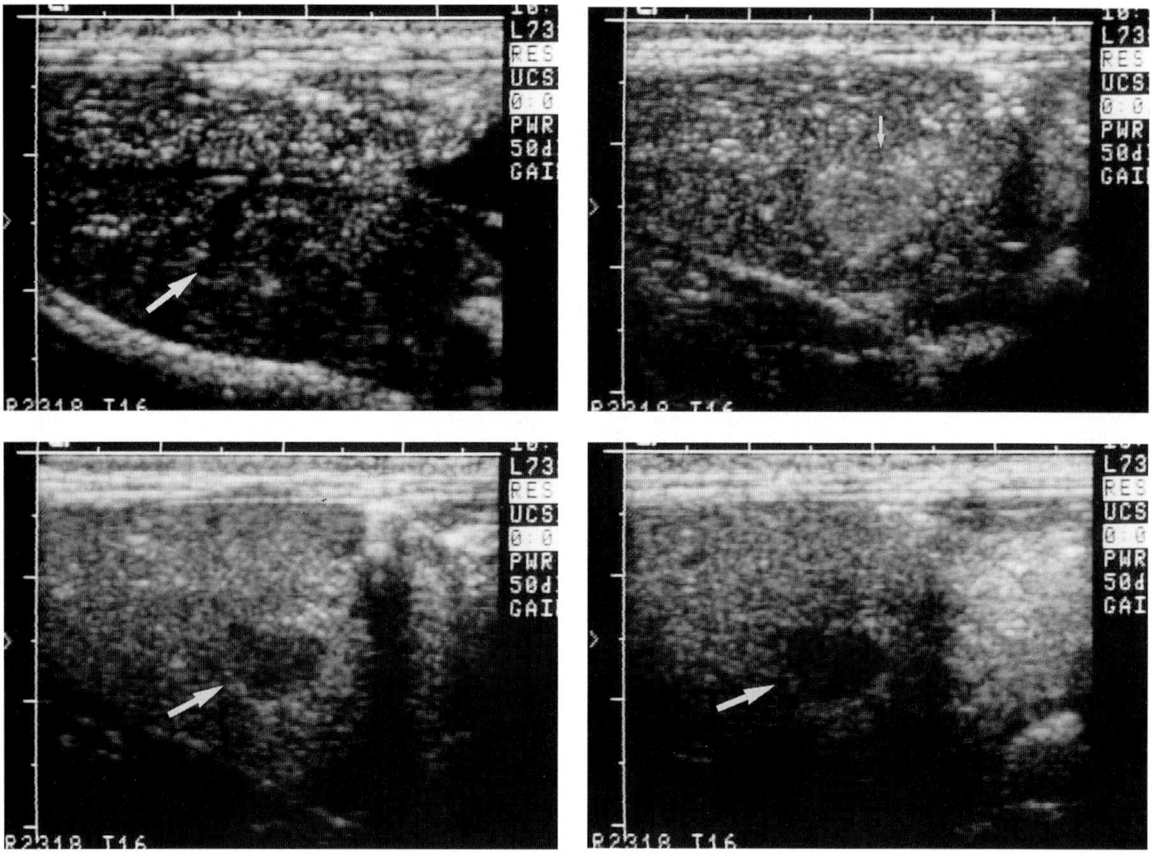

Fig. 32.6 a–d. An example of a small tumor not seen precontrast, depicting the triple-phase enhancement pattern following the injection of 0.5 ml of AF0145. Precontrast (**a**) the Vx2 tumor is essentially invisible posterior to the intrahepatic vessels (*arrow*). During the arterial phase (**b**), the liver enhances slightly; however, the vascular tumor rim enhances significantly more than liver (*small arrow*). The tumor center is enhanced on this image because it is not yet necrotic. During the portal phase (**c**), approximately 20 s later, the liver has become essentially isoechoic with the tumor rim and more echogenic than the tumor center (*arrow*). One minute later (**d**), during the parenchymal phase, the liver is markedly more echogenic than the entire tumor (*arrow*), and attenuation can be observed in the far field. (From GIRARD et al. 1998a)

tumor that was not seen precontrast, but demonstrated the typical enhancement dynamics following the administration of 0.5 ml of AF0145. When evaluating the time-intensity curve of the liver, tumor rim, and tumor center, the enhancement of the vascular tumor rim occurred earlier and was more transient than the enhancement of the liver (GIRARD et al. 1998a).

32.4 Contrast-Specific Imaging

There are several techniques that have been described that could allow the assessment of tissue perfusion. Several of these techniques utilize color or power Doppler because they utilize the standard circuitry and software of available instruments. As discussed elsewhere in this book, the specificity of the techniques to microbubbles results from the fact that they rely on bubble destruction, which occurs with the first pulse and is detected by the second pulse. As color pixels are assigned to voxels where bubbles have been lost, color assignment has no meaningful directional information. The color display appears as a mosaic of reds and blues. Since color carries no physiologic data, the lookup table can be in gray-scale rather than color.

The harmonic imaging techniques are bubble-specific because bubbles generate harmonics of the fundamental frequency that are of greater amplitude than those generated by tissues. It should also be noted that bubble destruction produces harmonics as well (BURNS et al. 1995). The aim of harmonic imaging, using either second harmonic or wideband techniques, is to decrease signal from regions con-

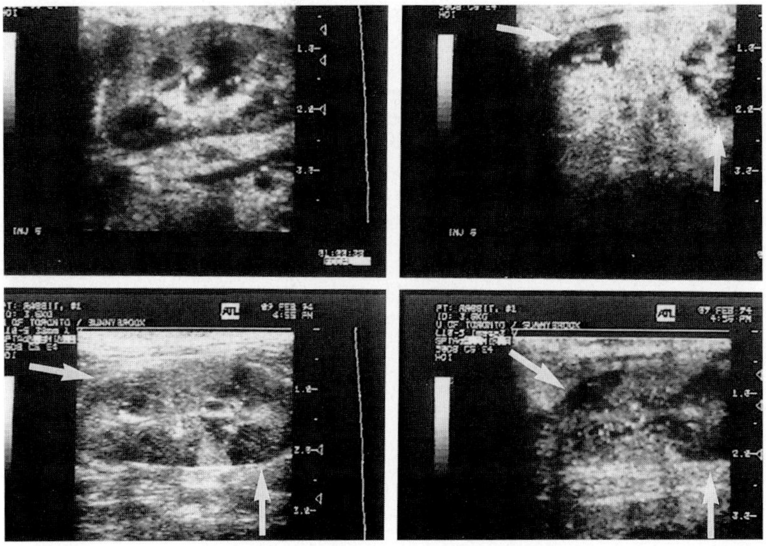

a,b

c,d

Fig. 32.7. Longitudinal scans of a rabbit kidney with multiple infarction (*arrows*) are shown before (**a**) and after 0.5-ml of AF0150 (**b–d**). The baseline second harmonic image is normal (**a**). At peak enhancement (**b**) with the second harmonic technique, two perfusion defects are clearly seen (*arrows*). Thirty seconds later, when imaged with the standard technique (**c**), the contrast between the infarctions and normal tissue is diminished. **d** Image contrast increased again when the instrument was switched back to second harmonic imaging approximately 30 s after **c** indicating that the loss of contrast in **c** with standard imaging is due to the imaging technique, not time delay

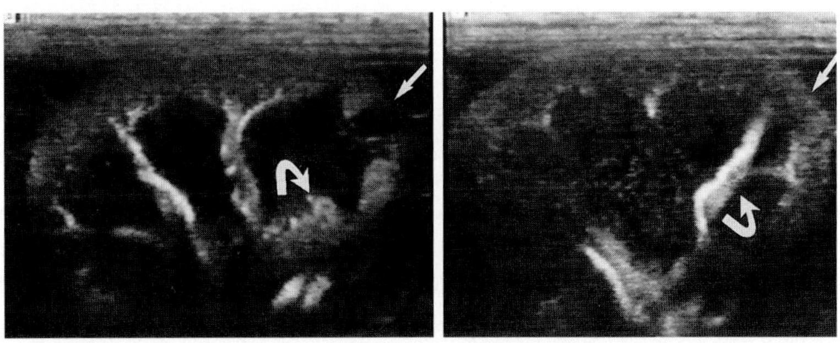

a b

Fig. 32.8. Longitudinal scans of a rabbit kidney obtained with the wideband harmonic imaging technique along the anterior (**a**) and posterior (**b**) circulation 24 h following the embolization of the renal artery with a single 1-mm bead. Note that the small infarction along the lower pole is clearly depicted (*arrow* in **a**), along the anterior circulation, while the comparable tissue supplied by normal posterior circulation is normal (*arrow* in **b**). Also note that, because the wideband technique shows intraparenchymal vessels, the occluded vessel in the anterior circulation (*curved arrow* in **a**) and its normal counterpart in the posterior circulation (*curved arrow* in **b**) are clearly depicted. This technique allows the assessment of vessels and their perfusion bed. (From Mattrey et al. 1998)

taining no contrast media, or less contrast media than the region of interest. Further, if bubbles are elastic, they have the potential to generate a second harmonic signal that is greater than that generated at the fundamental frequency. Therefore, image contrast between bubble-containing regions and background would be expected to increase. Using a rabbit model with renal infarction as an internal standard, we showed that B-mode second harmonic imaging is capable of nearly doubling image contrast and contrast duration, as compared with the standard B-mode technique (Girard et al. 1998b) (Fig. 32.7). Although the effect of wideband harmonic imaging on image contrast has not been evaluated, we would expect that, with its superior tissue suppression, image contrast would be greater than that of the second harmonic technique. However, because of its greater sensitivity to velocity, intraparenchymal vessels are well visualized. This feature allows the assessment not only of perfusion but also of the integrity of the vascular bed (Fig. 32.8). For further discussion, please refer to the chapter on contrast-specific imaging.

32.5 Potential for Quantitation of Tissue Perfusion

Although it is important to detect infarcted regions that heretofore have remained undetectable, the detection of differences in perfusion in order to diagnose arterial stenoses is even more critical. There is no vascular bed that is more important to evaluate

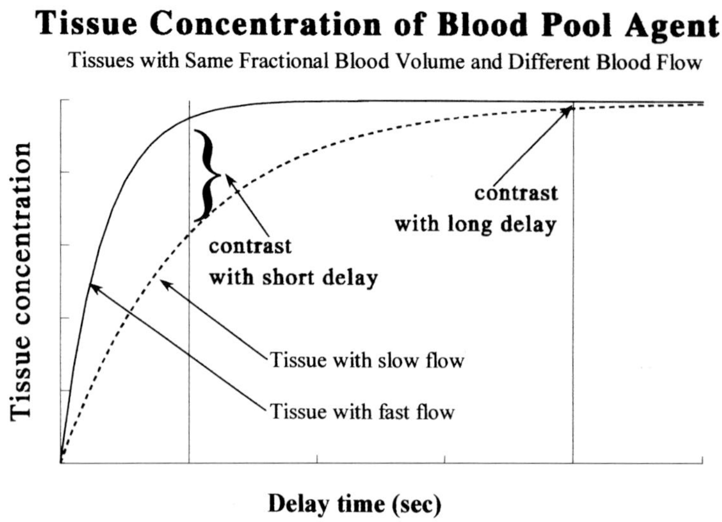

Fig. 32.9. Change in bubble concentration over time following the bolus injection of a blood pool agent. Tissue concentration grows exponentially with a time constant equal to the ratio of blood volume to blood flow, and reaches a plateau that is dependent upon the fractional blood volume of the tissue. Greater contrast is achieved between two regions with different flow rates and similar blood volume if the delay time between frames is short. This is because the blood space is nearly completely filled for the tissue with rapid flow and partially filled for the tissue with slow flow

than the coronary circulation. Several studies have attempted to assess coronary stenosis by assessing relative enhancement of the myocardium at risk as compared with normal regions, and some have attempted to quantitate blood flow (OHMORI et al. 1997; WEI et al. 1998). Although it is possible to measure videointensity (SCHWARZ et al. 1998), the relationship of echogenicity to contrast concentration is complex and multifactorial, as discussed earlier, particularly when adding the influence of bubble destruction on enhancement. To estimate myocardial perfusion, these authors reverted to intermittent imaging. For further discussion on myocardial blood flow as assessed by contrast media please refer to Chap. 33.

Intermittent imaging is a powerful technique that circumvents image contrast loss due to bubble destruction. It also allows the visualization of bubbles in vascular beds with very slow flow. The acquired frame is triggered either by an external pulse, such as the R wave of an electrocardiogram, or by an internal pulse that is software controlled. The degree of enhancement and contrast on the triggered image is dependent upon fractional blood volume, blood flow, and delay time between frames (SIRLIN et al. 1997, 1998; OHMORI et al. 1997; WEI et al. 1998). The relationship among these three factors is an exponential growth curve, where the fractional blood volume is the plateau of the curve and the time constant is the ratio of the fractional blood volume to flow rate (Fig. 32.9). The time delay will, therefore, control the contrast generated by controlling the number of bubbles delivered to each voxel. Short delay times do not allow the entire vascular space to fill, thus emphasizing flow rate differences between regions. Long delay times de-emphasize flow rate, as the entire vascular space will have been replaced by new blood with unexposed bubbles. Therefore, image contrast reflects fractional blood volume (Fig. 32.10).

By incrementing the delay time between frames, a growth curve can be reconstructed that will define the growth constant and the plateau, providing both relative blood flow and relative fractional blood volume between two regions. To truly quantitate blood flow and volume, all bubbles must be destroyed before the delay period begins. Otherwise, the residual bubbles will overestimate accumulation on the next frame. Complete bubble destruction can be assured with multiple consecutive high power pulses following the first frame and before the delay period begins.

Should bubble destruction not be complete, then the resultant image contrast, assuming constant bubble blood concentration, will be an equilibrium between the number of bubbles destroyed per frame and the number of bubbles accumulated during the delay period. Although not quantitative, this technique is still useful, as it provides a visual index of relative blood volume and blood flow between two regions. Using a similar technique, it was possible to differentiate hepatocellular carcinoma in the liver (high flow rate and low blood volume) from hemangioma (low flow rate and high blood volume) (MORIYASU et al. 1998).

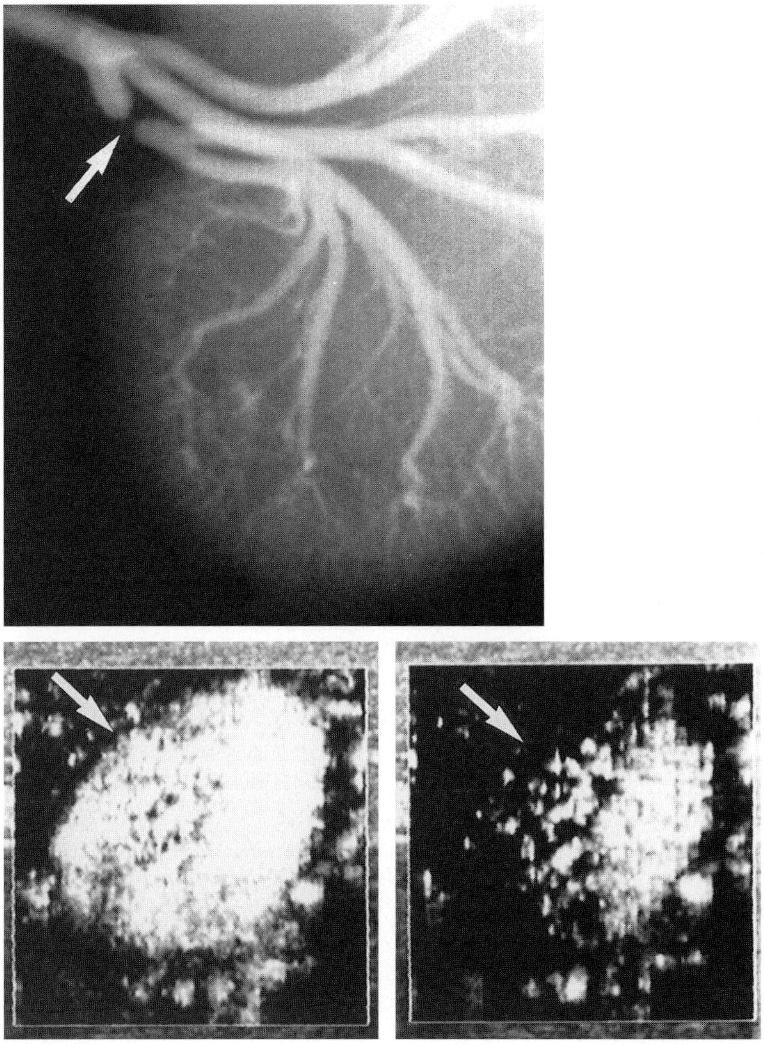

a b c

Fig. 32.10. Following a tight stenosis of a branch of the renal artery supplying the lower pole of a dog kidney (**a**), intermittent imaging was performed at 1 frame/5 s (**b**) and 1 frame/10 s (**c**) during a 1 ml/min infusion of AF0150. Note that when imaging was performed at 1 frame/5 s (**b**) the region with slow flow (*arrow*) did not enhance to the same degree as the normal region. The region with slow flow was nearly isoechoic with the normally perfusion region at 1 frame/10 s

32.6 Summary

The enhancement of perfused tissues on gray-scale has the potential to impact sonography, just as contrast media have impacted CT and MRI. The ability to distinguish vascular from nonvascular structures should make it easy to distinguish solid lesions from complex cysts, inflammation from abscess formation, hypervascular from hypovascular tumors, and so on. Further, with alteration in transmit power, image contrast can be manipulated to display vessels or tissue enhancement. The use of intermittent imaging will allow the manipulation of image contrast to display differences in blood flow rates or differences in blood volume, thereby permitting recognition of regions with high blood flow, such as tumor rim, or high blood volume, such as hemangiomas. These capabilities may prove superior to those of CT and MRI and will be available at the bedside or intraoperatively. Therefore, gray-scale enhancement of tissues with contrast media should add significantly to the clinical utility of sonography.

Acknowledgement. This work was supported in port by a grant from NIH-R01-CA36799 and Alliance Pharmaceutical Corp.

References

Bahr A, Wrigley RH (1997) Evaluation of Imagent US as an ultrasound contrast agent in normal livers and alcohol induced lesions in large dogs (abstract). J Ultrasound Med 16(Suppl):S36–S37

Barentsz JO, Jager GJ, van Vierzen PB, et al. (1996) Staging urinary bladder cancer after transurethral biopsy: value of fast dynamic contrast-enhanced MR imaging. Radiology 201:185–193

Burns PN, Fritzsch T, Weitschies W, Uhlendorf V, Hope-Simpson D, Powers JE (1995) Pseudo-Doppler shifts from stationary tissues due to the stimulated emission of ultrasound from a new microsphere contrast agent. Radiology 197(P):402

Forsberg F, Liu JB, Merton DA, Rawool NM, Goldberg BB (1995) Parenchymal enhancement and tumor visualization using a new sonographic contrast agent. J Ultrasound Med 14:949–957

Forsberg F, Goldberg BB, Liu J, Merton DA, Fujimoto M, Johnson DK (1997) Detection of Hepatic Vx-2 tumors in rabbits with ultrasound contrast and induced acoustic emission. Radiology 205(P):279

Fujita T, Ito K, Choji T, Honjo K, Arita T, Matsunaga N (1996) Hepatic parenchymal changes after ethanol injection in rabbits: correlation of conventional and dynamic MR imaging with pathologic findings. J Magn Reson Imaging 6:156–161

Girard MS, Baker KG, Steinbach GC, Deiranieh LH, Peterson TM, Mattrey RF (1998a) Assessment of liver and kidney enhancement using perfluorocarbon vapor-stabilized ultrasound contrast agent. Acad Radiol (in press)

Girard MS, Mattrey RF, Baker KG, Peterson T, Deiranieh LH, Steinbach GC (1998b) Comparison of standard and second harmonic b-mode sonography in the detection of renal infarction with ultrasound contrast in a rabbit model. J Ultrasound Med (in press)

Mattrey RF, Nemcek AA Jr., Shelton R, André MP, Mitten RM, Peterson T (1990) In vivo estimation of perfluorooctyl bromide concentration in tissues. Invest Radiol 25:915–921

Mattrey RF, Wrigley R, Steinbach GC, Schutt EG, Evitts DP (1994) Gas emulsions as ultrasound contrast agents. Preliminary results in rabbits and dogs. Invest Radiol 29:S139–S141

Mattrey RF, Steinbach G, Lee Y, Wilkening W, Lazenby J (1998) High-resolution harmonic gray-scale imaging of normal and abnormal vessels and tissues in animals. Acad Radiol 5(Suppl 1):S63–S65

Moriyasu F, Kono Y, Kamiyama N, et al. (1998) Flash echo imaging of liver tumors using ultrasound contrast agent and intermittent color doppler scanning (abstract). J Ultrasound Med 17:S63

Ohmori K, Cotter B, Kwan OL, Mizushige K, DeMaria AN (1997) Relation of contrast echo intensity and flow velocity to the amplification of contrast opacification produced by intermittent ultrasound transmission. Am Heart J 134:1066–1074

Schneider M, Broillet A, Bussat P, Ventrone R (1994) The use of polymeric microballoons as ultrasound contrast agents for liver imaging. Invest Radiol 29(Suppl 2):S149–S151

Schwarz KQ, Chen X, Steinmetz S (1998) Methods for quantifying ultrasound backscatter and two-dimensional video intensity: implications for contrast-enhanced sonography. J Am Soc Echocardiogr 11:155–168

Sehgal CM, Arger PH, Pugh CR (1995a) Sonographic enhancement of renal cortex by contrast media. J Ultrasound Med 14:741–748

Sehgal CM, Arger PH, Pugh CR (1995b) Influence of postprocessing curves on contrast-echographic imaging: preliminary studies. J Ultrasound Med 14:735–740

Sirlin CB, Girard MS, Steinbach GC, Baker KG, Broderdorf SK, Hall LA, Mattrey RF (1997) Effect of ultrasound transmit power on liver enhancement with imagent(r) US, a PFC-stabilized microbubble contrast agent. Int J Imaging Systems Technol 8:82–88

Sirlin CB, Girard MS, Baker KG, Steinbach GC, Deiranieh LH, Mattrey RF (1998) Effect of acquisition rate on liver and portal vein enhancement with microbubble contrast. J Ultrasound Med Biol (in press)

Unger EC, Fritz TA, Gertz E, Manspeaker P, Kaul S (1997) Assessment of myocardial infarct with a new ultrasound contrast agent (abstract). Radiology 205(P):419

Wei K, Jayaweera AR, Firoozan S, Linka A, Skyba DM, Kaul S (1998) Quantification of myocardial blood flow with ultrasound-induced destruction of microbubbles administered as a constant venous infusion. Circulation 97:473–483

33 Cardiac Applications

B. Cotter and A.N. DeMaria

CONTENTS

33.1 Introduction

The concept of contrast echocardiography has been applied since 1968, when Gramiak and Shah reported improved delineation of aortic root structures by M-mode echocardiography (Gramiak and Shah 1968; Gramiak et al. 1969). Other authors observed that the intracardiac injection of saline and indocyanine green dye resulted in dense ultrasonic reflectances (Feigenbaum et al. 1970). It was soon observed that similar ultrasonic densities could be produced by injecting almost any fluid. Moreover, intravenous injections were successful at opacifying the right-sided cardiac chambers, but not the left, owing to filtering of contrast by the lungs.

Contrast echocardiography soon achieved a clinical role in identifying the endocardial surfaces of the right-sided chambers. Moreover the failure to opacify left-sided chambers following intravenous injection led to the recognition of intracardiac shunts (Valdes-Cruz and Sahn 1984). Accordingly, visualization of contrast densities in the left-sided structures could only result from an abnormal communication, such as atrial or ventricular septal defects. Identification of a patent foramen ovale in patients with cerebral ischemic events of unknown etiology continues to be a major clinical application of contrast echocardiography (Fig. 33.1) (Lechat et al. 1988). Videodensitometric analysis was employed to quantitate the contrast effect and it was possible to obtain indicator dilution-type curves following contrast injections, which could be related to cardiac output and ejection fraction (DeMaria et al. 1984; Rovai et al. 1987). However, variability in contrast intensity from injection to injection limited the implementation of quantitative techniques. It was clear that, for contrast echocardiography to achieve prominence in clinical cardiology, new agents would have to be developed which yielded intense and reproducible signals and would opacify the left-sided cardiac chambers following an intravenous injection.

In order to develop new ultrasonic contrast agents, it was necessary to delineate the mechanism by which intravascular injection of a variety of fluids produced ultrasonic signals. Many different explanations were entertained; however, the ability to produce contrast signals by injection of the patient's own blood negated most possibilities. It was subsequently demonstrated that the origin of the contrast signals was microscopic gas bubbles injected into the circulation. As opposed to liquid and solid interfaces, which have a backscatter efficiency of approximately twofold, gaseous interfaces produced a backscatter efficiency of approximately ten to the twelfth power (10^{12}). Indeed, studies by Meltzer et al. (1980) clearly established that ultrasonic contrast was produced only by injections of fluids containing microbubbles. Thereby it was established that even microscopic quantities of gas were capable of producing abundant ultrasonic signals, and such small quantities of gas were unlikely to be associated with side-effects. Accordingly, the search for microbubble ultrasonic contrast agents suitable for application in humans began.

B. Cotter, MD, Assistant Professor of Medicine, Division of Cardiology, UCSD Medical Center, 200 West Arbor Drive, San Diego, CA 92103-8411, USA
A.N. DeMaria, MD, Professor of Medicine, Chief of Cardiovascular Medicine, Division of Cardiology, UCSD Medical Center, 200 West Arbor Drive, San Diego, CA 92103-8411, USA

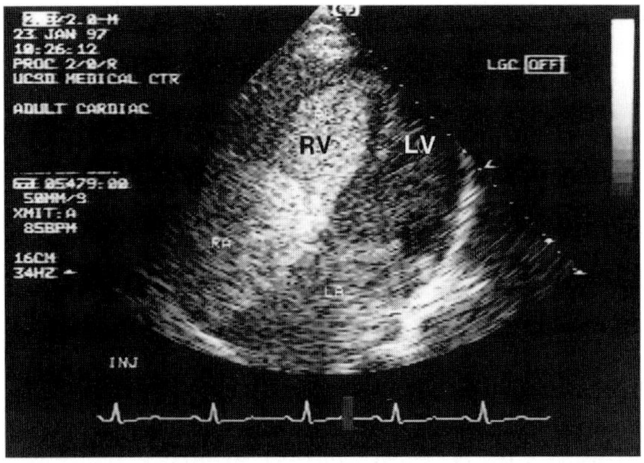

Fig. 33.1. The appearance of ultrasonic contrast in the left ventricle (*LV*) due to a patent foramen ovale in a patient with chronic pulmonary hypertension. Dense ultrasonic reflections produced by the contrast agent fill the right ventricle (*RV*), while a small number of bubbles pass through the patent foramen ovale into the left ventricle

33.2 First-Generation Ultrasonic Contrast Agents

Nearly all early clinical contrast echocardiographic studies performed utilized hand-agitated normal saline or dextrose in water. Typically, the agents were prepared by utilizing two syringes connected by a stopcock and rapidly transferring the saline from one syringe to the other prior to injection. Although this technique universally resulted in dense ultrasonic opacifications of the right-sided cardiac chambers, some variability in intensity continued. Importantly, enhancement of left-sided cardiac chambers remained impossible. The explanation for the inability to opacify the left-sided cardiac chambers soon became apparent. For a gas bubble to be sufficiently small to cross the pulmonary microcirculation it would require a diameter of approximately 6 µm. However, the surface tension of room air microbubbles of 6 µm diameter is such that they persist as bubbles in blood for approximately one-tenth of a second prior to dissolving. Therefore, to use room air as an ultrasonic contrast agent, some technique was necessary to alter the surface tension and enhance the life span of the bubble.

Several approaches have been implemented to increase the longevity of room air microbubbles following an intravenous injection. The new agents have employed additional substances such as albumin or galactose to alter the surface tension of the bubbles and increase the life span. The most successful approach to stabilizing room air microbubbles for clinical use employed albumin coating by sonication of human serum albumin and resulted in the commercially available agent Albunex (Mallinckrodt Inc., St. Louis, Mo., USA). The injection of Albunex produced dense opacification of both right- and left-sided cardiac chambers in approximately two-thirds of the patients, which was sustained for 15–30 s. A large multicenter study documented the ability of Albunex to improve the identification of the endocardial border delineation of the left ventricle (Crouse 1992; Crouse et al. 1993).

Another agent which recently gained regulatory approval in Europe is Levovist (Schering AG, Berlin, Germany). This ultrasonic contrast agent is a stable mixture of 99.9% specially manufactured microcrystalline galactose particles and 0.1% palmitic acid. Upon reconstitution with sterile water for injection, the galactose disaggregates and yields a fluid containing microbubbles with an estimated median diameter of 1.8 µm. Stabilization of the resulting air microbubbles takes place when they become coated with palmitic acid, separating the air to liquid interface and slowing their dissolution. These microbubbles are highly echogenic and are sufficiently stable to transit through the pulmonary circulation.

The development of Albunex and Levovist clearly established the ability of ultrasonic contrast agents to opacify the left-sided cardiac chambers following an intravenous injection. Utilization of these agents proved to be of value in identifying left ventricular endocardial border delineation and therefore in assessing left ventricular cavity size, wall thickness, and wall motion. This has been of benefit in stress echocardiography. The ability of these agents to enhance Doppler velocity signals has been used in conjunction with color Doppler flow imaging of the jets as well as in pulsed and continuous wave Doppler recordings of jet velocities (Terasawa et al. 1993; von Bibra et al. 1993, 1995). Importantly, these agents have proved to be extremely safe in the clinical setting. However, the microbubbles produced are somewhat fragile and may be destroyed either in the process of withdrawal and injection or at high left ventricular pressures. Despite their aforementioned applications, these ultrasonic contrast agents were found to be of little clinical value because opacification of the left-sided cardiac chambers was incomplete in one-third of the patients, and typically persisted only for 15–30 s. However the most important limitation of these ultrasonic contrast agents was the inability to produce, in conventional B-mode, contrast enhancement of the left ventricular myocardium.

33.3 Myocardial Opacification

Opacification of the left ventricular myocardium was first achieved in 1980, when Echovist, a galactose-based precursor of Levovist, was injected directly into the coronary arteries of dogs. Following intracoronary administration of Echovist, the left ventricular myocardium was uniformly enhanced with bright ultrasonic intensities. Opacification of the myocardium was found to faithfully reflect the distribution of coronary blood flow, and to be capable of delineating the area of risk from an occlusion of a given coronary artery (Smith et al. 1983). Myocardial contrast echocardiography was subsequently extended to humans by means of the direct intracoronary injection of radiographic contrast agents which had undergone sonication. Using sonicated radiographic agents, myocardial contrast echocardiography in conjunction with cardiac catheterization has been utilized in patients to discern evidence of coronary collateral flow (Sabia et al. 1992), a finding which is predictive of myocardial viability, and to delineate the "no-reflow" phenomenon following reperfusion of occluded vessels in patients with acute myocardial infarction (Ito et al. 1996).

Although it was clear that myocardial contrast echocardiography had the potential to provide valuable clinical information regarding the spatial distribution of coronary blood flow and the existence of coronary collateral circulation, the agents used required direct intracoronary administration. Clearly, an ultrasonic contrast agent which could achieve myocardial enhancement following intravenous injection would be of great potential clinical value. Therefore, a renewed intensive effort at developing ultrasonic contrast agents with enhanced capabilities has begun.

33.4 New Ultrasonic Contrast Agents

The development of new or second-generation ultrasonic contrast agents has been based upon the concept that superior production, completeness, persistence, and myocardial distribution of enhancement can be achieved by agents with extended survival as microbubbles in blood. Accordingly, the determinants of the persistence of a bubble prior to dissolving in blood have been defined and analyzed for potential approaches to prolongation.

The determinants of the persistence of the microbubble in blood are shown in the equation:

Table 33.1. Maneuvers to prolong microbubble persistence

– Increase size
– Increase density
– Decrease diffusion
– Decrease solubility

$$T = r_0^2 \cdot \varrho / 2D \cdot C_s,$$

where r = radius of bubble, ϱ = density of gas, C_s = concentration of saturation, and D = diffusivity of gas.

Thus, the longevity of a bubble is directly increased by its radius and the density of the gas inside the bubble. Persistence is inversely related to or is decreased by the diffusivity, or the potential of the gas to diffuse into blood, as well as the saturation constant of the gas in blood. In regard to this latter concept, a constant exists for any bubble dispersed in blood, which relates movement of the gas from the bubble to blood, as well as from blood into the bubble. The lower concentration at which blood is saturated with the gas, the more likely the gas will be to remain in the bubble, rather than dissolve. In light of the foregoing, it is clear that the persistence of a microbubble contrast agent can be prolonged by increasing either the size of the bubble or the density of the gas, or by decreasing either the diffusivity or the saturation concentration (solubility) of the gas (Table 33.1). Given the constraints of the microcirculation, microbubble size cannot exceed 6–8 µm without embolization. Therefore, one of the major approaches to the creation of a microbubble with prolonged persistence has been to utilize a gas with increased density, decreased diffusivity, and a low saturation concentration. Thus far, the gases which have proven to be most suitable in this regard have been the fluorocarbons. These compounds fulfil all three of the aforementioned criteria; in addition the gases themselves are well tolerated by humans and have been administered in large quantity as blood substitutes for their oxygen binding capacity without adverse effects. A number of new ultrasonic contrast agents with the ability to produce intense myocardial as well as left ventricular opacification following intravenous injection are currently under development. Many of them have passed through "phase 3" clinical trials, and one has recently been approved for clinical use by the Food and Drug Administration. Most of them employ fluorocarbons as their gases (Cotter et al. 1994a; Dittrich et al. 1995; Grauer et al. 1996; Grayburn et al. 1995; Porter et al. 1993a,b; Kaul and Jayaweera 1993).

Another way to prevent a gas such as air from diffusing out and going back into solution in the blood is to modify the "shells" which stabilize the microbubbles and thereby increase the longevity of the microbubble in the blood. Several agents have been introduced which have employed polymer shells with either nitrogen or perfluorocarbon gas to achieve prolonged bubble persistence. The thickness and elasticity of the shell can be varied to produce bubbles of different fragility and resonance characteristics.

The first new (so-called second-generation) ultrasonic contrast agent approved by the Food and Drug Administration was Optison. This ultrasonic contrast agent was developed by Molecular Biosystems Inc. (San Diego, Calif., USA) and is produced by heat treatment and sonication of human albumin using octafluoropropane as a gas. Each milliliter contains 5.0–8.0 × 10^8 particles, the mean diameter ranging from 2.5 to 4.5 µm. This agent has been demonstrated not to cause any alteration in myocardial blood flow, left ventricular wall thickening, pulmonary gas exchange, cardiac output, or systemic hemodynamics when injected in dogs (Dittrich et al. 1995). Its safety in humans has also been demonstrated. *Optison* produces intense left ventricular cavity and myocardial opacification (Fig. 33.2). Visualization of the myocardium using B-mode has been reported to persist for 20–30 s and conforms to the transit time of flow through the myocardium.

EchoGen (SONUS Pharmaceutical Inc., Bothell, Wash., USA) was the first agent to demonstrate myocardial opacification following intravenous injection (DeMaria et al. 1993). This contrast agent is an emulsion of dodecafluoropentane droplets which undergoes a phase shift following hypobaric activation (negative pressure created by syringe suction) and intravenous administration to become a dispersion of microbubbles with an average diameter of 5–7 µm. This agent has been shown to delineate myocardial perfusion defects and areas at risk following intravenous injection (Fig. 33.3). (Grayburn et al. 1995; Cotter et al. 1994b). EchoGen exhibits prolonged myocardial enhancement and is unique among the ultrasonic contrast agents in that the

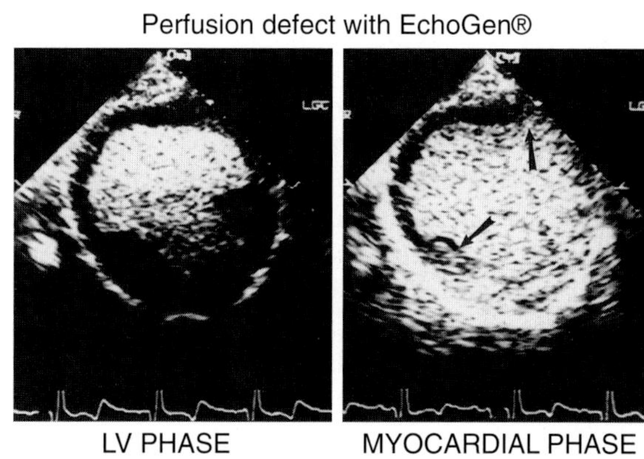

Fig. 33.3. A perfusion defect is well delineated following the injection of EchoGen after the occlusion of a coronary artery in an animal model. The *left panel* shows the contrast in the left ventricle. The *right panel* shows a perfusion defect from approximately 7 to 1 o'clock (*arrows*) while the rest of the myocardium shows homogeneous enhancement

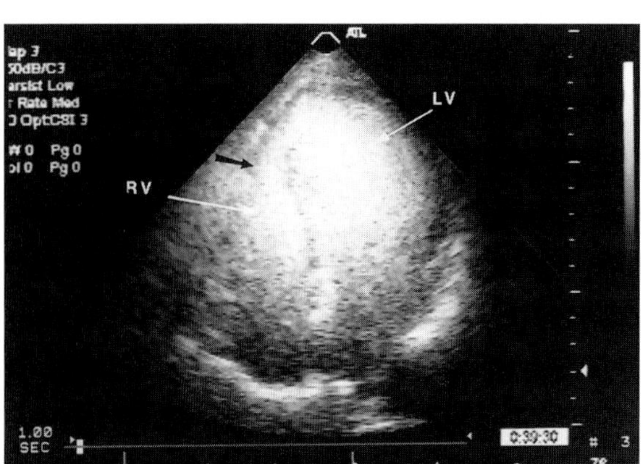

Fig. 33.2. Apical four-chamber view of a patient undergoing echocardiography. Dense opacification of the right (*RV*) and left (*LV*) ventricles can be seen following an intravenous injection of Optison. Homogeneous enhancement of the myocardium (*arrow*) can also be observed

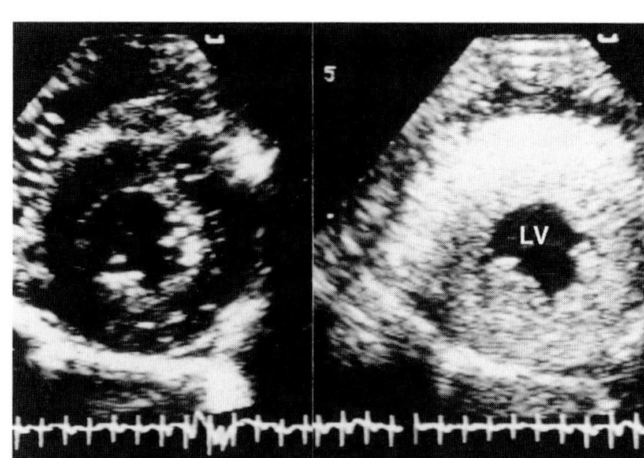

Fig. 33.4. Opacification of the myocardium following intravenous injection of EchoGen in an animal model. The *left panel* shows the short-axis view prior to contrast injection. The *right panel* shows the same view 5 min after the injection of the agent. Dense and homogeneous opacification of the myocardium is observed after the disappearance of most of the contrast agent from the left ventricle (*LV*)

myocardial enhancement persists beyond that of cavity opacification. Very high doses in animals yielded opacification for up to 20 min (Fig. 33.4). The precise mechanism responsible for the prolonged myocardial persistence of enhancement by EchoGen is unknown. Studies of the microcirculation by GE et al. (1995) have demonstrated that the agent is nonocclusive, but is slower in velocity as it transits through the microcirculation than are red blood cells.

QW7437 or SonoGen is a new ultrasonic contrast agent also developed by SONUS. It is also an emulsion of dodecafluoropentane droplets which undergoes a phase shift following hypobaric activation and intravenous injection to become a dispersion of microbubbles. QW7437 has a negatively charged surfactant to stabilize the microbubble. Studies in our laboratory have shown that QW7437 produces an intense myocardial opacification following an intravenous injection (Fig. 33.5). The time-intensity curve shows that the contrast peaks at approximately 2 min and returns to baseline after 8 min (Fig. 33.6). This agent was shown to cause no alterations in myocardial blood flow, left ventricular thickening, pulmonary gas exchange or cardiac and systemic hemodynamics when injected intravenously in dogs (COTTER et al. 1996a). Myocardial perfusion defects and areas at risk can also be detected following acute occlusion of a coronary artery (MAIN et al. 1997). Here again, the precise mechanism for the prolonged myocardial enhancement is unknown. Studies of the microcirculation in our laboratory by YASU et al. using fluorescent labeled microbubbles of QW7437 have demonstrated a transient adhesion (0.1–120 s)

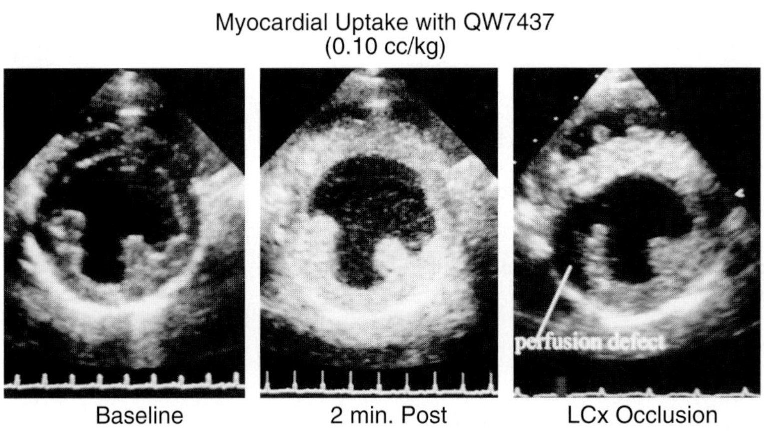

Fig. 33.5. Opacification of the myocardium following intravenous injection of QW7437 in an animal model. The *left panel* shows the short-axis view prior to contrast injection. The *middle panel* shows the same view 2 min after the injection of the contrast. Dense and uniform opacification is observed after the disappearance of the contrast agent from the left cavity. The *right panel* shows a myocardial perfusion defect due to the occlusion of the circumflex coronary artery

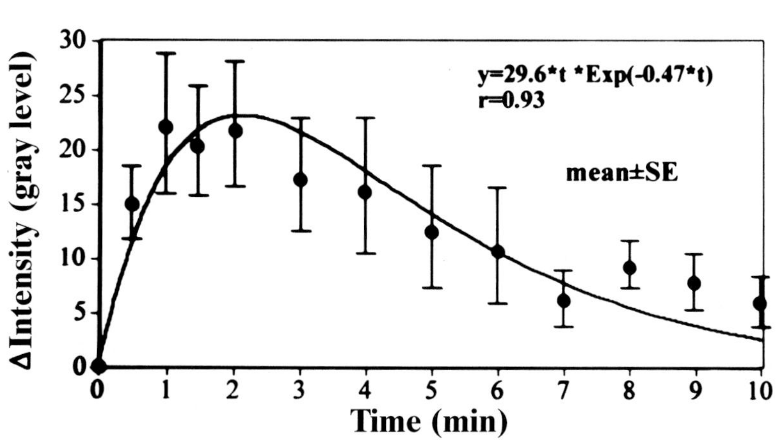

Fig. 33.6. Time-intensity curve derived from the left ventricular myocardium following intravenous injection of QW7437. The y-axis represents the delta change in intensity expressed in gray levels. As can be seen, the intensity peaks at approximately 2 min and gradually washes out after 10 min

Table 33.2. Ultrasonic contrast agents

Name	Type	Manufacturer
Albunex	Sonicated human albumin Mean diameter 4 µm	Mallinckrodt
Optison	Octafluoropropane microspheres Sonication of human albumin Mean diameter: 2.5–4.5 µm	Mallinckrodt
Echovist	Galactose-based microbubble	Schering
Levovist	Galactose-based microbubble stabilized with coating of fatty acid Median diameter: 1.8 µm	Schering
SHU 563A	Air-filled microspheres Cyanacrylate polymer shell Mean diameter: 1 µm	Schering
EchoGen	Emulsion of dodecafluoropentane Hypobaric activation Mean diameter: 2–4 µm	Sonus Pharm.
QW7437	Emulsion of dodecafluoropentane Negatively charged surfactant Hypobaric activation Mean diameter: 2–4 µm	Sonus Pharm.
Aerosomes (DMP115, MRX115)	Phospholipid coating Perfluoropropane gas Mean diameter: 2.5 µm	Dupont Merck
Imagent US	Perfluorohexane vapor Reconstituted with water Median diameter: 5 µm	Alliance Pharm.
NC100100	Perfluorocarbon microbubble Provided as dry power	Nycomed
BR1	Sulfur hexafluoride gas Phospholipid and polyethylene particles Mean diameter: 2–3 µm	Bracco
Quantison	Air-filled microcapsules Coated with heat-linked human serum Mean diameter: 3.2 µm	Andaris Ltd.
Quantison Depot	Air-filled microcapsules Coated with heat-linked human serum Mean diameter: 12 µm	Andaris Ltd.
Acusphere	Gas entrapped in 2-µm microspheres Stealth coated with polyethylene glycol Dry powder with water reconstitution	Acusphere Inc.
BiSphere	Double-walled, 3–5 µm Outer Biopolymer shell about 0.1 µm Inner structural polymer shell about 0.1 µm	PointBiomedical
Pesda	Perfluoropropane as gas Sonication of dextrose and albumin	University of Nebraska

of some microbubbles to the microvascular endothelium, especially in postcapillary venules (YASU et al. 1997). This transient adhesion neither obstructs nor slows the flow of red blood cells, nor does the size of the bubbles change during the period in which they are stationary.

Table 33.2 lists the approved ultrasonic contrast agents and those under development. They all can be injected through a peripheral vein, can cross the pulmonary circulation, and have been shown to produce myocardial opacification and to be safe in humans.

Almost immediately after the initial development of second-generation contrast agents, experimental studies demonstrated their ability to produce dense myocardial opacification after intravenous injection in dogs. In addition, coronary occlusions were observed to manifest readily visible perfusion defects on myocardial contrast echocardiography (MCE), the size of which correlated with risk area measurements obtained by a variety of methods. It was therefore assumed that these results would be easily extended to humans in the clinical setting. However, the initial attempts to use MCE to delineate perfusion defects due to coronary occlusions yielded only modest myocardial opacification, often with difficulties in visualizing abnormalities. Therefore, extension of intravenous MCE to patients required additional advances in instrumentation and recording techniques.

33.5 Advances in Instrumentation

Perhaps the most significant advance in ultrasonic instrumentation for contrast echocardiography has been of second harmonic imaging. Second harmonic imaging is based on the emission of harmonic signals due to the nonlinear resonation of microbubbles which pulsate in an ultrasonic field (MILLER 1981; SCHROPE et al. 1992; SCHROPE and NEWHOUSE 1993). A gas microbubble exposed to an ultrasonic field will resonate at a given frequency, that is the bubbles expand and contract with the oscillations of pressure caused by the incident sound. The resonance, or alternating expansion and contraction of the microbubble, depends on the bubble radius, the composition of the microbubble shell, the resonant frequency, the acoustic pressure and velocity, and the composition and the pressure of the surrounding medium. Microbubbles undergoing resonant oscillations have the ability to reflect significant ultrasonic energy at both the fundamental frequency of the ultrasonic beam transmitted and the frequency which results from the interaction between the transmitted signal and the resonating bubble. In this manner, imaging at a second harmonic frequency to the transmitted signal can amplify the reflections from microbubbles relative to that from tissue. With the harmonic mode, the signal from blood is enhanced but that from the tissue is reduced, reversing the contrast between tissue and blood (Fig. 33.7). For most of the new agents, the resonating characteristics during normal physiological conditions within the circulation result in a significant reflection of ultrasonic energy at the second harmonic of the transmitted frequency. However, not all agents display such a nonlinear response. Key factors in the harmonic response of an agent are likely to be the size distribution of the bubbles and the mechanical properties of the bubble capsule (a stiff capsule, for example, will dampen the oscillations and attenuate the nonlinear response).

The recognition of linear intramyocardial signals, rather than a diffuse myocardial blush, in response to the intravenous injection of ultrasonic contrast agents was initially reported by MULVAGH et al.

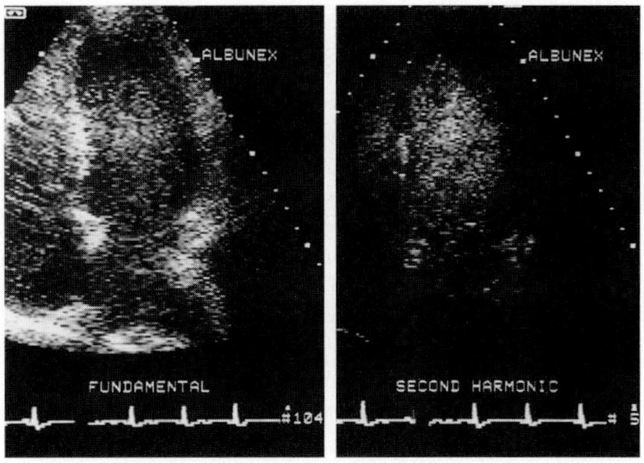

Fig. 33.7. The effect of second harmonic imaging upon contrast opacification of the left ventricular cavity produced by Albunex. The *left panel* shows the opacification of the left ventricle in a patient undergoing diagnostic echocardiography at a fundamental frequency of 2.5 MHz. The *right panel* shows the same patient while imaging at the second harmonic of 5 MHz. As can be seen, harmonic imaging produces a selected amplification of the contrast signal relative to the myocardium

(1996). These authors reported that, following the injection of AF0145 (Alliance Pharmaceutical Corp., San Diego, Calif., USA) during second harmonic imaging, long linear structures could be observed within the myocardium. These structures were seen to branch and were accompanied by punctuate signals consistent with linear structures imaged in cross-section; the authors were able to demonstrate that the structures in question were actually intramyocardial coronary arteries. Studies in our laboratory using AF0150 yielded the same results (COTTER et al. 1996b). Using second harmonic imaging we were able to observe linear structures that were comparable in size to intramyocardial vessels. Doppler recordings from within these structures yielded flow signals which were predominantly diastolic in velocity and which increased nearly two- to threefold after intravenous injection of dipyridamole (Fig. 33.8). We also concluded, therefore, that these structures clearly represent coronary vessels. These observations pointed to the importance of the interaction of microbubbles with ultrasound, and the potential role of ultrasonic bubble destruction.

The mechanisms by which intramyocardial vascular structures are visualized following intravenous injection remain uncertain. However, many studies have shed light upon this topic. It is now well recognized that ultrasonic energy can produce microbubble destruction and diminish contrast signals (OHMORI et al. 1997; WEI et al. 1997). It was soon discovered that imaging the heart one frame

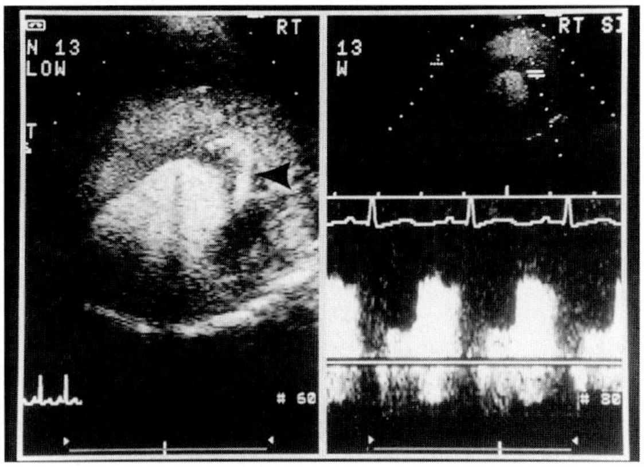

Fig. 33.8. Echocardiographic images obtained following intravenous injection of Imagent US in an animal model. The *left panel* shows contrast within the right and left ventricles, as well as discrete linear (*arrowhead*) and punctuate signals within the interventricular septum consistent with vascular structures. The *right upper panel* shows the position of a pulsed Doppler sample volume within one vessel. The *right lower panel* shows Doppler velocity recording from this structure and the predominant diastolic flow consistent with coronary blood flow

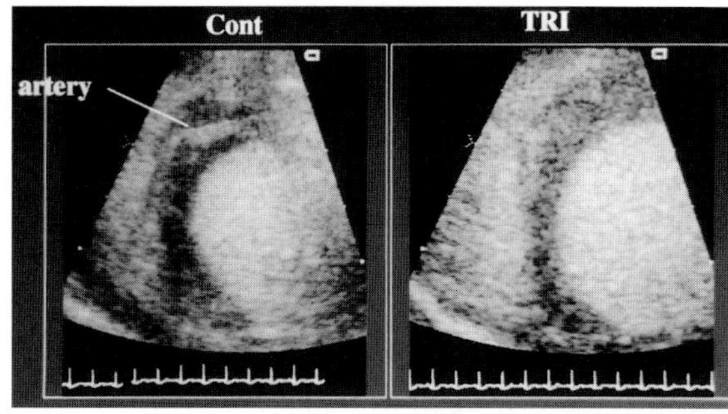

Fig. 33.9. Echocardiographic short-axis view from an animal model following intravenous injection with Imagent US. The *left panel* represents the left ventricle during continuous imaging. As can be seen, almost no contrast is present within the myocardium and a coronary artery is clearly seen. The *right panel* represents the same view obtained during intermittent (ECG-triggered) imaging. A diffuse myocardial blush can be observed within the myocardium, masking the intramyocardial coronary artery

per cardiac cycle resulted in contrast intensity which was significantly higher than that obtained by continuous imaging at 20–30 frames per second. It was reasoned that microbubbles with a slow transit rate would be affected to a greater extent than those with high velocity, since the slower moving bubbles would replace those destroyed in the imaging field to a lesser extent, and also be exposed to more ultrasound energy pulses. It was therefore a common sense step to use triggered imaging for myocardial perfusion, a technique referred to as "intermittent" or "transient" imaging (Porter and Xei 1995). Ultrasonic energy would destroy bubbles within the slow-flowing microcirculation to a greater extent than those with a high flow velocity in larger vessels. In this regard studies in our laboratory have demonstrated that rapid switching from continuous to intermittent imaging during injection of AF0150 yields a diffuse myocardial blush which can envelop and veil the linear and punctuate structures (Fig. 33.9) (Cotter et al. 1996b). This observation is consistent with the role of destruction by ultrasonic energy in the generation of the appearance of vascular structures.

Subsequently, Wei et al. (1998) utilized ultrasound destruction of microbubbles to quantify blood flow velocity. Using a pair of ultrasound pulses, one to destroy all microbubbles in the imaging field and the other, with a delay from the first, to evaluate the reappearance of contrast intensity in the imaging field, they obtained curves relating pulsing interval and videointensity during a constant intravenous infusion of contrast agent and observed that the rate of increase per increase in pulsing interval was closely related with myocardial blood flow velocity. They proposed that this relation could provide the basis for the estimation of myocardial blood flow velocity from contrast echocardiography. Studies in our laboratory by Ohmori et al. (unpublished work) demonstrated that comparison of intensity during transient and continuous exposure imaging yielded useful estimates of blood flow velocity, and could be applied to bolus injections of agents.

Using the combination of second harmonic transient imaging, myocardial opacification was achieved more reliably in patients. In fact, contrast echocardiography was demonstrated to be of value in delineating coronary stenosis in patients. To assess the feasibility of employing contrast echocardiography to identify coronary artery disease, Kaul et al. (1997) performed a study using Optison with intermittent harmonic imaging, to compare contrast echocardiography at rest and after the injection of dipyridamole with rest and stress technetium-99m sestamibi single-photon emission computed tomography (SPECT). They found a 92% concordance between the SPECT studies and contrast echocardiography for discriminating between normal perfusion and reversible or irreversible defects. Similar data have been reported by Porter et al. (1996, 1997) using Pesda.

Myocardial contrast echocardiography by intravenous injection has opened the door to important clinical applications. Perfusion defects should delineate the myocardial risk area associated with coronary occlusion and myocardial infarction. Moreover, disappearance of the defect after coronary recanalization should be a marker of successful reperfusion, while continued presence should signify the no-reflow phenomenon. MCE should be of value in identifying the presence of coronary collaterals and myocardial viability. It is anticipated that MCE in conjunction with vasodilator stress drugs will provide an alternative to radionuclide techniques for the diagnosis of coronary artery disease. Contrast microbubbles may even have therapeutic importance as a vehicle to deliver such agents as thrombolytic drugs and genes.

Although many clinical studies have shown the ability of MCE to produce myocardial opacification, many questions remain unanswered regarding the best technique for MCE. It is not clear whether all ultrasonic contrast agents differ in their ability to achieve myocardial opacification, and the optimal dose for these agents also remains uncertain. Although transient harmonic imaging appears to yield the greatest contrast intensity, it is not clear that imaging at fundamental frequencies cannot produce myocardial enhancement. Furthermore, the preferred phase (systole versus diastole) and frequencies of gating of cardiac cycle (every one, two, four, etc.) have still to be defined. No agreement exists regarding the instrument settings (gain, dynamic range, etc.) which produce the highest quality of images. The power setting (mechanical index) which achieves the best balance between contrast amplitude recorded and microbubble destruction produced remains speculative. So far, nearly all reported studies on MCE have utilized gray-scale tissue imaging, but application of power Doppler recordings may provide significantly better visualization of myocardial enhancement. Finally, controversies continue regarding the best methods for quantitative analysis of contrast echo data, while the range of normal findings and specific criteria by which to identify abnormalities remain undefined.

33.6 Conclusion

The past several years have seen a virtual explosion of new ultrasonic contrast agents and innovation in instrumentation to record the signals from these agents. It is now clear that opacification of both the left ventricular cavity and myocardium can be

Table 33.3. Current applications of contrast echocardiography

- Enhancement of left ventricular endocardial borders
- Suboptimal stress echocardiography
- Detection of patent foramen ovale
- Confirmation of atrial septal defect
- Enhancement of tricuspid regurgitation jet
- Enhancement of aortic stenosis jet

Table 33.4. Future directions of contrast echocardiography

- Detection of myocardial infarction
- Determination of infarct size, area at risk, and myocardial viability
- Distribution and quantification of coronary blood flow
- Drug and gene delivery
- Examination of endothelial function
- Tissue-specific imaging

achieved by intravenous injection of these agents, which have proven to be safe in humans. Several studies have demonstrated the ability to evaluate the spatial distribution of myocardial perfusion by contrast echocardiography. The extent of at risk and necrotic myocardial areas has been assessed by contrast echocardiography after coronary occlusion, and the findings have been accurate and reproducible from injection to injection. Additionally, since the new ultrasonic contrast agents are exclusively limited to the intravascular compartment, contrast echocardiography may permit measurements of coronary blood flow. Because it is noninvasive, inexpensive, and repeatable, contrast echocardiography should have important clinical applications in diagnosing and risk-stratifying cardiac diseases, in understanding the pathophysiology of coronary artery disease, and in elucidating the mechanism of action of various pharmacological agents. Table 33.3 shows the current applications of contrast echocardiography.

Early studies suggest that in the future contrast echocardiography may be used to assess endothelial function (Villanueva et al. 1997, 1998), and that contrast agents could be used as a vehicle for thrombus detection, sonothrombolysis, and drug and gene delivery (Table 33.4).

References

Cotter B, Kwan OL, Cha YM, Dittrich H, Bhargava V, DeMaria AN (1994a) Dose-response characteristics, time-course, and hemodynamic response to QW3600, an ultrasonic contrast agent capable of myocardial opacification by intravenous injection. J Am Coll Cardiol 23:393A

Cotter B, Kriett J, Perricone T, et al. (1994b) Detection of coronary artery occlusion by decreased myocardial opacification following intravenous injection of QW3600 (EchoGen®). Circulation 90:I-67

Cotter B, Duong A, Ohmori K, Kwan OL, DeMaria AN (1996a) Evaluation of QW7437, a third generation ultrasonic contrast agent capable of myocardial opacification: dose-response characteristics, time-course, hemodynamic response and detection of coronary occlusion (abstract). Circulation 94(Suppl I):I-319

Cotter B, Duong A, Kwan OL, Wheeler K, Nozaki S, DeMaria AN (1996b) Visualization of intramyocardial coronary vessels by contrast echocardiography, observations using AF0150 (Imagent® US) during second harmonic imaging. J Am Coll Cardiol 27:298A

Crouse LJ (1992) Sonicated serum albumin in contrast echocardiography: improved segmental wall motion depiction and implications for stress echocardiography. Am J Cardiol 69:42H–45H

Crouse LJ, Cheirif J, Hanly DE, et al. (1993) Opacification and border delineation improvement in patients with suboptimal endocardial border definition in routine echocardiography: results of the phase III Albunex multicenter trial. J Am Coll Cardiol 22:1494–1500

DeMaria AN, Bommer W, Kwan OL, Riggs K, Smith M, Waters J (1984) In vivo correlation of thermodilution cardiac output and videodensitometric indicator-dilution curves obtained from contrast two-dimensional echocardiograms. J Am Coll Cardiol 3:999–1004

DeMaria AN, Dittrich H, Kwan OL, Kimura B (1993) Myocardial opacification produced by peripheral venous injection of a new ultrasonic contrast agent. Circulation 88:I-401

Dittrich HC, Bales GL, Kuvelas T, Hunt RM, McFerran BA, Greener Y (1995) Myocardial contrast echocardiography in experimental coronary artery occlusion with a new intravenously administered contrast agent. J Am Soc Echocardiogr 8:465–474

Feigenbaum H, Stone JM, Lee DA, Nasser WK, Chang S (1970) Identification of ultrasound echoes from the left ventricle by use of intracardiac injections of indocyanine green. Circulation 41:615–621

Ge S, Giraud G, Shiota T (1995) Microcirculatory flow dynamics during peripheral intravenous injection of EchoGen: microscopic visualization of mesenteric microcirculatory flow with simultaneously transthoracic echo imaging in cats. J Am Coll Cardiol 23:293A

Gramiak R, Shah PM (1968) Echocardiography of the aortic root. Invest Radiol 3:356–366

Gramiak R, Shah PM, Kramer DH (1969) Ultrasound cardiography: contrast studies in anatomy and function. Radiology 92:939–948

Grauer SE, Xu J, Pantely GA, et al. (1996) MRX 115, an echocardiographic contrast agent, produces myocardial opacification after intravenous injection in primates: studies before and after occlusion of left anterior descending coronary artery. Acad Radiol 3 Suppl 2:S405–S406

Grayburn PA, Erickson JM, Escobar J, Womack L, Velasco CE (1995) Peripheral intravenous myocardial contrast echocardiography using a 2% dodecafluoropentane emulsion: identification of myocardial risk area and infarct size in the canine model of ischemia. J Am Coll Cardiol 26:1340–1347

Ito H, Maruyama A, Iwakura K, et al. (1996) Clinical implications of the "no reflow" phenomenon. A predictor of complications and left ventricular remodeling in reperfused anterior wall myocardial infarction. Circulation 93:223–228

Kaul S, Jayaweera AR (1993) Myocardial contrast echocardiography has the potential for the assessment of coronary microvascular reserve [editorial; comment]. J Am Coll Cardiol 21:356–358

Kaul S, Senior R, Dittrich H, Rava U, Khattar R, Lahiri A (1997) Detection of coronary artery disease with myocardial contrast echocardiography: comparison with ^{99m}Tc-sestamibi single-photon emission computed tomography. Circulation 96:785–792

Lechat P, Mas JL, Lascualt G (1988) Prevalence of patent foramen ovale in patients with stroke. N Engl J Med 318:1148–1152

Main ML, Escobar JF, Hall SA, Grayburn PA (1997) Safety and efficacy of QW7437, a new fluorocarbon-based echocardiographic contrast agent. J Am Soc Echocardiogr 10:798–794

Meltzer RS, Tickner EG, Sahines TP, Popp RL (1980) The source of ultrasound contrast effect. JCU J Clin Ultrasound 8:121–127

Miller DL (1981) Ultrasonic detection of resonant cavitation bubbles in a flow tube by their second-harmonic emissions. Ultrasonics 19:217–224

Mulvagh SL, Foley DA, Aeschbacher BC, Klarich KK, Seward JB (1996) Second harmonic imaging of an intravenously administered echocardiographic contrast agent: visualization of coronary arteries and measurement of coronary blood flow. J Am Coll Cardiol 27:1519–1525

Ohmori K, Cotter B, Kwan OL, Mizushige K, DeMaria AN (1997) Relation of contrast echo intensity and flow velocity to the amplification of contrast opacification produced by intermittent ultrasound transmission. Am Heart J 134:1066–1074

Porter TR, Xie F (1995) Transient myocardial contrast after initial exposure to diagnostic ultrasound pressures with minute doses of intravenously injected microbubbles. Demonstration and potential mechanisms. Circulation 92:2391–2395

Porter TR, D'Sa A, Pesko L, et al. (1993a) Usefulness of myocardial contrast echocardiography in detecting the immediate changes in anterograde blood flow reserve after coronary angioplasty. Am J Cardiol 71:893–896

Porter TR, D'Sa A, Turner C, et al. (1993b) Myocardial contrast echocardiography for the assessment of coronary blood flow reserve: validation in humans [see comments]. J Am Coll Cardiol 21:349–355

Porter TR, Kricsfeld A, Deligonul U, Xie F (1996) Detection of regional perfusion abnormalities during adenosine stress echocardiography with intravenous perfluorocarbon-exposed sonicated dextrose albumin. Am Heart J 132(1 Pt 1):41–47

Porter TR, Li S, Kricsfeld D, Armbruster RW (1997) Detection of myocardial perfusion in multiple echocardiographic windows with one intravenous injection of microbubbles using transient response second harmonic imaging. J Am Coll Cardiol 29:791–799

Rovai D, Nissen SE, Elion JE (1987) Contrast echo washout curves from the left ventricle: application of basic principles of indicator-dilution theory and calculation of ejection fraction. J Am Coll Cardiol 10:125–134

Sabia PJ, Powers ER, Jayaweera AR, Ragosta M, Kaul S (1992) Functional significance of collateral blood flow in patients with recent acute myocardial infarction. A study using myocardial contrast echocardiography. Circulation 85: 2080–2089

Schrope B, Newhouse VL (1993) Second harmonic ultrasonic blood perfusion measurement. Ultrasound Med Biol 19:567–579

Schrope B, Newhouse VL, Uhlendorf A (1992) Simulated capillary blood flow measurement using a non line ultrasonic contrast agent. Ultrason Imaging 14:134–158

Smith MK, Kwan OL, Reiser J, DeMaria AN (1983) Superior intensity and reproducibility of SHU-454, a new right heart contrast agent. J Am Coll Cardiol 3:992–998

Terasawa A, Miyatake K, Nakatani S, Yamagishi M, Matsuda H, Beppu S (1993) Enhancement of Doppler flow signals in the left heart chambers by intravenous injection of sonicated albumin. J Am Coll Cardiol 21:737–742

Valdes-Cruz L, Sahn DJ (1984) Ultrasonic contrast studies for the detection of cardiac shunts. J Am Coll Cardiol 3:978–985

Villanueva FS, Jankowski RJ, Manaugh C, Wagner WR (1997) Albumin microbubble adherence to human coronary endothelium: implications for assessment of endothelial function using myocardial contrast echocardiography. J Am Coll Cardiol 30:689–693

Villanueva FS, Jankowski RJ, Klibanov S, et al. (1998) Microbubbles targeted to intercellular adhesion molecule-1 bind to activated coronary artery endothelial cells. Circulation 98:1–5

von Bibra H, Becher H, Firschke C, Schlief R, Emslander HP, Schomig A (1993) Enhancement of mitral regurgitation and normal left atrial color Doppler flow signals with peripheral venous injection of a saccharide-based contrast agent. J Am Coll Cardiol 22:521–528

von Bibra H, Sutherland G, Becher H, Neudert J, Nihoyannopoulos P (1995) Clinical evaluation of left heart Doppler contrast enhancement by a saccharide-based transpulmonary contrast agent. The Levovist Cardiac Working Group. J Am Coll Cardiol 25:500–508

Wei K, Skyba DM, Firschke C, Jayaweera AR, Lindner JR, Kaul S (1997) Interactions between microbubble and ultrasound: in vitro and in vivo observations. J Am Coll Cardiol 29:1081–1088

Wei K, Jayaweera AR, Firoozan S, Linka A, Skyba DM, Kaul S (1998) Quantification of myocardial blood flow with ultrasound-induced destruction of microbubbles administered as a constant venous infusion. Circulation 97:785–792

Yasu T, Schmid-Schoenbein GW, Cotter B, DeMaria AN (1997) Intravital microscopic study of QW7437, a new dodecafluoropentane contrast agent: potential for prolonged myocardial enhancement (abstract). Circulation 96(Suppl I):I-214

34 Targeting and Delivery of Drugs with Ultrasound Contrast Agents

E.C. Unger

CONTENTS

34.1 Background

There are many possibilities for targeting ultrasound contrast media and for using acoustically active materials for drug delivery. In this chapter I will review some of the background behind the use of ultrasound for therapy and drug delivery. I will touch upon some of the exciting new developments in ultrasound contrast media, drug and gene delivery.

Ultrasound increases the permeability of the skin to drugs and has been used for transcutaneous drug delivery (Mitragotri et al. 1995a,b; Machluf and Kost 1993; Bommannan et al. 1992). Recently, low-frequency ultrasound, e.g., 20–60 kHz, was found to be more effective than higher frequencies (e.g., 1 MHz) at increasing penetration of drugs across the skin (Mitragotri et al. 1996). Ultrasound could have applications for transcutaneous delivery of macromolecules, peptides, and other drugs that normally are not possible to deliver topically.

Ultrasound has been used for some time in therapy (Lindholm et al. 1987; Fry and Johnson 1978; Fosmire et al. 1993; Waterman and Hoh 1995). Therapeutic ultrasound has been used to heat tissues and more recently for thermal ablation (Hynynen et al. 1993). Generally, lower frequency ultrasound transducers are used for ultrasound hyperthermia than for diagnostic imaging (Hynynen et al. 1987). For example, 0.5- or 1.0-MHz ultrasound is used for therapeutic ultrasound, although higher and lower frequencies can also be employed. Low frequencies, e.g., 1 MHz, have better tissue penetration than higher frequencies, which are more rapidly attenuated within the tissues (Curry et al. 1990). In ultrasonic hyperthermia, the goal is generally to maintain tumor temperature over 43°C for a sufficient time to achieve a tumoricidal effect (Lin et al. 1992; Lalonde and Hunt 1995). Usually hyperthermia will not be sufficient on its own to destroy the tumor, but hyperthermia is synergistic with radiation and chemotherapy. (Li and Hahn 1978; Ben-Yosef and Kapp 1993; Moros et al. 1995; Harrison et al. 1996).

High-energy focussed ultrasound may be used to directly ablate tissues (e.g., tumor tissue) (Hynynen et al. 1987; Dorr and Hynynen 1992). The energy employed for tissue ablation is higher than in ultrasonic hyperthermia (Hynynen et al. 1987). Temperatures as high as 70°–80°C may be reached in the tissue within the focal zone in as little as a few seconds (Hynynen et al. 1987, 1993). High-energy focussed ultrasound can be performed under magnetic resonance (MR) imaging (Darkazanli et al. 1993). As the temperature in the tissue increases, T1 is prolonged and the signal intensity decreases on T1-weighted MR images (Darkazanli et al. 1993). Necrosis is visualized well on MR as a region of increased signal intensity (Darkazanli et al. 1993).

Ultrasonic hyperthermia has been used in concert with systemically administered chemotherapy for drug delivery (Rosberger et al. 1994; Saad and Hahn 1992). Temperature-sensitive carriers can be made to release their contents as they enter the region of elevated temperature (Ning et al. 1994). Liposomes which have been developed for drug delivery have been studied as temperature-sensitive drug carriers (Chelvi and Ralhan 1995; Ma et al. 1987; Ono et al. 1995; Inoue 1974). As the lipids in

E.C. Unger, MD, Professor of Radiology, Director of Cross Sectional Imaging, The University of Arizona Health Sciences Center, 1501 N. Campbell Avenue, Tucson, AZ 85724-5067, USA and President and CEO, ImaRx Pharmaceutical Corp., Tucson, Ariz., USA liposomes pass through the phase transition from gel state to liquid crystalline, the bilayers become particularly permeable (Ono et al. 1994; Chan and Magin 1989). Increased permeability of the bilayers causes drugs to be released more rapidly by the liposomes (Papahadjopoulos et al. 1973; Singer 1979, 1981). Careful selection of the materials can produce liposomes with lipids that undergo the phase transition at selected temperatures (e.g., at 43°C for use with hyperthermia). Following intravascular injection, the liposomes will circulate throughout the vasculature, and drugs are released locally by the liposomes as they enter the region of increased temperature. Polymeric carriers can also be formulated as temperature-sensitive microspheres for drug delivery (Agrawal et al. 1994; Kost and Langer 1992).

Until recently, prior work on ultrasound for drug delivery and therapy has not utilized acoustically active carrier vehicles. The acoustic impedance or prior art systems has been near that of water. By incorporating gas or gaseous precursor material into a drug carrier, we can change its acoustic impedance and make it acoustically active. Acoustically active carriers should increase the efficacy of ultrasound-mediated therapy and drug delivery.

34.2 Acoustically Active Agents for Targeting and Drug Delivery

Why use acoustically active agents for targeting and drug delivery? In the past, ultrasound has already been used with temperature-sensitive liposomes. Why should acoustically active agents perform any better with ultrasound? Acoustically active materials, such as bubbles, do amazing things when they encounter ultrasound waves (Suslick et al. 1990). Not only do they reflect sound, highly useful for imaging, bubbles also absorb sound energy (Forsberg 1997). Furthermore, bubbles are ruptured by sound energy (Walker 1997). Ultrasound can also be used to manipulate microbubbles (Fowlkes et al. 1995, 1997). Sonic energy can be applied so as stop microbubbles flowing within a vessel and to change their direction of movement (Fowlkes et al. 1997).

Given that microbubbles can be manipulated and ruptured with ultrasound, how is it that ultrasound contrast agents can be used therapeutically? As I shall discuss, there are therapeutic applications for acoustically active materials carrying drugs, prodrugs and genes.

Naked microbubbles, coated bubbles (including gas-filled microspheres), perfluorocarbons, and gaseous precursor materials can all be used as potentiators for ultrasonic hyperthermia (US patents 5149319 and 5209720). As shown in Fig. 34.1, a solution exposed to therapeutic ultrasound which contains gas microbubbles has a higher rate of heating than a solution without the extra microbubbles. In separate experiments, which we performed several years ago, we suspended CO_2 microbubbles and gas-filled liposomes in beakers of saline and showed that the liquid containing the microbubbles had a higher rate of heating (US patents 5149319 and 5209720). We hypothesized that microbubbles could be used for therapeutic ultrasound to increase efficacy for

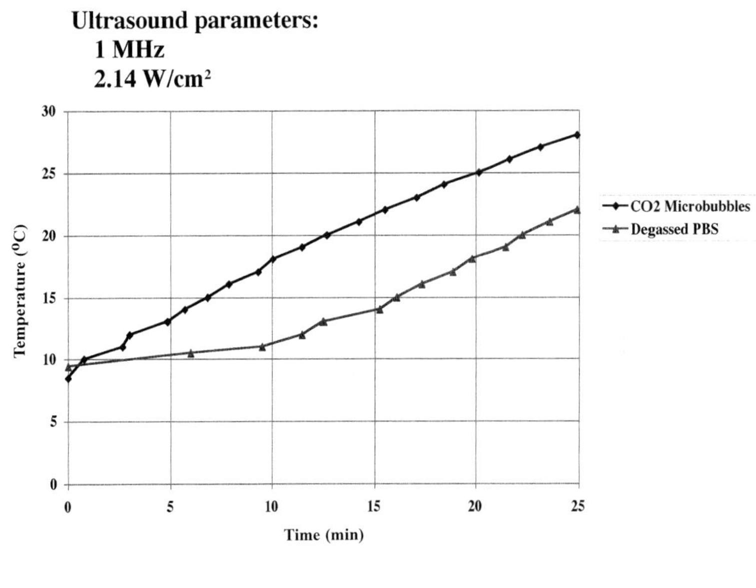

Fig. 34.1. Heating of a liquid with and without microbubbles with 1.0-MHz therapeutic ultrasound. A faster rate of heating is observed in the sample containing microbubbles until the microbubbles are destroyed

treating tumors and other conditions (US patents 5149319 and 5209720). It is also possible to use microbubbles to lower the cavitation threshold for procedures such as lithotripsy (US patent 5380411). Recent ultrasound-mediated experiments assessed heating in gels which contained microbubbles (WATMOUGH et al. 1993). These experiments showed similar increases in heating as in our experiments in liquid. In these latter experiments, the investigators hypothesized that cavitation was responsible for the higher rate of heating in the gels containing microbubbles.

What is the mechanism responsible for increased heating in suspensions containing microbubbles? Microbubbles have a markedly different acoustic impedance from fluids and tissues (BALEN et al. 1994; GOLDBERG et al. 1994). The acoustic impedance mismatch between microbubbles and surrounding fluid/tissue increases absorption of ultrasound energy and conversion into mechanical energy and heat. Cavitation is an important mechanism underlying microbubble rupture and local conversion of ultrasound into thermomechanical energy (HYNYNEN 1991). At high ultrasound energies (e.g., 10 W), cavitation can be a violent event transferring large amounts of energy to local biological tissues and fluids (HYNYNEN 1991). Cavitation can take a variety of forms (IERNETTI et al. 1996). Stable cavitation occurring within an ultrasonic field can even produce fluorescence. Depending upon conditions, bubbles can be made to resonate and oscillate in a stable pattern by sound waves. The frequency of bubble oscillation will depend upon ultrasound frequency, pulse repetition rate, and intensity of the sound energy. Cavitation is commonly thought of as a violent event which results in catastrophic destruction of the bubble. Cavitation may enhance a range of bubble phenomena, extending from stable pulsation to bubble collapse and rupture. Although increased heating in ultrasonic hyperthermia may be due to cavitation, other mechanisms may also be important.

In our early experiments with ultrasonic hyperthermia, we noted that the bubbles were destroyed by the ultrasound. The increase in rate of heating occurred only while the bubbles were present. After the microbubbles had been destroyed, the rate of heating was the same as for solutions without microbubbles.

We hypothesized that gaseous precursors, perfluorocarbons, and other materials that create an acoustic mismatch would also increase the efficiency of ultrasonic hyperthermia (US patents 5149319 and 5209720). Recently uncoated perfluoropentane microbubbles were shown to increase the rate of clot dissolution during sonolysis (NISHIOKA et al. 1966). High sonication power was required, and high blood and tissue temperatures were necessary, in order to achieve effective sonolysis in this model.

34.3 Aerosomes

Although acoustically active materials can potentiate local delivery of ultrasonic energy, we recognized that bubble destruction might also be used as a delivery vehicle (US patents 5542935, 5580575, and 5585112). We might imagine two different forms of delivery using ultrasound contrast agents. The first we might refer to as carrier-mediated targeting. In this form of targeting, we might modify the surface chemistry of the microbubble or other acoustically active material to increase its affinity for a particular receptor or target. We have incorporated antibodies, antibody fragments, carbohydrates, peptides, and other ligands into the wall-forming materials of Aerosomes (phospholipid-coated microbubbles) (MCCREERY et al. 1997; UNGER and FRITZ 1997). As shown in Fig. 34.2, in vitro targeted microbubbles

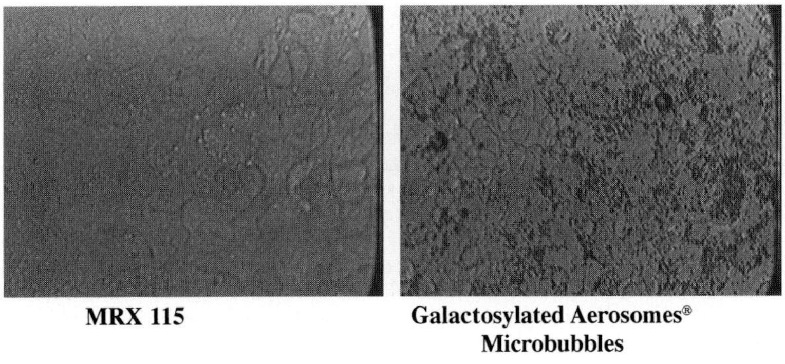

Fig. 34.2. Image of cultured human hepatocytic cells before and after incubation with galactosylated Aerosomes. The galactosylated Aerosomes bind avidly to the hepatocytes. Studies with control Aerosomes (MRX 115) without targeting ligand do not show any binding

bind avidly to cellular targets. In vivo, however, the capillary fenestration might make it more difficult for 1 μm-sized bubbles to seek extravascular targets. Endothelial and vascular targets might be more accessible to targeted microbubbles. Partly for this reason, and also partly because of the large clinical problem, we have focused some of our efforts on developing thrombus-specific microbubbles (Unger and Fritz 1997).

We have synthesized lipids bearing peptides that bind to the GPIIBIIIA receptor of activated platelets. These targeted lipids have been incorporated into the wall-forming materials of Aerosomes. As shown in Fig. 34.3, this thrombus-specific ultrasound contrast agent increases the echogenicity and visibility of thrombus. Shadowing is evident below the clot secondary to large concentrations of microbubbles. Control studies with nontargeted Aerosomes fail to enhance thrombus.

Given that we can selectively target thrombosis, how might this be used clinically? Firstly, if we improve clot detection, this may improve diagnosis and management of vascular thrombosis. Secondly, we may use the targeted microbubbles to enhance ultrasound-mediated clot lysis. As noted above, free microbubbles increased clot lysis with sonication. Recall that cavitation is a local thermomechanical phenomenon. Ideally ultrasound imaging will be performed in concert with sonothrombolysis to monitor cavitation and clot lysis. We anticipate that imaging for therapy will take advantage of subharmonic and ultraharmonic frequencies, as these will monitor cavitation more closely than the fundamental frequency (US patent 5 558 092).

Cavitation nuclei (e.g., thrombus-specific microbubbles) should be expected to increase the efficiency of clot lysis with ultrasound. Co-administration of targeted microbubbles with thrombolytic drugs should further increase the efficiency of sonolysis.

In the second form of targeting, using acoustically active materials, we may use ultrasound to "pop" the bubbles, or activate the gaseous precursor materials for local drug or therapeutic delivery. Note that it is possible to use both methods of targeting together. As shown above, we have used targeting ligands to bind clot and proposed using sound for clot therapy. A further extension is to incorporate drugs into acoustically active materials and use ultrasound to release and/or activate drugs at the target tissue.

How can we then incorporate drugs into acoustically active materials for therapy? There are many approaches. First, the acoustically active material should have sufficient in vivo stability to circulate as a blood pool agent. Polymeric microspheres can be filled with drugs and gas to create ultrasound-sensitive delivery vehicles (Fig. 34.4). Drugs can be incorporated into or onto the wall-forming materials of microbubbles. Pro-drugs can be synthesized to improve incorporation of the therapeutic com-

a

b

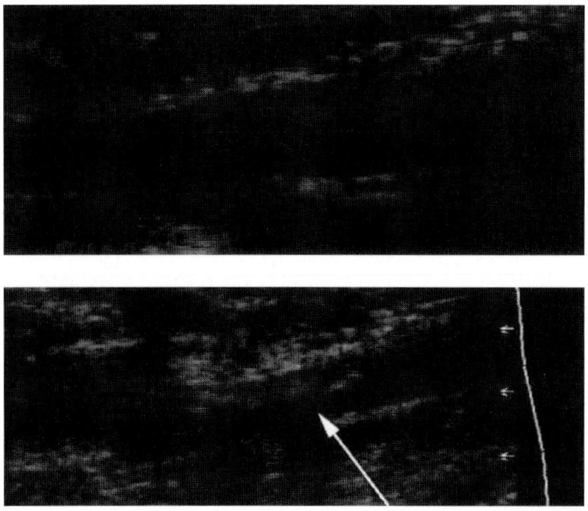

Fig. 34.3. **a** Pre- and **b** post-contrast images of intra-arterial thrombus in the iliac artery of a dog after intravenous administration of Aerosomes targeted to GPIIBIIIA receptor of activated platelets. The postcontrast image shows increased echogenicity of clot and shadowing (*arrow*). Control Aerosomes without targeting ligand do not enhance clot

a b c

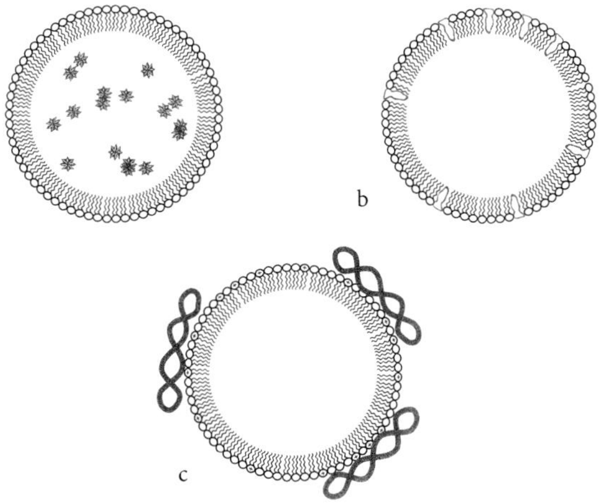

Fig. 34.4 a–c. Schematic diagrams of acoustically active carriers containing drugs are shown. Three of the potential means of delivering drugs with acoustically active carriers are shown. **a** Drugs are entrapped within the interior of gas-filled microspheres. **b** Hydrophobic drugs or pro-drugs are incorporated into the membranes surrounding the microbubbles. **c** Charged materials are incorporated into the membrane stabilizing the microbubble. For example, cationic lipids can be used to bind genetic materials

pounds into the membrane coating the microbubble. Similar and varying approaches can be used to prepare emulsions and microparticles containing acoustically active gaseous precursors.

With phospholipid-coated microbubbles as the delivery vehicle, we might use active drugs that do not require a large amount for efficacy and incorporate the drug into or onto the membrane surrounding the microbubble. We have focused some of our efforts on dexamethasone, a highly active anti-inflammatory drug requiring milligram systemic doses for efficacy. Pressure-stable Aerosomes with up to 30 mole percent dexamethasone have been prepared (McCreery et al. 1998). The pro-drug is biologically active and is released from the Aerosomes by sonication. Although in vivo tests are ongoing at this time, we envision many potential applications for microbubbles bearing dexamethasone. Following intravenous injection, therapeutic ultrasound can be applied to the target tissue to release the drug locally at the desired site. This technique might be used to treat joints, skin, and other tissues afflicted by inflammatory processes. Following intravenous injection, ultrasound might be applied to the thymus to decrease T-cell-mediated hypersensitivity.

34.4 Gene Therapy

Clearly, one of the most exciting areas in biomedicine is the emerging field of gene therapy. How might acoustically active materials be used for gene therapy? It turns out that there are many potential applications for acoustically active materials in gene therapy. Ultrasound energy increases the efficiency of gene expression following transfection (Fritz et al. 1997), and certain acoustically active materials also increase gene expression.

Cationic liposomes have been developed as gene delivery agents for research studies in the laboratory and have also been tested in a number of human clinical trials for gene therapy (Gao and Huang 1995; Felgner 1993; Schreier and Sawyer 1996; Lasic and Templeton 1996). In our development of cationic Aerosomes as gene delivery agents, we discovered that ultrasound energy increases the efficiency of gene expression (Unger et al. 1997a).

Figure 34.5 shows the effect on gene expression of 1-MHz ultrasound applied to cell culture after liposomal transfection with the chloramphenicol acetyltransferase (CAT) gene. Application of ultrasound energy 1 h after transfection results in increased gene expression. The amount of ultrasound energy required to do this is probably more than is used for most diagnostic studies, although levels employed in Doppler ultrasound might be sufficient to enhance gene expression. The level of energy required is certainly below the threshold for lethal cell damage. We have observed ultrasound-enhanced gene expression in multiple different cell lines. As shown in Fig. 34.5, the effects appear most striking in cell lines which only achieve low levels of gene expression following conventional liposomal transfection. After application of ultrasound, high levels of gene expression are observed even in hard to transfect cells. Ultrasound-enhanced gene expression could have important clinical applications. In ex vivo therapy, the efficiency of gene expression following transfection could be increased with ultrasound. Therapeutic genes could be inserted and expressed in autologous or donor cells and then administered to the patient. In vivo, after gene therapy, ultrasound might be applied to the target tissue to enhance gene expression.

The mechanism underlying ultrasound-enhanced transfection is uncertain. Transfection experiments with cationic liposomes demonstrate that most liposomal DNA is degraded within intracellular endosomes. The steps limiting gene expression in these experiments appeared not to be cellular uptake, but release from the endosome and passage to the cell nucleus. Perhaps ultrasound stimulates release of DNA from the endosomes and passage to the nucleus. Clearly more experiments are necessary to explore these mechanisms.

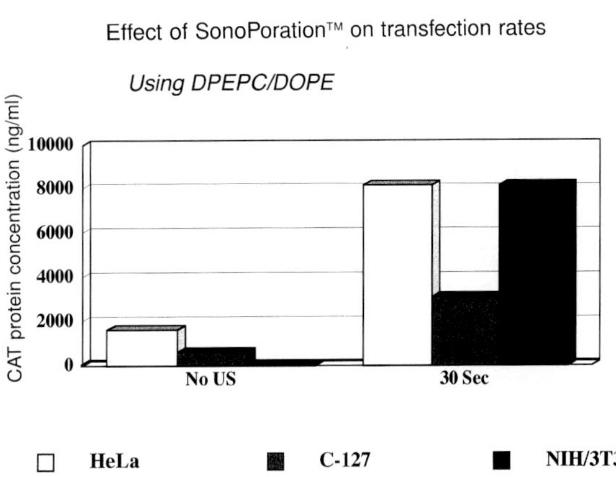

Fig. 34.5. Effect of ultrasound on gene expression (chloramphenicol acetyltransferase, *CAT*) in HeLa, C-127, and NIH/3T3 cells after liposomal transfection. Ultrasound (1 MHz 0.5 W/cm^2 with 100% duty cycle) was applied for 30 s to in vitro cell cultures. Increased gene expression is attained when ultrasound is applied to the cells after transfection

In our efforts to develop acoustically active gene delivery agents, we prepared cationic lipid delivery vehicles from a variety of different lipids, gases, and gaseous precursor materials. We discovered that halocarbons, and especially perfluorocarbons (UNGER et al. 1997b; SWEITZER et al. 1997), greatly enhance the efficiency of gene expression from transfection (Fig. 34.6). Gene expression is further augmented by the application of ultrasound. The preferred halocarbons for enhanced transfection, bromononafluorobutane and perfluorohexane, are liquids at room temperature. A wide variety of fluorinated compounds improve the transfection efficiency of cationic lipids.

We believe the liquid perfluorocarbons reside within the center of the liposomes as a fluorinated core. Perfluoropentane and other perfluorocarbons can also be activated into a gas by agitation, temperature, or pressure. We have then created an acoustically active gene delivery agent, designated FluoroGene. Both with and without ultrasound, these FluoroGene vehicles have many potential applications in gene therapy. As shown in Fig. 34.7, ultrasound application might also be used following vascular or interstitial administration to cause local cavitation and cellular delivery of the genetic material.

34.5 Summary

A variety of potential applications await for targeting and drug delivery with ultrasound contrast agents. Ligands can be used to direct acoustically active

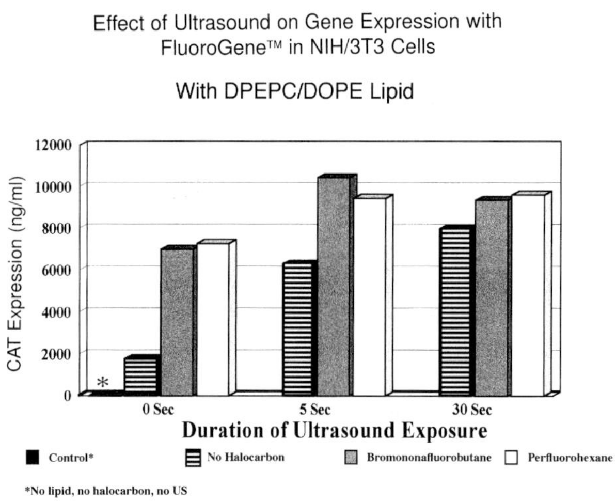

Fig. 34.6. Halocarbons, including bromononafluorobutane and perfluorohexane, greatly enhance the efficiency of gene expression from transfection. Gene expression is further augmented by the application of ultrasound. We define FluoroGene as proprietary formulations of acoustically active, synthetic, gene delivery vehicles with a halocarbon core

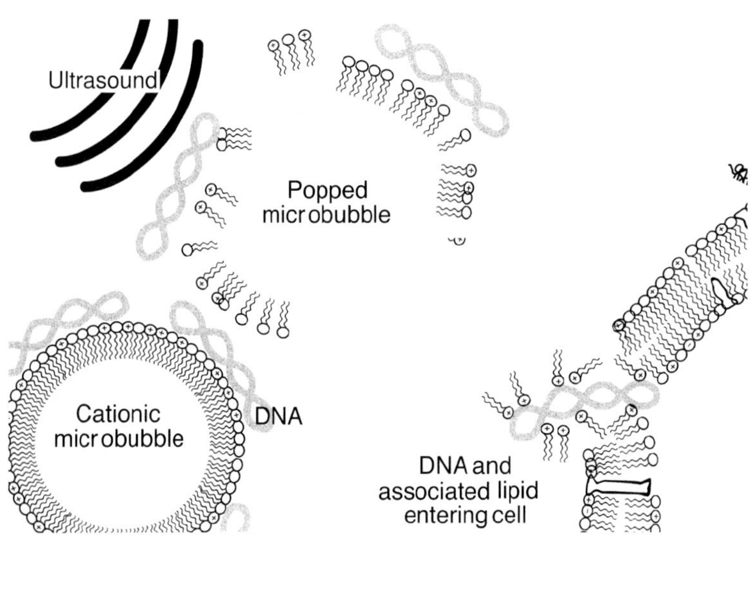

Fig. 34.7. Schematic diagram of acoustically active carrier binding DNA as it is "popped" by ultrasound delivering genes to selected cells

materials to vascular and cellular targets. Hyperthermia and sonolysis can be potentiated by bubbles circulating as blood pool agents, and perhaps even more efficiently by acoustically active materials directed by ligands to the target tissue. Drugs carried by microbubbles and gaseous precursors can be delivered by ultrasound-mediated gas activation and bubble rupture. High-efficiency, acoustically active gene delivery vectors may enhance transfection for gene therapy.

References

Agrawal CM, Kennedy ME, Micallef DM (1994) The effect of ultrasound irradiation on a biodegradable 50–50% copolymer of polylactic and polyglycolic acids. J Biomed Materials Res 28:851–859

Balen FG, Allen CM, Lees WR (1994) Ultrasound contrast agents. Clin Radiol 49:77–82

Ben-Yosef R, Kapp DS (1993) Prognostic factors in metastatic malignant melanoma treated with combined radiation therapy and hyperthermia. Int J Hyperthermia 9:767–781

Bommannan D, Okuyama H, Stauffer P, Guy RH (1992) Sonophoresis. I. The use of high-frequency ultrasound to enhance transdermal drug delivery. Pharm Res 9:559–564

Chan H-C, Magin RL (1989) Characterization of temperature-dependent drug release from liposomes using electron spin resonance. J Pharm Sci 78:311–313

Chelvi TP, Ralhan R (1995) Designing of thermosensitive liposomes from natural lipids for multimodality cancer therapy. Int J Hyperthermia 11:685–695

Curry TS, Dowdey JE, Murry RC (1990) Ultrasound. In: Curry TS, Dowdey JE, Murry RC (eds) Christensen's physics of diagnostic radiology, 4th edn. Lea and Febiger, Philadelphia, pp 323–371

Darkazanli A, Hynynen K, Unger EC, Schenck JF (1993) Online monitoring of ultrasonic surgery with MR imaging. J Magn Reson Imaging 3:509–514

Dorr LN, Hynynen KL (1992) The effects of tissue heterogeneities and large blood vessels on the thermal exposure induced by short high-power ultrasound pulses. Int J Hyperthermia 8:45–59

Felgner PL (ed) (1993) Issue on cationic lipids. J Liposome Res 3:3–106

Forsberg F (1997) Physics of ultrasound contrast agents. In: Goldberg BB (ed) Ultrasound contrast agents. Martin Dunitz, London, pp 9–20

Fosmire H, Hynynen K, Drach GW, Stea B, Swift P, Cassady R (1993) Feasibility and toxicity of transrectal ultrasound hyperthermia in the treatment of locally advanced adenocarcinoma of the prostate. Int J Radiat Oncol Biol Phys 26:253–259

Fowlkes JB, Gardner EA, Carson PL, Ivey JA, Rubin JM (1995) Acoustic interruption of ultrasound contrast agents for blood flow evaluation. J Ultrasound Med 14:513

Fowlkes JB, Sirkin DW, Rhee R, Rubin JM, Carson PL (1997) In vivo interruption of contrast agents for temporally short arterial bolus production. J Ultrasound Med 16:S71

Fritz T, Unger EC, Sutherland G, Sahn D (1997) Phase I clinical trials of MRX 115: a new ultrasound contrast agent. Invest Radiol 32:735–740

Fry FJ, Johnson LK (1978) Tumor irradiation with intense ultrasound. Ultrasound Med Biol 4:337–341

Gao X, Huang L (1995) Cationic liposome-mediated gene transfer. Gene Ther 2:710–722

Goldberg BB, Liu J, Forsberg F (1994) Ultrasound contrast agents: a review. Ultrasound Med Biol 20:319–333

Harrison GH, Balcer-Kubiczek EK, Gutierrez PL (1996) In vitro action of continuous-wave ultrasound combined with adriamycin, X rays or hyperthermia. Radiat Res 145:98–101

Hynynen K (1991) The threshold for thermally significant cavitation in dog's thigh muscle in vivo. Ultrasound Med Biol 17:157–169

Hynynen K, Roemer R, Anhalt D, Johnson C, Xu ZX, Swindell W, Cetas T (1987) A scanned, focused, multiple transducer ultrasonic system for localized hyperthermia treatments. Int J Hyperthermia 3:21–35

Hynynen K, Darkazanli A, Unger EC, Schenck JF (1993) MRI guided noninvasive ultrasound. Med Phys 20:107–115

Iernetti G, Ciuti P, Calligaris F, Francescutto A, Dezhkunov NV (1996) Cavitation threshold dependence on the rate of the transducer voltage variation. Ultrasonics 34:193–195

Inoue K (1974) Permeability properties of liposomes prepared from dipalmitoyllecithin, dimyristoyllecithin, egg lecithin, rat liver lecithin and beef brain sphingomyelin. Biochim Biophys Acta 339:390–402

Kost J, Langer R (1992) Responsive polymer systems for controlled delivery of therapeutics. Tibtech 10:127–131

Lalonde RJ, Hunt JW (1995) Optimizing ultrasound focus distributions for hyperthermia. IEEE Trans Biomed Eng 42:981–990

Lasic DD, Templeton NS (1996) Liposomes in gene therapy. Adv Drug Del Rev 20:221

Li GC, Hahn GM (1978) Ethanol-induced tolerance to heat and to adriamycin. Nature 274:699–701

Lin WL, Roemer RB, Moros EG, Hynynen K (1992) Optimization of temperature distributions in scanned, focused ultrasound hyperthermia. Int J Hyperthermia 8:61–78

Lindholm CE, Kjellen E, Nilsson P, Hertzman S (1987) Microwave-induced hyperthermia and radiotherapy in human superficial tumours. Int J Hyperthermia 3:393–411

Ma LD, Magin RL, Dunn F (1987) Effects of divalent cations on the ultrasonic absorption coefficient of negatively charged liposomes (LUV) near their phase transition temperature. Biochim Biophys Acta 902:183–192

Machluf M, Kost J (1993) Ultrasonically enhanced transdermal drug delivery. Experimental approaches to elucidate the mechanism. J Biomater Sci Polymer Edn 5:147–156

McCreery TP, Sweitzer RH, Shen D, Wu G, Unger EC (1997) A novel ultrasound contrast agent for the detection of thrombosis. Ultrasound Contrast Research Symposium, San Diego, Calif., 7–9 February 1997, p 21

McCreery TP, Sweitzer RH, Vielhauer G, Wu G, Shen D, Yellowhair D, Unger EC (1998) A novel ultrasound contrast agent with therapeutic properties. Acta Radiol 5 (Suppl 1): S247–S249

Mitragotri S, Edwards D, Blankschtein D, Langer R (1995a) A mechanistic study of ultrasonically enhanced transdermal drug delivery. J Pharm Sci 84:697–706

Mitragotri S, Blankschtein D, Langer R (1995b) Ultrasound-mediated transdermal protein delivery. Science 269:850–853

Mitragotri S, Blankschtein D, Langer R (1996) Transdermal drug delivery using low-frequency sonophoresis. Pharm Res 13:411–420

Moros EG, Straube WL, Klein EE, Yousaf M, Myerson RJ (1995) Simultaneous delivery of electron beam therapy and ultrasound hyperthermia using scanning reflectors: a feasibility study. Int J Radiat Oncol Biol Phys 31:893–904

Ning S, Macleod K, Abra RM, Huang AH, Hahn GM (1994) Hyperthermia induces doxorubicin release from long-circulating liposomes and enhances their anti-tumor efficacy. Int J Radiat Oncol Biol Phys 29:827–834

Nishioka T, Luo H, Fishbein MC, et al. (1996) In vivo ultrasonic clot disruption by combination of dodecafluoropentane and transcutaneous ultrasound. Circulation 94(8 Suppl 5):499

Ono A, Yamaguchi M, Horikoshi I, Shintani T, Ueno M (1994) Calcein release from temperature-sensitive liposome with or without stirring. Biol Pharm Bull 171:166–168

Ono A, Horikoshi I, Ueno M (1995) Study on hepatic artery chemoembolization using temperature-sensitive liposome or Lipiodol emulsion. Biol Pharm Bull 18:279–83

Papahadjopoulos D, Jacobson K, Nir S, Isaac T (1973) Phase transitions in phospholipid vesicles. Fluoroscence polarization and permeability measurements concerning the effect of temperature and cholesterol. Biochim Biophys Acta 311:330–348

Rosberger DF, Coleman DJ, Silverman R, Woods S, Rondeau M, Cunningham-Rundles S (1994) Immunomodulation in choroidal melanoma: reversal of inverted CD4/CD8 ratios following treatment with ultrasonic hyperthermia. Biotechnol Ther 5:59–68

Saad AH, Hahn GM (1992) Ultrasound-enhanced effects of adriamycin against murine tumors. Ultrasound Med Biol 18:715–723

Schreier H, Sawyer SM (1996) Liposomal DNA vectors for cystic fibrosis gene therapy. Current applications, limitations, and future directions. Adv Drug Del Rev 19:73–87

Singer M (1979) Interaction of small molecules with phospholipid bilayer membranes: permeability studies. Chem Phys Lipids 25:15–28

Singer M (1981) Permeability of phosphatidylcholine and phosphatidylethanolamine bilayers. Chem Phys Lipids 28:253–267

Suslick KS, Doktycz SJ, Flint EB (1990) On the origin of sonoluminescence and sonochemistry. Ultrasonics 28:280–290

Sweitzer RH, McCreery TP, Unger EC (1997) Ultrasound-enhanced lipofection. Ultrasound Contrast Research Symposium, San Diego, Calif., 7–9 February 1997

Unger EC, Fritz TA (1997) Phase I/II clinical trials of MRX-115: A new ultrasound contrast agent. American Institute of Ultrasound in Medicine, San Diego, Calif., 23–26 March 1997

Unger EC, McCreery TP, Sweitzer RH (1997a) Ultrasound enhances gene expression of liposomal transfection. Invest Radiol 32:723–727

Unger EC, McCreery TP, Sweitzer RH (1997b) Ultrasound enhancement of gene expression from liposomal transfection. Radiology 205 (Suppl 5):724

US patents 5 149 319. Methods for providing localized therapeutic heat to biological tissues and fluids. Unger, Issued Sept 22, 1992

US patents 5 209 720. Methods for providing localized therapeutic heat to biological tissues and fluids using gas filled liposomes. Unger, Issued May 11, 1993

US patents 5 380 411. Ultrasound or shock wave work process and preparation for carrying out same. Schlief, Issued Jan 10, 1995

US patents 5 542 935. Therapeutic delivery systems related applications. Unger, Fritz, Matsunaga, Ramaswami, Yellowhair, Wu, Issued Aug 6, 1996

US patents 5 558 092. Methods and apparatus for performing diagnostic and therapeutic ultrasound simultaneously. Unger, Yellowhair, Issued Sept 24, 1996

US patents 5 580 575. Therapeutic drug delivery systems. Unger, Fritz, Matsunaga, Ramaswami, Yellowhair, Wu, Issued Dec 3, 1996

US patents 5 585 112. Method of preparing gas and gaseous precursor-filled microspheres. Unger, Fritz, Matsunaga, Ramaswami, Yellowhair, Wu, Issued Dec 17, 1996

Walker K (1997) Bubble destruction with ultrasound. Invest Radiol

Waterman FM, Hoh LL (1995) A recommended revision in the RTOG thermometry guidelines for hyperthermia administered by ultrasound. Int J Hyperthermia 11:121–130

Watmough DJ, Lakshmi R, Ghezzi F, et al. (1993) The effect of gas bubbles on the production of ultrasound hyperthermia at 0.75 MHz: a phantom study. Ultrasound Med Biol 19: 231–241

35 Can the Presence of Contrast Media Promote Ultrasound Bioeffects?

C.C. Church and A.A. Brayman

CONTENTS

35.1 Introduction

Diagnostic ultrasound interacts with biological tissue in many ways. The most useful is the backscattering from tissue interfaces and inhomogeneities that allows visualization of internal body structures. In addition, tissue absorbs ultrasound, limiting the depth at which images may be obtained. Absorption also heats the tissue involved, and thermal mechanisms are a well-known cause of ultrasound bioeffects. Other, nonthermal mechanisms also may induce bioeffects. The most common of the nonthermal mechanisms is cavitation. Miller and Thomas (1995) define acoustic cavitation as "any interaction between an ultrasound field and any gaseous inclusion in the medium," and note that, by this definition, "cavitation occurs . . . whenever bubble-based contrast agents are exposed to ultrasound."

Most ultrasound contrast media are suspensions of micrometer-sized gas bubbles that are stabilized against dissolution by surfactants, such as lipids or other surface-active molecules, or by shells of partially denatured proteins or synthetic polymers. The use of relatively insoluble gases, e.g., perfluorocarbons (PFCs), tends to increase the lifetime of these microbubbles even more. Microbubbles respond to exposure to ultrasonic waves by pulsating radially, and it is these pulsations that are the source of much of the increased backscatter responsible for the contrast effect. As the intensity of the acoustic wave increases, so does the magnitude of the bubble response. High-amplitude bubble pulsation, or inertial cavitation, is known to be responsible for various adverse bioeffects in vitro. Thus the injection and subsequent ultrasonic exposure of microbubbles in humans may alter the general perception of the absolute safety of diagnostic ultrasonography.

A substantial literature exists on nonthermal ultrasound bioeffects in "normal" media, i.e., media to which no contrast agents have been added. Gas bubble contrast agents have been available for a relatively short time, and consequently, knowledge of the influence of contrast agents on such phenomena is extremely limited. Most of the information now available was obtained from in vitro studies. In many of the bioeffect studies discussed here, the acoustic pressures used were sufficiently large to ascribe the observed bioeffects to inertial cavitation.

35.2 Theoretical Studies

35.2.1 Physical Properties of the Materials

The many different contrast agents commercially available or under development may be sorted into a few general classes. These are shown in Table 35.1, along with one or two examples of each. It is desirable to characterize the physical nature of each class of microbubble, and more specifically the nature of each of the components of microbubbles in each class, in order to be able to predict and understand the potential responses of each to impinging ultrasonic waves.

C.C. Church, PhD, Acusphere, Inc., University Park at MIT, 38 Sidney Street, Cambridge, MA 02139, USA
A.A. Brayman, PhD, Department of Obstetrics and Gynecology, School of Medicine and Dentistry, The University of Rochester, Rochester, NY 14642, USA

Table 35.1. Classes of microbubble contrast agents

Class	Example
Free bubbles	Agitated saline
Surfactant-coated	Aerosomes
	BR1
	EchoGen
	Imagent US
	SonoGen
Galactose "shell"	Echovist
	Levovist
Stiff-shell, protein	Albunex
	Optison
	Quantison
Stiff-shell, polymer	NC100100
	Sonovist

Table 35.2. Physical properties of microbubble components

Property	Free bubble	Surfactant-coated	Stiff-shell
Shell			
Material	None	Surfactant	Denatured protein
Stiffness	None	"Negative"	Very high
Viscosity	None	Low	Very high
Gas			
Material	Air	C_5F_{12}	Air
Solubility	Medium	Very low	Medium
Diffusivity	Medium	Very low	Medium
Heat capacity	Medium	Very high	Medium

Generally, contrast microbubbles are composed of two major components, the shell (defined here as any material at the gas-liquid interface) and the gas within. The relative values of the most important physical properties of these components are given in Table 35.2 for surfactant-coated bubbles and for protein-encapsulated, or "stiff-shell" bubbles. The values for free bubbles, such as agitated saline, are given for comparison.

Several features of these tables are worth noting. The stiffness of a bubble is provided by the pressure of the gas within the bubble. This is given by the sum of the atmospheric and Laplace pressures, which is proportional to the surface tension. Because the surfactants on surfactant-coated microbubbles reduce surface tension, these bubbles may be said to have a "negative" stiffness, i.e., they are less stiff than free air bubbles of the same size. By contrast, the protein shells surrounding stiff-shell bubbles greatly increase the stiffness of these microbubbles. In general, bubbles with a higher stiffness have higher resonance frequency and lower pulsation amplitude than less stiff bubbles. The effective viscosity in the material of a shell will dampen the response of a microbubble to an ultrasonic wave and thus reduce the magnitude of the response to the wave.

The nature of the gas within a bubble has two important effects on its ultrasonic activity. The first is to determine the lifetime of the microbubble. As surface tension produces an increase in the gas pressure within the bubble, small bubbles tend to dissolve relatively rapidly, and particularly so in liquids undersaturated with gas, e.g., venous blood. By replacing the relatively soluble gases of air, primarily nitrogen and oxygen, with less soluble and less easily diffusible gases such as PFCs, surfactant-coated microbubbles will persist for a much greater time than similarly sized air bubbles. Use of lower molecular weight PFC gases also increases bubble lifetime, but to a lesser extent than the relatively heavy PFC gases. The protein shell encapsulating a stiff-shell microbubble also provides some resistance to the tendency to dissolution, but this is not as effective as gas substitution. The greater intravascular persistence of PFC-containing microbubbles will increase their exposure to ultrasonic waves, increasing the probability for cavitation and its consequent biological effects.

The second important effect of gas composition is related to their heat capacity, the final property listed in Table 35.2, which lessens the potential for adverse events by reducing or eliminating excessive heating and therefore free radical formation, one of the major mechanisms by which cavitation acts. The very high heat capacity of PFC gases means that the surfactant-coated bubble, and bubbles of similar composition, are much less likely to generate free radicals when (and if) they undergo inertial cavitation. This is discussed in more detail below.

35.2.2 Equations for Bubble Dynamics

The first theoretical investigation of the responses to diagnostic ultrasound of microbubbles encapsulated by an elastic solid protein shell was developed by DE JONG et al. (1992) and DE JONG and HOFF (1993), who modeled the effects of the shell's stiffness and viscosity by ad hoc additions to the Rayleigh-Plesset equation. Later, CHURCH (1995) developed a more rigorous mathematical model. This model related important acoustic quantities, such as backscatter and attenuation coefficients, to the values of physical parameters, such as the thickness and rigidity of the encapsulating shell. This model, which consists of a nonlinear Rayleigh-Plesset-like equation for the case of a spherical gas bubble encapsulated by molecules that behave collectively as a continuous, incompressible, damped elastic solid, has the form:

$$\begin{aligned} & R_1 U_1^{\acute{Y}} \left[1+\left(\frac{\varrho_L-\varrho_S}{\varrho_S}\right)\frac{R_1}{R_2}\right]+U_1^2 \\ & \left[\frac{3}{2}+\left(\frac{\varrho_L-\varrho_S}{\varrho_S}\right)\left(\frac{4R_2^3-R_1^3}{2R_2^3}\right)\frac{R_1}{R_2}\right] \\ & =\frac{1}{\varrho_S}\left[P_{G,eq}\left(\frac{R_{01}}{R_1}\right)^{3\kappa}-P_\infty(t)-\frac{2\sigma_1}{R_1}-\frac{2\sigma_2}{R_2}\right. \\ & \left.-\frac{4U_1}{R_1}\left(\frac{V_s\mu_s+R_1^3\mu_L}{R_2^3}\right)-\frac{4V_sG_s}{R_2^3}\left(1-\frac{R_{e1}}{R_1}\right)\right], \end{aligned} \quad (35.1)$$

where R_1 is the radius of the gas-filled cavity, U_1 is the radial velocity of interface 1 (i.e., the interface between the gaseous interior and the encapsulating solid), R_2 is the exterior radius of the encapsulating material, ϱ_L is the density of the surrounding liquid, ϱ_S is the density of the encapsulating shell, $P_{G,eq}$ is the equilibrium gas pressure within the bubble, R_{01} is the initial radius of the gas-filled cavity, $P_\infty(t)$ is the pressure at infinity (including the acoustic driving pressure), σ_1 and σ_2 are the interfacial tensions at the gas-shell and shell-liquid interfaces, respectively, μ_1 and μ_2 are the effective viscosity of the shell and the surrounding liquid, $V_S = R_2^3 - R_1^3$ (assumed constant), G_S is the rigidity (i.e., the stiffness) of the shell, and R_{e1} is the unstrained equilibrium position of the gas-shell interface. As noted above, the presence of an encapsulating shell can greatly restrict the microbubble's pulsation amplitude, resulting in decreased backscatter and attenuation coefficients relative to those found for similarly sized, free gas bubbles.

In contrast to microbubbles encapsulated by elastic solids, free gas bubbles or those stabilized by surfactants are not much restricted in terms of their radial pulsation amplitudes. Although several Rayleigh-Plesset-like equations have been developed to account for various aspects of the behavior of surfactants at the gas-liquid interfaces of microbubbles (Glazman 1983; Atchley 1988), the strong acoustic radiation produced by such bubbles is better modeled by an equation correct to higher order in the Mach number U/C. One such equation which has been found to be surprisingly accurate when compared with "exact" computations (Prosperetti and Lezzi 1986), is Gilmore's equation (Gilmore 1952):

$$\begin{aligned} & R\left(1-\frac{U}{C}\right)\frac{dU}{dt}+\frac{3}{2}\left(1-\frac{U}{3C}\right)U^2 \\ & =\left(1+\frac{U}{C}\right)H+\frac{U}{C}\left(1-\frac{U}{C}\right)R\frac{dH}{dt}, \end{aligned} \quad (35.2)$$

where C is the speed of sound in the liquid at the bubble wall, and H is the enthalpy of the liquid. For the case of surfactant-coated microbubbles, Eq. 35.2 is used by simply assuming a lower-than-water value for the surface tension.

While the equations for bubble dynamics may be used to predict those acoustic properties of microbubbles important to their efficacy as ultrasound contrast agents, the equations also may be used to predict the bubbles' potential for producing adverse biological effects. This potential is directly related to the intensity of the individual bubbles' responses to the impinging ultrasonic waves. The greater the response, the more likely is the production of adverse effects.

35.2.3 Results and Predictions

There are two general modes of bubble response, noninertial and inertial cavitation, which may be distinguished by the bubble's pulsation amplitude. The former is characterized by lower amplitude, repetitive pulsations, whereas the latter involves marked bubble expansion, followed by violent collapse with subsequent production of intense radiated pressure waves, high temperatures, and chemically reactive free radicals. The transition from noninertial to inertial cavitation is marked by a relatively sharp threshold that is dependent on the pressure amplitude and frequency of the ultrasonic wave and on the physical properties of the surrounding material. Examples are presented here to illustrate the mechanisms important to the production of biological effects due to each mode of bubble response for the three examples of bubble classes detailed in Table 35.2, and the transitions between them.

When microbubbles are exposed to lower amplitude ultrasound in long tone bursts or continuous wave form, the response is the stable pulsation of noninertial cavitation. Because there is a phase difference between the ultrasonic wave and that of the bubble volume oscillation, the bubble experiences a net force in the direction of propagation of the wave.

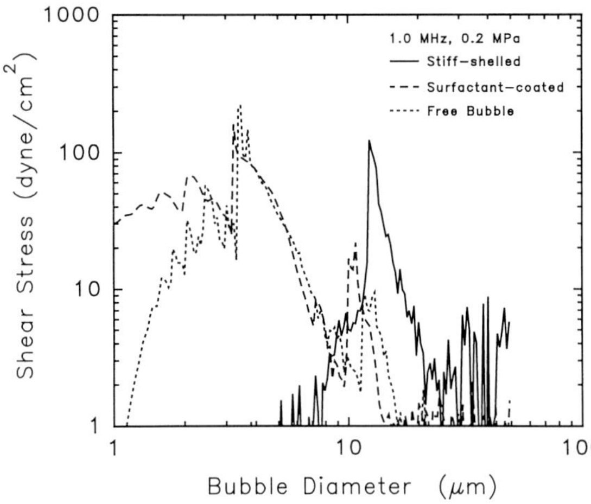

Fig. 35.1. Calculated shear stress produced in the fluid surrounding a microbubble driven by 1.0-MHz, 0.2-MPa continuous wave ultrasound

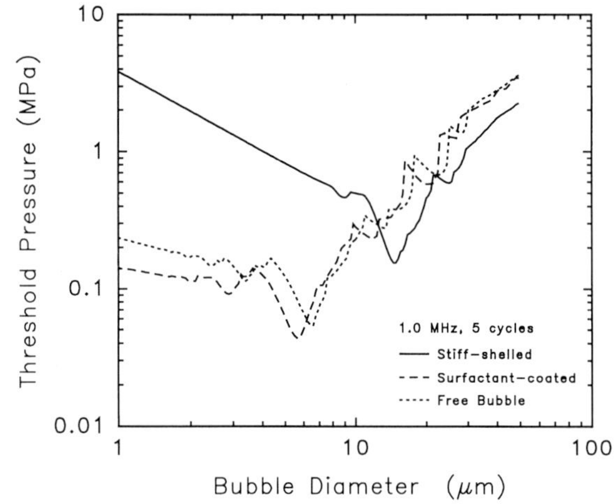

Fig. 35.2. Predictions of thresholds for inertial cavitation of microbubbles exposed to 5-cycle-long pulses of 1.0-MHz ultrasonic waves

This force pushes the bubble along with the wave, and the fluid in the bubble's path must flow around it. The velocity of this flow is greater near the bubble and less farther away. The differential flow produces a shearing action in the fluid, with the amplitude of the shear increasing with the intensity of the ultrasonic wave. Biological cells positioned close to passing bubbles may be caught in this shearing flow and be lysed (i.e., ruptured) by it. Figure 35.1 shows the calculations of shear stress in the fluid (assumed to be water) surrounding each of the three representative microbubbles when exposed to 1.0-MHz, 0.2-MPa continuous wave ultrasound. Notice that, while the position of the maximum shear stress differs due to the different resonance frequencies of the three bubble types, the expected magnitude for all three is approximately the same, i.e., a few hundred dyne/cm^2. Measurements of the critical shear stress for the lysis of red blood cells shows that the threshold for cell destruction by this means is $\sim 10^4$ dyne/cm^2 (Williams et al. 1970; Blackshear and Blackshear 1987), indicating that this mechanism may not be operative in vivo.

As noted above, the transition between lower amplitude, noninertial cavitation and high-amplitude, inertial cavitation is delineated by a relatively sharp threshold. The nature of this threshold differs for the different classes of bubbles. For free bubbles and surfactant-coated bubbles, the threshold may be defined as the acoustic pressure required to cause the bubble to expand to at least twice its initial diameter (Flynn 1975). For bubbles encapsulated by protein shells, it is necessary to break the shell before inertial cavitation may occur. Experimental determinations of the cavitation threshold for Albunex indicate that the shells on encapsulated bubbles must experience a tensile stress of about 100 MPa before they will rupture (Roy et al. 1990; M.W. Miller et al. 1995). Figure 35.2 shows the calculations of the threshold for inertial cavitation for acoustic pulses 5 cycles long. The minima in each curve are caused by bubble resonances. The lowest thresholds for all three bubble types occur at those diameters resonant with the driving frequency, 1.0 MHz, with both larger and smaller bubbles requiring higher pressures to induce inertial cavitation. Note that the minimum in the encapsulated bubble curve occurs at a substantially larger bubble size than for the surfactant-coated or free bubbles, an effect due to the increase in resonance size produced by the added stiffness of the elastic solid shell.

Microbubbles that experience inertial cavitation expand greatly, collapse violently to very small diameters, and then rebound. Two consequences of this phenomenon are important to studies of ultrasound bioeffects. In the first, and the one apparently responsible for many of the biological effects usually studied, the pressure within the collapsed bubble becomes very high, with the consequence that, immediately following the collapse, the rebounding bubble may radiate intense pressure waves. These pressures can generate very high stresses in nearby biological materials, which can lyse individual cells and disrupt tissues. Figure 35.3 shows the calculations of the pressures within bubbles at the point of maximum collapse. The values for the free bubble

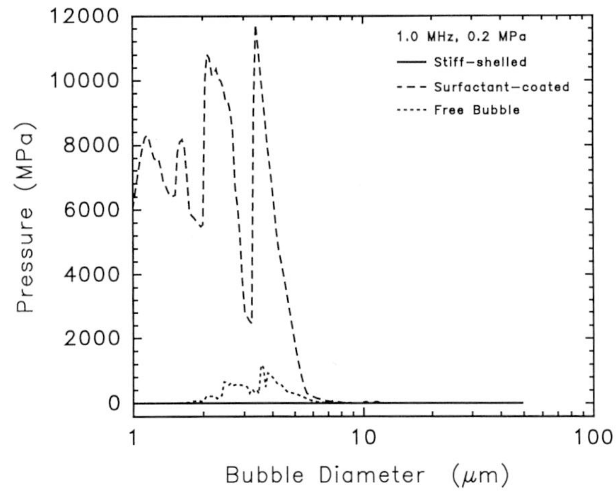

Fig. 35.3. Calculated maximum pressures within microbubbles driven to inertial cavitation by 1.0-MHz, 0.2-MPa continuous wave ultrasound

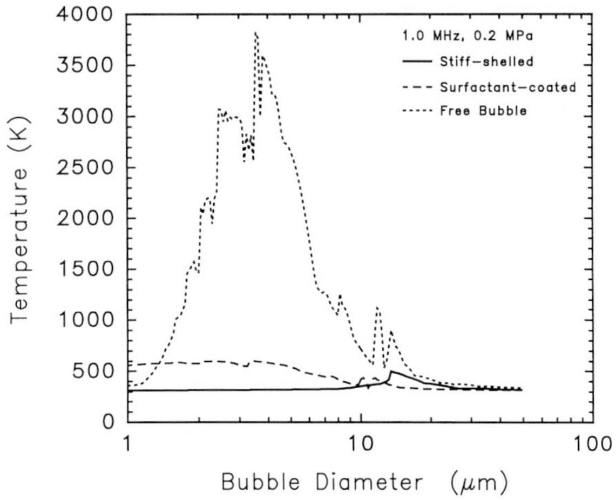

Fig. 35.4. Calculated maximum temperatures within microbubbles driven to inertial cavitation by 1.0-MHz, 0.2-MPa continuous wave ultrasound

reach a peak of more than 1000 MPa at the diameter resonant with the impinging ultrasonic wave, whereas the curve for stiff-shell bubbles is nearly flat, indicating that these bubbles cannot undergo inertial cavitation while still encapsulated. If its shell is broken, however, it is reasonable to assume that an Albunex microbubble will behave much like a free air bubble. The curve for surfactant-coated microbubbles indicates that they, like the free bubble, may experience biologically destructive inertial collapse (although the very high values shown in the figure are probably an artifact of the computational method).

The second important consequence of inertial cavitation is the generation of extremely high temperatures in the gas within the bubble at the point of its maximum collapse (Fig. 35.4). Interestingly, the temperatures within the free air bubble are much greater than for the other two classes, with a maximum of over 3700 K. Such high temperatures generate chemically reactive free radicals, which are known to damage biological materials (Kondo and Kano 1988; Riesz and Kondo 1992). Stiff-shell bubbles do not attain high internal temperatures, again because the encapsulating shell does not permit inertial cavitation. The temperature within surfactant-coated PFC bubbles also remains relatively low because the gas has a very high heat capacity (see Table 35.2), allowing the gas to "absorb" most of the energy of the collapse without a significant change in temperature. The ability of PFCs to limit the maximum temperatures within microbubbles experiencing inertial collapse is a general feature of PFC gases (Suslick and Kemper 1993). Thus even the very low level mutagenic ability of continuous wave ultrasound (Doida et al. 1990) may be effectively suppressed by use of PFC gases in ultrasound contrast agents. Regardless of gas composition, however, any microbubble undergoing inertial cavitation appears to be capable of producing cell lysis.

35.3 Experimental Studies

35.3.1 Effect of Contrast Agents on Cavitation Thresholds

Holland and Apfel (1990) explored the effect of Albunex on the pressure threshold for inertial cavitation using a passive cavitation detector. Cavitation thresholds in water ranged from 1.94 to 2.43 MPa at frequencies of 0.757–2.3 MHz. With Albunex, the threshold at 0.757 MHz was reduced about threefold. Miller and Thomas (1995) also studied the promotion of inertial cavitation by contrast agents, using sonochemically produced H_2O_2 as the endpoint. At 2.17 MHz and 0.82 MPa, no measurable H_2O_2 was produced in plain saline. With either Levovist or Albunex added, H_2O_2 was detected at ~0.4 MPa. They also found that in all test fluids, the acoustic pressure required to cause cavitation decreased with decreasing frequency. At 3.8 MHz, no cavitation occurred in these materials, even at a pressure amplitude of 1.16 MPa. At 2.95 MHz, cavitation in saline-containing contrast occurred at about 0.6 MPa, and at 2.17 MHz, the threshold was about 0.4 MPa. Thus, microbubble contrast agents can lower significantly the threshold acoustic pressures required for inertial cavitation inception. This result has potentially important consequences for the occurrence of non-thermal bioeffects in vivo.

35.3.2 Potentially Undesirable Bioeffects

Hemolysis is the best-studied contrast agent-enhanced bioeffect of ultrasound. WILLIAMS et al. (1991) insonated human erythrocyte suspensions with continuous wave ultrasound at 0.75 MHz and at 0.5 W/cm^2 spatial average temporal average (SATA). Suspensions had different hematocrits (Hcts) and different Echovist concentrations. Lysis was dependent on both Hct and Echovist concentration. In the absence of Echovist, ~33% of the cells suspended at 0.5% Hct lysed when exposed to ultrasound. With 8 mg Echovist/ml present, hemolysis increased to ~60%. WILLIAMS et al. (1991) observed, as have others, that the fraction of cells lysed decreased as Hct increased, with no lysis detectable in most samples at Hcts >5%. This observation is relevant to the issue of cavitation-related hemolysis in vivo, and thus warrants discussion.

For a given ultrasound exposure, a large fraction of cells in suspension may be lysed when the cell concentration (or Hct) is "low," but only a small or undetectable fraction may be lysed when the cell concentration is "high," suggesting that the latter condition either inhibits or eliminates inertial cavitation. However, M.W. MILLER et al. (1995) noted that although the fraction of cells lysed by ultrasound with Albunex present decreased with increasing Hct, the number of cells lysed remained roughly constant. Similar results were reported for cell lysis produced by stable pulsations of trapped microbubbles (D.L. MILLER 1988). These observations suggest that cell lysis is not abolished by increasing cell concentration, but rather merely represents a decreasing fraction of the cells present in the sample. BRAYMAN et al. (1996b) examined this issue, and found that although relative sonolytic yield declines as Hct increases, the absolute extent of lysis increases rather than decreases, albeit nonlinearly. Their results indicate that in vitro sonolysis of cells at high cell densities is limited by the number of microbubbles available, and/or by the number of cells a bubble may encounter before being "inactivated" by the formation of cell aggregates around pulsating bubbles.

M.W. MILLER et al. (1995) used Albunex at concentrations of 0–41 µl/ml in human erythrocyte suspensions having Hcts of 1%–20%. These were exposed or sham-exposed to continuous wave, 1-MHz ultrasound of 1–5 W/cm^2 (I_{SPTP}) for 60–120 s with or without exposure vessel rotation. Hemolysis in 1% Hct suspensions sonicated at 5 W/cm^2 I_{SP} increased from 28% to ~50% when Albunex was added at concentrations within the range 1.3–41 µl/ml. At 1 W/cm^2 there was no differential associated with the presence of Albunex; at higher intensities, Albunex significantly increased sonolysis. With or without Albunex, the fraction of cells lysed decreased as Hct increased. BRAYMAN et al. (1995) evaluated human erythrocyte sonolysis in the presence or absence of 35 µl/ml Albunex using pulsed ultrasound (P^+ = 4.7, P^- = −2.7 MPa). They found that without Albunex, sonication produced statistically significant levels of hemolysis only at 1% Hct, while with Albunex, significant hemolysis was observed at all tested Hcts, and the number of cells lysed per sample remained more or less constant over the 5%–40% range of Hcts.

BRAYMAN et al. (1996a) examined the acoustic pressure and pulse length dependence of hemolysis produced by 1-MHz ultrasound in the presence of Albunex. Human erythrocyte suspensions of 40% Hct containing 3.6 V% Albunex were exposed to pulsed, 1 MHz ultrasound. Acoustic pressures ranged from 0 to 7.39 MPa (P^+), and 0–4.00 MPa (P^-). The duty factor was 0.01, and pulse duration varied between 5 and 1000 µs. When the data were adjusted for the level of spontaneous hemolysis in sham-exposed control samples, hemolysis was observed in all insonated samples, including those exposed to the lowest acoustic pressure/intensity at the shortest pulse duration tested (0.5 MPa, 5-µs pulses). At constant pulse duration, there was a clear dose-response relationship between ultrasound intensity and hemolysis. At constant intensity hemolysis increased generally with increasing pulse duration.

The frequency dependence of hemolysis produced by pulsed ultrasound exposure in the presence of 3.6 V% Albunex was investigated by BRAYMAN et al. (1997), using 40% Hct erythrocyte suspensions. Samples were exposed to ultrasound pulses with center frequencies of 1.02, 2.24, and 3.46 MHz at peak negative pressures of 0.0–3.0 MPa. At low acoustic pressures, hemolysis depended weakly on frequency, but the apparent frequency dependence became sharper as acoustic pressure increased. The finding that hemolysis decreases with increasing frequency is encouraging, as most diagnostic ultrasound equipment operates in the 2- to 7-MHz range. However, BRAYMAN et al. (1997) noted that, under worst case conditions during an echocardiographic examination with Albunex, it might be possible to lyse a small percent of the erythrocytes in the body. Support for this conclusion has been obtained experimentally by DALECKI et al. (1997), as discussed below. Moreover, sonicated Albunex suspensions retain the ability to nucleate inertial cavitation and lyse red cells despite apparent ultrasonic destruction of the microspheres (BRAYMAN and MILLER 1997). Thus, with continued insonation, enhanced cavitation activity may persist for some time.

MILLER and THOMAS (1996) used whole canine blood (50% Hct) to study the effect of Albunex on hemolysis. A lithotripter ($P^+ \sim 24$, $P^- \sim 5$ MPa) and 1.3 MHz, high-intensity focused ultrasound (HIFU) sources were used. HIFU was applied in continuous or burst mode, with burst lengths of 20, 100, or 1000 µs and pressure amplitudes ranging from 1 to 18 MPa. Albunex concentrations ranged from 0 to 10 V%. The presence of Albunex in samples exposed to the lithotripter shocks decreased the number of shocks required to observe greater hemolysis than in the shams, but did not significantly affect the extent of hemolysis with a large number of shocks. Acoustic pressure thresholds for hemolysis varied with exposure duration and presence or absence of Albunex. Compared to blood without or with 0.1% Albunex that had no effect on hemolysis, 1% and 10% Albunex decreased equally the threshold pressure required to achieve hemolysis at all exposures. However, at very high acoustic pressures (e.g., ~18 MPa), hemolysis occurred in all insonated samples, regardless of the presence or absence of Albunex, with the exception of those exposed to 20-µs bursts without Albunex, in which there was none. Hemolysis increased with increasing burst length (20 µs, 100 µs, or 1000 µs), and was greater with Albunex than without at suprathreshold acoustic pressures.

Erythrocytes are not the only blood cells susceptible to sonolysis. At comparable cell concentrations, human erythrocytes and lymphocytes are lysed in roughly equivalent numbers by ultrasound exposures above the cavitation threshold. However, the white cells are somewhat more sensitive to lysis than the red cells, apparently because white cells are larger and mechanically more fragile (MILLER and BRAYMAN 1997).

There are very few reports dealing with in vivo bioeffects arising in the presence of microbubble contrast agents. DALECKI et al. (1997) used a murine model to study ultrasonic hemolysis in relation to the presence or absence of Albunex. Albunex or plain saline solution was injected intravenously into mice, and their hearts were then exposed to pulsed ultrasound (10 ms pulse duration, 100 Hz pulse repetition frequency, 1.2 or 2.4 MHz; pressure amplitudes as high as 10 MPa). Blood was then collected and hemolysis assayed. At 1.2 MHz the apparent pressure threshold, at the level of the heart, for hemolysis was ~3 MPa P^+, 1.9 MPa P^-. At 10 MPa P^+, there was an approximately tenfold increase in hemolysis (3% vs 0.3%) associated with Albunex treatment relative to saline control. At 2.4 MHz and 10 MPa P^+, there was no significant difference in hemolysis between Albunex- or saline-injected treatment groups, indicating a very sharp frequency dependence for hemolysis at high acoustic pressures, as discussed previously.

RAEMAN et al. (1997) tested the hypothesis that ultrasonic lung hemorrhage results from inertial cavitation activity within the pulmonary capillaries by injecting Albunex or saline intravenously into mice, followed by insonation of the lung (10 ms pulse duration, 100 Hz pulse repetition frequency, 5 min, 2 MPa P^+). There was no significant difference in the surface area of hemorrhage between the two treatment groups, suggesting that the inertial cavitation within the pulmonary capillaries is not the primary mechanism by which ultrasonic lung hemorrhage arises.

PRAT et al. (1991) explored the effect of microbubble contrast agent injections on hepatic lesion formation in rabbits exposed to lithotripter fields having amplitudes comparable to those used to disintegrate kidney stones. Some animals were injected with saline as a control and were exposed to 500 shocks, whereas others were injected only with microbubbles (Plasmion), and a third group was injected with microbubbles and exposed to 500 shocks. With 500 shocks, animals given saline had a small number of hepatic lesions while those given microbubbles had more and larger lesions.

35.3.3 Potentially Useful Bioeffects

A number of papers have been published in which ultrasound has been reported to enhance the effectiveness of certain anticancer drugs, apparently via nonthermal mechanisms (YUMITA et al. 1987, 1989, 1990; SAAD and HAHN 1989; LOVEROCK et al. 1990;

Umemura et al. 1990; Harrison et al. 1991; Kessel et al. 1994). The use of ultrasound microbubble contrast agents to deliberately nucleate cavitation as a means of directly disrupting tissues, or as an adjunct to ultrasound-drug interactions, is a relatively recent development. Space considerations permit discussion of just a few representative reports here. For additional discussion please refer to Chap. 36.

Lipid-coated microbubbles (LCMs) have been shown to accumulate in tumor tissue to a much greater extent than in surrounding tissues (Simon et al. 1992, 1993; Barbarese et al. 1995), thus presenting the possibility of therapeutic intervention by the induction of inertial cavitation in LCM-enriched tumor tissues. Simon et al. (1993) tested this idea using Walker-256 tumors implanted subcutaneously in rats. Although insonation did not affect tissue temperature within the limits of detection of their instruments (±0.5°C), continuous wave, 4.5 MHz ultrasound applied at a SATA intensity of 250 mW/cm^2 for 8 min caused a consistent elevation of tumor necrosis in animals pretreated with LCMs relative to either the controls or the ultrasound-only treatment group.

A similar approach was tried by Prat et al. (1993). These workers implanted tumors in the abdomens of rats, and used an electrohydraulic lithotripter (250–500 shocks, P^+ ~60 MPa) to induce cavitation while the abdomens were being infused with air-filled, gelatin-encapsulated microbubbles. This treatment was tried with and without co-treatment with fluorouracil. The drug alone was 100% effective only at high doses that compromised the liver. While shock waves and microbubbles without drug cured about half of the animals, they cured all animals when combined with low-dose fluorouracil.

Jeffers et al. (1995) explored ultrasound-induced cavitation of stabilized microbubbles as a potential tool to aid in the destruction of tumors. The goal was to enhance the membrane-damaging effect of the polar solvent and tumoricidal drug *N,N*-dimethylforamide (DMF), by ultrasound in a very localized tissue volume, such that systemic drug doses might be reduced to avoid liver toxicity effects while still producing tumoricidal activity. The related drugs monomethylforamide and dimethylsulfoxide were also tested. Membrane damage of HL-60 human promyelocytic leukemia cell suspension, assessed by measurement of lactate dehydrogenase activity in the supernatant, was detected only when sonicated in the presence of albumin-stabilized microbubbles as compared with vehicle controls (i.e., no bubbles). Membrane damage produced by the ultrasound+bubbles treatment increased with increasing ultrasound intensity, reaching ~35% at the highest exposure level. Membrane damage increased further when DMF was added to the suspension prior to insonation. Qualitatively similar results were obtained at constant ultrasound intensity with the other drugs tested, i.e., their cytotoxic effect was marked when present during insonation with microbubbles, while insonation alone or the drugs alone had no appreciable effect. Cell membrane damage in the ultrasound+DMF+bubbles and the ultrasound+bubbles treatments was strongly correlated with the subharmonic emission amplitude measured during sample insonation, indicating that inertial cavitation was responsible for the effect. When cells were added and incubated in preinsonated suspension of microbubbles with or without DMF, no membrane damage was detected, suggesting that any effective sonochemicals produced by the insonation were short-lived. Other assessments indicated that the presence of DMF did not increase cavitation activity relative to DMF-free controls, nor did DMF sensitize the cells to damage by shear forces applied to the cells by nonacoustic means. When taken together, the observations that (1) there was no bulk heating of the insonated suspensions, (2) enhancement of DMF cytotoxicity was proportional to inertial cavitation activity, and (3) the DMF did not affect the occurrence of cavitation or the susceptibility of the cells to rupture by shear forces generated by nonacoustic means, suggest that free radicals or other short-lived sonochemicals, rather than the sonomechanical forces produced by inertial cavitation, were responsible for the effect.

35.4 Summary

In this chapter we have presented the current knowledge of the potential for bioeffects when microbubble contrast agents are used in diagnostic ultrasound. We can conclude that the presence of contrast media increases the opportunity for cell lysis or tissue damage to occur. For damage to occur, data indicate that the ultrasound energy needs to be greater and the frequency lower than those currently used with diagnostic ultrasound. Therefore the probability of inducing detectable ultrasound bioeffects is low.

In therapeutic applications, on the other hand, where high energy and low frequency can be used, microbubbles can enhance the ultrasonic effect, which can be exploited to lyse clots or treat solid tumors.

References

Atchley AA (1988) The Blake threshold of a cavitation nucleus having a radius-dependent surface tension. J Acoust Soc Am 85:152–157

Azadniv M, Doida Y, Miller MW, Brayman AA, Meltzer RS (1995) Temporality in ultrasound-induced cell lysis in vitro. Echocardiography 13:45–55

Barbarese E, Ho SY, D'Arrigo JS, Simon RH (1995) Internalization of microbubbles by tumor cells in vivo and in vitro. J Neuro-Oncol 26:25–34

Blackshear PL, Blackshear GL (1987) Mechanical-hemolysis. In: Skalak R, Chien S (eds) Handbook of engineering. McGraw-Hill, New York, pp 15.1–15.19

Brayman AA, Miller MW (1997) Acoustic cavitation nuclei survive the apparent ultrasonic destruction of Albunex microspheres. Ultrasound Med Biol 23:793–796

Brayman AA, Doida Y, Miller MW (1992) Apparent contribution of respiratory gas exchange to the in vitro "cell density effect" in ultrasonic cell lysis. Ultrasound Med Biol 18:701–714

Brayman AA, Azadniv M, Makin IRS, et al. (1995) Effect of a stabilized microbubble contrast agent on hemolysis of human erythrocytes exposed to high-intensity pulsed ultrasound. Echocardiography 12:13–22

Brayman AA, Azadniv M, Cox C, Miller MW (1996a) Hemolysis of Albunex-supplemented, 40% hematocrit human erythrocytes in vitro by 1 MHz pulsed ultrasound: acoustic pressure and pulse length dependence. Ultrasound Med Biol 22:927–938

Brayman AA, Church CC, Miller MW (1996b) Re-evaluation of the concept that high cell concentrations "protect" cells in vitro from ultrasonically-induced lysis. Ultrasound Med Biol 22:497–514

Brayman AA, Strickler PS, Luan H, Barned SL, Raeman CH, Cox C, Miller MW (1997) Hemolysis of 40% hematocrit, Albunex-supplemented human erythrocyte suspensions by intense pulsed ultrasound: frequency, duty factor, pulse length and sample rotation dependence. Ultrasound Med Biol 13:1237–1250

Carstensen EL, Kelly P, Church CC, Brayman AA, Child SZ, Raeman CH, Schery L (1993) Lysis of erythrocytes by exposure to CW ultrasound. Ultrasound Med Biol 19: 147–165

Church CC (1995) The effects of an elastic solid surface layer on the radial pulsations of gas bubbles. J Acoust Soc Am 97:1510–1521

Dalecki D, Raeman CH, Child SZ, Cox C, Francis CW, Meltzer RS, Carstensen EL (1997) Hemolysis in vivo from exposure to pulsed ultrasound. Ultrasound Med Biol 23:307–313

de Jong N, Hoff L (1993) Ultrasound scattering properties of Albunex microspheres. Ultrasonics 31:175–181

de Jong N, Hoff L, Skotland T, Bom N (1992) Absorption and scatter of encapsulated gas filled microspheres: theoretical considerations and some measurements. Ultrasonics 30:95–103

Doida Y, Miller MW, Cox C, Church CC (1990) Confirmation of an ultrasound-induced mutation in two in-vitro mammalian cell lines. Ultrasound Med Biol 16:699–705

Flynn HG (1975) Cavitation dynamics. II. Free pulsations and models for cavitation bubbles. J Acoust Soc Am 58:1160–1170

Gilmore FR (1952) The collapse and growth of a spherical bubble in a viscous compressible liquid. California Institute of Technology Hydrodynamics Laboratory, Report 26-4. California Institute of Technology, Pasadena, Calif

Glazman RE (1983) Effects of adsorbed films on gas bubble radial oscillations. J Acoust Soc Am 74:980–986

Harrison GH, Balcer-Kubiczek EK, Eddy HA (1991) Potentiation of chemotherapy by low-level ultrasound. Int J Radiat Biol 59:1453–1466

Holland CK, Apfel RE (1990) Thresholds for transient cavitation in a controlled nuclei environment. J Acoust Soc Am 88:2059–2069

Inoue M, Miller MW, Church CC (1990) An alternative explanation for a postulated non-thermal non-cavitational ultrasound mechanism of action on in vitro cells at hyperthermic temperature. Ultrasonics 28:185–189

Jeffers RJ, Feng RQ, Fowlkes JB, Hunt JW, Kessel D, Cain CA (1995) Dimethylforamide as an enhancer of cavitation-induced cell lysis in vitro. J Acoust Soc Am 97:669–676

Kessel D, Jeffers RJ, Fowlkes JB, Cain CA (1994) Porphyrin-induced enhancement of ultrasound cytotoxicity. Int J Radiat Biol 66:221–228

Kondo T, Kano E (1987) Enhancement of hyperthermic cell killing by non-thermal effect of ultrasound. Int J Radiat Biol 51:157–166

Kondo T, Kano E (1988) Effect of free radicals induced by ultrasonic cavitation on cell killing. Int J Radiat Biol 51:475–486

Loverock P, ter Haar G, Omerod MG, Imrie PR (1990) The effect of ultrasound on the cytotoxicity of adriamycin. Br J Radiol 63:542–546

Makin IRS, Everbach EC, Porter T, Xie F, Meltzer RS (1995) Comparison of cavitational activity of echocontrast agents filled with different gases. Circulation 92 (Suppl I):I-192

Miller DL (1988) The influence of hematocrit on hemolysis by ultrasonically activated gas-filled micropores. Ultrasound Med Biol 14:293–297

Miller DL, Thomas RM (1995) Ultrasound contrast agents nucleate inertial cavitation in vitro. Ultrasound Med Biol 21:1059–1065

Miller DL, Thomas RM (1996) Contrast agent gas-bodies enhance hemolysis induced by lithotripter shockwaves and high-intensity focused ultrasound in whole blood. Ultrasound Med Biol 22:1089–1095

Miller MW, Brayman AA (1997) Comparative sensitivity of human erythrocytes and lymphocytes to sonolysis by 1 MHz ultrasound. Ultrasound Med Biol 23:635–638

Miller MW, Azadniv M, Doida Y, Brayman AA (1995) Effect of a stabilized microbubble contrast agent on CW ultrasound-induced red blood cell lysis in vitro. Echocardiography 12:1–12

Prat F, Ponchon T, Burger F, Chapelon JY, Gagnon P, Cathignol D (1991) Hepatic lesions in the rabbit induced by acoustic cavitation. Gastroenterology 100:1345–1350

Prat F, Chapelon JY, el Fadil FA, Theillere Y, Ponchon T, Cathignol D (1993) In vivo effects of cavitation alone or in combination with chemotherapy in a peritoneal carcinomatosis in the rat. Br J Cancer 68:13–17

Prosperetti A, Lezzi A (1986) Bubble dynamics in a compressible liquid. Part 1. First-order theory. J Fluid Mech 168:457–478

Raeman CH, Dalecki D, Child SZ, Meltzer RS, Carstensen EL (1997) Albunex does not increase the sensitivity of the lung to pulsed ultrasound. Echocardiography 14:553–557

Riesz P, Kondo T (1992) Free radical formation induced by ultrasound and its biological implications. Free Radic Biol Med 13:247–270

Roy RA, Church CC, Calabrese A (1990) Cavitation produced by short pulses of ultrasound. In: Hamilton MF, Blackstock DA (eds) Frontiers of nonlinear acoustics: proceedings of the 12th ISNA. Elsevier, London, pp 476–481

Saad AH, Hahn GM (1989) Ultrasound-enhanced drug toxicity on Chinese hamster ovary cells in vitro. Cancer Res 49:5931–5934

Simon RH, Ho SY, Perkins CR, D'Arrigo JS (1992) Quantitative assessment of tumor enhancement by ultrastable lipid-coated microbubbles as a sonographic contrast agent. Invest Radiol 27:29–34

Simon RH, Ho SY, Lange SC, Uphoff DF, D'Arrigo JS (1993) Applications of lipid-coated microbubble contrast to tumor therapy. Ultrasound Med Biol 19:123–125

Suslick KS, Kemper KA (1993) The effect of fluorocarbon gases on sonoluminescence: a failure of the electrical hypothesis. Ultrasonics 31:463–465

Umemura S, Yumita N, Nishigaki R, Umemura K (1990) Mechanism of cell damage by ultrasound in combination with hematoporphyrin. Jpn J Cancer Res 81:962–966

Williams AR, Hughes DE, Nyborg WL (1970) Hemolysis near a transversely oscillating wire. Science 169:971–973

Williams AR, Kubowicz G, Cramer E, Schlief R (1991) The effects of the microbubble suspension SHU 454 (Echovist) on ultrasonically-induced cell lysis in a rotating tube exposure system. Echocardiography 8:423–433

Yumita N, Okumura A, Nishigaki R, Umemura K, Umemura S (1987) The combination treatment of ultrasound and antitumor drugs on Yoshida sarcoma. Jpn J Hypertherm Oncol 3:175–182

Yumita N, Nishigaki R, Umemura K, Umemura S (1989) Hematoporphyrin as a sensitizer of cell-damaging effect of ultrasound. Jpn J Cancer Res 80:219–222

Yumita N, Nishigaki R, Umemura K, Umemura S (1990) Synergistic effect of ultrasound and hematoporphyrin on Sarcoma 180. Jpn J Cancer Res 81:304–308

IV
Radiopharmaceuticals (Nuclear Medicine)

36 Imaging Techniques and Existing Agents

H.-Y. Oei, D.J. Kwekkeboom, and E.P. Krenning

CONTENTS

H.-Y. Oei, MD, PhD, Department of Nuclear Medicine, University Hospital Rotterdam, Dijkzigt, P.O. Box 2040, 3000 CA Rotterdam, The Netherlands
D.J. Kwekkeboom, MD, PhD, Department of Nuclear Medicine, University Hospital Rotterdam, Dijkzigt, P.O. Box 2040, 3000 CA Rotterdam, The Netherlands
E.P. Krenning, MD, PhD, Professor, Department of Nuclear Medicine, University Hospital Rotterdam, Dijkzigt, P.O. Box 2040, 3000 CA Rotterdam, The Netherlands

36.1 Introduction

Although the images obtained with nuclear medicine techniques have a poor resolution, these techniques often have a significant role in the decision tree for the management of particular pathological conditions. The high sensitivity in identifying the presence of disease and the noninvasiveness of nuclear medicine techniques are important advantages that render them the methods of choice in the search for these conditions. Another important advantage is the negligible adverse reactions observed. Table 36.1 lists the imaging techniques employed in daily nuclear medicine practice; the list includes applications in all organ systems as well as in oncology and the localization of inflammatory processes.

Most radiopharmaceuticals are formulated as aqueous, sterile, and apyrogenic injections and are administered to patients for diagnostic or therapeutic purposes. In this respect they are no different from conventional parenteral medicines in the requirements for purity or efficiency. Standards of quality and purity have been devised for these materials and dispensed products should be tested

Table 36.1. Imaging techniques and existing agents

Investigation	Radiopharmaceutical (dose in MBq)
1. *Bone and joints*	
Bone imaging	^{99m}Tc-HDP, ^{99m}Tc-MDP (400–800)
2. *Cardiovascular*	
First-pass ventriculography	^{99m}Tc-DTPA (750)
Gated cardiac blood pool imaging	^{99m}Tc-erythrocytes (500)
Myocardial perfusion imaging	^{99m}Tc-MIBI, ^{99m}Tc-tetrofosmin (350–700)
	^{201}Tl-thallous chloride (100)
Myocardial infarct imaging	^{99m}Tc-pyrophosphate (400)
Evaluation of left-to-right shunt	^{99m}Tc-DTPA (750)
Evaluation of right-to-left shunt	^{99m}Tc-MAA (100)
Radionuclide angiography (first-pass study)	^{99m}Tc-DTPA (750)
Regional distribution of blood flow	^{99m}Tc-MIBI (750), ^{201}Tl-thallous chloride (100)
Radionuclide venography	^{99m}Tc-MAA (80/extremity)
Lymphoscintigraphy	^{99m}Tc-nanocolloid (20/injection site)
3. *Endocrine*	
Thyroid gland imaging	^{99m}Tc-pertechnetate (80), ^{123}I-sodium iodide (20)
Imaging of parathyroid adenoma	^{99m}Tc-MIBI (400)
Imaging of adrenocortical tumors	^{131}I-iodomethylnorcholesterol, ^{75}Se-selenomethylnorcholesterol (20)
4. *Gastrointestinal*	
Salivary gland imaging	^{99m}Tc-pertechnetate (100)
Evaluation of esophageal transit	^{99m}Tc-colloid (5–20)
Evaluation of esophageal reflux	^{99m}Tc-colloid (10)
Gastric emptying study	^{99m}Tc-colloid, ^{99m}Tc-DTPA, ^{111}In-DTPA (10)
Liver and spleen imaging	^{99m}Tc-colloid, ^{99m}Tc-phytate (80)
Imaging of liver hemangioma	^{99m}Tc-erythrocytes (500)
Hepatobiliary imaging	^{99m}Tc-IDA derivatives (80)
Evaluation of gastrointestinal bleeding	^{99m}Tc-erythrocytes, ^{99m}Tc-colloid (700)
Imaging of Meckel's diverticulum	^{99m}Tc-pertechnetate (200)
Peritoneovenous shunt-patency study	^{99m}Tc-MAA (175–350)
5. *Genitourinary*	
Renography	^{99m}Tc-MAG3 (80), ^{99m}Tc-DTPA (150), ^{123}I-OIH (20)
Static renal imaging	^{99m}Tc-DMSA (80), ^{99m}Tc-GHA (150)
Renal perfusion imaging (first-pass study)	^{99m}Tc-DTPA (350)
Evaluation of acute scrotal pain	^{99m}Tc-pertechnetate (350)
Imaging of varicocele	^{99m}Tc-erythrocytes (350)
6. *Hematology*	
Bone marrow imaging	^{99m}Tc-nanocolloid (350–700)
Spleen imaging	^{99m}Tc-denaturated erythrocytes (80)
7. *Neurology*	
Cerebral perfusion imaging	^{99m}Tc-HMPAO, ^{99m}Tc-ECD (500)
Cerebrospinal fluid imaging	^{111}In-DTPA (20)
Dopamine D2 receptor imaging	^{123}I-iodobenzamide (185)
Benzodiazepine receptor imaging	^{123}I-iomazenil (185)
8. *Pulmonary*	
Perfusion scintigraphy	^{99m}Tc-MAA (100)
Ventilation scintigraphy	^{81m}Kr gas, ^{133}Xe gas, ^{99m}Tc-aerosols, ^{99m}Tc-carbon
9. *Localization of inflammatory disease*	
Gallium scintigraphy	^{67}Ga citrate (40–150)
Radiolabelled leukocyte imaging	^{111}In-labeled leukocytes (30), ^{99m}Tc-labeled leukocytes (500)
10. *Oncology*	
Imaging of malignant processes	^{67}Ga citrate (150)
	^{201}Tl-thallous chloride (80–200)
	^{99m}Tc-MIBI (400)
Imaging of pheochromocytoma and neuroblastoma	^{123}I-MIBG (300), ^{131}I-MIBG (30)
Somatostatin receptor scintigraphy	^{111}In-pentetreotide (200)
Sentinel node imaging	^{99m}Tc-nanocolloid (10/injection site)

Abbreviations as defined in the text.

to ensure compliance with these standards as described in the pharmacopoeias and the instruction leaflet for the product (KARESH 1996; THEOBALD 1994).

As radiopharmaceuticals are unsealed radioactive substances, radiation hazard may occur through ingestion, inhalation, or absorption through the skin. It is necessary, therefore, to follow protocols regarding the safety of the patient and the personnel. Most countries have legislation on the handling, use, storage, administration, disposal, and transportation of radiopharmaceuticals. Such legislation may require that a person should be nominated to advise on and supervise radiological protection. In the absence of local legislation, users should comply with internationally recognized standards such as those promulgated by the International Atomic Energy Agency and the International Commission on Radiological Protection (LAZARUS 1994).

All operations involving radiopharmaceuticals should be carried out in restricted areas by persons trained and authorized in their handling and administration to humans. Working protocols should be adopted to prevent contamination with radioactivity during handling, to guarantee the radiopharmaceutical quality, and to safeguard the sterility. All radioactive sources, including prepared radiopharmaceuticals, should be clearly identified with the radionuclide, activity, chemical form, reference time and date, and batch number where appropriate. Relevant tests of the quality of generators, radionuclides, and prepared radiopharmaceuticals should be performed. Radioactive waste and disposal should comply with local rules and guidelines (LAZARUS 1994).

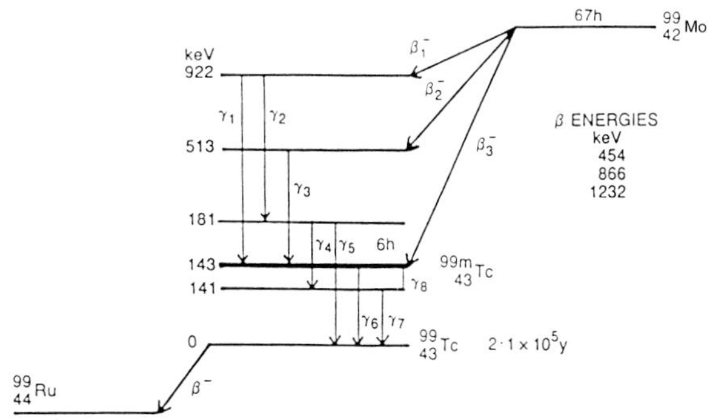

Fig. 36.1. Decay scheme for ^{99}Mo/^{99m}Tc (adapted from SHORT 1994)

36.2 Technetium-Labeled Radiopharmaceuticals

36.2.1 Cold Kits

Due to the availability and advantageous physical properties of technetium-99m, most tracers applied in nuclear medicine are ^{99m}Tc labeled. ^{99m}Tc, a metastable state, is a daughter product of molybdenum-99. The decay scheme is shown in Fig. 36.1. The preparation of technetium-labeled tracers usually involves the simple addition of sodium pertechnetate eluate to the vial containing the unlabeled kit. Subsequent agitation and a short period of incubation are all that is required to obtain the final product. An additional heating step is required for some products. Cold kits are supplied in vials as a freeze-dried mixture of the ligand and excipients, which are essential for the formulation of the kit. They are sterile, pyrogen-free, and sealed under nitrogen. The instruction leaflets include a description of the contents of the kit, the labeling procedure, the properties of the reconstituted solution, the methods for quality control of the agent, and the radiation dosimetry. Also, the indications, dosage, pharmacodynamics, contraindications, adverse reactions, precautions, and warnings are listed. Provided the manufacturer's instructions are strictly adhered to, particularly with regard to maximum activity and volumes of ^{99m}Tc-pertechnetate which should be added, the final product is guaranteed as a diagnostically effective product. Reconstituted kits are usually stable for 6–8 h although for some this period can be shorter. The freeze-dried cold kits themselves have a long shelf-life, usually of more than 1 year if stored at the indicated temperature (KARESH 1996).

Several components can be added to the ligand during the formation of cold kits: reductant, antioxidant, buffer, transfer ligand, solutionizing agent, and filler. Reductant lowers the oxidation state of pertechnetate, which is essential for the formation of Tc-complexes. Due to its practical properties, stannous salt is the most frequently used reductant and almost all currently available cold kits contain it as reductant (NOWOTNIK 1994).

A common problem which limits the postlabeling shelf-life of technetium radiopharmaceuticals is the oxidation of complexed reduced technetium to pertechnetate. Oxidation may occur when air enters the vial when a patient dose is withdrawn from a reconstituted vial or when a patient dose is redispensed or held in the syringe for a long time. To prevent oxidation, antioxidant such as ascorbic acid, gentisic acid, or *p*-aminobenzoic acid is added.

Since the pH of technetium eluate may vary between generators from different suppliers and the radiochemical purity of Tc-complexes or the predominant product of complex formation is pH dependent, the presence of a buffer is of importance. However, since some ligands act as buffer, such addition is not always necessary.

Adding transfer ligand permits the formation of the desired complex. Solubilizing agents or surfactants are used in kits of lipophilic tracers, also to prevent particle aggregation. Fillers, such as mannitol or sodium chloride, are necessary to achieve the appropriate particle size of the freeze-dried solids of a cold kit. The fine particle size makes possible rapid solubilization after addition of the technetium eluate (Karesh 1996; Nowotnik 1994).

36.2.2 ^{99m}Tc-Sodium Pertechnetate

Technetium-99m is obtained from a generator, which consists of ^{99}Mo adsorbed onto a sterile aluminum oxide column. Although the column is shielded with lead or depleted uranium, it is necessary to use secondary shielding to reduce radiation to desirable levels. The ^{99m}Tc is eluted from the column with sterile 0.9% sodium chloride solution. The generator is a sterile system which will be used over a period of 1–2 weeks. The storage and elution of the generator should occur under conditions which will maintain the sterility of the column and also protect operators from radiation and radioactivity released from the system. Elution should be done in accordance with the manufacturer's instructions, using the eluting solvent and collection vials provided (Hojelse et al. 1994).

The radionuclide purity specification of ^{99m}Tc eluted from a generator depends on the source of the parent ^{99}Mo. In the case of nonfission pertechnetate, in which ^{99}Mo is produced by neutron bombardment of ^{98}Mo, not more than 0.1% of the total radioactivity is due to the parent ^{99}Mo, and not more than 0.01% of all other radionuclidic impurities. With fission pertechnetate, where the ^{99}Mo is extracted from uranium fission products, the radionuclidic impurities are: ^{99}Mo (0.1%), iodine-131 (0.005%), ruthenium-103 (0.005%), strontium-89 (0.00006%), strontium-90 (0.000006%), and alpha-emitting impurities (0.0000007%) (Theobald 1994).

In both sources an unspecified quantity of the long-lived isotope ^{99}Tc resulting from decay of the ^{99m}Tc is present. It should be noted that high levels of ^{99}Tc can interfere with the labeling efficiency of a number of newer kits through isotopic dilution and competition for binding sites on the ligands. Manufacturers may specify a maximum regrowth time for ^{99m}Tc in a generator (i.e., maximum time between elutions) to limit subsequent eluant content of ^{99}Tc and thus maintain the apparent efficiency of radiolabeling (Theobald 1994).

Another problem for all technetium radiopharmaceuticals is that of radiolysis. It is well known that ionizing radiation will decompose water molecules to give hydrogen peroxide and free radicals. Oxidants can accumulate on the columns of technetium generators, and be eluted with ^{99m}Tc-pertechnetate. This build-up of oxidants is particularly severe during the period between generator production and first elution; therefore it is generally recommended not to use the first eluate obtained from a new generator for the preparation of technetium radiopharmaceuticals (Molinkski 1982).

In conclusion, care must be taken in following the manufacturer's recommended protocols in order to ensure satisfactory performance of the radiopharmaceutical.

36.2.2.1 *Thyroid Gland Imaging*

Technetium-99m obtained directly from the generator can be used to image the thyroid gland. ^{99m}Tc is far cheaper than ^{123}I and has excellent availability. In the thyroid ^{99m}Tc is trapped by the follicular cells, but is not organified. Generally, the thyroid scan performed with ^{99m}Tc shows the same distribution as the iodine scan, although in some instances a cold nodule on the iodine scan is hot on the technetium scan. ^{99m}Tc is also taken up in salivary glands and to a lesser extent in the buccal mucosa. Due to excreted activity, the esophagus can be visualized and this can be reduced by letting the patient swallow some water (Park 1996).

36.2.2.2 *Salivary Gland Imaging*

Salivary gland imaging (SGI) is indicated in assessing functional impairment of salivary glands as can occur in Sjögren's syndrome. As SGI is both a functional and a morphological test, it may be indicated in malignancy of the gland. Like iodine, technetium is accumulated in the epithelial cells of intralobar ducts. In a patient with normal salivary glands, both the parotid and the submandibular glands are normally seen within 1 min, with peak activity at 5–10 min. After 10 min, the excretory phase begins and lasts up to 30 min. Following salivary gland stimulation, there is a complete discharge of the activity from the salivary glands in most cases. The uptake in the parotid and submandibular glands is equal to or greater than that in the thyroid (PILBROW et al. 1990; SHIRAZI 1996).

36.2.2.3 Imaging of Meckel's Diverticulum

Technetium-99m can also be used for detecting ectopic gastric mucosa in a Meckel's diverticulum, an etiology of gastrointestinal bleeding, particularly in children. The pertechnetate anion is accumulated selectively by the surface cells of gastric mucosa and then secreted into the bowel lumen. To increase the uptake, pentagastrin is given subcutaneously. The uptake is inhibited by perchlorate. After intravenous administration approximately 25% of the ^{99m}Tc localizes in the wall of the stomach and 20% is rapidly eliminated by the kidneys. Ectopic gastric mucosa is visualized as a hot spot. Radioactivity in the genitourinary system is a source of false-positive findings (PIEPSZ et al. 1991; TREVES and GRAND 1995).

36.2.2.4 First-Pass Study

First-pass study or scintiangiography can be performed by a bolus (intravenous) injection of ^{99m}Tc. First-pass ventriculography is the method of choice for the assessment of right ventricular ejection fraction and is indicated in patients with chronic obstructive pulmonary disease or valvular heart disease. A left-to-right shunt can also be identified with a first-pass technique. In normal cases, the lung curve is similar in configuration to that of the superior vena cava (SVC). In the case of a significant left-to-right shunt, there is early recirculation of tracer in the pulmonary region. Using the data from the SVC and the pulmonary region of interest, a process known as gamma-variate analysis can be used to quantify the shunt (GERMANO et al. 1996; MURPHY and PORT 1996).

Scintiangiography may also be valuable as a screening technique in assessing arterial and graft patency. This method can accurately demonstrate the status of the arterial system of the extremities to the levels of the midcalf and the wrist. Although individual arteries of the hands and feet are rarely visualized, blood flow in these vessels can be assessed by comparing the gross vascularity of the area with that of similar areas in the contralateral extremity or adjacent digits (SIEGEL and STEWART 1996; WILSON and O'MARA 1996).

First-pass study of the kidneys can demonstrate the vascularity of renal masses, further arteriovenous fistulae of the kidneys, aortic aneurysms, and other extrarenal abnormalities. Methods have been developed in the analysis of the time-activity curves of the kidney and the aorta or iliac artery for semiquantitative estimation of the renal blood flow and have been applied in the evaluation of the transplanted kidney (BLAUFOX 1991).

In acute scrotal pain this technique can be applied to differentiate acute epididymitis from testicular torsion (BELTRAN 1996).

36.2.3 Radiopharmaceuticals for Bone Imaging

Technetium-99m methylenediphosphonate (MDP, medronate) and ^{99m}Tc-hydroxymethylenediphosphonate (HDP, oxidronate) are the radiopharmaceuticals of choice for bone imaging. ^{99m}Tc-pyrophosphate was initially used for this purpose but is now applied only for myocardial infarct imaging, or in vivo pretinning for red cell labeling with ^{99m}Tc (SPENCER et al. 1996). The structure of these compounds is demonstrated in Fig. 36.2.

36.2.3.1 Bone Imaging

Bone scanning is indicated in patients with bone pain. In this category of patients bone scintigraphy is very sensitive and can show abnormalities earlier

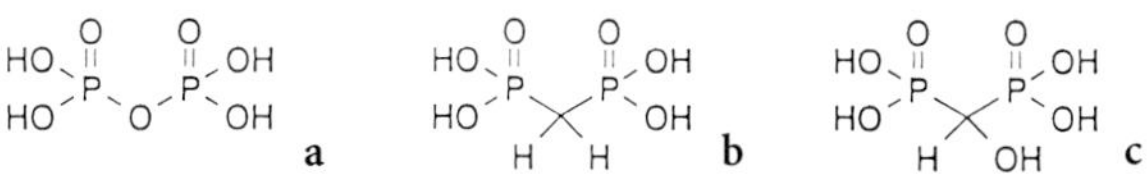

Fig. 36.2. Chemical structures of pyrophosphate (**a**), methylenediphosphonate (**b**), and hydroxymethylenediphosphonate (**c**)

than other imaging modalities, but it is not specific. Benign as well as malignant disorders are visualized as areas with increased uptake. False-negative results can be observed in purely lytic lesions, or due to altered blood supply. In patients with malignancies the bone scan can demonstrate or exclude bone metastases, which may be essential for treatment planning. In patients with sympathetic reflex dystrophy, Paget's disease, and fibrous dysplasia the distribution pattern on the bone scan is quite characteristic and may have additional value in establishing the diagnosis (Brown et al. 1993; Fogelman and Maisey 1994).

Following i.v. injection, the radiopharmaceuticals exchange rapidly with extracellular fluid; simultaneously, bone uptake and urinary excretion are both taking place. Skeletal imaging is usually performed 2–4 h p.i.; by then about 30% of MDP and 40% of HDP will be localized in skeletal bone in the normal adult. Unbound compounds are excreted by the kidneys; this amounts to approximately 60% in the first 24 h. Consequently, the radiation dose is lower if the patient voids frequently. Therefore a high intake of fluid is recommended. Pyrophosphate, which displays lower bone uptake than MDP or HDP, shows a lower target to background ratio (Spencer et al. 1996).

Autoradiographic studies have shown that bone-seeking agents mainly localize in the mineral phase of skeletal bone, especially at the sites of reactive bone formation. Bone uptake is thought to result from the interaction of the diphosphonates with the surface of the hydroxyapatite crystal. Absorption of the diphosphonate complexes into immature calcium phosphates at the calcifying front is significantly greater than into mature crystalline hydroxyapatite. Increased uptake in pathological processes reflects increased vascularity and relatively rapid turnover of bone tissue (Francis et al. 1980; Guillemart et al. 1978).

36.2.3.2
Myocardial Infarct Imaging

The most appropriate use of infarct-avid imaging is in the study of patients with suspected acute myocardial infarctions when the diagnosis remains unclear after a review of all the available clinical information. Factors that can complicate the diagnosis of infarction include: left bundle branch block, immediate postoperative period, postcardioversion, evidence of previous infarcts on the electrocardiogram, and subendocardial (non-Q-wave) myocardial infarcts. The basis of myocardial infarct visualization is the accumulation of pyrophosphate in the necrotic myocardium. In irreversibly damaged myocardial cells calcium is deposited in crystalline and subcrystalline form, for which pyrophosphate has high affinity. Irreversible cellular damage from almost any cause, including trauma, cardioversion, and invasive tumors, can result in pyrophosphate uptake (Corbett et al. 1996).

36.2.4
Radiopharmaceuticals for Cerebral Perfusion Imaging

At present there are two commercially available radiopharmaceuticals used for single-photon emission computerized tomography (SPECT) imaging of cerebral perfusion: ^{99m}Tc-hexamethylpropylene amine oxime (HMPAO, exametazime) and ^{99m}Tc-ethylcysteinate dimer (ECD, bicisate). The structures of both ligands are shown in Fig. 36.3.

Cerebral perfusion imaging is frequently performed to identify local reductions in flow due to changes in perfusion pressure, such as in stroke or ischemic situations. However, changes in blood flow will not be detected by changes in tracer distribution until compensation mechanism limits are exceeded. Most patients who are asymptomatic will have unremarkable or minimal changes in flow if no intervention or challenge is used. Therefore, to evaluate the hemodynamic consequences of carotid stenosis or cerebral vascular disease these studies are performed with concomitant use of a cerebral vasodilator such as acetazolamide. Other applications are classification of dementia, documentation of ictal sources, confirmation of brain death, and, in psychiatry, classification of certain diseases (Burt 1996).

1. ^{99m}Tc-HMPAO is a neutral lipophilic complex. After intravenous injection, HMPAO is cleared

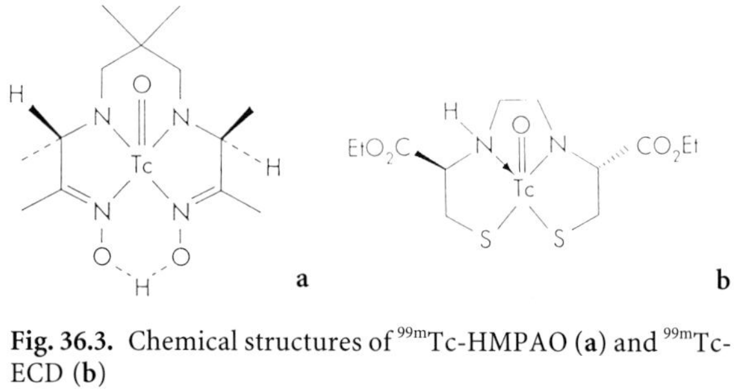

Fig. 36.3. Chemical structures of ^{99m}Tc-HMPAO (**a**) and ^{99m}Tc-ECD (**b**)

rapidly from the blood. Peak brain activity is reached within 10 min following intravenous injection, at which time 3.5%–7% of the total tracer dose is localized in the brain. Within the first 2 min, 15% of the dose initially absorbed may wash back from the brain. After reaching its plateau, redistribution of HMPAO within the brain does not occur for at least 8 h, and washout is only 0.4%/h (Babich 1991; Suess et al. 1991).

The mechanism of retention of HMPAO in the brain is conversion to a second, more hydrophilic complex that cannot diffuse back out of the brain. The formation of the hydrophilic complex that is trapped in the brain is thought to be the result of a simple chemical reaction with glutathione, which is present in a millimolar concentration in brain cells, although other mechanisms have been proposed. The activity not accumulated in the brain is distributed throughout the body, particularly in muscle and soft tissue. About 30% of the injected dose is found in the liver and gastrointestinal tract immediately after injection and about 50% of this is excreted through the gut over 48 h. Within 48 h about 40% of the dose is excreted in the urine (Babich 1991; Suess et al. 1991; Burns and Gibson 1996).

2. ^{99m}Tc-ECD is also a neutral, lipophilic complex. This compound is stable in vitro, whereas HMPAO is chemically instable. After intravenous injection ECD is rapidly cleared from the blood. Peak brain activity reaches more than 6% of the injected dose by 5 min and is followed by a slow cerebral washout of about 6%/h during the first 6 h. The rate of decrease in brain activity is the same for all regions of the brain and should have a minimal effect on image quality (Léveillé et al. 1992). ECD rapidly enters the brain via passive diffusion. After entering the brain, selective enzyme-catalyzed hydrolysis of one of the ester groups to a carboxylic acid results in the formation of a negatively charged complex, which cannot diffuse across the blood-brain barrier, thus preventing washout from the brain. Since retention of this tracer in the brain involves enzymatic hydrolysis, the distribution of ECD in the brain reflects both regional CBF and enzymatic activity. When enzymatic activity and blood flow are coupled, the distribution of this tracer correlates with blood flow. The enzyme responsible for this hydrolysis has not yet been identified. Retention of this complex in the brain is species specific: it occurs in monkeys and man but not in rats or rabbits (Walovitch et al. 1989, 1994). Clearance of ECD from the body is primarily through the kidneys, with about 49% of the dose being present in urine by 2 h and 71.5% by 24 h. Excretion through the hepatobiliary system is 11.5% ±4.8% of the dose at 48 h after injection. The rapid metabolism of ECD to polar mono- and di-acid products may explain the rapid elimination of the tracer from structures other than the brain. By about 5 min after injection metabolites account for 75% of the blood activity. The rapid washout from facial muscles and from the salivary glands results in higher brain to soft tissue ratios than HMPAO at comparable times after injection (Burns and Gibson 1996; Pupi et al. 1994).

36.2.5 Radiopharmaceuticals for Myocardial Perfusion Imaging

Two Tc-labeled agents commercially available are ^{99m}Tc-methoxyisobutylisonitrile (MIBI) and ^{99m}Tc-tetrofosmin. The structures of both ligands are shown in Fig. 36.4. ^{99m}Tc-teboroxime, which was not popular, is now no longer available commercially.

a,b

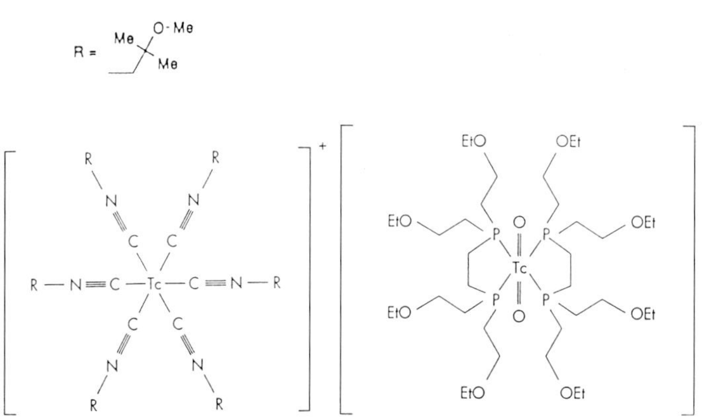

Fig. 36.4. Chemical structures of ^{99m}Tc-MIBI (**a**) and ^{99m}Tc-tetrofosmin (**b**)

1. MIBI myocardial uptake is not dependent on an Na-K-ATPase system. The fractional extraction by the myocardium is approximately 40%. Intracellular MIBI is associated with mitochondria as a free cationic complex. The distribution of MIBI in the myocardium following administration during coronary occlusion correlates with flow and can delineate the regions at risk. Necrotic areas do not retain this compound; thus its uptake indicates myocardial viability. At rest the myocardial uptake is approximately 1.2%, and after exercise about 1.5%. Within 48 h, about 33% of the injected dose is excreted via the hepatobiliary system and 27% through the kidneys (Jones et al. 1984).

2. Tetrofosmin, a diphosphine, which belongs to the class of lipophilic compounds, also shows good myocardial uptake and slow myocardial clearance. This compound has the advantage of an easier labeling procedure and more rapid liver excretion. By 10 min blood activity is <5% of the injected dose, and by 60 min liver activity is <4.5% (Jain et al. 1993; Kelly et al. 1993). As myocardial clearance of these compounds from both ischemic and non-ischemic regions is minimal, separate injections are needed for rest and exercise images. Because for some patients returning on the second day (2-day protocol) is a problem, a 1-day protocol has been employed (AHA/ACC Task Force Report 1995; Taillefer 1990).

36.2.5.1
Myocardial Perfusion Imaging

Myocardial perfusion imaging (MPI) allows the diagnosis of obstructive coronary artery disease and differentiation between myocardial infarction and ischemia. MPI is performed in conjunction with physical exercise or pharmacological stress, because a decrease in coronary flow during exercise is already observed in a 50% stenosis, whereas at rest coronary blood flow is not reduced until the stenosis exceeds 90%. Exercise can be done on a bicycle or treadmill. In patients who are unable to exercise due to physical inability, perfusion imaging is performed with pharmacological stress testing by administering dipyridamole, adenosine, or dobutamine. Each mode of stress tests coronary flow reserve by increasing myocardial oxygen demand (exercise and dobutamine) and/or direct coronary vasodilation (adenosine, dipyridamole, and dobutamine) (AHA/ACC Task Force Report 1995; Iskandrian et al. 1994; Udelson 1995).

Single-photon emission computerized tomographic images obtained with MIBI or tetrofosmin are certainly better than tomographic slices obtained with thallium. MIBI and tetrofosmin provide sufficient count rates to permit ECG-gated SPECT acquisition. Using this technique, quantification can be applied on end-diastolic images which may reduce artifacts and partial volume errors related to heart motion. Moreover indices of left ventricular function can be obtained simultaneously (Berman et al. 1995; Van Train et al. 1995).

36.2.5.2
Imaging of Parathyroid Adenoma and Malignancies

Other applications of MIBI are the localization of parathyroid adenomas and as a tumor-seeking agent, in particular for the detection of breast cancer and its metastases in axillary lymph nodes. The exact mechanism of MIBI uptake by tumor cells has not been defined. Many of the proposed mechanisms are derived from studies of myocardial tissue; therefore, extrapolation to tumor cells is speculative. In contrast to the involvement of active transport in thallium accumulation within the myocardium, the fundamental mechanism of myocellular accumulation of MIBI most likely involves passive diffusion across the sarcolemmal and mitochondrial membranes in response to transmembrane potentials. MIBI is considered a lipophilic cation which is greatly influenced by the negative charges on the mitochondria and the increased mitochondrial density that is present in tumors. As with thallium accumulation in the myocardium or in tumors, adequate blood flow must be present for uptake to occur. Thus, in tumors, as in the myocardium, limitation of blood supply may result in decreased MIBI uptake. Extraction, however, appears to be dependent upon the transmembrane potential difference developed by tumors as well as mitochondrial density (Waxman 1996).

Retention of the radiopharmaceutical in the delayed image indicates parathyroid localizations. However, "false-positive" retention may occur in multinodular goiter (Chen et al. 1995; Staudenherz et al. 1995; Taillefer et al. 1992).

As in the case of thallium-201 imaging, scintigraphy with MIBI has been performed in patients with malignancies such as sarcomas, lung cancer, and in particular breast cancer. SPECT acquisition may increase the sensitivity of the procedure and has more precise localizing properties (Waxman 1996).

36.2.5.3 Regional Distribution of Blood Flow

The distribution of intravenously administered MIBI in skeletal muscle reflects the fractional distribution of cardiac output and is thus related to regional blood flow. The images obtained permit evaluation of the effect of arterial pathology on the perfusion at the microcirculation level. The perfusion is proportional to muscle mass, with relative hypoperfusion of nonmuscular structures such as the knees and ankles. A significant increase in the muscular-to-nonmuscular perfusion ratio is observed during exercise (Siegel and Stewart 1996).

36.2.6 Radiopharmaceuticals for Renal Studies

There are four Tc-labeled radiopharmaceuticals for renal studies: ^{99m}Tc-diethylene triamine pentaacetic acid (DTPA, pentetate), ^{99m}Tc-mercaptoacetyltriglycine (MAG3, mertiatide), ^{99m}Tc-dimercaptosuccinic acid (DMSA, succimer), and ^{99m}Tc-glucoheptonic acid (GHA, gluceptate). DTPA and MAG3 are used for renography, DMSA for static renal imaging, and GHA for both of these studies. The structures of these compounds are demonstrated in Fig. 36.5.

1. DTPA penetrates capillary walls to enter the extravascular space within 4 min after intravenous administration. Equilibration with the extracellular fluid occurs within a matter of hours and takes longer in the presence of edema. Due to its lipid insolubility and negative charge, DTPA does not enter the cells. DTPA is removed from the circulation solely by glomerular filtration in the kidneys. Its renal clearance is unaffected by urine flow or the administration of probenecid. DTPA can also be applied for first-pass study. Due to its rapid clearance, DTPA is considered preferable to ^{99m}Tc-sodium pertechnetate (Chervu and Blaufox 1989; Eshima and Fritzberg 1996).

2. MAG3 is the radiopharmaceutical of choice for renography. This compound is excreted mainly by tubular secretion. Because of its more efficient extraction, MAG3 provides better images than DTPA, particularly in patients with impaired renal function. About 90% of the plasma activity is bound to plasma proteins. The unbound 10% is subjected to glomerular filtration. Although the renal extraction of MAG3 is 60% of that for *ortho*-iodohippurate (OIH), in a normal person 70% of the injected dose of MAG3 is excreted into the urine in 30 min, essentially the same as for OIH. The secretory mechanism is the usual one for carboxylic acids and can be blocked with probenecid in rats and *para*-aminohippurate (PAH) in humans. Liver uptake is greater for MAG3 than for OIH, and the gallbladder is sometimes seen (Chervu and Blaufox 1989; Eshima and Fritzberg 1996).

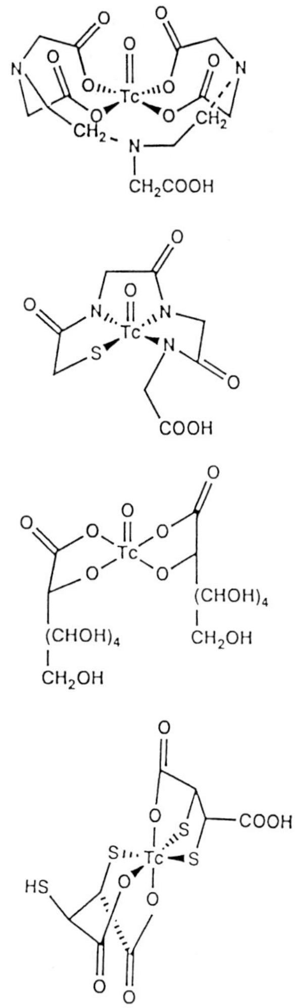

a b c d

Fig. 36.5. Chemical structures of ^{99m}Tc-DTPA (**a**), ^{99m}Tc-MAG3 (**b**), ^{99m}Tc-GHA (**c**), and ^{99m}Tc-DMSA (**d**)

3. DMSA is an excellent renal cortical imaging agent. After intravenous injection of DMSA, most of the circulating activity is bound to plasma proteins. Its renal clearance of 34 ml/min is lower than for the filtered agents. Most of the activity removed from the blood is retained in the renal cortex, about a third

passing unchanged into the urine. Kidney uptake amounts to 40% in the two kidneys at 3 h, comparable to the uptake of chlormerodrin, and is unaffected by probenecid and PAH. Urinary excretion is increased in the presence of renal tubular acidosis, probably by tubular reabsorption. In the presence of renal failure, DMSA activity can be seen in liver, gallbladder, and gut (Eshima and Fritzberg 1996; Taylor 1989).

4. GHA is mainly filtrated glomerularly; 30%–40% of the injected dose is excreted into the urine within the first hour. Only 10%–15% of the dose remains firmly bound to the tubular cells. Since half of the plasma activity is bound to protein, and only the unbound fraction can be filtered, some tubular secretion or uptake accounts for the observed rate of excretion. Further evidence for tubular secretion is the finding that PAH and probenecid decrease the accumulation of GHA in rats. Delayed imaging with GHA provides similar visualization of the renal cortex to that offered by DMSA images, although DMSA tends to be preferred. A disadvantage of GHA is its hepatobiliary excretion, which may interfere with the interpretation (Eshima and Fritzberg 1996; Taylor 1989).

36.2.6.1
Renography

Renography is a dynamic renal study performed after i.v. injection of a radiopharmaceutical which is excreted by the kidneys. In a normal study there is a practically symmetrical appearance of the kidneys. In the 2nd minute there is a good delineation of the renal cortex. Appearance of activity in the collecting system and renal pelves begins in the 3rd or 4th minute. Shortly thereafter the activity will reach the ureter and the bladder. Both renal curves show a symmetrical appearance with times to peak between 3 and 5 min. The most important indications for this study are diagnosis of renovascular hypertension, diagnosis of urinary tract obstruction, and calculation of the ratio between the left and right kidney function. The examination is also often carried out for the monitoring of post-transplant course and in patients who have undergone intervention of the renal artery or upper urinary tract. During renography, glomerular filtration rate or effective renal plasma flow can be estimated. Furthermore renal transit times can be determined. For the diagnosis of urinary tract obstruction, stimulation of urine flow rate by intravenous administration of frusemide is mandatory. In renovascular hypertension the sensitivity and specificity of renography are higher when the examination is performed after administration of captopril (Oei 1994, O'Reilly et al. 1996; Taylor and Nally 1995; Taylor et al. 1996).

36.2.6.2
Static Renal Imaging

The main objective of static renal imaging is to visualize foci of acute pyelonephritis. Several reports have shown the DMSA scan to be significantly more sensitive than other imaging modalities. Other indications are the identification of an ectopic kidney and the differentiation of renal masses such as prominent columns of Bertin from true pathology. The availability of other techniques with superior resolution has relegated this examination to a secondary role in the diagnosis of space-occupying lesions. SPECT is more sensitive than planar scintigraphy in detecting renal foci of acute pyelonephritis; however, SPECT introduces more false-positive findings (Goldraich and Goldraich 1995; Majd and Rushton 1992; Mackenzie 1996).

36.2.7
Radiopharmaceuticals for Gastrointestinal Motility Studies

Gastrointestinal motility studies include the evaluation of esophageal transit, diagnosis of esophageal reflux, and measurement of gastric emptying rate. ^{99m}Tc-sulfur colloid, which is not absorbed or degraded by gastric juice, is a perfect marker for this purpose. Studies have indicated that ^{99m}Tc-DTPA or indium-111 DTPA are also suitable. Important in these studies is the choice of an appropriate test meal, in which the marker has to be mixed thoroughly.

36.2.7.1
Evaluation of Esophageal Transit

This study allows the assessment of the completeness of bolus ingestion, observation of the progression of the bolus through the esophagus, and identification of bolus retention in any portion of the esophagus. The principal indication for esophageal transit study is the assessment of the effectiveness of medical or surgical treatment in disorders such as achalasia, scleroderma, diffuse esophageal spasm, or nonspecific motor disorders. It can also provide additional information about the underlying causes of delayed transit in secondary motor disturbances of esophageal motility or in other conditions (URBAIN et al. 1996). To evaluate esophageal transit, water is the most common medium employed and is usually given in the form of a bolus of 10–20 ml mixed with ^{99m}Tc-sulfur colloid; in achalasia a larger volume of 150 ml should be applied (OEI et al. 1986). To avoid interference, the esophageal transit test should be performed after a fast and after withdrawal of any medication which may influence esophageal function (MALMUD and FISHER 1981; O'CONNOR et al. 1988).

36.2.7.2 Evaluation of Esophageal Reflux

Gastroesophageal reflux scintigraphy is indicated to identify reflux and to assess the effectiveness of medical and surgical treatment. The test has gained wide acceptance in pediatric practice because of its physiological and noninvasive character. It is less often performed in adults since the introduction of 24-h pH monitoring, which is more accurate. After an overnight fast, the patient is studied in the supine position to avoid the counterreflux effect of gravity. Additional aggravants of reflux such as an acid load to the stomach and increasing the pressure gradient across the lower esophageal sphincter are used to enhance the sensitivity of the test (URBAIN et al. 1996). In adults 300 ml of acidified orange juice is used as a test meal (MALMUD and FISCHER 1981). In infants and children, the study is performed with milk or pudding (WYNCHANK et al. 1995).

36.2.7.3 Gastric Emptying Study

Gastric emptying study is indicated to identify diabetic gastroparesis and to demonstrate abnormal gastric emptying patterns occurring, for instance, after surgical procedures or in patients with systemic sclerosis or gastroesophageal reflux. Also, the effects of gastrokinetic agents can be demonstrated by testing with and without medication (URBAIN et al. 1996).

There is as yet no consensus in the literature regarding the use of a standardized test meal for the scintigraphic evaluation of gastric emptying. Numerous solid foods including whole eggs, egg whites, in vitro labeled chicken liver, liver paté, hamburgers, fibers, and nondigestible particles have been used. The test meal used by URBAIN et al. (1996) is an egg sandwich (one scrambled egg labeled with ^{99m}Tc-sulfur colloid, and 100 g regular white bread) and 150 ml of tap water. This meal contains approximately 230 calories with 35% fat, 47% carbohydrates, and 18% protein. For dual-isotope solid-liquid emptying studies, water is labeled with ^{111}In-DTPA. In the author's institution porridge and pancake are used as a test meal (AKKERMANS et al. 1984).

36.2.8 Radiopharmaceuticals for Hepatobiliary Imaging

Hepatobiliary imaging is indicated in the diagnosis of cholecystitis and to a lesser extent for the evaluation of cholestatic jaundice. In neonates this technique is indicated if biliary atresia is suspected. At present the evaluation of hepatobiliary function is performed with Tc-labeled iminodiacetic acid (IDA) derivatives. Several derivatives are commercially manufactured: ^{99m}Tc-dimethyl iminodiacetic acid (HIDA = hepatic IDA, lidofenin), ^{99m}Tc-diisopropyl IDA (DISIDA, disofenin), ^{99m}Tc-trimethyl bromo IDA (BRIDA, mebrofenin), ^{99m}Tc-diethyl IDA (EHIDA, etifenin), and ^{99m}Tc-diethyl iodo IDA (IODIDA, iodofenin). Only the first three compounds have received FDA approval. Their structures are shown in Fig. 36.6.

Upon introduction into the blood, IDA is weakly associated with serum albumin. After reaching the space of Disse, dissociation occurs. Free IDA then contacts the hepatocyte surface. Hepatic uptake of IDA compounds is facilitated by carrier-mediated, non-sodium-dependent, organic anioinic pathways similar to those responsible for bilirubin uptake. After entering the hepatocyte, IDA is excreted unchanged. From this point, the elimination process is relatively passive, essentially following the flow of bile through the biliary tree. Progression of the compound is influenced primarily by the tone of the sphincter of Oddi and the patency of the bile ducts. Depending on intrabiliary pressures, some portion of the injected dose will enter the gallbladder through the cystic duct, whereas the remainder will bypass the gallbladder, travel through the common bile duct, and empty into the small bowel. The radioactivity proceeds through the gastrointestinal tract and is eliminated in the feces (HLADIK and NORENBERG 1996a).

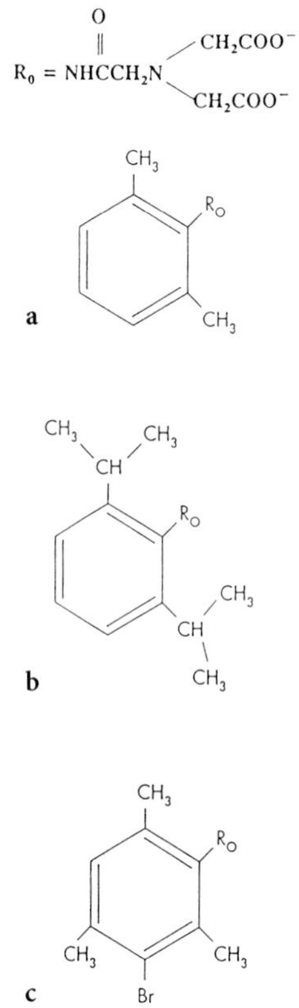

Fig. 36.6. Chemical structures of lidofenin (**a**), disofenin (**b**), and mebrofenin (**c**)

Table 36.2. Hepatic uptake and excretion measured at 24 h

	% dose in blood	% dose in urine	% dose in liver
HIDA	0.6 ± 0.1	15.5 ± 2.7	83.9
DISIDA	0.9 ± 0.2	11.1 ± 1.5	88.0
BRIDA	0.4 ± 0.01	1.5 ± 0.3	98.1

Abbreviations as defined in the text.

In healthy individuals, the liver is typically seen within the first minute after injection, and hepatic activity peaks at approximately 10 min. The gallbladder and common bile duct appear as early as 10–20 min after injection, and the bowel is visualized shortly thereafter. Overall liver activity should be significantly decreased 60–90 min after administration of the tracer. Data obtained at 24 h are shown in Table 36.2. These data indicate that mebrofenin is the superior agent; it has the highest amount eliminated in the bile and the lowest amount excreted in the urine (Hladik and Norenberg 1996a; Krishnamurthy and Krishnamurthy 1989).

Since bilirubin is handled by the same hepatocyte transport system as the IDA compounds, the presence of bilirubin in the serum can have a profound effect on the biodistribution of these agents. However, even at very high levels of serum bilirubin, IDA derivatives are always extracted to some extent by the hepatocytes. This may be due to the fact that these compounds are taken up by the fatty acid and conjugated acid pathways in addition to the organic anion transport system. Studies have shown that mebrofenin is the most resistant to the effects of bilirubin. Mebrofenin maintains a hepatic uptake of approximately 70% even at bilirubin levels of 20 mg%, and the renal excretion is only minimally increased. Therefore, in patients with moderately to markedly elevated bilirubin levels, the images obtained with mebrofenin are superior to those obtained with the other two agents. However, these advantages may not be readily apparent in patients with normal bilirubin levels (Hladik and Norenberg 1996a; Krishnamurthy and Krishnamurthy 1989).

36.3 Radiolabeled Blood Cells

36.3.1 Red Blood Cells

Labeled red blood cells (RBCs) are used as a radiopharmaceutical in the following studies: gated cardiac blood pool imaging, evaluation of gastrointestinal bleeding, imaging of liver hemangioma, and imaging of varicocele. For spleen imaging RBCs that have been damaged by heating are used. Labeling of RBCs may be performed in vitro, in vivo, or by a combination of both methods. The choice of the labeling method depends on the clinical study to be done.

All the methods of labeling RBCs with ^{99m}Tc involve treating the cells with a reducing agent, usually stannous chloride, followed by administration of pertechnetate. The stannous chloride is necessary because pertechnetate freely diffuses in and out of the RBCs, whereas if it is reduced within the cells it becomes bound to the beta-chain of hemoglobin and is retained by the cell. It is also important to remove any surplus extracellular stannous ions before the pertechnetate is added, because it could reduce the pertechnetate to a form which is unable to penetrate the cells, resulting in lower labeling efficiency (Danpure and Osman 1994).

1. The procedure of in vitro labeling includes:

collecting heparinized blood, separation of the erythrocytes, and addition of stannous chloride to give an approximate final concentration of 0.006 µg tin/ml erythrocytes. After a 5-min incubation freshly eluted pertechnetate is added. The labeled cells are then washed and resuspended with ice-cold saline before administration. Using this procedure, the highest labeling efficiency will be achieved, although the procedure is time-consuming and requires a sterile environment (Danpure and Osman 1994). An in vitro kit technique (UltraTag RBC kit, Mallinckrodt Medical) was developed and refined to achieve simplicity and convenience comparable with the in vivo method. Using this method the mean labeling yield was 97.4% ±1.6% and the blood radioactivity levels remained unchanged over 3 h after administration (Srivastava and Straub 1990; Wilson and Hung 1992).

2. The in vivo method simply involves injecting two solutions intravenously: first a solution of stannous chloride followed by ^{99m}Tc-pertechnetate. Pretinning can be done with a cold kit containing stannous tin such as pyrophosphate. With this method, it is not possible to remove the excess stannous ions, so it is important to ensure that the amount of tin is kept low. Although methods vary, 10–20 µg stannous ions per kilogram body weight should be satisfactory. The RBCs incorporate the tin given in vivo so that when the pertechnetate is subsequently injected it is taken up by the RBCs, reduced by the tin, and retained by the cells. The problem with this method is that the labeling efficiency is variable (Danpure and Osman 1994).

3. During the combination of the in vitro and in vivo methods, the RBCs are tinned in vivo but labeled in vitro to allow accurate measurement of labeling efficiency and to enable any unincorporated technetium to be washed from the cells before they are reinjected into the patient. This method also prevents pertechnetate distributing in the extracellular fluid compartment. Using this method a high labeling efficiency of erythrocytes can be achieved (Danpure and Osman 1994).

36.3.1.1 Gated Cardiac Blood Pool Imaging

Initially, ^{99m}Tc-labeled human serum albumin was used as an intravascular tag in gated cardiac blood pool imaging. However, because of the large amount of albumin sequestered in the pulmonary tree, the use of labeled albumin was virtually replaced in the late 1970s by ^{99m}Tc-labeled RBCs, which show a much more favorable target-to-background ratio compared with labeled albumin, resulting in better image quality (Murphy and Port 1996; Strauss et al. 1979). Gated cardiac blood pool imaging permits noninvasive measurements of left ventricular ejection fraction, regional wall motion, ventricular size and volume, and the diastolic performance parameters of peak ventricular filling rate and time to peak filling rate. Identification of abnormal systolic function following chemotherapy presages the clinical development of symptoms of either congestion or low output. In coronary artery disease this technique assesses the functional consequences of perfusion abnormalities (Dilsizian et al. 1990; Rocco et al. 1989).

36.3.1.2 Evaluation of Gastrointestinal Bleeding

The basis of this study is the identification of a small fraction of injected radiopharmaceutical agent extravasated at the site of active bleeding. A study indicates gastrointestinal bleeding if it demonstrates a focal area of extravasated RBCs with a subsequent movement within the intraluminal space. Extravasated blood is a bowel irritant, producing peristaltic contractions that cause the blood to move freely within the bowel in both retrograde and antegrade directions. Use of ^{99m}Tc-labeled RBCs takes advantage of the 20-h intravascular half-life to depict intermittent bleeding. The study quality is directly influenced by the labeling technique used. The in vivo method of labeling autologous RBCs is suboptimal due to the amount of free pertechnetate activity. Free pertechnetate is concentrated and secreted by the gastric mucosa and excreted via the kidneys and into the bladder, interfering with accurate study interpretation (Lecklitner 1986; Kostamo 1996).

Technetium-99m colloid can also be used for this study. Extravasated colloid provides a high target-to-background ratio because it is cleared by the reticuloendothelial system of the liver, spleen, and bone marrow and not absorbed by the bowel. The $T_{1/2}$ within the vascular system is 2–6 min with the majority cleared within 15 min. In cases of chronic gastrointestinal bleeding, heparin can be used as a provocative aid to induce bleeding (Lecklitner 1986; Kostamo 1996; Lecklitner and Hughes 1986).

36.3.1.3
Imaging of Liver Hemangioma

Hemangiomas are the most frequent benign tumors of the liver, which are usually asymptomatic and are detected as incidental findings on ultrasound or CT studies. Characteristic of these lesions is their large blood volume. Increased uptake on the delayed blood pool image following intravenous administration of RBCs is quite specific for hemangioma. SPECT images are superior to planar images in identifying small hemangiomas (OPPENHEIM 1996).

36.3.1.4
Imaging of Varicocele

Varicoceles, which usually occur on the left side, are painless dilatation of the pampiniform plexus and may cause infertility in men. Rapid dynamic and static images are performed in the upright position. Retrograde blood flow and abnormal blood pool indicate the presence of a varicocele (FREITAS et al. 1996; MALI et al. 1986a,b).

36.3.1.5
Spleen Imaging

Spleen-specific imaging is performed when looking for accessory spleens or in cases where radiocolloid in the liver may interfere with visualization of a potential lesion in the spleen. It is well known that senescent erythrocytes are destroyed by the spleen, and the resulting cellular debris is sequestered by the macrophages of this organ. Taking advantage of this natural process, scintiphotos of the spleen can be obtained following the administration of radiolabeled RBCs that have been purposely damaged with heat (SRIVASTAVA and STRAUB 1990; SPENCER 1996).

36.3.2
White Blood Cells

Granulocytes and mixed leukocytes are labeled with gamma-emitting radionuclides for the study and detection of inflammation and infection. Labeling of white blood cells (WBCs) was initially done with ^{111}In-oxinate; subsequently it was performed with ^{111}In-tropolonate and ^{99m}Tc-HMPAO (Fig. 36.7). The transport of the complex into the cells supposedly

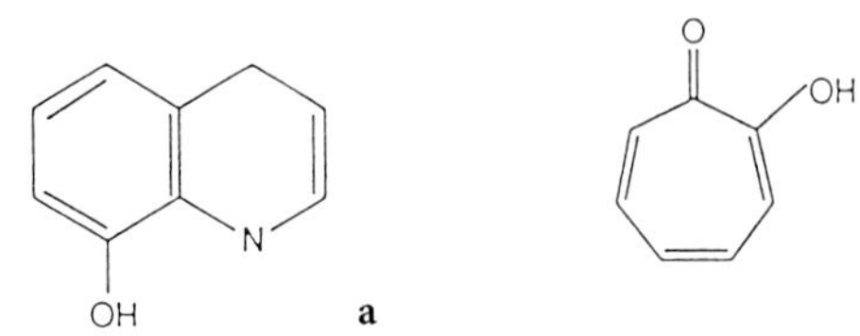

a b

Fig. 36.7. Chemical structures of oxine (**a**) and tropolone (**b**)

follows a lipophilic mechanism. Although ^{99m}Tc-HMPAO gives excellent images, the stability of ^{99m}Tc-HMPAO in blood cells is lower than that of ^{111}In and this results in some loss of ^{99m}Tc from the labeled leukocytes after they have been reinjected into the patient. This eluted ^{99m}Tc accumulates in the kidneys, bladder, gallbladder, and bowel and may impair the interpretation of the images (DANPURE and OSMAN 1994; SRIVASTAVA and STRAUB 1990).

Since for radiolabeling of WBCs nonselective agents which indiscriminately label all types of blood cells are used, to label a particular type of blood cell it is essential to isolate those cells first from the whole blood. Separation of pure granucolytes from mixed WBCs can be achieved using iso-osmotic Percoll (Pharmacia). The granulocytes are then washed free from Percoll with cell-free plasma containing Hespan, which can be separated by centrifugation (DANPURE and OSMAN 1994). As recently described, pure neutrophils (>90%) can also be obtained from whole blood using a double-gradient separation method. This method does not require prior collection of mixed leukocytes. The pure granulocytes or mixed leukocytes resuspended in ACD-plasma are then ready for labeling using freshly prepared ^{99m}Tc-HMPAO, ^{111}In-tropolonate, or ^{111}In-oxinate. Estimation of labeling efficiency should be performed before reinjection of the labeled cells into the patient (DANPURE and OSMAN 1994). Health and safety aspects of any study involving human blood are very important with the known risks of contracting hepatitis and acquired immune deficiency syndrome. It is therefore imperative that all personnel who work with blood are fully aware of the dangers and are carefully instructed in the safe handling and disposal of blood samples.

Radiolabeled WBCs are used to localize foci of acute infections. The inflammatory conditions successfully diagnosed include Crohn's disease, osteomyelitis, infected orthopedic implants, infected vascular prostheses, and fever of unknown origin. Labeled WBCs will leave the vessels and penetrate an infection-invaded area directed by chemotactic factors, amongst others. Normal accumulation of radioactivity is seen in the liver, spleen, and bone marrow. With ^{99m}Tc-labeled WBCs, bowel activity is not uncommon. At 4 h p.i. blood pool activity and activity in the lung capillary bed are usually seen. Advantages of ^{99m}Tc-labeled cells are the better quality of the images and the low radiation dose to the patient, but ^{111}In-labeled leukocytes have the advantage of absence of bowel activity and the opportunity for delayed imaging. Although there is still controversy over the subject, purified granulocytes do not seem to have much advantage over mixed leukocytes for labeling. WBCs are less successful in chronic infections. In these conditions, gallium-67 scintigraphy is more appropriate (Arndt et al. 1993; Neumann and McAfee 1996; Forstrom 1996; Peters 1996; Prats et al. 1994).

36.4 Technetium-Labeled Particles

36.4.1 Macroaggregates

Radiopharmaceuticals used for diagnostic studies which belong to this group are all technetium labeled and supplied as cold kits. Depending on the size of the particles, these agents can be divided into three groups: (a) ^{99m}Tc-macroaggregated albumin (MAA, macrosalb); (b) ^{99m}Tc-colloid; (c) ^{99m}Tc-nanosized colloid. MAA is prepared from human serum albumin and used mainly for lung perfusion study. The particle size ranges mainly between 10 and 50 μm. Particles with diameters in excess of 10 μm cannot pass through the smallest capillaries and are therefore filtered out of circulation on arrival at these vessels. Intravenous injection results in the particles becoming trapped in the arterioles and capillaries of the pulmonary circulation. Arterial injection results in trapping within the capillaries of the perfused organ, e.g., injection into the hepatic artery leads to entrapment in the liver. During lung scanning approximately 250 000 particles are intravenously injected. These particles will occlude a part of the capillary lung bed (generally less than 0.1%). In the lung capillary MAA will undergo degradation and phagocytosis. After lung scanning, MAA has an effective half-life of 2–6 h according to the product information from various suppliers. The mechanism by which MAA is removed from the lungs is simple mechanical erosion or fragmentation of the particles. Several factors influence the rate of MAA clearance. Larger particles clear slower than smaller particles. Softer particles are more easily fractured and leave the lung faster than the harder particles of equivalent size. ^{99m}Tc is released from the degraded particles as pertechnetate and will be accumulated in the thyroid gland, and eliminated via the kidneys. Maximal activity in the thyroid has been observed at approximately 2 h post injection and in the intestine at 24 h. Some activity seen in the liver can be clarified by the fact that the radiolabeled degraded particles are taken up by the RES. Cumulative urinary excretion of radioactivity following the administration of MAA averages 20%–40% at 24 h.

36.4.1.1 Lung Perfusion Scintigraphy

The major indications for perfusion scintigraphy are: pulmonary embolism, preoperative assessment of differential lung function, and quantification of perfusion abnormalities in patients with vascular malformations. To diagnose pulmonary embolism this study is performed in conjunction with a ventilation study. Perfusion imaging is performed after the injection of ^{99m}Tc-MAA, given when the patient is in supine position and breathing moderately deeply, in order to ensure an even distribution in the pulmonary vascular bed. The container with the radiopharmaceutical should be agitated before filling the syringe, and the syringe agitated before injection into the patient in order to avoid clumping of the radiopharmaceutical. For the same reason no blood should be aspirated into the syringe prior to the injection. Pulmonary embolism will result in filling defects on the perfusion scintigrams (Spies 1996).

36.4.1.2 Radionuclide Venography

Radionuclide venography is indicated if contrast venography is contraindicated or uninterpretable. This study is frequently performed in conjunction with perfusion study of the lung in patients with suspected pulmonary embolism and for venous pathology of the lower limbs. MAA is administered into both dorsal pedal veins while moderately tight tourniquets are placed just above the ankles to direct the tracer towards the deep venous system. Radionuclide venography is excellent for detecting a thrombus at or proximal to the popliteal veins and is less accurate for detecting thrombi in the calves. Signs of venous occlusion are an abrupt cut-off of flow with collateral flow, or significant focal narrowing (ZIFFER et al. 1988).

36.4.1.3 Evaluation of Intracardiac Shunt

The presence of a right-to-left shunt can be identified by the injection of MAA, which is commonly used for lung scanning. If a right-to-left shunt is present, some tracer will pass into the systemic circulation. The percent of total activity outside the lung fields is proportional to the degree of the right-to-left shunt (GELFAND and HANNON 1987).

36.4.1.4 Peritoneovenous Shunt-Patency Study

The method of choice for evaluation of shunt patency is the intraperitoneal administration of a lung perfusion agent. MAA is administered by needle injection into the ascites. Patency of the shunt is indicated by the prompt visualization of lung activity within 10 min of intraperitoneal injection. Most patients with delayed lung visualization have a significant obstruction of their peritoneovenous shunt. Complete absence of lung and shunt activity by 60 min suggests that the shunt is totally occluded (SINGH 1996).

36.4.2 Colloids and Nanocolloids

Commercially available colloids and nanocolloids are prepared from organic (human serum albumin) or inorganic material (antimony, tin, sulfur, rhenium). Agents for liver and spleen imaging contain predominantly colloids with particle sizes between 0.4 and 1 µm. Nanocolloids with a particle diameter of less than 0.08 µm are used for bone marrow imaging and studies of the lymphatic system. After intravenous administration, particles in the upper size range of this group tend to clear from the circulation more rapidly and predominantly go to the liver. The smaller size range, i.e., 10 nm or less, clears more slowly and a larger proportion will be found in the spleen and bone marrow. Two mechanisms have been proposed to account for the removal of colloids from the vascular compartment, in accordance with particle size and composition.

1. The mechanism of clearance of small particles (<0.1 µm) is that of phagocytosis, which is a property possessed by cells of the reticuloendothelial system (RES). Optimal phagocytosis of colloid particles is dependent on proper coating of these particles with specific serum proteins called opsonins. If these serum opsonins become depleted, owing to a disease or the injection of too many colloid particles, the ability of the RES to phagocytize colloid diminishes. The particles, whether opsonized or not, are then recognized by receptors on the phagocytic cell surface. Perhaps other receptors are responsible for the recognition of an unopsonized foreign surface. Phagocytized particles are probably stored in the cytoplasm of Kupffer cells and transferred to successive replacement cells. Inert particles may remain in the cell for long periods. Degradable particles, e.g., albumin, will be broken down and the components are released (HLADIK and NORENBERG 1996b).

2. Larger particles (0.1–1.0 µm), used for liver and spleen imaging, will predominantly leave the vascular space through slits between endothelial cells and are lodged in the space of Disse. Particles trapped in the space of Disse will be drained slowly into the nearby lymphatics. Both albumin colloid and sulfur colloid clear from the blood with a half-life of 2–3 min. In the first 10–15 min albumin colloid disappears from the blood faster than sulfur colloid, but by 30 min blood levels of each radiopharmaceutical are essentially equal. In healthy subjects, 80%–90% of an injected dose of either ^{99m}Tc-albumin colloid or ^{99m}Tc-sulfur colloid distributes to the liver, 5%–10% to the spleen, and the remainder to the bone marrow. Localization of these radiocolloids in the liver and spleen is virtually complete by 15 min, at which time static imaging can start. The effective half-lives of albumin colloid and sulfur colloid in the liver are approximately 4 and 6 h, respectively. After liver scanning with sulfur colloid, 3% of the administered dose is eliminated in the feces and 4% in the urine. After administration of albumin colloid, which is biodegradable, 4%–30% of the activity is excreted in the urine within 24 h (HLADIK and NORENBERG 1996b).

3. Another agent used to image the liver is ^{99m}Tc-sodium phytate (Fig. 36.8). Sodium phytate is a water-soluble compound which forms an insoluble colloid (calcium phytate) by chelating blood calcium. Colloidal calcium phytate undergoes reticuloendothelial trapping in the liver and, to a lesser extent, in the spleen and bone marrow. Intravenously injected ^{99m}Tc-sodium phytate clears from the

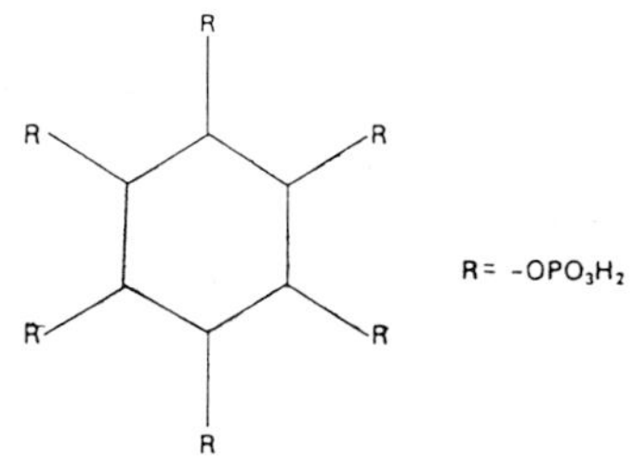

Fig. 36.8. Chemical structure of phytic acid

blood rapidly. Maximum uptake in the liver is reached about 15 min post injection. The biological half-life is 13.5 days and the effective half-life in the body is 5.8 h. The cumulative urinary excretion at 2 h post injection reaches 3.5% (Arzoumanian et al. 1977; Subramanian et al. 1973).

4. Particles injected interstitially for lymphoscintigraphy are opsonized and engulfed by the phagocytic cells of the lymph nodes. The kinetics of clearance have been extensively studied by Bergqvist et al. (1983), who examined different agents. The fate of interstitially injected material is strongly dependent on particle size. Particles not larger than a few nanometers will mostly be exchanged through blood capillaries. Larger particles with diameters up to a few tens of nanometers will be absorbed into the lymph capillaries by passage through junctions between the endothelial cells and/or transport in vesicles through the cells by pinocytosis. Large particles with diameters of hundreds of nanometers will spend a long time trapped in the interstitial spaces.

36.4.2.1 Liver and Spleen Imaging

Radiocolloid imaging of the liver is an effective method to evaluate the presence or absence of neoplastic disease, both metastatic and primary. It was once a very common study, but has been largely supplanted by ultrasonography, CT, and MRI. The technique may be useful in the diagnosis and follow-up of diffuse liver disorders such as hepatic cirrhosis or portal hypertension. The biodistribution pattern is related to the blood flow rates (volumes) through the organs as well as the functional capacity of the phagocytic cells. In disease states where one or both of these parameters may be reduced, for example in cirrhosis, the concentration of radiocolloid in the liver will be decreased, whereas activity in the spleen and bone marrow will be increased. This phenomenon is referred to as a colloid shift (Sylvester 1996).

36.4.2.2 Bone Marrow Imaging

Bone marrow imaging may help in localizing the diseased sites for marrow sampling in patients with a nonuniform marrow distribution. In patients with sickle cell disease, marrow scintigraphy in conjunction with bone imaging has been used in the evaluation of bone and joint complaints. At present nanocolloid is the only commercially available agent used for bone marrow imaging. Reticuloendothelial activity generally corresponds to erythroblastic activity in normal and pathological states. In normal adults about 15%–20% of the injected activity will be distributed in the reticuloendothelial cells of the marrow. The presence of activity in the liver and spleen prevents optimal visualization of the marrow in the lower thoracic and upper lumbar spine region (Kim et al. 1996).

36.4.2.3 Lymphoscintigraphy

For lymphoscintigraphy a dynamic study is performed after subcutaneous injection of the nanosized radiocolloid in the interdigital web spaces or in the dorsum of the feet or hands. If the spontaneous transport of the tracer is delayed or impaired, images are obtained after exercise, which normally will promote tracer transit. This technique allows identification of the presence (or absence) of lymphatic channels (Vaqueiro et al. 1986; Weissleder and Thrall 1989).

36.4.2.4 Sentinel Node Imaging

To image the sentinel node(s), nanocolloid is injected into the peritumoral area. In melanoma, the presence of metastasis in these nodes significantly alters the extent of surgery performed. In some centers this technique is also applied to localize the internal mammary lymph node chain for radiation therapy planning in patients with breast cancer (Giuliano et al. 1995; Slingluff et al. 1994; Uren et al. 1993, 1995; van der Veen et al. 1994).

36.5 Gases and Aerosols for Ventilation Imaging

Ventilation imaging is mostly performed in combination with perfusion scintigraphy using ^{99m}Tc-MAA when there is suspicion of pulmonary embolism. This study can be carried out with radioactive gases, aerosols, or Technegas, as shown in Table 36.3.

36.5.1 Krypton-81m

Krypton-81m is obtained from a generator and is eluted with moist air. The short half-life of 13 s does not present a waste disposal problem. Since the generator must be sited next to the gamma camera so that the ^{81m}Kr-loaded air can be passed directly from the generator to the patient, extra shielding around the generator is required. The generator is only available for a single day due to the short half-life of rubidium-81 (4.6 h), the parent radionuclide of ^{81m}Kr. Since the photon energy of ^{81m}Kr is higher than that of ^{99m}Tc, the ventilation study can be performed after the perfusion scintigrams; thus the ventilation study can be done optionally in cases with abnormal perfusion scans. In ^{81m}Kr studies, areas with abnormal ventilation will show as defects. Because of the short half-life of ^{81m}Kr, washout images cannot be obtained. Other disadvantages of ^{81m}Kr in comparison with xenon-133 are the high cost and the limited use of the generator. However, the images are superior to those obtained with ^{133}Xe (Loken 1987; Lowe and Sostman 1994; Norenberg and Hladik 1996).

36.5.2 Xenon-133

Xenon-133 is available in vials and can be kept in stock for use when required. Its use needs dedicated equipment, i.e., a closed spirometer system, to trap the exhaled air. With ^{133}Xe ventilation studies should be performed before perfusion imaging because of the lower photon energy of ^{133}Xe compared with ^{99m}Tc used for perfusion imaging. In ventilation studies using xenon, areas with abnormal ventilation will appear as defects on the equilibrium images and as areas with retention of radioactivity during washout. ^{127}Xe, with higher photon energy than ^{133}Xe, resulting in better images, is no longer available commercially (Loken 1987; Lowe and Sostman 1994; Norenberg and Hladik 1996).

Table 36.3. Radiopharmaceuticals for ventilation imaging. Half-lifes and energy data of the radionuclides are adopted from ICRP Publication 38 (1983)

Radiopharmaceutical	Half-life	Energy (keV)
^{81m}Kr	13 s	190
^{133}Xe	5.24 days	81
^{99m}Tc-aerosol	6.02 h	140
^{99m}Tc-carbon	6.02 h	140

36.5.3 ^{99m}Tc-Aerosols

Since ^{81m}Kr is available only at intervals and ^{133}Xe has the disadvantage that one has to dispose of the exhaled air contaminated with the isotope, radioactive aerosols of technetium have been developed. Radioactive aerosols are prepared from ^{99m}Tc-DTPA or ^{99m}Tc-colloids, in a machine for the generation of aerosols, which is manufactured by several commercial suppliers. After loading ^{99m}Tc-DTPA into the nebulizer, air under pressure is passed through the solution. The generated radioactive aerosol droplets are inhaled by the patient through a mouthpiece. Droplets larger than those required for the ventilation study will settle in the reservoir bag. Exhaled radioactivity is trapped by a filter. One-way flap valves ensure the unidirectional flow of the aerosols. All parts of the system are disposable. The whole system is enclosed in lead shielding. Advantages of aerosols are the day-to-day availability, the low cost, and the favorable imaging characteristics of ^{99m}Tc. A disadvantage is that bronchial depositions may occur, especially in patients with chronic obstructive pulmonary disease (Lowe and Sostman 1994; Norenberg and Hladik 1996).

36.5.4 ^{99m}Tc-Carbon

A newer development in the preparation of a ^{99m}Tc radiopharmaceutical for ventilation imaging is the introduction of Technegas. This radiopharmaceutical consists of ultra-fine dispersion of ^{99m}Tc-labeled carbon, and is generated by heating ^{99m}Tc-pertechnetate in a graphic crucible at 2500°C in an atmosphere of pure argon using dedicated commercially available equipment (LOWE and SOSTMAN 1994; NORENBERG and HLADIK 1996).

36.6 Commercially Prepared Radiopharmaceuticals

Commercially prepared radiopharmaceuticals are purchased in vials as a sterile solution appropriate for intravenous injection or other routes of administration. No pharmaceutical manipulations are required before administration to the patient. These preparations can be single dose or multidose. They often do not contain a preservative. Successive doses can be removed under aseptic conditions, and the remainder returned to stock after resterilization when possible. Occasionally the volume required to provide an individual dose can be very small, making dilution necessary. For this purpose the diluent must be appropriate and should be of the desired quality as stated in the instruction leaflet. If the radiopharmaceutical contains a preservative, this may be diluted to below its effective concentration and inclusion of a preservative in the diluent may be necessary (LAZARUS 1994). The physical properties of the radionuclides used to label these agents are shown in Table 36.4.

36.6.1 Gallium [^{67}Ga] Citrate

After intravenous administration ^{67}Ga is bound to transferrin. Most of the ^{67}Ga uptake in tumors is transferrin receptor mediated. However, part of the uptake is also transferrin receptor independent. In inflamed tissues ^{67}Ga binds to lactoferrin which is released from granulocytes, and also to bacterial products. In chronic infection, binding of ^{67}Ga-lactoferrin to macrophages is supposed to be involved. Within the first 24h, 15%–20% of the injected dose is excreted in the urine; thereafter the liver becomes the main route of excretion, resulting in elimination of another 15%–20% with the feces. The normal pattern of radioactivity distribution in man includes uptake in the liver, spleen, bone, and bone marrow, and also in female breasts, salivary and lacrimal glands, mucosa of the nose, and genitals. Salivary gland uptake can be increased after radiotherapy. Uptake in children may include the thymus, skull base, and epiphyses. Recent surgical wounds may also be visualized.

Gallium-67 imaging is used for staging and follow-up of lymphomas, especially in Hodgkin's disease and non-hodgkin's lymphoma. ^{67}Ga scintigraphy may also be used for the imaging of melanoma, hepatoma, and lung carcinoma.

To localize infection sites in patients with fever of unknown origin this technique has been proposed as the first choice. The high uptake in bone and excretion in the bowel, however, hamper image interpretation. Therefore, labeled leukocytes are preferred by many. In chronic infections, the sensitivity of ^{67}Ga is higher than that of labeled leukocytes. The same holds true for the investigation of the diabetic foot (NEUMANN et al. 1996; NEUMANN and MCAFEE 1996; PETERS 1994).

Table 36.4. Half-life and photon energy (keV) of radionuclides applied in commercially prepared agents. Data are adopted from ICRP Publication 38 (1983)

Radionuclide	Half-life	Energy (keV)
Gallium-67	3.26 days	93, 184, 300
Selenium-75	119.8 days	136, 265
Indium-111	2.83 days	171, 245
Iodine-123	13.1 h	159
Iodine-131	8.04 days	364
Thallium-201	73.0 h	70, 167

36.6.2 ^{111}In-Diethylene Triamine Penta-acetic Acid (DTPA, Pentetate)

Indium-111-DTPA is the most commonly utilized radiopharmaceutical for cerebrospinal fluid (CSF) imaging. CSF imaging is a functional test to demonstrate the flow of CSF. Another application is to localize a fistula in suspected CSF leak. CSF tracers are usually introduced into the CSF area via lumbar puncture. Another possibility is direct introduction into the cisterna magna or the ventricular system. Only 20%–35% of the injected tracer will reach the basilar cisterns for imaging; the majority will remain in the lumbar cul-de-sac for more than 48h. The flow of radiopharmaceutical continues along the base of the brain to the frontal poles and the Sylvian fissure, and diffuses over the cerebral hemispheres. By 24h, the majority of the tracer is localized along the sagittal sinus with decreasing activity in the basilar cisterns. In most normal patients, no significant reflux of tracer occurs into the ventricular system, although occasionally transient ventricular reflux is seen. ^{111}In-DTPA is absorbed with the CSF from the subarachnoid space into the blood through the arachnoid granulations. Maximal blood concentration is reached between 2 and 6h post administration. Approximately 65% of the dose is excreted in the urine within the first 24h. The target-to-nontarget ratio is high due to the continued blood clearance of DTPA by the kidneys. Alternatively ^{99m}Tc-DTPA can be used, but its obvious benefits of higher availability, lower cost, and improved tissue dosimetry are offset by the lack of physical half-life needed for imaging beyond 24h (BOLES 1996; LAWRENCE et al. 1996).

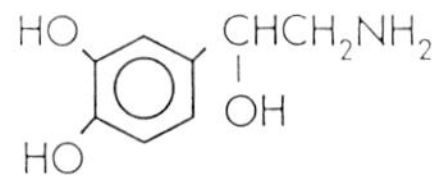
a

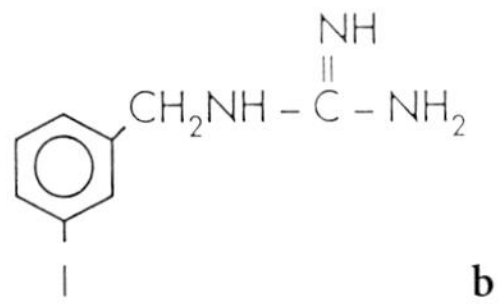
b

Fig. 36.9. Chemical structures of norepinephrine (**a**) and MIBG (**b**)

36.6.3 ^{123}I- and ^{131}I-Sodium Iodide

^{123}I- and ^{131}I-sodium iodide are used for thyroid imaging. The main indications for thyroid imaging using iodine isotope are assessment of the nature of thyrotoxicosis, differentiation of hot or cold nodules, assessment of retrosternal extension of goiters, measurement of thyroid uptake, and diagnosis of metastatic spread of differentiated thyroid carcinoma. For identification of metastatic spread of thyroid carcinoma, the highest sensitivity can be achieved with imaging performed after administration of a therapeutic dose of ^{131}I.

Iodide is actively transported into the thyroid; subsequently the trapped iodide is oxidized, bound to thyroglobulin in the thyroid follicular cells, and organified in thyroid hormone. Normally 10%–35% of the administered iodine is taken up in the thyroid at 24h. The half-time of iodide elimination from the thyroid is estimated at 80 days. Approximately 35%–75% is excreted via the kidney, while fecal excretion is about 1%. Iodine uptake is also seen in salivary glands, in gastric mucosa, and to lesser extent in buccal mucosa.

Although ^{131}I is cheaper than ^{123}I and has a better availability due to the longer half-life, ^{131}I is less used due to the unfavorable photon energy, which results in poor image quality, and the higher radiation dose to the patient. At present thyroid scintigraphy is usually performed with ^{99m}Tc, although measurement of uptake at 24h is not possible since this isotope is not organified (HURLEY and BECKER 1996; PARK 1996; SANDLER et al. 1996).

36.6.4 ^{123}I- and ^{131}I-Metaiodobenzylguanidine (MIBG, Iobenguane)

Metaiodobenzylguanidine is the radiopharmaceutical of choice in the diagnosis and follow-up of patients with pheochromocytoma and neuroblastoma. It has also been applied in other neuroendocrine tumors, but the results are disappointing, and the sensitivity is significantly lower than with ^{111}In-pentetreotide (KRENNING et al. 1995). MIBG is structurally (Fig. 36.9) related to norepinephrine and in pheochromocytoma and neuroblastoma is actively accumulated via the amine uptake mechanism into the chromaffin granules. Tracer uptake is affected by some drugs, such as labetalol, reserpine, and tricyclic antidepressants. Normal uptake is seen in salivary glands, heart, liver, spleen, and lung. Faint visualization of the normal adrenals is commonly observed. After 24h about 64% is excreted unchanged in the urine and only 0.06%–1.68% is excreted in the feces. For imaging both ^{123}I-MIBG and ^{131}I-MIBG can be applied. Advantages of ^{123}I-MIBG are the lower radiation burden and the more favorable energy emission, resulting in better image quality. Advantages of ^{131}I-MIBG are lower cost, wider availability, and longer shelf-life (GORDON et al. 1990; HOEFNAGEL 1994; NAKAJO et al. 1983).

36.6.5 ^{123}I-*ortho*-Iodohippurate (OIH, Hippuran)

Along with ^{99m}Tc-MAG3 and ^{99m}Tc-DTPA, OIH is used for renography. OIH has the highest extraction fraction by the kidney, resulting in excellent images. Because the normal human kidney removes most of the OIH from plasma entering the renal artery, the rate of OIH excretion is a measure of effective renal plasma flow, which is slightly less than that obtained with *para*-aminohippurate. Figure 36.10 shows the structures of both compounds. About two-thirds of the OIH in plasma is bound reversibly to plasma proteins. The unbound fraction is subject to glomerular filtration, the remainder being actively secreted in the proximal tubule. The secretory

a
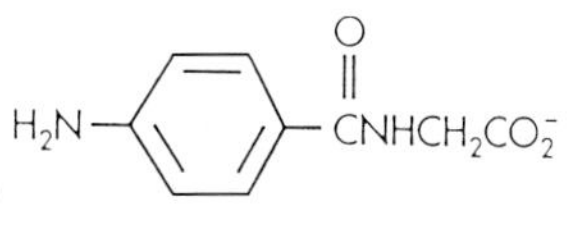

b
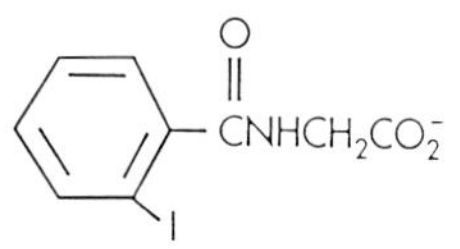

Fig. 36.10. Chemical structures of *p*-aminohippurate (**a**) and *o*-iodohippurate (**b**)

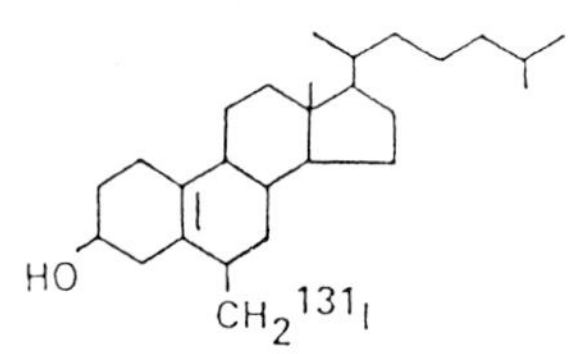
a

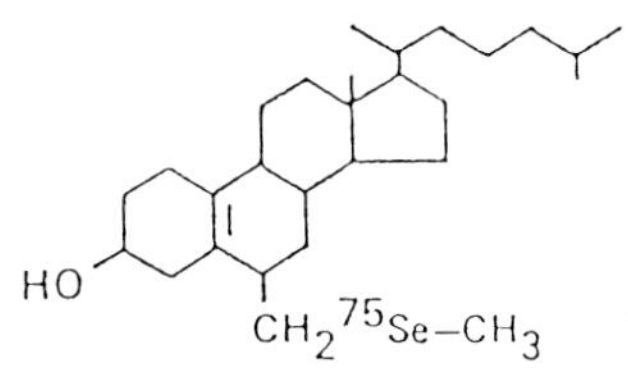
b

Fig. 36.11. Chemical structures of ^{131}I-iodomethylnorcholesterol (**a**) and ^{75}Se-selenomethylnorcholesterol (**b**)

mechanism is the usual one for carboxylic acids; therefore, drugs such as probenecid will interfere with the secretion of OIH, as will doses of carrier OIH in excess of the tubular maximum. Hepatic excretion is less than 2% of the injected dose; however, in patients with renal disease, the proportion excreted by the liver increases. The use of ^{123}I-OIH is hampered by the expense and by logistic problems; to date this agent is not available commercially in the United States. Because of the undesirable physical properties of ^{131}I, ^{131}I-OIH should not be used (CHERVU and BLAUFOX 1989; ESHIMA and FRITZBERG 1996).

36.6.6 ^{131}I-Iodomethylnorcholesterol and ^{75}Se-Selenomethylnorcholesterol

The structures of ^{131}I-iodomethylnorcholesterol and ^{75}Se-selenomethylnorcholesterol are shown in Fig. 36.11. Both agents show comparable effectiveness for adrenocortical imaging. Major indications for scintigraphy with radiolabeled cholesterol are the differential diagnosis of Cushing's syndrome and the demonstration of aldosteronomas in Conn's syndrome. For this last indication the study is performed under dexamethasone suppression. After intravenous administration radiocholesterol binds to plasma lipoprotein, chiefly low-density lipoprotein (LDL), and in the first 48 h is widely distributed throughout the body and taken up by the tissues identical to that of native LDL. After between 2 and 6 days the adrenal cortex shows the highest concentration. Uptake is increased by adrenocorticotropic hormone (ACTH), and suppressed by dexamethasone or other glucocorticoids. Several drugs such as oral contraceptives, diuretics, corticosteroids, and aldactone may interfere with the uptake of radiolabeled cholesterol, and should be discontinued. In contrast to the native compound, radiolabeled cholesterol is esterified but is not further metabolized and retained in the adrenals. The estimated effective half-life of the compound in the adrenals varies within the range of 25–105 days. Normally both adrenals are visualized, the right adrenal somewhat more intensely because of overprojection of liver activity. Due to excretion, radioactivity can be observed in the gallbladder and the colon (GROSS et al. 1989; HAY et al. 1996).

36.6.7 Thallous [^{201}Tl] Chloride

Before the introduction of ^{99m}Tc-MIBI, ^{201}Tl was the radiopharmaceutical of choice for myocardial perfusion imaging. Thallium uptake on these images indicates myocardial viability. Upon intravenous injection, thallous ion in low concentrations follows a pathway analogous to that followed by potassium ions. It is rapidly cleared from the blood, accumulating actively in viable myocardial muscle to a greater extent than in the surrounding tissue. Its similarity to potassium implies active accumulation in all viable muscle tissue and in the kidneys. Transient accumulation occurs in organs with a large blood pool and a high metabolic activity such as the thyroid and the liver. Normally ^{201}Tl also accumulates in the salivary and lacrimal glands. Thallium is transported across the myocyte cell membrane via the Na-K-ATPase pump. The first-pass extraction by the myocardium is approximately 85%. After 30 min 3%–4% of the injected dose accumulates in the myocardium. The distribution in the myocardium is in proportion to myocardial blood flow. Redistribution occurs within the following 12–18 h. Both uptake and clearance from myocytes in the hypoperfused myocardium are slower than normal (Gibson and Burns 1996; AHA/ACC Task Force Report 1995; Udelson 1995).

Other applications of ^{201}Tl include the localization of parathyroid adenomas, using the dual-isotope subtraction technique, and in oncology. For the detection of parathyroid adenoma the use of ^{99m}Tc-MIBI without the time-consuming subtraction technique is more popular (Freitas and Freitas 1996). In oncology ^{201}Tl is used to differentiate between benign and malignant lesions and to assess the grade of malignancy of a tumor; however, the role of thallium in oncology is still to be established (Waxman 1996).

36.7 Radiopharmaceuticals for Receptor Imaging

36.7.1 [^{111}In-DTPA-D-Phe^{1}]-Octreotide (Pentetreotide)

[^{111}In-DTPA-D-Phe^{1}]-octreotide, a chelated somatostatin analog, is used to demonstrate somatostatin receptor-positive tumors and diseases. Studies have demonstrated its high sensitivity for the detection of neuroendocrine tumors, such as carcinoid tumor, gastrinoma, paraganglioma, and small cell lung carcinoma. For medullary thyroid carcinoma, insulinoma, and pheochromocytoma the detection rate is lower. Other tumors, such as breast and brain tumors, can also be visualized. Furthermore the extent of diseases in which activated leukocytes play a role, such as Hodgkin's disease, non-Hodgkin's lymphoma, sarcoidosis, and tuberculosis, can be assessed by this technique.

Pentetreotide, which is eight amino acids long (Fig. 36.12), binds to somatostatin receptors on both tumorous and nontumorous tissues. This agent, which is produced as a cold kit, can be labeled easily with ^{111}In-chloride. Pentetreotide is mainly excreted by the kidneys. Studies in humans demonstrate that 85% to more than 90% of the injected dose is excreted within the first 24 h and 48 h respectively. Less than 2% of the dose is found in feces collected until 72 h after injection (Krenning et al. 1992). Because of its relatively long effective half-life, pentetreotide can be used to visualize the pathology efficiently after 24 and 48 h, when interfering background radioactivity is minimized by renal clearance. Physiological uptake is observed in the pituitary, thyroid gland, spleen, liver, and kidneys. Therefore, SPECT is mandatory in seeking small foci of pathology in the pancreatic region. Patients on octreotide treatment show a diminished accumulation of radioligand in the spleen. Due to excretion the urinary bladder is clearly visualized. Some excretion via the gallbladder is responsible for its visualization and also the presence of intestinal radioactivity (Krenning et al. 1995).

a Ala-Gly-Cys-Lys-Asn-Phe-*Phe-Trp-Lys-Thr*-Phe-Thr-Ser-Cys

b ^{111}In-DTPA-D-Phe-Cys-*Phe-D-Trp-Lys-Thr*-Cys-Thr(ol)

Fig. 36.12. Chemical structures of somatostatin (**a**) and ^{111}In-pentetreotide (**b**)

36.7.2 ^{123}I-Iodobenzamide (IBZM)

Iodobenzamide is a dopamine D2 receptor antagonist (Fig. 36.13). Preliminary studies indicate that its application might be of value in schizophrenic patients and in diseases with a change in D2 receptor density in the basal ganglia, such as parkinsonism. After intravenous administration the total brain uptake is approximately 3.7% of the dose, but it washes out rapidly to 0.7% at 20 h. Therefore SPECT imaging is optimally performed at between 60 and 120 min. The maximum ratio of striatum to cortex is 2.48; this ratio decreases with age. Iodobenzamide is also accumulated in the lung, liver, and kidneys. Urine excretion is more than 40% of the dose at 24 h and more than 60% at 48 h. Between 5 and 6 h after injection 10% of the dose is excreted via the hepatobiliary system (Saha et al. 1994; Verhoef 1993).

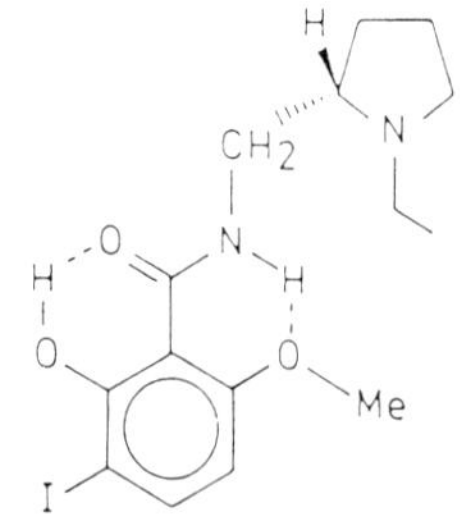

Fig. 36.13. Chemical structure of iodobenzamide

36.7.3
^{123}I-Iomazenil

Iomazenil, an analog of flumazenil, is a benzodiazepine antagonist (Fig. 36.14). Benzodiazepine receptor binding is diminished in epileptogenic foci and may be visualized as decreased activity on the SPECT images acquired with iomazenil. Due to its lipophilicity this compound distributes rapidly in the brain. After a maximum reached at 10–15 min post injection, the blood flow-dependent image turns to an image of the benzodiazepine receptors. At 90 min 7% of the injected dose is located in the brain and is predominantly bound to receptors in the cerebral cortex. The total brain radioactivity declines with a half-time of approximately 3.5 h. Receptor binding is impaired by benzodiazepine derivatives; therefore these should be discontinued several days before the examination. No other major organ systems show significant uptake of iomazenil. The compound is excreted through the renal and enterohepatic routes. Within 24 h approximately 85%–90% of the dose is found in the urine and 10%–15% in the feces (Dey et al. 1994; Saha et al. 1994; Verhoef 1993).

36.8
Causes of Defects in Radiopharmaceuticals

The quality of the radiopharmaceutical has a significant impact on the accuracy of the diagnosis. Therefore, it should be routinely tested whether radiopharmaceuticals fulfil the specifications cited in the product information or the official pharmacopoieas. For material used in research and clinical trials, where established standards may not be available, limits of purity may need to be specifically established for the product in question. Table 36.5 shows the frequencies of quality control testing recommended by the Dutch Society of Nuclear Medicine. The parameters to be tested include: radionuclide purity, radiochemical purity, specific activity, particle size (if appropriate), pH, and sterility or apyrogenicity, as well as the appearance (Oei and Blokland 1993).

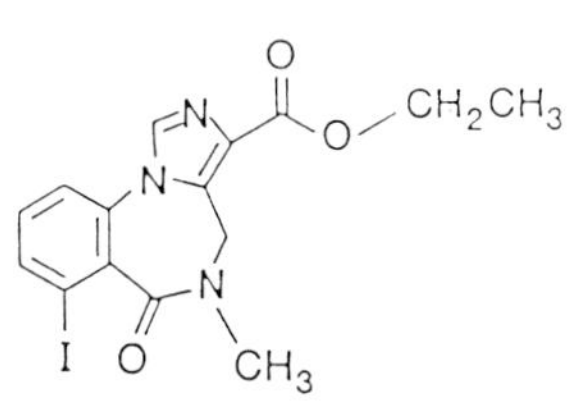

Fig. 36.14. Chemical structure of iomazenil

If the obtained images indicate the possibility of a defective radiopharmaceutical, samples from the same batch should be immediately quality tested. Defects in radiopharmaceuticals are usually recognized as an unexpected biodistribution in the patient. Other presentations of defects include fever or reactions due to microbial or pyrogen contamination. If the material is found to be defective, the obtained images may be inappropriate for inter pretation. If the quality testing indicates that the radiopharmaceutical fulfils the specifications, then the possibility of drug interference or faulty handling techniques should be considered (Hojelse et al. 1994).

In this section examples of causes of defective products are given. Also examples of faulty handling techniques are described. It is not the intention to present all possible causes of defects; rather the most frequently observed deficiencies are described.

36.8.1
Technetium Generators

The defect most frequently reported is reduced elution efficiency. Generators from different manufacturers can be involved and the problems can range from complete lack of elution to reduced technetium yield in the presence of a normal elution volume. Most of the problems can be easily explained, e.g.,

Table 36.5. Frequency of quality controls

	Batch control or random control	Every preparation
^{99m}Tc-generator		
Absence of aluminum	+	
Elution yield		+
Molybdenum breakthrough		+
Radiochemical purity	+	
radionuclidic purity	+	
Sterility (in retrospect)	+	
^{99m}Tc-labeled radiopharmaceuticals		
Appearance		+
pH	+	
Labeling yield	+	
Sterility	+	
Commercial prepared agents		
Appearance		+
Labeling yield	+	
Radionuclidic purity	+	

blockage in tubing inside the generator or freezing of the generator due to low temperatures during transport (EANM 1996).

Another problem is the so-called Monday effect, where problems sometimes arise after labeling with eluate from a generator that has not been eluted for several days. This problem has been reduced to some extent by the use of generators that are in a dry state between elutions. Other methods include the use of oxidants in the eluate (e.g., sodium nitrate) or copper salts on the column (Hojelse et al. 1994).

Another source of problems is the presence of tracer metal impurities. It has been shown that it is essential to prepare ^{99m}Tc-exametazime using eluate that is not more than 2 h old owing to the build-up of impurities in older eluates. The addition of small amounts of sodium iodide to the generator eluates immediately after elution enables them to be used up to at least 6 h after elution, with no adverse effect on the radiochemical purity (Hojelse et al. 1994).

Another possible impurity in the generator eluate is aluminum. The quantity found is usually very low but excess aluminum has been shown to cause flocculation of colloids and their subsequent deposition in the lungs (Vinberg 1980).

36.8.2 Instability of the Radiopharmaceutical

The radiochemical purity of a radiopharmaceutical can often influence its biodistribution. The most common occurrence is the release of unbound radionuclide from the labeled compound. Examples are iodide in iodinated compounds and free pertechnetate in ^{99m}Tc-labeled products. Technetium-labeled compounds are normally stable for several hours. However, introduction of air can lead to oxidation with the release of free pertechnetate. This is observed in the patient as uptake in the salivary glands, thyroid, and stomach (Hojelse et al. 1994).

Several reports have described DTPA to be stable only if the vial is unopened; if air is introduced during the removal of doses, the radiochemical purity markedly decreases. Moreover, DTPA has been shown to be markedly unstable if it is diluted or if there is a lengthy delay before injecting the patient (Hojelse et al. 1994).

It has also been reported that the sensitivity of ^{99m}Tc-HMPAO to radiolytic induced decomposition rapidly reduces the radiochemical purity after reconstitution. High specific activity and high concentration exacerbate this problem (Tubergen et al. 1991).

36.8.3 Volumes of Reagents

Experience has shown that the purity of a number of products may depend on the accuracy of volumes of the solution used for their preparation. Different brands of injection syringes may have differing dead volumes and inaccuracy can easily occur during preparation. An example where accuracy in volume is important is the radiolabeling of leukocytes, where a high labeling efficiency of, for instance, exametazime is dependent on a small volume as well as a high concentration of ^{99m}Tc-exametazime (Sampson 1991).

36.8.4 Heat

A number of kits require heat for the labeling. These include the isonitriles for imaging the myocardium and mercaptoglycine for renal studies. It is essential to heat according to the manufacturer's instructions to obtain an appropriate labeling yield (Hojelse et al. 1994).

36.8.5 Radionuclide Purity

There are few published reports of radionuclide impurities affecting the visual appearance of a scintigram. An example is the prolonged use of a ^{123}I product where the radionuclide is prepared by the (p,2n) procedure. Preparations of this type may contain the impurity ^{124}I with a half-life of 4.2 days. The percentage of ^{124}I will increase in time and this may affect the quality of the scan due to the high photon energy emitted (Hojelse et al. 1994).

36.8.6 Change in pH

Carrier-free solutions may be sensitive to changes in pH which can occur by simple dilution of unbuffered solutions. Adjustment of pH and addition of carrier may be needed in these instances. Changes in pH can also produce colloid formation in ^{111}In-chloride solutions and this can affect the labeling of blood cells and antibodies (Hojelse et al. 1994).

36.8.7 Contamination and Cross-contamination

Radiopharmaceuticals are, almost universally, dispensed in multidose vials and do not usually contain bacteriostatic agents. Their use should therefore be limited to a short time and preparations should be routinely stored in a refrigerator to prevent bacterial contamination.

Potential problems are related to the radiolabeling of blood products, where the blood may be contaminated with, for example, hepatitis B or HIV. Further, there is risk of cross-contamination between blood samples. This can be prevented by strict separation of the samples (Danpure and Osman 1994).

36.8.8 Swabbing of Vials During Dispensing

Excessive swabbing of the rubber septum of a multidose vial can cause pooling of antiseptic on the surface of the septum followed by injection of droplets into the vial, which may result in the formation of a colloidal complex. This was observed after contamination of DMSA with centrimide and chlorohexidine (Murray 1986).

It has been reported that an iodinated antiseptic was responsible for the formation of free pertechnetate in technetium-labeled radiopharmaceuticals and that chlorohexidine may have caused the aggregation of sulfur colloid particles, resulting in accumulations of aggregated colloids (larger particles) in the lung (Hojelse et al. 1994). Also reported was an effect of ethyl alcohol on generator vials which may have impaired elution efficiency. It is therefore essential that swabbing should be performed only by the system recommended by the manufacturer (Hojelse et al. 1994).

36.8.9 Adhesion

Radiopharmaceuticals are characterized by very small amounts of chemical substances used both in the original kit and in the final product. Also, the volumes administered to the patient are usually small. Any reduction in dose volume could therefore result in a marked underdosage to the patient and poor scan quality. Another frequently reported etiology of underdosage of radiopharmaceuticals is adhesion to the syringe or to the inside of the container. ^{99m}Tc-macroaggregates are known to stick to the glass vial as well as the syringe. Gallium citrate adheres to most qualities of glassware and siliconizing largely reduces this tendency. Siliconizing of the glass vial of ^{201}Tl is also necessary to reduce adhesion (Hojelse et al. 1994).

36.8.10 Interactions with Syringes or Catheters

The administration of radiopharmaceuticals via heparinized catheters occasionally produces defects. For example, when a heparinized catheter is used for in vivo RBC labeling with pyrophosphate, diminished cardiac activity and increased renal activity have been observed (Hegge et al. 1978). A few reports have been published of cases where the radiopharmaceutical reacted in some way with the components of a syringe or needle (Hojelse et al. 1994).

36.8.11 Faulty Injection Technique

Extravascular injection of a significant part of the dose makes the study inappropriate for interpretation. Moreover the local radiation dose at the injection site is significantly higher. This is particularly true for ^{201}Tl, which may cause radiation "burn" due to the emission of Auger electrons (Castronovo et al. 1988). Another example of faulty handling is the withdrawal of un-anticoagulated blood in the syringe with ^{99m}Tc-MAA, which may result in hot spots on the lungs (Preston and Greenlaw 1970).

36.9 Adverse Reactions to Radiopharmaceuticals

36.9.1 Definition

In a recent publication the Pharmacopoeia Committee of the Society of Nuclear Medicine defined an adverse reaction associated with the use of radiopharmaceuticals as follows: "An adverse drug reaction is any response to a drug which is noxious and unintended following the administration of a radiopharmaceutical or nonradioactive adjunct pharmaceutical. The reaction is unanticipated from the known pharmacologic action of the nonradioactive pharmaceutical, is not the result of an overdose, is not the result of injury caused by poor injection technique, and is not caused by a vasovagal response" (SILBERSTEIN and RYAN 1996).

36.9.2 Prevalence

Using this definition, the Pharmacopoeia Committee conducted a 5-year prospective study with the aim of ascertaining the prevalence of adverse reactions to radiopharmaceutical and interventional drugs. Eighteen institutions that perform a high volume of nuclear medicine procedures participated in this study. All reported the number of radiopharmacological administrations as well as the number of observed adverse reactions. Adverse drug reactions which were to be reported included: (a) untoward effects, whether observed frequently or rarely, following administration of the radiopharmaceutical, (b) life-threatening reactions requiring hospitalization or fatal reactions from nonradiopharmaceuticals (i.e., interventional drugs), (c) reactions unanticipated from the known pharmacological action of a nonradioactive pharmaceutical, and (d) anaphylactoid or allergic reactions. Excluded were reactions due to overdosage, vasovagal response, injury from poor injection technique, and deterministic effects from therapy with unsealed sources (SILBERSTEIN and RYAN 1996).

In this study, which took place between 1989 and 1994, the total number of radiopharmaceutical and adjunct nonradioactive drug injections was 783 525 and 67 835, respectively. The total number of adverse reactions for radiopharmaceuticals and adjunct nonradioactive drugs observed was 18 and 4, respectively. Thus, the incidence of adverse reactions for radiopharmaceuticals and adjunct nonradioactive drug injections was 0.0023% and 0.0059%, respectively. These incidence rates are 1000 times lower than those reported for x-ray contrast media and for drugs administered in a hospital setting. In the same period the Task Group on Radiopharmaceuticals of the European Association of Nuclear Medicine registered 201 (Table 36.6) adverse reactions, including vasovagal response, which was excluded by the SNM Pharmacopoeia Committee (EANM 1990, 1992a,b, 1994, 1995).

Table 36.6. Adverse reactions to radiopharmaceuticals reported in 1989–1993

Radiopharmaceutical	Number	Type of reaction[a]			
		A	B	C	D
^{51}Cr-EDTA	1				×
^{51}Cr-erythrocytes	1		×		
^{111}In-oxinate	2		×	×	
^{111}In-monoclonal antibodies	1	×			×
^{111}In-leukocytes	2		×		×
^{123}I-MIBG	10	×	×		×
^{123}I-sodium iodide	3	×			×
^{131}I-hippuran	5	×	×		
^{131}I-MIBG	1	×			
^{131}I-monoclonal antibodies	2	×			
^{131}I-sodium iodide	4	×			×
^{131}I-norcholesterol	1		×		
^{99m}Tc-albumin colloid	10	×	×	×	
^{99m}Tc-diethyliodo-IDA	1	×			
^{99m}Tc-erythrocytes	5	×	×		×
^{99m}Tc-exametazime	6	×	×		
^{99m}Tc-leukocytes	2	×			
^{99m}Tc-immunoglobulin	2	×			
^{99m}Tc-MAA	18	×	×		×
^{99m}Tc-MAG3	14	×	×		×
^{99m}Tc-microspheres	1	×			
^{99m}Tc-phosphonates	58	×	×	×	×
^{99m}Tc-DTPA	31	×	×		×
^{99m}Tc-pertechnetate	5	×		×	
^{99m}Tc-pyrophosphate	1	×	×		
^{99m}Tc-MIBI	6		×		×
^{99m}Tc-DMSA	5	×			×
^{99m}Tc-stannous colloid	1	×			
^{89}Sr-chloride	1			×	
^{201}Tl-thallous chloride	1				×
Total	201				

Abbreviations as defined in the text.
[a] A, Allergic; B, vasovagal; C, local; D, other.

Although the numbers reported to the EANM Task Group in the years 1994 and 1995 (EANM 1995, 1996) show some increase to 73 and 64 respectively, the prevalence observed by the Committees of both societies is significantly lower than in the previous publication of KEELING (1994), in which a prevalence of 1 per 4000 administrations was mentioned.

36.9.3 Types of Reaction

The symptoms of the adverse reactions reported are generally mild or moderate and can be divided into four categories: allergic, vasovagal, local, and other reactions. The frequencies of each of these symptoms as reported by the EANM Task Group are demonstrated in Table 36.6. In the majority of reports, the problems observed were minor and often resolved without medical intervention. In many cases, the reporter considered that the association between administration of the radiopharmaceutical and the symptoms was not proven.

Serious allergic reactions were reported in connection with ^{99m}Tc-albumin colloid, ^{99m}Tc-DTPA, ^{99m}Tc-diethyl IDA, ^{99m}Tc-exametazime, ^{131}I-monoclonal antibodies, and ^{99m}Tc-microspheres. Other serious reactions were reported in connection with ^{99m}Tc-MAA, ^{99m}Tc-MAG3 and ^{99m}Tc-DMSA. Phosphonates were the most commonly reported causative agents; allergic reactions can occur following administration of unlabeled kits as part of the RBC labeling procedure. Symptoms reported following administration of DTPA included fainting, itching, and tightness in the chest, whilst those reported for MAA included fainting, edema of the neck and throat, and vomiting (EANM 1990, 1995).

Three allergic reactions were reported following reinjection of labeled autologous leukocytes. Two labelings were performed with technetium exametazime and one with indium oxinate. Symptoms included rash, pruritis, and a feeling of suffocation and cyanosis. In each of these cases, plasma volume expanders had been used to increase erythrocyte sedimentation and the possibility exists that such agents may be involved in provoking the reaction (EANM 1993).

One report of a neurological complication following intrathecal administration of ^{99m}Tc-DTPA was received. Although details of the formulation of the radiopharmaceutical are still not known, paralysis following intrathecal administration of the pentasodium salt of DTPA has previously been described (EANM 1994).

One of the recurrent reports during 1994 was pain upon injection of ^{123}I-MIBG. There was no evidence to suggest extravasation of the injection or that it had been given excessively quickly. The symptoms were described as intense tingling in the injection arm, and in pediatric patients a severe irritation at the injection site was observed. This was not seen when saline was injected prior to and following MIBG. The reports were received from three centers, using material obtained from more than one manufacturer. It is possible that the pain is associated with components of the formulation other than MIBG itself (EANM 1995).

Although there were no indications that the causes of two fatal cases were connected directly with the administration of radiopharmaceuticals, two deaths due to cardiac arrest were observed in 1990 in Europe: one after ^{99m}Tc-MIBI and another after ^{99m}Tc-MAG3 which were administered 3 h and 1.5 min beforehand, respectively (EANM 1992a). In 1991, too, two fatal cases were reported, which were not directly attributable to the administered radiopharmaceuticals. Both patients underwent lung studies using ^{99m}Tc-MAA; one patient had cardiac arrest 55 min thereafter and the other died suddenly on the way back to the ward (EANM 1992b). During the years 1992–1994 no fatalities were reported. One serious reaction was observed 2 min after repeated administration of MAA in 1993. The patient stopped breathing and became pulseless; however, the patient recovered after immediate resuscitation (EANM 1993, 1994, 1995). In 1995, again, two fatal cases were reported, one involving medronate and the other MAA. In each case a thorough investigation indicated that death had not occurred as a result of radiopharmaceutical administration. The patient who received MAA was a 77-year-old male who was rapidly deteriorating at the time of injection. Images were suggestive of massive pulmonary emboli and the patient died 40 min later (EANM 1996).

During the 5-year study of the SNM committee no fatal case was reported. Ten of the 18 adverse reactions reported in this study were rashes. None of the patients exhibiting an adverse reaction to the radiopharmaceutical required hospitalization. Interventional pharmaceuticals used as an adjunct to the nuclear medicine procedure rarely lead to temporary hospitalization. Their prevalence is about 6 per 100 000 injections. None of these patients exhibited any sequelae (Silberstein and Ryan 1996).

36.9.4 Conclusions

Unlike drugs given for therapeutic purposes, radiopharmaceuticals rarely cause adverse reactions. The explanation for the safety of radiopharmaceuticals lies not only in the very small mass of drug injected, usually in the microgram range, but also in the fact that radiopharmaceuticals are typically administered only once or a very limited number of times to any given patient. The use of a radiopharmaceutical is not based upon its ability to produce a pharmacological effect, but rather on differences in the distribution and pharmacokinetics of the agent between normal and abnormal physiological processes. It can be concluded that the use of radiopharmaceuticals is extremely safe, that the incidence of adverse reactions to radiopharmaceuticals is extremely low, and that in general the usually mild symptoms are often resolved without medical intervention.

References

AHA/ACC Task Force Report (1995) Guidelines for clinical use of cardiac radionuclide imaging. Circulation 91:1278–1303

Akkermans LMA, Jacobs F, Smout AJPM, Oei HY, Wittebol P (1984) Radionuclide measurement of normal and disturbed gastric motility. Scand J Gastroentol 19(Suppl 96):19–26

Arndt JW, van der Sluys Veer A, Blok D, et al. (1993) Prospective comparative study of technetium-99m-WBCs and indium-III-ganulocytes for the examination of patients with inflammatory bowel disease. J Nucl Med 34:1052–1057

Arzoumanian A, Rosenthall L, Seto H (1977) Clinical comparison of ^{99m}Tc-labelled preformed phytate colloid and sulfur colloid: concise communication. J Nucl Med 18:118–120

Babich JW (1991) Technetium-99m-HMPAO retention and the role of glutathione. J Nucl Med 32:1981–1983

Beltran MR (1996) Testicular imaging. In: Henkin RE et al. (eds) Nuclear medicine, vol 2. Mosby, St. Louis, pp 1110–1122

Berman D, Kiat H, Germano G, et al. (1995) ^{99m}Tc sestamibi SPECT. In: Gordon DePuey E, et al. (eds) Cardiac SPECT imaging. Raven Press, New York, pp 121–146

Bergqvist L, Strand S-E, Persson BRR (1983) Particle sizing and biokinetics of interstitial lymphoscintigraphic agents. Semin Nucl Med 13:9–19

Blaufox MD (1991) Procedures of choice in renal nuclear medicine. J Nucl Med 32:1301–1309

Boles MA (1996) Cerebrospinal fluid imaging. In: Henkin RE et al. (eds) Nuclear medicine, vol 2. Mosby, St. Louis, pp 1313–1330

Brown ML, Collier D, Fogelman I (1993) Bone scintigraphy: part 1. Oncology and infection. J Nucl Med 34:2236–2240

Burns HD, Gibson RE (1996) Radiopharmaceuticals for cerebral imaging. In: Henkin RE et al. (eds) Nuclear medicine, vol 2. Mosby, St. Louis, pp 1273–1288

Burt RW (1996) Cerebral perfusion imaging. In: Henkin RE et al. (eds) Nuclear medicine, vol 2. Mosby, St. Louis, pp 1289–1312

Castronovo FP (1988) The infiltrated radiopharmaceutical injection: dosimetric considerations. Eur J Nucl Med 14:93–97

Chen CC, Skarulis MC, Fraker DL, et al. (1995) Technetium-99m-sestamibi imaging before reoperation for primary hyperparathyroidism. J Nucl Med 36:2186–2191

Chervu LR, Blaufox MD (1989) Radiopharmaceuticals for the measurement of glomerular filtration rate and renal plasma flow. In: Blaufox MD (ed) Evaluation of renal function and disease with radionuclides: the upper urinary tract, 2nd edn. Karger, Basel, pp 28–59

Corbett JR, Parkey RW, Bonte FJ, Buja LM, Willerson JT (1996) Infarct avid imaging. In: Henkin RE et al. (eds) Nuclear medicine, vol 1. Mosby, St. Louis, pp 742–759

Danpure HJ, Osman S (1994) Radiolabelling of blood cells-methodology. In: Sampson CB (ed) Textbook of radiopharmacy, theory and practice, 2nd edn. Gordon and Breach, Yverdon, Switzerland, pp 75–86

Dey HM, Seibyl JP, Stubbs JB, et al. (1994) Human biodistribution and dosimetry of the SPECT benzodiazepine receptor radioligand iodine-123-iomazenil. J Nucl Med 35:399–404

Dilsizian V, Rocco TP, Bonow RO, et al. (1990) Cardiac blood-pool imaging. II. Applications in noncoronary heart disease. J Nucl Med 31:10–22

EANM (1990) European system for reporting of adverse reactions and drug defects. Seventh report: 1989. Eur J Nucl Med 17:A14–A16 (Suppl)

EANM (1992a) European system for reporting of adverse reactions and drug defects. Eighth report: 1990. Eur J Nucl Med 19:A11–A12 (Suppl)

EANM (1992b) European system for reporting of adverse reactions and drug defects. Ninth report: 1991. Eur J Nucl Med 19:A10–A11 (Suppl)

EANM (1993) European system for reporting of adverse reactions to and defects in radiopharmaceuticals: annual report 1992. Eur J Nucl Med 20:A22–A26 (Suppl)

EANM (1994) European system for reporting of adverse reactions to and defects in radiopharmaceuticals: annual report 1993. Eur J Nucl Med 21:BP29–BP34 (Suppl)

EANM (1995) European system for reporting of adverse reactions to and defects in radiopharmaceuticals: annual report 1994. Eur J Nucl Med 22:BP29–BP33 (Suppl)

EANM (1996) European system for reporting of adverse reactions to and defects in radiopharmaceuticals: annual report 1995. Eur J Nucl Med 23:BP27–BP31 (Suppl)

Eshima D, Fritzberg AR (1996) Radiopharmaceuticals for renal imaging. In: Henkin RE et al. (eds) Nuclear medicine, vol 2. Mosby, St. Louis, pp 1055–1064

Fogelman I, Maisey M (1994) Bone. In: Fogelman I, Maisey MN, Clarke SEM (eds) An atlas of clinical nuclear medicine, 2nd edn. Martin Dunitz, London, pp 1–110

Forstrom L (1996) Indium-111 labelled leucocyte imaging in the diagnosis of infection and inflammatory disease. In: Henkin RE et al. (eds) Nuclear medicine, vol 2. Mosby, St. Louis, pp 1619–1635

Francis MD, Ferguson DL, Tofe AJ, et al. (1980) Comparative evaluation of three diphosphonates: in vitro adsorption (C-14 labelled) and in vivo osteogenic uptake (Tc-99m labeled complexed). J Nucl Med 21:1185–1189

Freitas JE, Freitas AE (1996) Parathyroid scintigraphy. In: Henkin RE et al. (eds) Nuclear medicine, vol 1, Mosby, St. Louis, pp 877–885

Freitas JE, Nagle CE, Freitas AE (1996) Scrotal imaging. In: Sandler MP et al. (eds) Diagnostic nuclear medicine, 3rd edn, vol II. Williams and Wilkins, Baltimore, pp 1233–1242

Gelfand MJ, Hannon DW (1987) Pediatric nuclear cardiology. In: Gerson MC (ed) Cardiac nuclear medicine. McGraw-Hill, New York, pp 437–474

Germano G, Van Train K, Kiat H, Berman DS (1996) Digital techniques for the acquisition, processing, and analysis of nuclear cardiology images. In: Sandler MP et al. (eds) Diagnostic nuclear medicine, 3rd edn, vol I. Williams and Wilkins, Baltimore, pp 347–385

Gibson RE, Burns HD (1996) Radiopharmaceutical agents for cardiac imaging. In: Henkin RE et al. (eds) Nuclear medicine, vol 1. Mosby, St. Louis, pp 613–625

Giuliano AE, Dale PS, Turner RR, et al. (1995) Improved axillary staging of breast cancer with sentinel lymphadenectomy. Ann Surg 222:394–401

Goldraich NP, Goldraich IH (1995) Update on dimercaptosuccinic acid renal scanning in children with urinary tract infection. Pediatr Nephrol 9:221–226

Gordon I, Peters AM, Gutman A, et al. (1990) Skeletal assessment in neuroblastoma – the pitfalls of iodine-123-MIBG scans. J Nucl Med 31:129–134

Gross MD, Shapiro B, Thrall JH, Freitas JE, Beierwaltes WH (1989) The scintigraphic imaging of endocrine organs. Endocrine Rev 5:221–281

Guillemart A, Besnard JC, Le Pape A, et al. (1978) Skeletal uptake of pyrophosphate labeled with technetium-

95m and technetium-96, as evaluated by autoradiography. J Nucl Med 19:895–899
Hay RV, Shapiro B, Gross MD (1996) Scintigraphy imaging of the adrenals and neuroectodermal tumors. In: Henkin RE et al. (eds) Nuclear medicine, vol 1. Mosby St. Louis, pp 855–876
Hegge FN, Hamilton GW, Larson SM (1978) Cardiac chamber imaging: a comparison of red blood cells labelled with Tc-99m in vitro and in vivo. J Nucl Med 19:129–134
Hladik WB III, Norenberg JP (1996a) Radiopharmaceuticals for hepatobiliary imaging. In: Henkin RE et al. (eds) Nuclear medicine, vol 2. Mosby, St. Louis, pp 986–996
Hladik WB III, Norenberg JP (1996b) Radiopharmaceuticals for liver and spleen imaging. In: Henkin RE et al. (eds) Nuclear medicine, vol 2. Mosby, St. Louis, pp 966–976
Hoefnagel CA (1994) Metaiodobenzylguanidine and somatostatin in oncology: role in the management of neural crest tumours. Eur J Nucl Med 21: 561–581
Hojelse C, Kristensen K, Sampson CB (1994) Factors which affect the integrity of radiopharmaceuticals. In: Sampson CB (ed) Textbook of radiopharmacy, theory and practice, 2nd edn. Gordon and Breach, Yverdon, Switzerland, pp 145–151
Hurley JR, Becker DV (1996) Treatment of thyroid cancer with radioiodine. In: Sandler MP et al. (eds) Diagnostic nuclear medicine, 3rd edn, vol II. Williams and Wilkins, Baltimore, pp 959–989
ICRP Publication 38 (1983) Radionuclide transformations; energy and intensity of emissions. Pergamon Press, Oxford
Iskandrian AS, Verani MS, Heo J (1994) Pharmacologic stress testing: mechanisms of action, hemodynamic responses, and results in detection of coronary artery disease. J Nucl Cardiol 1:94–111
Jain D, Wackers FJT, Mattera J, et al. (1993) Biokinetics of technetium-99m-tetrofosmin: myocardial perfusion imaging agent: implications for a one-day imaging protocol. J Nucl Med 34:1254–1259
Jones AG, Adrams MJ, Davison A, et al. (1984) Biological studies of a new class of technetium complexes: the hexakis-(alkylisonitrile)-technetium (I) cations. Int J Nucl Med Biol 11:225–234
Karesh SM (1996) Principles of radiopharmacy. In: Henkin RE et al. (eds) Nuclear medicine, vol 1. Mosby, St. Louis, pp 334–349
Keeling DH (1994) Adverse reactions and untoward events associated with the use of radiopharmaceuticals. In: Sampson CB (ed) Textbook of radiopharmacy, theory and practice, 2nd edn. Gordon and Breach, Yverdon, Switzerland, p 285
Kelly JD, Forster AM, Higley B, et al. (1993) Technetium-99m-tetrofosmin as a new radiopharmaceutical for myocardial perfusion imaging. J Nucl Med 34:222–227
Kim CK, Reske SN, Alavi A (1996) Bone marrow scintigraphy. In: Henkin RE et al. (eds) Nuclear medicine, vol 2. Mosby, St. Louis, pp 1223–1249
Kostamo KL (1996) Evaluation of gastrointestinal bleeding by nuclear medicine techniques. In: Henkin RE et al. (eds) Nuclear medicine, vol 2. Mosby, St. Louis, pp 1016–1022
Krenning EP, Bakker WH, Kooij PPM, et al. (1992) Somatostatin receptor scintigraphy with indium-111-DTPA-D-Phe-1-octreotide in man: metabolism, dosimetry and comparison with iodine-123-Tyr-3-octreotide. J Nucl Med 33:652–658
Krenning EP, Kwekkeboom DJ, Pauwels S, Kvols LK, Reubi JC (1995) Somatostatin receptor scintigraphy. In: Freeman LM (ed) Nuclear medicine annual 1995. Raven Press, New York, pp 1–50
Krishnamurthy S, Krishnamurthy GT (1989) Technetium-99m-iminodiacetic acid organic anions: review of biokinetics and clinical application in hepatology. Hepatology 9:139–153
Lawrence SK, Sandler MP, Partain CL, James AE Jr (1996) Cerebrospinal fluid imaging. In: Sandler MP et al. (eds) Diagnostic nuclear medicine, 3rd edn, vol II. Williams and Wilkins, Baltimore, pp 1163–1176
Lazarus CR (1994) Techniques for dispensing of radiopharmaceuticals. In: Sampson CB (ed) Textbook of radiopharmacy, theory and practice, 2nd edn. Gordon and Breach, Yverdon, Switzerland, pp 59–68
Lecklitner ML (1986) Pitfalls of gastrointestinal bleeding studies with ^{99m}Tc-labeled RBCs. Semin Nucl Med 16:151–154
Lecklitner ML, Hughes JJ (1986) Pitfalls of gastrointestinal bleeding studies with ^{99m}Tc sulfur-colloid. Semin Nucl Med 16:155–156
Léveillé J, Demonceau G, Walovitch RC (1992) Intrasubject comparison between technetium-99m-ECD and technetium-99m-HMPAO in healthy human subjects. J Nucl Med 33:480–484
Loken MK (ed) (1987) Pulmonary nuclear medicine. Appleton & Lange, Norwalk, Connecticut
Lowe VJ, Sostman HD (1994) Pulmonary embolism. In: Murray IPC, Ell PJ (eds) Nuclear medicine in clinical diagnosis and treatment. Churchill Livingstone, Edinburgh, pp 29–46
Mackenzie JR (1996) A review of renal scarring in children. Nucl Med Commun 17:176–190
Majd M, Rushton HG (1992) Renal cortical scintigraphy in the diagnosis of acute pyelonephritis. Semin Nucl Med 22:98–111
Mali WPTM, Oei HY, Arndt JW, et al. (1986a) Hemodynamics of the varicocele. Part I. Correlation among the clinical, phlebographic and scintigraphic findings. J Urol 135:483–488
Mali WPTM, Oei HY, Arndt JW, et al. (1986b) Hemodynamics of the varicocele. Part II. Correlation among the results of renocaval pressure measurements, varicocele scintigraphy and phlebography. J Urol 135:489–493
Malmud LS, Fisher RS (1981) The evaluation of gastroesophageal reflux before and after medical therapies. Semin Nucl Med 11:205–215
Molinkski VJ (1982) A review of ^{99m}Tc generator technology. Int J Appl Radiat Isotop 33:811–819
Murphy PB, Port SC (1996) Radionuclide evaluation of left ventricular function. In: Sandler MP et al. (eds) Diagnostic nuclear medicine, 3rd edn, vol I. Williams and Wilkins, Baltimore, pp 403–442
Murray T (1986) Formation of labelled colloid in Tc-99m DMSA due to the presence of bactericidal fluid. Nucl Med Commun 7:505–510
Nakajo M, Shapiro B, Copp J, et al. (1983) The normal and abnormal distribution of the adrenomedullary imaging agent *m*-[I-131] iodobenzylguanidine (I-131 MIBG) in man: evaluation by scintigraphy. J Nucl Med 24:672–682
Neumann RD, McAfee JG (1996) Gallium-67 imaging in infection. In: Sandler MP et al. (eds) Diagnostic nuclear medicine, 3rd edn, vol II. Williams and Wilkins, Baltimore, pp 1493–1507
Neumann RD, Kemp JD, Weiner RE (1996) Gallium-67 imaging for detection of malignant disease. In: Sandler MP et al. (eds) Diagnostic nuclear medicine, 3rd edn, vol II. Williams and Wilkins, Baltimore, pp 1243–1260
Norenberg JP, Hladik III WB (1996) Radiopharmaceuticals for pulmonary imaging. In: Henkin RE et al. (eds) Nuclear medicine, vol 2. Mosby, St. Louis, pp 1362–1381

Nowotnik DP (1994) Physico-chemical concepts in the preparation of technetium radiopharmaceuticals. In: Sampson CB (ed) Textbook of radiopharmacy, theory and practice, 2nd edn. Gordon and Breach, Yverdon, Switzerland, pp 29–49

O'Connor MK, Byrne PJ, Keeling P, et al. (1988) Esophageal scintigraphy: applications and limitations in the study of esophageal disorders. Eur J Nucl Med 14:131–136

Oei HY (1994) Dynamic and static renal imaging. In: Murray IPC, Ell PJ (eds) Nuclear medicine in clinical diagnosis and treatment. Churchill Livingstone, Edinburgh, pp 213–227

Oei HY, Blokland JAK (1993) Aanbevelingen nucleair geneeskundige diagnostiek (An official publication of the Dutch Society of Nuclear Medicine). Eburon, Delft

Oei HY, Akkermans LMA, Bogaard JW, Smout AJPM, ten Thije OJ (1986) Assessment of esophageal function in achalasia with small and large test volumes. In: Schmidt HAE et al. (eds) Nuklearmedizin in Forschung und Praxis. Schattauer, Stuttgart, pp 249–251

Oppenheim BE (1996) Liver imaging. In: Sandler MP et al. (eds) Diagnostic nuclear medicine, 3rd edn, vol I. Williams and Wilkins, Baltimore, pp 749–758

O'Reilly P, Aurell M, Britton K, et al. (1996) Consensus on diuresis renography for investigating the dilated upper urinary tract. J Nucl Med 37:1872–1876

Park H-M (1996) The thyroid gland. In: Henkin RE et al. (eds) Nuclear medicine, vol 1. Mosby, St. Louis, pp 830–854

Peters AM (1994) Occult fever. In: Murray IPC, Ell PJ (eds) Nuclear medicine in clinical diagnosis and treatment. Churchill Livingstone, Edinburgh, pp 141–151

Peters AM (1996) Imaging inflammation and infection Tc-99m HMPAO labeled leucocytes. In: Henkin RE et al. (eds) Nuclear medicine, vol 2. Mosby, St. Louis, pp 1636–1655

Piepsz A, Gordon I, Hahn K (1991) Paediatric nuclear medicine. Eur J Nucl Med 18:41–66

Pilbrow WJ, Brownless SM, Cawood JI, et al. (1990) Salivary gland scintigraphy – a suitable substitute for sialography? Br J Radiol 63:190–196

Prats E, Banzo J, Abos MD, et al. (1994) Diagnosis of prosthetic vascular graft infection by technetium-99m-HMPAO-labeled leukocytes. J Nucl Med 35:1303–1307

Preston DF, Greenlaw RH (1970) "Hot spots" in lung scans. J Nucl Med 11:422–425

Pupi A, Castagnoli A, De Cristofaro MTR, Bacciottini L, Petti AR (1994) Quantitative comparison between ^{99m}Tc-HMPAO and ^{99m}Tc-ECD: measurement of arterial input and brain retention. Eur J Nucl Med 21:124–130

Rocco TP, Dilsizian V, Fischman AJ, Strauss HW (1989) Evaluation of ventricular function in patients with coronary artery disease. J Nucl Med 30:1149–1165

Saha GB, MacIntyre WJ, Go RT (1994) Radiopharmaceuticals for brain imaging. Semin Nucl Med 24:324–349

Sampson CB (1991) Tc-99m exametazime labelled leucocytes: effect of volume and concentration of exametazime on labelling efficiency, and clinical protocol for high efficiency multi-dose radiolabelling. Nucl Med Commun 12:719–723

Sandler MP, Martin WH, Powers TA (1996) Thyroid imaging. In: Sandler MP et al. (eds) Diagnostic nuclear medicine, 3rd edn, vol II. Williams and Wilkins, Baltimore, pp 911–942

Shirazi P (1996) Salivary glands. In: Henkin RE et al. (eds) Nuclear medicine, vol 2. Mosby, St. Louis, pp 933–947

Short MD (1994) Basic principles of radionuclide physics. In: Sampson CB (ed) Textbook of radiopharmacy, theory and practice, 2nd edn. Gordon and Breach, Yverdon, Switzerland, pp 1–17

Siegel ME, Stewart CA (1996) Peripheral vascular disease: arterial and venous. In: Henkin RE et al. (eds) Nuclear Medicine, vol 1. Mosby, St. Louis, pp 798–827

Silberstein EB, Ryan J and the Pharmacopoeia Committee of the Society of Nuclear Medicine (1996) Prevalence of adverse reactions in nuclear medicine. J Nucl Med 37:185–192

Singh A (1996) Peritoneovenous shunts: patency studies. In: Henkin RE et al. (eds) Nuclear medicine, vol 2. Mosby, St. Louis, pp 1041–1052

Slingluff CL Jr, Stidham KR, Ricci WM, et al. (1994) Surgical management of regional lymph nodes in patients with melanoma. Experience with 4682 patients. Ann Surg 219:120–130

Spencer RP (1996) Spleen imaging. In: Sandler MP et al. (eds) Diagnostic nuclear medicine, 3rd edn, vol II. Williams and Wilkins, Baltimore, pp 865–874

Spencer RP, Weiner R, Hosain F (1996) Bone imaging radiopharmaceuticals. In: Henkin RE et al. (eds) Nuclear medicine, vol 2. Mosby, St. Louis, pp 1125–1140

Spies WG (1996) Ventilation/perfusion scintigraphy. In: Henkin RE et al. (eds) Nuclear medicine, vol 2. Mosby, St. Louis, pp 1382–1439

Srivastava SC, Straub RF (1990) Blood cell labeling with ^{99m}Tc: progress and perspectives. Semin Nucl Med 20:41–51

Staudenherz A, Telfeyan D, Steiner E, et al. (1995) Scintigraphic pitfalls in giant parathyroid glands. J Nucl Med 36:467–469

Strauss HW, McKusick KA, Boucher CA, et al. (1979) Of linens and lases - the eight anniversary of the gated blood pool scan. Semin Nucl Med 9:296–308

Subramanian G, McAfee JG, Mellter A (1973) ^{99m}Tc-stannous phytate: a new in vivo colloid for imaging the reticuloendothelial system. J Nucl Med 14:459

Suess E, Malessa S, Ungersbock K, et al. (1991) Tc-99m-d,l-hexamethylpropyleneamine oxine (HMPAO) uptake and glutathione content in brain tumors. J Nucl Med 32:1675–1681

Sylvester JM (1996) Liver and spleen imaging. In:Henkin RE et al. (eds) Nuclear medicine, vol 2. Mosby, St. Louis, pp 977–985

Taillefer R (1990) Technetium-99m sestamibi myocardial imaging: same-day rest-stress studies and dipyridamole. Am J Cardiol 66:80E–84E (Suppl)

Taillefer R, Boucher Y, Potvin C, Lambert R (1992) Detection and localization of parathyroid adenomas in patients with hyperparathyroidism using a single radionuclide imaging procedure with technetium-99m-sestamibi (double-phase study) J Nucl Med 33:1801–1807

Taylor A Jr (1989) Radiopharmaceuticals for the measurement of "functioning renal mass" In: Blaufox MD (ed) Evaluation of renal function and disease with radionuclides: the upper urinary tract, 2nd edn. Karger, Basel, pp 60–83

Taylor A Jr, Nally JV (1995) Clinical applications of renal scintigraphy. AJR 164:31–41

Taylor A, Nally J, Aurell M, et al. (1996) Consensus report on ACE inhibitor renography for detecting renovascular hypertension. J Nucl Med 37:1876–1882

Theobald AE (1994) Quality control of radiopharmaceuticals. In: Sampson CB (ed) Textbook of radiopharmacy, theory and practice, 2nd edn. Gordon and Breach, Yverdon, Switzerland, pp 103–144

Treves ST, Grand RJ (1995) Gastrointestinal bleeding. In: Treves ST (ed) Pedriatic nuclear medicine, 2nd edn. Springer Verlag, New York, pp 453–465

Tubergen K, Corlya M, Volkert WA, Holmes RA (1991) Sensitivity of technetium-99m-*d,l*-HMPAO to radiolysis in aqueous solutions. J Nucl Med 32:111–115

Udelson JE (1995) Choosing a thallium-201 or technetium-99m sestamibi imaging protocol. J Nucl Cardiol 1:S99–108

Urbain J-LC, Vekemans M-CM, Malmud LS (1996) Esophageal transit and reflux and gastric emptying. In: Henkin RE et al. (eds) Nuclear medicine, vol 2. Mosby, St. Louis, pp 948–965

Uren RF, Howman-Giles RB, Shaw HM, et al. (1993) Lymphoscintigraphy in high-risk melanoma of the trunk: predicting draining node groups, defining lymphatic channels and locating the sentinel node. J Nucl Med 34:1435–1440

Uren RF, Howman-Giles RB, Thompson JF, et al. (1995) Mammary lymphoscintigraphy in breast cancer. J Nucl Med 36:1775–1780

van der Veen H, Hoekstra OS, Paul MA, et al. (1994) Gamma-probe guided sentinel node biopsy to select patients with melanoma for lymphadenectomy. Br J Surg 81:1769–1770

Vaqueiro M, Gloviczki P, Fisher J (1986) Lymphoscintigraphy in lymphedema: an aid to microsurgery. J Nucl Med 27:1125–1130

Van Train KF, Garcia EV, Cooke CD, Areeda J (1995) Quantitative analysis of SPECT myocardial perfusion. In: Gordon DePuey EG et al. (eds) Cardiac SPECT Imaging. Raven Press, New York, pp 49–74

Verhoef NPLG (1993) Neuroreceptor ligand imaging by single photon emission computerised tomography, Thesis, University of Amsterdam, Amsterdam

Vinberg N (1980) Fission Mo-99/Tc-99m generators – a study of their performance. Eur J Nucl Med 5:435–438

Walovitch RC, Hill TC, Garrity ST, et al. (1989) Characterization of Tc-99m-L,L-ECD for brain perfusion imaging. J Nucl Med 30:1892–1901

Walovitch RC, Cheesman EH, Maheu LJ, Hall KM (1994) Studies of the retention mechanism of the brain perfusion imaging agent ^{99m}Tc-bicisate (^{99m}Tc-ECD). J Cereb Blood Flow Metab 14:S4

Waxman AD (1996) Thallium chloride and ^{99m}Tc methoxyisobutyl isonitrile (MIBI) in nuclear oncology. In: Sandler MP et al. (eds) Diagnostic nuclear medicine, 3rd edn, vol II. Williams and Wilkins, Baltimore, pp 1261–1274

Weissleder R, Thrall JH (1989) The lymphatic system: diagnostic imaging studies. Radiology 172:315–317

Wilson ME, Hung JC (1992) Evaluation of heparin and anticoagulant citrate dextrose in the preparation of technetium-99m-red blood cells with UltraTag^{r} RBC kit. J Nucl Med 33:306–308

Wilson GA, O'Mara RE (1996) Peripheral vascular imaging. In: Sandler MP et al. (eds) Diagnostic nuclear medicine, 3rd edn, vol I. Williams and Wilkins, Baltimore, pp 567–583

Wynchank S, Mann MD, Guillet J (1995) Gastro-oesophageal reflux in children and nuclear medicine. Presse Med 24:1595–1597

Ziffer JA, Hull JE, Alspaugh JP, et al. (1988) Radionuclide venography in the evaluation of deep venous thrombosis: assessment of specific interpretive criteria. J Nucl Med 29:825

37 New and Future Trends in Radiopharmaceuticals

M.D. Blaufox and J.K. Moran

CONTENTS

37.1 Introduction

Among all of the diagnostic imaging specialties, none is so dependent on the development of new agents as nuclear medicine. Changes in instrumentation lead to dramatic improvements in the diagnostic capabilities of radiographic devices including ultrasound and magnetic resonance. Similar developments in instrumentation have a very profound effect on nuclear medicine performance as well, but only if the appropriate diagnostic agents are available.

During the past decade, two radioisotopic labels have achieved preeminence in clinical nuclear medicine. These are technetium-99m for conventional nuclear medicine imaging and fluorine-18 for positron emission tomography (PET). Other radioisotopes, including those of indium and gallium, also play an important role in nuclear medicine but they are eclipsed by the multitude of procedures which are made possible by the availability of ^{99m}Tc and ^{18}F. Radioiodine continues to play a small, but important role. Such is the preeminence of ^{99m}Tc that virtually all general diagnostic nuclear medicine equipment is designed to optimize performance at the energy level of this isotope.

The other characteristic of nuclear medicine which again sets it apart from general radiology is the strong interrelationship between function and imaging. Many nuclear medicine procedures are performed solely for the evaluation of function and even for those procedures which are carried out to obtain morphologic detail, proper interpretation is only possible with a full appreciation of the functional characteristics of the agent.

It is possible to organize a discussion of future trends in the development of most nuclear medicine agents according to the organ for which they are used. Many agents such as those used for immunoimaging, receptor imaging, and PET have uses in multiple organ systems and diseases and are best discussed under broad functional categories. This chapter consequently will review each of the major organ systems with a commentary on future trends and then will provide some insight into broader categories such as immunoimaging and their prospects for impact on future practice. To exemplify the diversity of radionuclides and labeling procedures used in nuclear medicine, three new radiopharmaceuticals incorporating the most commonly used radioisotopes are shown in Fig. 37.1.

37.2 Imaging of the Central Nervous System

The study of the brain in nuclear medicine rivals the kidney in terms of the diversity of radiopharmaceuticals available for study and the complexity of

M.D. Blaufox, MD, PhD, Professor and Chairman, Department of Nuclear Medicine, Albert Einstein College of Medicine and Montefiore Medical Center, Montefiore Medical Park, 1695A Eastchester Road, Bronx, NY 10461, USA
J.K. Moran, PhD, Assistant Professor, Director of the Radiochemistry Laboratory, Department of Nuclear Medicine, Albert Einstein College of Medicine and Montefiore Medical Center, Montefiore Medical Park, 1695A Eastchester Road, Bronx, NY 10461, USA

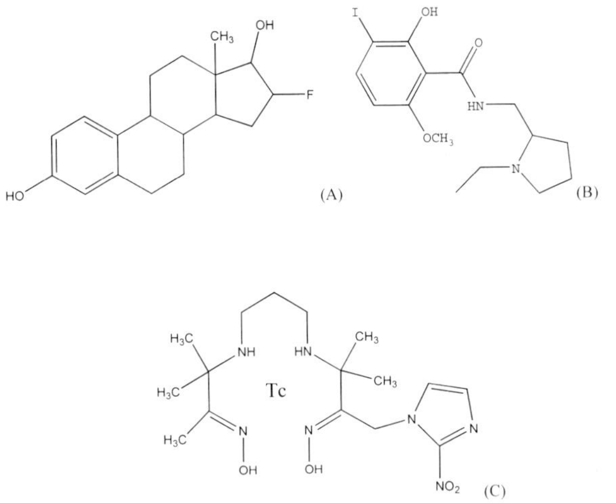

Fig. 37.1 A–C. Comparison of new tracers in nuclear medicine. **A** 16α-^{18}F-fluoro-17β-estradiol (FES). FES is labeled with ^{18}F and is used to image both primary and metastatic breast cancers by PET. Accumulation of FES within metastatic lesions of breast carcinoma is a receptor-mediated process. **B** 2-Hydroxy-3-iodo-6-methoxy-*N*-((-ethyl-2-pyrrolidnyl)methyl) benzamide (IBZM). IBZM is labeled with [123]I. Its mechanism of uptake is not completely understood. It is believed that IBZM binds to melanin within the cell. IBZM is primarily used to study neuropsychiatric disorders including schizophrenia and Parkinson's disease. Recently, it has been used to detect melanoma. **C** Propylene amine oxime-1,2-nitroimidazole (BMS-181321). BMS-181321 is labeled with [99m]Tc. It undergoes reduction within cells, forming reactive intermediates depending on the intracellular oxygen concentration. It is used to image hypoxic but potentially salvageable myocardium

the functions measured. Many new developments in brain imaging relate to the application of ^{18}F-labeled agents which are specific for brain receptors. These are discussed in the section on PET imaging. A number of agents have been developed which can be used in conventional single-photon emission computerized tomography (SPECT). Planar imaging of the brain, which was at one time the single most widely utilized nuclear medicine procedure, has almost completely passed into history.

The considerable interest in the diagnosis of Parkinson's disease, especially before it is fully developed, has resulted in exploration of a number of new compounds. Among these is iodine-123-β-CIT, which binds to dopamine and seratonin. This agent promises to be of help in quantitating dopamine transporters in the brain (Seibyl et al. 1996; Marek et al. 1996).

A new agent which can be used with SPECT imaging in patients with drug-resistant epilepsy is ^{123}I-iomazenil. This agent images benzodiazepine receptors and is used in epileptic patients in whom a focal defect may be found using SPECT imaging. It has been suggested that ^{123}I-iomazenil provides better diagnostic information than the clinically approved agent ^{99m}Tc-hexamethylpropylene amine oxime (HMPAO), which is in routine clinical use (Sjoholm et al. 1995). Another radiopharmaceutical which has been utilized in the brain, as well as for kidney studies, is *N,N'*-1,2-ethylene-diylbis-l-cysteine diethylester dihydrochloride (Otte et al. 1996). This agent has been used to evaluate cerebral perfusion and the cited reference reports its value in demonstrating bilateral parieto-occiptal hypoperfusion in patients with whiplash injury.

37.3 Pulmonary Imaging

The major developments in lung imaging relate to the potential availability of new thrombus imaging agents and the use of fluorodeoxyglucose in the differential diagnosis of pulmonary cancer from benign lesions. These agents are discussed respectively in Sects. 37.7 and 37.10. Unfortunately, the currently available agents for the differential diagnosis of pulmonary embolism leave us with the very unsatisfactory three-way decision-making process of probable, intermediate or indeterminate, and low probability scans. A positive thrombus imaging agent should have a profound effect on the value and reliability of the lung scan. One of the promising agents for ventilation perfusion lung imaging is Technegas (Bellomo et al. 1994), which, although it promises to be an improvement over the currently used technetium-DTPA aerosols, has not yet been approved for routine use in the United States.

37.4 Cardiac Imaging

The field of cardiovascular nuclear medicine appears to have attained a degree of maturity so that the bulk of the studies are now being directed toward evaluation of the significance of various findings rather than the development of new techniques. In fact it is quite interesting to see the ubiquitous use of ^{99m}Tc-sestamibi and thallium in a variety of other noncardiac clinical situations. It seems likely that in the future sestamibi will serve not only as a cardiac imaging agent but also will be accepted as a routine parathyroid imaging agent for the endocrine system. It also seems likely that thallium will fall by the wayside even though relatively successful attempts have been made to utilize it instead of sestamibi in these extracardiac conditions as well. The use of these two agents in differentiating various malignant forms of tumors also seems likely to give way to the far more sensitive and specific tests available with PET.

Some new agents are being developed commercially for cardiac evaluation but these appear to be more "me too" agents than significant new developments. Fatty acid analogues continue to be explored with the disadvantage that they have to be labeled with ^{123}I rather than ^{99m}Tc and data are lacking in showing any great advantage over current techniques for the evaluation of cardiac perfusion and metabolism. It has been suggested (TAMAKI et al. 1996) that a disparity in uptake between 15-iodophenyl-3-*R*,*S*-methyl pentadecanoic acid (BMIPP) and thallium may be a predictor for future cardiac events. However, further information is required to elucidate the relationship of these agents in differentiating perfusion and function and their significance (TAKI et al. 1995).

One of the major goals of therapy for myocardial infarction and unstable angina is the preservation of ischemic but viable myocardium. Nitroimidazoles are used to indicate the state of tissue oxygenation, and have been labeled with ^{18}F (SHELTON et al. 1989) and ^{131}I (MARTIN et al. 1993). Recently, a new ^{99m}Tc nitroimidazole analog has been developed, i.e., BMS-181321 (Fig. 37.1C), and is currently undergoing animal studies (KAZUKI et al. 1996).

Several labeled antibodies have been developed for cardiac imaging. Recently, Myoscint has been approved for use in the United States. Myoscint is an IgG2A Fab fragment labeled with indium-111 that recognizes cardiac myosin. Myoscint can detect transmural myocardial infarction with a sensitivity of 91%. It is less sensitive with nontransmural myocardial infarction, with an overall sensitivity of 88% (AZRIN 1992).

37.5 Renal Imaging

The search for improved renal agents has been a prolonged and frustrating experience for many of us. The primary agents which are currently available do a very adequate job but are not perfect by any means. ^{99m}Tc-labeled mercaptoacetyltriglycine (MAG3) has become extremely popular as a tubular imaging agent. More recently several related agents have been reported in the literature. ^{99m}Tc mercaptoacetylglycyl-D-alanylglycine (BORMANS et al. 1992) has been studied and reported to have superior excretion characteristics to MAG3 but requires high-performance liquid chromatography purification and is unlikely to become a primary agent. Use of another interesting agent, L,L-ethylene dicysteine (VAN NEROM et al. 1993), was reported in healthy human volunteers in 1993. This agent has significant differences in handling from MAG3, being only about 31% plasma protein bound as compared to 88% for MAG3 and with a similar urinary excretion. It is also reported to have a somewhat higher renal clearance and may have some useful role (SURMA et al. 1994; STOFFEL et al. 1994). However, the difference does not seem dramatic enough to supplant MAG3.

Technetium-99m cysteine has been suggested as an agent which would allow measurement of renal morphology and function and perhaps have advantages over glucoheptonate. It has been reported to produce superior renal images to glucoheptonate but work on this is limited (MISRA et al. 1994).

Attesting to the ubiquitous utilization of ^{99m}Tc-sestamibi, at least one report has appeared suggesting its potential role in the diagnosis of renovascular disease (HURWITZ et al. 1994).

37.6 Imaging of the Gastrointestinal Tract

There has been little development in gastroenterologic imaging during the last few years with the exception of techniques for the detection of cancer utilizing immunoimaging and peptide imaging, which are discussed in Sect. 37.9.

37.7 Vascular Imaging

A number of thrombus detection agents have been introduced which appear promising and will be useful in the detection of thrombophlebitis and perhaps pulmonary embolism. Human recombinant fibrin binding domain labeled with ^{111}In (ROSENTHALL and LECLERC 1995) has been studied successfully in 62 patients, yielding positive images of blood clots. Another similar agent (BUTLER et al. 1996), ^{99m}Tc-modified recombinant tissue plasminogen activator, has also been used to detect deep vein thrombosis with a reported sensitivity for proximal vein disease of 93% and a specificity of 92%. For calf vein thrombosis, the sensitivity was 86% with a specificity of

93%. Yet another thrombus imaging agent is ^{99m}Tc-labeled activated platelet receptor binding peptide (LISTER-JAMES et al. 1996), which shows a high affinity for in vivo thrombus imaging (MUTO et al. 1995). An interesting new agent is ^{123}I-iodoazomycinarabinoside (AL-ARAFAJ et al. 1994). Using this agent, a correlation is observed between impaired oxygen tension in tissue and increased tracer uptake. ^{123}I-iodoazomycinarabinoside has been suggested as an agent for helping to manage diabetes with impaired vascular supply. Several new peptide-based thrombus imaging agents are currently being developed and will be discussed in Sect. 37.9.

37.8 Endocrinology

Many of the most exciting developments in endocrinology are discussed below in Sect. 37.9. However, there has been a dramatic effort in endocrinology to apply the cardiac imaging agents to patients with endocrine disease. Many authors have reported on the use of ^{99m}Tc-sestamibi in imaging the parathyroid with very good results. This is turning out to be the agent of choice and is most useful in patients in whom reexploration of the neck is considered (MARTINEZ et al. 1995; LEE et al. 1995; BENARD et al. 1995; CHEN et al. 1995; CAIXAS et al. 1995). Thallium has also been utilized in this situation but does not appear to offer any great advantage over sestamibi and has the disadvantage of a less desirable emission energy (DEREBEK et al. 1996). In the general rush to apply cardiac agents to parathyroid imaging, the use of ^{99m}Tc-tetrofosmin has also been attempted (AIGNER et al. 1996).

Other than these new applications of well-established agents, no dramatic new approaches to the endocrine system have been developed utilizing standard imaging techniques.

37.9 Immunoimaging and Receptor Imaging

The utilization of radiolabeled antibodies is at a transitional stage in its development and application to nuclear medicine. In Europe there is extensive utilization of radiolabeled antibodies for diagnostic studies. However, approval of radiolabeled antibodies for oncologic diagnosis by the Food and Drug Administration in the United States has been slower. Currently, four radiolabeled antibodies have been approved by the Food and Drug Administration (ZUCKIER and DENARDO 1997). OncoScint (B72.3) was the first radiolabeled antibody approved for use in the United States. OncoScint is labeled with ^{111}In using the chelating agent diethylene triamine pentaacetic acid (DTPA). B72.3 is a murine IgG1 whole antibody that recognizes the TAG-72 epitope and is currently approved for imaging colorectal and ovarian carcinoma. It is also undergoing phase II clinical trials for breast carcinoma and axillary lymph nodes. Since antibody fragments have faster blood clearance than whole antibodies, it is possible to label these smaller molecules with shorter half-life radionuclides. CEA-Scan (IMMU-4) is a murine IgG1 Fab′ fragment that is labeled with ^{99m}Tc and targets the 200-kDa colorectal cancer tumor marker CEA (carcinoembryonic antigen). In addition, CEA-Scan is undergoing phase II and III clinical trials for breast and lung carcinoma respectively. Verluma (NR-LU-10) was approved in 1996 for imaging small cell lung cancer. Verluma is a murine IgG2b Fab fragment labeled with ^{99m}Tc using a diamide dimercaptide chelating agent, and recognizes a 40-kDa cell surface glycoprotein. Phase III clinical trials have just recently finished on the use of Verluma for non-small cell lung cancer. The most recently approved radiolabeled antibody is ProstaScint (7E11-C5.3), which is a whole murine IgG1 that targets a 100-kDa glycoprotein from the cytoplasmic membrane-rich fragment of LNCaP cells. It is labeled with ^{111}In using DTPA.

Yet another immunoimaging agent is ^{111}In-labeled monoclonal antibody Mab 1A3, which has been used for colorectal disease. This agent provided a positive predictive value of 83% for nonhepatic tumors but the liver continues to be a problem (PHILPOTT et al. 1994). ^{99m}Tc-labeled monoclonal antifibrin antibodies has had some successful trials in the evaluation of arterial thrombosis (STRATTON et al. 1994).

A somewhat unusual approach for antibody imaging has been the use of monoclonal antibodies directed against E-selectin in an effort to image vascular endothelial activation. Preliminary results with this agent suggest that it may be effective in evaluating inflammatory disease (KEELAN et al. 1994; CHAPMAN et al. 1994).

Therapeutic utilization of radiolabeled antibodies, although still held out as a hope, has not yet achieved its anticipated application. However, there have been some promising early trials. The improve-

Table 37.1. Radionuclides with favorable characteristics for therapeutic applicatons

Radionuclide	Half-life (days)	Beta energy (MeV)	Gamma energy (keV)
^{131}I	8.04	0.606	364 (81%)
^{90}Y	2.67	2.28	
^{67}Cu	2.58	0.570	93 (31%), 185 (48%)
^{177}Lu	6.71	0.497	208 (11%)
^{186}Re	3.77	1.08	137 (10%)
^{64}Cu	0.53	0.573	Positron (19%)

ments in the therapeutic use of radiolabeled antibodies have been mainly in the radiolabel attached to the antibody. The first therapeutic radionuclide used to label antibodies was ^{131}I. However, the half-life of ^{131}I (8.04 days) is considerably longer than the antibody-antigen half-life (2–3 days), making it a suboptimal radionuclide for labeling. The search for the ideal therapeutic radionuclide is still underway, but several promising candidates have emerged (Table 37.1). The use of unusual radiometals for labeling antibodies has precipitated the need for the development of chelating agents which form more stable complexes in vivo (MEARES et al. 1991). The pure beta emitter yttrium-90 has been used by several groups (PRESS et al. 1993; DENARDO et al. 1995). One drawback with pure beta emitters is that to do imaging, it is necessary to label the antibody with an additional gamma-emitting isotope. To avoid this problem several groups have examined the use of radionuclides that emit both beta particles for therapy and gamma photons for imaging. ^{131}I-labeled murine monoclonal antibody has been used in the treatment of metastatic colon carcinoma (DIVGI et al. 1995) and the use of deoxyspergualin was suggested in this particular study to reduce some of the side-effects of the antibody. Copper-67 has been used to label Lym-1, a murine antilymphoma IgG2a antibody, and is currently undergoing clinical trials (DENARDO et al. 1991). Rhenium-186 has been used to treat patients with squamous cell carcinoma of the head and neck using a variety of monoclonal antibodies (VAN GOG et al. 1996). Lutetium-177 labeled murine monoclonal antibody of the CC49 group also has been used in other trials of patients with advanced adenocarcinoma (^{177}Lu is an unusual label) (MULLIGAN et al. 1995). Small cell lung carcinoma has been treated with anti-GD2 ganglioside monoclonal antibody 3F8, again in an early pilot study, i.e., a great deal of work remains to be done (GRANT et al. 1996). The use of ^{99m}Tc-labeled IMMU-4 monoclonal antibody has been evaluated for recurrent pelvic carcinoma, but unfortunately was reported not to improve significantly on the sensitivity or specificity of CT (STOMPER et al. 1995). Numerous other antibodies are currently being investigated but it is too early to determine which will prove to have routine clinical value. In the United States a significant number of promising agents have "orphan drug" status because of their limited applicability (Table 37.2) (SWANSON 1996).

The slow pharmacokinetics of whole antibodies and the accumulation of radioactivity in the liver is a major concern, especially in diagnostic imaging. Pretargeting techniques provide an alternative method to achieve high selective tumor uptake with minimal nontarget tissue background (GOODWIN 1995). Pretargeting consists of initial administration of an unlabeled antibody to which has been conjugated an acceptor molecule that has high-affinity noncovalent binding sites. After localization of the antibody-conjugate at the tumor site, a clearing agent is administered to remove any unbound antibody-conjugate from the circulation. Finally, a small radiolabel effector molecule which has a high affinity for the acceptor molecule conjugated to the antibody is given. Pretargeting results in maximum tumor concentration and tumor-to-background ratios in 1–3 h after administration of the radiolabel. Several different acceptor/effector systems are currently being investigated, including avidin/biotin (PAGANELLI et al. 1991), enzyme/prodrug (SENTER 1990), and oligonucleotide/antisense oligonucleotide (BOS et al. 1994). The complexity of this procedure may be offset by the high target to background ratios that may be obtained.

The slow blood clearance, poor target to nontarget ratios, and potential production of human antimouse antibodies (HAMA) have limited the use of antibodies for diagnostic imaging. Antibody fragments have alleviated some but not all of these problems.

A rapidly growing area of utilization is receptor imaging, which has the advantage of potential for agents which are more specific than antibodies without the attendant immunologic reaction (for a list of the chelating agents most commonly used in nuclear medicine, see Table 37.3). The success of OctreoScan (pentetreotide), a cyclic octapeptide analog of human somatostatin labeled with ^{111}In via DTPA, in the imaging of somatostatin-positive tumors has spurred research in the use of labeled peptides. The

Table 37.2. Radiopharmaceuticals with orphan drug designation in the United States

Radiopharmaceutical	Indication	Sponsor
^{111}In and ^{90}Y murine MoAb (288-Mx-DTPA)	Treatment of non-Hodgkin's B-cell lymphoma	IDEC Pharmaceutics Corp, San Diego, Calif.
^{111}In murine MoAb FAB to myosin	Aid in diagnosis of myocarditis	Centocor, Inc, Malvern, Pa.
^{111}In Altumornab pentetate	Detection of suspected, previously unidentified tumor foci of recurrent colorectal carcinoma	Hybritech, Inc, San Diego, Calif.
^{131}I B1 MoAb	Treatment of non-Hodgkin's B-cell lymphoma	Coulter Corp, Miami, Fl.
^{131}I 6B-iodomethyl-19-norcholesterol	Adrenal cortical imaging	Univ. Michigan Med Ctr, Ann Arbor, Mich.
^{131}I-metaiodobenzylguanidine sulfate	Diagnostic adjunct in patients with pheochromocytoma	Univ. Michigan Med Ctr, Ann Arbor, Mich.
^{131}I murine MoAb IgGZA to B cells	Treatment of B-cell leukemia and B-cell hymphoma	Immunomedics, Inc, Morris Plains, N.J.
^{131}I murine MoAb to α-fetoprotein	Treatment of hepatocellular carcinoma and hepatoblastoma Treatment of α-fetoprotein-producing germ-cell tumors	Immunomedics, Inc, Morris Plains, N.J.
^{131}I murine MoAb to hCG	Treatment of hCG-producing tumors such as germ cell and trophoblastic cell tumors	Immunomedics, Inc, Morris Plains, N.J.
^{123}I murine MoAb to α-fetoprotein	Detection of hepatocellular carcinoma and hepatoblastoma Detection of α-fetoprotein-producing germ cell tumors	Immunomedics, Inc, Morris Plains, N.J.
^{123}I murine MoAb to hCG	Detection of hCG-producing tumors such as germ cell and trophoblastic cell tumors	Immunomedics, Inc, Morris Plains, N.J.
^{99M}Tc anti-melanoma murine MoAb	Detection of metastases of malignant melanoma	NeoRx Corp, Seattle, Wash.
^{99M}Tc murine MoAb (IgGZA) to B cells	Evaluation of disease extent in patients with histologically confirmed non-Hodgkin's B-cell lymphoma. acute B-cell lymphoblastic leukemia, or chronic B-cell lymphocytic leukemia	Immunomedics, Inc, Morris Plains, N.J.
^{99M}Tc murine MoAb to human α-fetoprotein	Detection of hepatocellular carcinoma and hepatoblastoma Detection of α-fetoprotein-producing germ cell tumors	Immunomedics, Inc, Morris Plains, N.J.
^{99M}Tc murine MoAb to hCG	Detection of hCG-producing tumors such as germ cell and trophoblastic cell tumors	Immunomedics, Inc, Morris Plains, N.J.

Data from the Office of Orphan Products Development.
MoAb, Monoclonal antibody.

Table 37.3. Chelating agents used in nuclear medicine

Chelating agent	Abbreviation	Donor atoms	Metals complexed	References
Diethylene triamine penta-acetic acid	DTPA	Nitrogen, oxygen	Universal chelator	PHILPOTT et al. (1994)
Mercaptoacetyltriglycine	MAG3	Nitrogen, oxygen, sulfur	Tc, Re	VAN GOG et al. (1996)
Hyrazine nicotinic acid	HYNIC	Nitrogen	Tc	BABICH et al. (1993)
Tetra-azadodecane tetra-acetic acid	DOTA	Nitrogen, oxygen	In, Y, Lu	DENARDO et al. (1995)
Tetra-azatetradecane tetra-acetic acid	TETA	Nitrogen, oxygen	Cu	ANDERSON et al. (1995)
Hexamethylpropylene amine oxime	HMPAO	Nitrogen	Tc	OYEN et al. (1996)
N,N'-2-ethylenediylbis-l-cysteine	EDC	Nitrogen, sulfur	Tc	VAN NEROM et al. (1993)

preclinical evaluation of two ^{99m}Tc-labeled somatostatin receptor binding peptides P587 and P829 (VALLABHAJOSULA et al. 1996) has been reported recently. These somatostatin analogs were labeled with ^{99m}Tc using a MAG3-like (N_3S) chelating agent. Although it is too early to tell whether these peptides will replace OctreoScan, they do have the advantage that they can be labeled with ^{99m}Tc.

Vasoactive intestinal peptide (VIP) scintigraphy has seen increasing use and has been applied for the diagnosis of intestinal adenocarcinomas as well as some endocrine tumors (VIRGOLINI et al. 1995). In the study cited, ^{123}I-VIP was used successfully for the detection of pancreatic adenocarcinoma in two patients, ileocecal carcinoid tumor in one patient, lymph node metastases in two patients, and lymph node metastases in two of three patients. Another study has shown a large number of human tumors which have VIP or somastosatin receptors and this study provides useful guidance for choosing those tumors which would be susceptible to this type of imaging (REUBI 1995). Among those with higher concentrations of receptors are breast cancer, ovarian cancer, and endometrial cancer, as well as prostate, bladder, lung, brain, and a variety of neuroendocrine tumors. Most of the tumors have receptors for both VIP and somatostatin but there are some disparities. For instance, in the aforementioned study, although 20 out of 24 patients with ovarian carcinoma had VIP-positive receptors, none had somatostatin receptors. In general the cross-reactivity between somatostatin and VIP is quite high.

Other new receptor agents include ^{131}I-labeled epidermal growth factor, which has been used for the localization of squamous cell lung carcinoma (CUARTERO-PLAZA et al. 1996). A receptor that is attracting a considerable amount of attention is the GPIIb/IIIa receptor, which is expressed on the surface of activated platelets. It is known that the peptide sequence arginine-glycine-aspartate (RGD) binds to the GPIIb/IIIa receptor with high affinity. Consequently several peptide analogs that mimic the RGD sequence have been synthesized and labeled with ^{99m}Tc. In preliminary studies the peptide P280, which contains two RGD mimics, had a faster blood clearance compared to ^{99m}Tc-HMPAO labeled platelets, but the uptake by thrombi was less, re sulting in similar thrombus to blood ratios (LISTER-JAMES et al. 1996). Several other peptides are currently undergoing animal studies, and it is too early to judge whether they will result in useful imaging agents.

37.10 Positron Emission Tomographic Scanning

Fluorodeoxyglucose has become as ubiquitous for PET scanning as ^{99m}Tc has become for general nuclear imaging. There are a number of encouraging new agents which are being studied for PET scanning, most of which are directed toward the brain and brain receptors. Among them is carbon-11 diprenorphine, which has been used to measure striatal opioid receptors in Parkinson's disease (BURN et al. 1995), ^{18}F-fluorodopa, which has been used to evaluate patients who have received grafts for Parkinson's disease (REMY et al. 1995), and a wide variety of other new receptor agents aimed specifically at brain function. Assessment of estrogen receptors in breast cancer has been studied utilizing 16α-^{18}F-fluoro-17β-estradiol (Fig. 37.1A) but it does not appear to have any significant advantage over fluorodeoxyglucose, which is more easily obtained and utilized (DEHDASHTI et al. 1995).

Carbon-11 methionine is a potential tumor-seeking agent for PET studies which reflects the amino acid metabolism in tumors. Studies comparing FDG and ^{11}C-methionine have shown the same overall sensitivity in detecting recurrent tumors after treatment (INOUE et al. 1996).

Two isotopes of copper that are currently being investigated as possible PET tracers are ^{62}Cu and ^{64}Cu. ^{62}Cu-PTSM is a generator-produced lipophilic complex that is highly extracted and retained in organs. It is being investigated for both brain and heart imaging (GREEN 1987; HERRERO et al. 1996). ^{64}Cu has been used to label the monoclonal antibody fragment 1A3-F(ab')$_2$ for imaging colorectal carcinoma (ANDERSON et al. 1995).

It appears that the trend in PET will be toward central radiopharmacies so that relatively long-lived isotopes like ^{18}F or those that can be generator produced are likely to dominate future clinical applications.

37.11 Miscellaneous

37.11.1 Hematology

Hematologic applications overlap with those cited above. Very little new work has been done specifically in areas of hematologic disease. There still remains a need for agents for the treatment of lymphomas, but this will probably be met through antibodies or nonradioactive agents.

37.11.2 Oncology

New developments in oncology are proceeding somewhat in parallel with the increasing utilization of PET for the detection of cancer; however, there are some compounds which are usable with SPECT and which do not fall into the group of agents listed above. Among these is ^{99m}Tc-sestamibi, which has received considerable interest for the evaluation of breast cancer (Khalkhali et al. 1995; Palmedo et al. 1996); however, although the high sensitivity and specificity are encouraging, the demands placed on a successful agent by a lesion which is potentially palpable and for which mammography is well established seem almost insurmountable.

There is increasing use of tomography for the performance of lymphoscintigraphy. This technique appears to be very promising when utilizing ^{99m}Tc-sulfur colloid in patients with melanoma (Mudun et al. 1996; Pijpers et al. 1995), and it has also been applied in cases of breast cancer. With the increasing interest in the occurrence of melanoma, techniques to detect its spread have taken on a new importance. A novel agent with single-photon characteristics is ^{123}I-labeled IBZM (Fig. 37.1B). This agent (2-hydroxy-3-iodo-6-methoxy-*N*-((1-ethyl-2-pyrrolidinyl)methyl)benzamide) has also been used to study neuropsychiatric disorders including schizophrenia and Parkinson's disease (Maffioli et al. 1994). In 11 patients with melanoma, six cutaneous lesions were detected with IBZM, as were five of six superficial lymph nodes, four of five pulmonary metastases, and one of two hepatic metastases.

37.11.3 Infection

One of the biggest problems with infection has been the nonspecific nature of gallium in infection and the difficulties of labeling white blood cells (WBCs). Almost any radiopharmaceutical can be used to image infection due to increased capillary permeability at sites of inflammation, resulting in good sensitivity, but very low specificity. In recent years, lipophilic complexes such as ^{111}In oxime and ^{99m}Tc-HMPAO have been used to label WBCs. Due to the physical properties of these complexes, all types of cells are labeled indiscriminately (Becker 1995). Therefore, leukocytes must first be separated from other blood cells before labeling. The in vitro labeling of leukocytes is associated with significant risks to both laboratory personnel and patients, particularly with the high incidence of HIV infection in hospitalized populations.

Studies have been conducted to evaluate radiolabeled antibodies which would have the advantage of being injected directly into the patient, labeling the WBCs in vivo, and then localizing in the site of infection, thereby avoiding the tedious and sometime difficult task of removing WBCs for separate labeling. The two main approaches for imaging infection with antibodies are those using: (a) murine monoclonal antibodies directed against the nonspecific cross-reacting antigen 95 (NCA-95) (Locher et al. 1986), and (b) nonspecific human polyclonal immunoglobulins (Corstens and Claessens 1992). Since little difference is seen between the two, the method of localization of both specific and nonspecific antibodies is most likely based on nonspecific, non-antigen-related uptake of free antibody due to an increased capillary permeability at the site of infection.

A considerable amount of work has been done investigating ^{99m}Tc-labeled polyclonal human immunoglobulins and their localization at sites of infection (Calame et al. 1995). It has been demonstrated that liposomes labeled with ^{111}In will localize at sites of infection (Boerman et al. 1995). The current generation of liposomes are rapidly cleared from the circulation, but work is being conducted to prolong circulation time, and further comparative studies are needed (Oyen et al. 1996).

Another method to label leukocytes in vivo is with chemotactic peptides. Chemotactic peptides bind to high-affinity receptors located on the surface of neutrophils. The high affinity coupled with rapid blood clearance should yield a radiopharmaceutical with high sensitivity and high specificity. To date chemotactic peptides have been labeled with ^{111}In (Fischman et al. 1991), ^{99m}Tc (Babich et al. 1993), and ^{18}F (Vaidyanathan and Zalutsky 1995). Before animal studies of these compounds can give way to human studies, certain biological side-effects, in particular neutropenia, must be overcome. A new technique of labeling leukocytes with colloidal ^{99m}Tc-SnF_2 has been suggested (Puncher and Blower 1995); however, this technique does not obviate the need for separation of the blood and numerous other disadvantages, including its direct effect on the WBCs, make it unlikely that it will replace currently available agents.

Antigranulocyte antibody has been used and compared with three-phase bone scan in patients with suspected osteomyelitis, and was reported to have a sensitivity of 100% and a specificity of 75% (Scheidler et al. 1994).

Anti-T-lymphocyte antibody (OKT-3) has been suggested for use in patients with rheumatic joint disease (Marcus et al. 1994).

37.12 Conclusion

It is not possible to review all of the agents currently under development in this brief space. We have attempted to highlight those which have advanced to preliminary human trials and which provide examples of new trends in application. The next 5–10 years of nuclear medicine will be a rapidly advancing and exciting era as these new agents and many others proceed from conceptualization to animal trials to human application.

References

Aigner RM, Fueger GF, Nicoletti R (1996) Parathyroid scintigraphy: comparison of technetium-99m methoxyisobutylisonitrile and technetium-99m tetrofosmin studies. Eur J Nucl Med 23:693–696

Al-Arafaj A, Ryan EA, Hutchison K, Mannan RH, Mercer J, Wiebe LI, McEwan AJB (1994) An evaluation of iodine-123 iodoazomycinarabinoside as a marker of localized tissue hypoxia in patients with diabetes mellitus. Eur J Nucl Med 21:1338–1342

Anderson CJ, Schwarz SW, Connett JM, et al. (1995) Preparation, biodistribution and dosimetry of copper-64-labeled anti-colorectal carcinoma monoclonal antibody fragments 1A3-F(ab′)$_2$. J Nucl Med 36:850–858

Azrin MA (1992) The use of antibodies in clinical cardiology. Am Heart J 124:753–768

Babich JW, Solomon H, Pike MC, et al. (1993) Technetium-99m-labeled hydrazino nicotinamide derivatized chemotactic peptide analogs for imaging focal sites of bacterial infection. J Nucl Med 34:1964–1974

Becker W, (1995) The contribution of nuclear medicine to the patient with infection. Eur J Nucl Med 22:1195–1211

Bellomo R, Low R, Pianko S, Korman A, Clarke K, White S, Wong C (1994) The 1-month outcome of patients with a low probability Technegas ventilation/perfusion lung scan. Nucl Med Commun 15:505–510

Benard F, Lefebvre B, Beuvon F, et al. (1995) Rapid washout of technetium-99m-MIBI from a large parathyroid adenoma. J Nucl Med 36:241–243

Boerman OC, Storm G, Oyen WJG, et al. (1995) Sterically stabilized liposomes labeled with indium-111 to image focal infection. J Nucl Med 36:1639–1644

Bormans GM, Cleynhen BJ, DeRoo MJK, Verbruggen AM (1992) Evaluation of the renal excretion characteristics of technetium-99m mercaptoacetylglycyl-D-alanylglycine in healthy volunteers. Eur J Nucl Med 19:271–277

Bos ES, Kuijpers WHA, Meesters-Winters M, et al. (1994) In vitro evaluation of DNA-DNA hybridization as a two-step approach in radioimmunotherapy of cancer. Cancer Res 54:3479–3486

Burn DJ, Rinne JO, Quinn NP, et al. (1995) Striatal opioid receptor binding in Parkinson's disease, striatonigral degeneration and Steele-Richardson-Olszewski syndrome: a [^{11}C]diprenorphine PET study. Brain 118:951–958

Butler SP, Boyd SJ, Parkes SL, et al. (1996) Technetium-99m-modified recombinant tissue plasminogen activator to detect deep venous thrombosis. J Nucl Med 37:744–748

Caixas A, Berna L, Piera J, et al. (1995) Utility of ^{99m}Tc-sestamibi scintigraphty as a first-line imaging procedure in the preoperative evaluation of hyperparathyroidism. Clin Endocrinol 43:525–530

Calame W, Welling M, Feitsma HIJ, et al. (1995) Contribution of phagocytic cells and bacteria to the accumulation of technetium-99m labelled polyclonal human immunoglobulin at sites of inflammation. Eur J Nucl Med 22:638–644

Chapman PT, Jamar F, Harrison AA, Binns RM, Peters A, Haskard DO (1994) Noninvasive imaging of e-selectin expression by activated endothelium in urate crystal-induced arthritis. Arthritis Rheum 37:1752–1756

Chen CC, Skarulis MC, Fraker DL, et al. (1995) Technetium-99m-sestamibi imaging before reoperation for primary hyperparathyroidism. J Nucl Med 36:2186–2191

Corstens FHM, Claessens RAMJ (1992) Imaging inflammation with human polyclonal immunoglobulin: not looked for, but discovered. Eur J Nucl Med 19:155–158

Cuartero-Plaza A, Martinez-Miralles E, Rosell R, et al. (1996) Radiolocalization of squamous lung carcinoma with ^{131}I labeled epidermal growth factor. Clin Cancer Res 2:13–20

Dehdashti F, Mortimer JE, Siegel BA, et al. (1995) Positron tomographic assessment of estrogen receptors in breast cancer: comparison with FDG-PET and in vitro receptor assays. J Nucl Med 36:1766–1774

DeNardo GL, DeNardo SJ, Meares CF, et al. (1991) Pharmacokinetics of copper-67 conjugated Lym-1, a potential therapeutic radioimmunoconjugate in mice and in patients with lymphoma. Antibody Immunoconjugates Radiopharmaceuticals 4:777–785

DeNardo SJ, Zhong GR, Salako Q, Li M, DeNardo GL, Meares CF (1995) Pharmacokinetics of chimeric l6 conjugated to indium-111 and yttrium-90-DOTA-peptide in tumor-bearing mice. J Nucl Med 36:829–836

Derebek E, Biberoglu S, Kut O, et al. (1996) Early and delayed thallium-201 scintigraphy in thyroid nodules: the relationship between early thallium-201 uptake and perfusion. Eur J Nucl Med 23:504–510

Divgi CR, Scott AM, Gulec S, et al. (1995) Pilot radioimmunotherapy trial with ^{131}I-labeled murine monoclonal antibody CC49 and deoxyspergualin in metastatic colon carcinoma. Clin Cancer Res 1:1503–1510

Fischman AJ, Pike MC, Kroon D, et al. (1991) Imaging of focal bacterial infection in rats with indium-111-labeled chemotactic peptide analogs. J Nucl Med 32:483–491

Goldberg SN, Palmer EL, Scott JA, Fischer R (1994) Pulmonary embolism: prediction of the usefulness of initial ventilation-perfusion scanning with chest radiographic findings. Radiology 193:801–805

Goodwin DA (1995) Tumor pretargeting: almost the bottom line. J Nucl Med 36:876–879

Grant SC, Kostakoglu L, Kris MG, et al. (1996) Targeting of small-cell lung cancer using the anti-GD2 ganglioside monoclonal antibody 3F8: a pilot trial. Eur J Nucl Med 23:145–149

Green MA (1987) A potential copper radiopharmaceutical for imaging the heart and brain copper-labeled pyrualkehyde bis(N^4-methylthiosemicarbazone). Nucl Med Biol 14:59–61

Herrero P, Hartman JJ, Green MA, et al. (1996) Regional myocardial perfusion assessed with generator-produced copper-62-PTSM and PET. J Nucl Med 37:1294–1300

Hurwitz GA, Ghali SK, Mattar AG, Gravelle DR, Husni M (1994) Dynamic renal imaging with technetium-99m-sestamibi in hypertension: potential for assessment of renovascular disorders. J Nucl Med 35:1959–1964

Inoue T, Kim EE, Wong FCL, et al. (1996) Comparison of fluorine-18-fluorodeoxyglucose and carbon-11-methionine PET in detection of malignant tumors. J Nucl Med 37:1472–1479

Kazuki F, Hideo K, Yosiyuki W, Fugiwara T, Nishimara T (1996) Ischemic and reperfused myocardium detected with technetium-99m-nitroimidizol. J Nucl Med 37:761–766

Keelan ETM, Harrison AA, Chapman PT, Binns RM, Peters AM, Haskard DO (1994) Imaging vascular endothelial activation: an approach using radiolabeled monoclonal antibodies against the endothelial cell adhesion molecule E-selectin. J Nucl Med 35:276–281

Khalkhali I, Cutrone J, Mona I, et al. (1995) Technetium-99m-sestamibi scintimammography of breast lesions: clinical and pathological follow-up. J Nucl Med 36:1784–1789

Lee VS, Wilkinson RH Jr, Leight GS Jr, et al. (1995) Hyperparathyroidism in high-risk surgical patients: evaluation with double-phase technetium-99m sestamibi imaging. Radiology 197:627–633

Lister-James J, Knight LC, Maurer AH, Bush LR, Moyer BR, Dean RT (1996) Thrombus imaging with a technetium-99m-labeled activated platelet receptor-binding peptide. J Nucl Med 37:775–781

Locher JT, Seybold K, Andres RY, et al. (1986) Imaging of inflammatory and infectious lesions after injection of radioiodinated monoclonal antigranulocyte antibodies. Nucl Med Commun 7:659–670

Maffioli L, Mascheroni L, Mongioj V, et al. (1994) Scintigraphic detection of melanoma metastases with a radiolabeled benzamide ([iodine-123]-(*S*)-IBZM) J Nucl Med 35:1741–1747

Marcus C, Thakur ML, Huyng TV, Louie JS, Leibling M, Minami C, Diggles L (1994) Imaging rheumatic joint diseases with anti-T lymphocyte antibody OKT-3. Nucl Med Commun 15:824–830

Marek KL, Seibyl JP, Zoghbi SS, et al. (1996) ^{123}Iβ-CIT/SPECT imaging demonstrates bilateral loss of dopamine transporters in hemi-Parkinson's disease. Neurology 46:231–237

Martin GV, Biskupiak JE, Caldwell JH, Rasey JS, Krohn KA (1993) Characterization of iodovinylmisonidazole as a marker for myocardial hypoxia. J Nucl Med 34:918–924

Martinez DA, King DR, Romshe C, et al. (1995) Intraoperative identification of parathyroid gland pathology: a new approach. J Pediatr Surg 30:1306–1309

Meares CF, Diril H, Kukis D, et al. (1991) Radiochemistry of antibodies: some recent advances. Antibody Imunoconjugates Radiopharmaceutical 4:389–398

Misra M, Sarkar HS, Chakravarty M, et al. (1994) ^{99}Tc^{m}-cystine, a renal function and imaging agent: a comparative study in dog with ^{131}I-hippurate and ^{99}Tc^{m}-glucoheptonate to evaluate its functional and imaging characteristics. Nucl Med Comm 15:878–885

Mudun A, Murray DR, Herda SC, et al. (1996) Early stage melanoma: lymphoscintigraphy, reproducibility of sentinel node detection, and efffectiveness of the intraoperative gamma probe. Radiology 199:171–175

Mulligan T, Carrasquillo JA, Chung Y, et al. (1995) Phase I study of intravenous ^{177}Lu-labeled CC49 murine monoclonal antibody in patients with advanced adenocarcinoma. Clin Cancer Res 1:1447–1454

Muto P, Lastoria S, Varrella P, et al. (1995) Detecting deep venous thrombosis with technetium-99m-labeled synthetic peptide P280. J Nucl Med 36:1384–1391

Otte A, Ettlin T, Fierz L, et al. (1996) Parieto-occipital hypoperfusion in late whiplash syndrome: first quantitative SPET study using technetium-99m bicisate (ECD). Eur J Nucl Med 23:72–74

Oyen WJG, Boerman OC, Storm G, et al. (1996) Detecting infection and inflammation with technetium-99m-labeled stealth liposomes. J Nucl Med 37:1392–1397

Paganelli G, Magnani P, Zito F, et al. (1991) Three step monoclonal antibody tumor targeting in carcinoembroyonic antigen-positive patients. Cancer Res 51:5960–5966

Palmedo H, Schomburg A, Grunwald F, et al. (1996) Technetium-99m-MIBI scintimammography for suspicious breast lesions. J Nucl Med 37:626–630

Philpott GW, Siegel BA, Schwarz SW, et al. (1994) Immunoscintigraphy with a new indium-111-labeled monoclonal antibody (MAb 1A3) in patients with colorectal cancer. Dis Colon Rectum 37:782–792

Pijpers R, Collet GJ, Meijer S (1995) The impact of dynamic lymphoscintigraphy and gamma probe guidance on sentinel node biopsy in melanoma. Eur J Nucl Med 22:1238–1241

Press OW, Eary JF, Appelbaum FR, et al. (1993) Radiolabeled antibody therapy of B-cell lymphoma with autologous bone marrow support. N Engl J Med. 329:1219–1224

Puncher MRB, Blower PJ (1995) Labelling of leucocytes with colloidal technetium-99m-SnF_2: an investigation of the labelling process by autoradiography. Eur J Nucl Med 22:101–107

Remy P, Samson Y, Hantraye P, et al. (1995) Clinical correlates of (^{18}F)fluorodopa uptake in five grafted parkinsonian patients. Ann Neurol 38:580–588

Reubi JC (1995) In vitro identification of vasoactive intestinal peptide receptors in human tumors: implications for tumor imaging. J Nucl Med 36:1846–1853

Rosenthall L, Leclerc J (1995) A new thrombus imaging agent: human recombinant fibrin binding domain labeled with In-111. Clin Nucl Med 20:398–402

Scheidler J, Leinsinger G, Pfahler M, Kirsch CM (1994) Diagnosis of osteomyelitis: accuracy and limitations of antigranulocyte antibody imaging compared to three-phase bone scan. Clin Nucl Med 19:731–737

Seibyl JP, Laruelle M, vanDyck CH, et al. (1996) Reproducibility of iodine-123-β-CIT SPECT brain measurement of dopamine transporters. J Nucl Med 37:222–228

Senter PD (1990) Activation of prodrugs by antibody-enzyme conjugates: a new approach to cancer therapy. FASEB J 4:188–193

Shelton ME, Dence CS, Hwang DR, Welch MJ, Bergmann SR (1989) Myocardial kinetics of fluorine-18 misonidazole: a marker of hypoxic myocardium. J Nucl Med 30:351–358

Sjoholm H, Rosen I, Elmqvist D (1995) Role of I-123-Iomazenil SPECT imaging in drug resistant epilepsy with complex partial seizures. Acta Neurol Scand 92:41–48

Stoffel M, Jamar F, VanNerom C, et al. (1994) Evaluation of technetium-99m-L,L-EC in renal transplant recipients: a comparative study with technetium-99m-MAG_3 and iodine-125-OIH. J Nucl Med 35:1951–1958

Stomper PC, D'Souza DJ, Bakshi SP, et al. (1995) Detection of pelvic recurrence of colorectal carcinoma: prospective, blinded comparison of Tc-99m-IMMU-4 monoclonal antibody scanning and CT. Radiology 197:688–692

Stratton JR, Cerqueira MD, Dewhurst TA, Kohler TR (1994) Imaging arterial thrombosis: comparison of technetium-99m-labeled monoclonal antifibrin antibodies and indium-111 platelets. J Nucl Med 35:1731–1737

Surma MJ, Wiewiora J, Liniecki J (1994) Usefulness of $^{99}Tc^{m}$-*N,N*-ethylene-1-dicysteine complex for dynamic kidney investigations. Nucl Med Commun 15:628–635

Swanson DP (1996) Radiopharmaceuticals as orphan drugs. Semin Nucl Med 26:91–95

Taki J, Nakajima K, Matsunari I, et al. (1995) Impairment of regional fatty acid uptake in relation to wall motion and thallium-201 uptake in ischaemic but viable myocardium: assessment with iodine-123-labelled beta-methyl-branched fatty acid. Eur J Nucl Med 22:1385–1392

Tamaki N, Tadamura E, Kudoh T, et al. (1996) Prognostic value of iodine-123 labelled BMIPP fatty acid analogue imaging in patients with myocardial infarction. Eur J Nucl Med 23:272–279

Vaidyanathan G, Zalutsky MR (1995) Fluorine-18 labeled chemotactic peptides: a potential approach for the PET imaging of bacterial infection. Nucl Med Bio 22:759–764

Vallabhajosula S, Moyer BR, Lister-James J, et al. (1996) Pre-clinical evaluation of technetium-99m labeled somatostatin receptor-binding peptides. J Nucl Med 37:1016–1022

van Gog FB, Visser GWM, Klok R, et al. (1996) Monoclonal antibodies labeled with rhenium-186 using the MAG3 chelate: relationship between the number of chelated groups and biodistribution characteristics. J Nucl Med 37:352–362

Van Nerom CG, Bormans GM, DeRoo MJ, Verbruggen AM (1993) First experience in healthy volunteers with technetium-99m L,L-ethylenedicysteine, a new renal imaging agent. Eur J Nucl Med 20:738–746

Virgolini I, Kurtaran A, Raderer M, et al. (1995) Vasoactive intestinal peptide scintigraphy. J Nucl Med 36:1732–1739

Zuckier LS, DeNardo GL, (1997) Trials and tribulations: oncologic antibody imaging comes to the fore. Semin Nucl Med 27:10–29

Subject Index

List of Contributors

R. Agati, MD
Servizio di Neuroradiologia
Ospedale Bellaria
Via Altura 3
I-40139 Bologna
Italy

Thomas Albrecht, MD, FRCR
Department of Radiology and Nuclear Medicine
Universitätsklinikum Benjamin Franklin
Freie Universität Berlin
Hindenburgdamm 30
D-12205 Berlin
Germany

Torsten Almén, MD, PhD
Professor emeritus
Institute of Diagnostic Radiology
Malmö University Hospital
S-20502 Malmö
Sweden

Isabelle Berry, MD, PhD
Department of Neuroradiology
University Hospital Purpan and
Department of Biophysics and Nuclear Medicine
University Hospital Rangueil
1, avenue Jean-Poulhès
F-31054 Toulouse Cédex
France

M. Donald Blaufox, MD, PhD
Professor and Chairman
Department of Nuclear Medicine
Albert Einstein College of Medicine and
Montefiore Medical Center
1695A Eastchester Road
Bronx, NY 10461
USA

Martin J.K. Blomley, MB, FRCR
Hammersmith Hospital and
Imperial College School of Medicine
du Cane Road
London W12 OH5
UK

H. Bosmans, PhD
Professor, Department of Radiology
University Hospitals Gasthuisberg
Catholic University of Leuven
Herestraat 49
B-3000 Leuven
Belgium

Andrew A. Brayman, PhD
Department of Obstetrics and Gynecology
School of Medicine and Dentistry
The University of Rochester
Rochester, NY
USA

William H. Bush, Jr., MD, FACR
Radiology Department
University of Washington School of Medicine
Box 357115
1959 NE Pacific Street
Seattle, WA 98195
USA

Carlo Catalono, MD
Università Degli Studi di Roma
"La Sapienza"
Istituto di Radiologia Cattedra II
Policlinico Umberto I
I-00161 Roma
Italy

Peter P. Chang, PhD
Research Scientist
Applied Physics Laboratory
University of Washington
1013 NE, 40th St.,
Seattle, WA 98105-6698
USA

Charles C. Church, PhD
Acusphere, Inc.
University Park at MIT
38 Sidney Street
Cambridge, MA 02139
USA

Michel Clanet, MD
Department of Neurology
University Hospital Purpan
Place du Docteur Baylac
F-31059 Toulouse
France

Richard H. Cohan, MD
Department of Radiology
University of Michigan Medical Center
1500 East Medical Center Drive
Ann Arbor, MI 48109-0030
USA

Brian Coley, MD
4370 Limerick Lane
Dublin, OH 43017
USA

David O. Cosgrove, BM, FRCR
Hammersmith Hospital and
Imperial College School of Medicine
du Cane Road
London W12 OH5
UK

Bruno Cotter, MD
Assistant Professor of Medicine
Division of Cardiology
UCSD Medical Center
200 West Arbor Drive
San Diego, CA 92103-8411
USA

Anthony N. DeMaria, MD
Professor of Medicine, Chief of Cardiovascular Medicine
Division of Cardiology
UCSD Medical Center
200 West Arbor Drive
San Diego, CA 92103-8411
USA

Jean Francois Desreux, PhD
Professor, Coordination and Radiochemistry
University of Liège
Sart Tilman (B6)
B-4000 Liège
Belgium

Robert J. Eckersley, PhD
Hammersmith Hospital and
Imperial College School of Medicine
du Cane Road
London W12 OH5
UK

James H. Ellis, MD
Department of Radiology
University of Michigan Medical Center
1500 East Medical Center Drive
Ann Arbor, MI 48109-0030
USA

Anne Kjersti Fahlvik, PhD
Nycomed Imaging AS
P.O. Box 4220 Torshov
N-0401 Oslo
Norway

Sigrid L. Fossheim, PhD
Nycomed Imaging AS
P.O. Box 4220 Torshov
N-0401 Oslo
Norway

Bo Frennby, MD, PhD
Department of Diagnostic Radiology
Malmö University Hospital
S-20502 Malmö
Sweden

Dominque Gilsoul, PhD
Coordination and Radiochemistry
University of Liège
Sart Tilman (B6)
B-4000 Liège
Belgium

Michael S. Girard, MD
c/o Robert F. Mattrey, MD
Department of Radiology
University of California, San Diego Medical Center
200 W. Arbor Drive
San Diego, CA 92109-8756
USA

Klaes Golman, PhD
Professor
Department of Experimental Research
Malmö University Hospital and
Nycomed Innovation AB
Ideon-Malmö
S-20512 Malmö
Sweden

Alina Greco, MD
Centre Hospitalier Princesse Grace
Magnetic Resonance Unit
Avenue Pasteur, BP No. 489
MC-98012 Monte Carlo Cédex
Monaco

Richard W. Katzberg, MD
Professor, Department of Radiology
School of Medicine
University of California, Davis
Sacramento, CA 95817
USA

A. Kornerup Hansen, DVM, Dr.Vet.Sci.
Professor, Department of Pharmacology and Pathobiology
Royal Veterinary and Agricultural University
13 Bülowsvej
DK-1870 Frederiksberg C
Denmark

Eric P. Krenning, MD
Professor, Department of Nuclear Medicine
Department of Nuclear Medicine
University Hospital Rotterdam, Dijkzigt
P.O.Box 2040
3000 CA Rotterdam
The Netherlands

Gabriel Paul Krestin, MD
Professor and Chairman
Department of Radiology
Academic Hospital
Erasmus University Rotterdam
Molewaterplein 40
3015 GD Rotterdam
The Netherlands

Dik J. Kwekkeboom, MD
Department of Nuclear Medicine
University Hospital Rotterdam, Dijkzigt
P.O.Box 2040
3000 CA Rotterdam
The Netherlands

Antonio L'Abbate, MD
CNR Clinical Physiology Institute
Via Paolo Savi 8
I-56126 Pisa
Italy

Andrea Laghi, MD
Università Degli Studi di Roma
"La Sapienza"
Istituto di Radiologia Cattedra II
Policlinico Umberto I
I-00161 Roma
Italy

Peter Leander, MD, PhD
Department of Diagnostic Radiology
Malmö University Hospital
SE-205 02 Malmö
Sweden

Marco Leonardi, MD
Professor and Chairman
Servizio di Neuroradiologia
Ospedale Bellaria
Via Altura 3
I-40139 Bologna
Italy

Massimo Lombardi, MD
C.N.R. Clinical Physiology Institute
Via Paolo Savi 8
I-56126 Pisa
Italy

Claude Manelfe, MD
Department of Neuroradiology
University Hospital Purpan
Place du Docteur Baylac
F-31059 Toulouse
France

Guy Marchal, MD, PhD
Professor, Department of Radiology
University Hospitals Gasthuisberg
Catholic University of Leuven
Herestraat 49
B-3000 Leuven
Belgium

Robert F. Mattrey, MD
Department of Radiology
University of California, San Diego Medical Center
200 W. Arbor Drive
San Diego, CA 92109-85756
USA

M.T. McNamara, MD
Centre Hospitalier Princesse Grace
Magnetic Resonance Unit
Avenue Pasteur, BP No. 489
MC-98012 Monte Carlo Cédex
Monaco

Justin K. Moran, PhD
Assistant Professor
Director of the Radiochemistry Laboratory
Department of Nuclear Medicine
Albert Einstein College of Medicine
and
Montefiore Medical Center
1695A Eastchester Road
Bronx, NY 10461
USA

Anne Nævestad, MSc
Department of Medical Chemistry
School of Pharmacy, P.O.Box 1177
Blindern, N-0316 Oslo
Norway

Hong-Yoe Oei, MD, PhD
Department of Nuclear Medicine
University Hospital Rotterdam, Dijkzigt
P.O. Box 2040
3000 CA Rotterdam
The Netherlands

Robert A. Older, MD
Professor of Radiology and Urology
University of Virginia
Health Sciences Center
Department of Radiology, Box 170
Charlottesville, VA 22908
USA

Paolo Pavone, MD
Università Degli Studi di Roma
"La Sapienza"
Istituto di Radiologia Cattedra II
Policlinico Umberto I
I-00161 Roma
Italy

Timothey Pelura, PhD
Alliance Pharmaceutical Corp.
3040 Science Park Road
San Diego, CA 92121
USA

Howard M. Pollack, MD, FACR
Professor Emeritus of Radiology and Urology
420 Miller Rd # 408
Scottsdale, AZ 85251
USA

Jean-Philippe Ranjeva, PhD
Department of Neuroradiology
University Hospital Purpan
Place du Docteur Baylac
F-31059 Toulouse
France

Peter A. Rinck, MD, PhD
Professor of Diagnostic Imaging
NMR Laboratory, Medical Image Processing Group
Faculty of Medicine and Pharmacy
University of Mons-Hainaut
24, Avenue du Champ de Mars
B-7000 Mons
Belgium
and
Centre Hospitalier Princesse Grace
Magnetic Resonance Unit
Avenue Pasteur, BP No. 489
MC-98012 Monte Carlo Cédex
Monaco

K. Kirk Shung, PhD
Professor of Bioengineering
Bioengineering Program
31 Hallowell Bldg.
The Pennsylvania State University
University Park, PA 16802
USA

Claude B. Sirlin, MD
c/o Robert F. Mattrey, MD
Department of Radiology
University of California, San Diego Medical Center
200 W. Arbor Drive
San Diego, CA 92109-8756
USA

Fulvio Stacul, MD
Institute of Radiology
University of Trieste
Ospedale di Cattinara
Strada di Fiume 447
I-34149 Trieste
Italy

Gregory C. Steinbach, MSBE
Department of Radiology
UCSD Medical Center
200 W. Arbor Drive
San Diego, CA 92103-8756
USA

Gunnar Sterner, MD, PhD
Division of Nephrology
Department of Vascular and Renal Diseases
Malmö University Hospital
S-20502 Malmö
Sweden

Irene M. Stilbo, MD
The Danish Medicines Agency
378 Frederikssundsvej
DK-2700 Brønshøj
Denmark

Ove Svendsen, DVM, PhD, Dr.med.Sci.
Professor, Department of Pharmacology and Pathobiology
Royal Veterinary and Agricultural University
13 Bülowsvej
DK-1870 Frederiksberg C
Denmark

Henrik S. Thomsen, MD
Department of Diagnostic Radiology
Copenhagen University Hospital at Herlev
Herlev Ringvej 75
DK-2730 Herlev
Denmark

Geir Torheim, MS
MR Center, Medical Section
University of Trondheim, Trondheim, Norway
and NMR Laboratory, Medical Image Processing Group
Faculty of Medicine and Pharmacy
University of Mons-Hainaut
24, Avenue due Champ de Mars
B-7000 Mons
Belgium

Robertson Towart, BSc, PhD
Department of Experimental Research
Malmö University Hospital and
Nycomed Innovation AB
Ideon-Malmö
S-20512 Malmö
Sweden

Evan C. Unger, MD
Professor of Radiology
Director of Cross-Sectional Imaging
Department of Radiology
The University of Arizona Health
Sciences Center
1501 N. Campbell Avenue
Tucson, AZ 85724-5067
USA
and
President and CEO
ImaRx Pharmaceutical Corp.
Tucson, AZ 85724
USA

Hanns-Joachim Weinmann, PhD
Research Laboratories of Schering AG
Fo KM für KST
D-13342 Berlin
Germany

Erik R. Wisner, DVM
Associate Professor and Head of Radiology
Department of Veterinary Clinical Sciences
College of Veterinary Medicine
Ohio State University
Columbus, OH 43210-1089
USA

Gerald L. Wolf, MD, PhD
Center for Imaging and Pharmaceutical Research
Massachusetts General Hospital
149 13th Street
Charlestown, MA 02129
USA

Medical Radiology
Diagnostic Imaging and Radiation Oncology

Titles in the series already published

Diagnostic Imaging

Innovations in Diagnostic Imaging
Edited by J.H. Anderson

Radiology of the Upper Urinary Tract
Edited by E.K. Lang

The Thymus - Diagnostic Imaging, Functions, and Pathologic Anatomy
Edited by E. Walter, E. Willich, and W.R. Webb

Interventional Neuroradiology
Edited by A. Valavanis

Radiology of the Pancreas
Edited by A.L. Baert, co-edited by G. Delorme

Radiology of the Lower Urinary Tract
Edited by E.K. Lang

Magnetic Resonance Angiography
Edited by I.P. Arlart, G.M. Bongartz, and G. Marchal

Contrast-Enhanced MRI of the Breast
S. Heywang-Köbrunner and R. Beck

Spiral CT of the Chest
Edited by M. Rémy-Jardin and J. Rémy

Radiological Diagnosis of Breast Diseases
Edited by M. Friedrich and E.A. Sickles

Radiology of the Trauma
Edited by M. Heller and A. Fink

Biliary Tract Radiology
Edited by P. Rossi

Radiological Imaging of Sports Injuries
Edited by C. Masciocchi

Modern Imaging of the Alimentary Tube
Edited by A. R. Margulis

Diagnosis and Therapy of Spinal Tumors
Edited by P. R. Algra, J. Valk, and J. J. Heimans

Interventional Magnetic Resonance Imaging
Edited by J. F. Debatin and G. Adam

Abdominal and Pelvic MRI
Edited by A. Heuck and M. Reiser

Orthopedic Imaging
Techniques and Applications
Edited by A.M. Davies and H. Pettersson

Radiology of the Female Pelvic Organs
Edited by E.K.Lang

Magnetic Resonance of the Heart and Great Vessels
Clinical Applications
Edited by J. Bogaert, A. J. Duerinckx, and F. E. Rademakers

Modern Head and Neck Imaging
Edited by S. K. Mukherji and J. A. Castelijns

Radiological Imaging of Endocrine Diseases
Edited by J. N. Bruneton in collaboration with B. Padovani and M.-Y. Mourou

Trends in Contrast Media
Edited by H. S. Thomsen, R. N. Muller, and R. F. Mattrey

Functional MRI
Edited by C. T. W. Moonen and P. A. Bandettini

Radiology of the Pancreas
2nd Revised Edition
Edited by A. L. Baert
Co-edited by G. Delorme and L. Van Hoe

Radiation Oncology

Lung Cancer
Edited by C.W. Scarantino

Innovations in Radiation Oncology
Edited by H.R. Withers and L.J. Peters

Radiation Therapy of Head and Neck Cancer
Edited by G.E. Laramore

Gastrointestinal Cancer – Radiation Therapy
Edited by R.R. Dobelbower, Jr.

Radiation Exposure and Occupational Risks
Edited by E. Scherer, C. Streffer, and K.-R. Trott

Radiation Therapy of Benign Diseases - A Clinical Guide
S.E. Order and S.S. Donaldson

Medical Radiology
Diagnostic Imaging and Radiation Oncology

Titles in the series already published

Radiation Oncology

Interventional Radiation Therapy Techniques - Brachytherapy
Edited by R. Sauer

Radiopathology of Organs and Tissues
Edited by E. Scherer, C. Streffer, and K.-R. Trott

Concomitant Continuous Infusion Chemotherapy and Radiation
Edited by M. Rotman and C.J. Rosenthal

Intraoperative Radiotherapy – Clinical Experiences and Results
Edited by F.A. Calvo, M. Santos, and L.W. Brady

Radiotherapy of Intraocular and Orbital Tumors
Edited by W.E. Alberti and R.H. Sagerman

Interstitial and Intracavitary Thermoradiotherapy
Edited by M.H. Seegenschmiedt and R. Sauer

Non-Disseminated Breast Cancer
Controversial Issues in Management
Edited by G.H. Fletcher and S.H. Levitt

Current Topics in Clinical Radiobiology of Tumors
Edited by H.-P. Beck-Bornholdt

Practical Approaches to Cancer Invasion and Metastases
A Compendium of Radiation Oncologists' Responses to 40 Histories
Edited by A.R. Kagan with the Assistance of R.J. Steckel

Radiation Therapy in Pediatric Oncology
Edited by J.R. Cassady

Radiation Therapy Physics
Edited by A.R. Smith

Late Sequelae in Oncology
Edited by J. Dunst and R. Sauer

Mediastinal Tumors. Update 1995
Edited by D.E. Wood and C.R. Thomas, Jr.

Thermoradiotherapy and Thermochemotherapy
Volume 1:
Biology, Physiology, and Physics
Volume 2:
Clinical Applications
Edited by M.H. Seegenschmiedt, P. Fessenden, and C.C. Vernon

Carcinoma of the Prostate
Innovations in Management
Edited by Z. Petrovich, L. Baert, and L.W. Brady

Radiation Oncology of Gynecological Cancers
Edited by H.W. Vahrson

Carcinoma of the Bladder
Innovations in Management
Edited by Z. Petrovich, L. Baert, and L.W. Brady

Blood Perfusion and Microenvironment of Human Tumors
Implications for Clinical Radiooncology
Edited by M. Molls and P. Vaupel

Radiation Therapy of Benign Diseases. A Clinical Guide
2nd Revised Edition
S.E. Order and S.S. Donaldson

Carcinoma of the Kidney and Testis, and Rare Urologic Malignancies
Innovations in Management
Edited by Z. Petrovich, L. Baert, and L.W. Brady

Progress and Perspectives in the Treatment of Lung Cancer
Edited by P. Van Houtte, J. Klastersky, and P. Rocmans